Functional Movement
Development
Across the Life Span

Second Edition

Functional Movement
Development
Across the Life Span

Donna J. Cech, MS, PT, PCS
Program Director and Associate Professor
Physical Therapy Program
Midwestern University
Downers Grove, Illinois

Suzanne "Tink" Martin, MACT, PT
Professor
Department of Physical Therapy
University of Evansville
Evansville, Indiana

SAUNDERS

An Imprint of Elsevier

SAUNDERS
An Imprint of Elsevier

The Curtis Center
Independence Square West
Philadelphia, Pennsylvania 19106

Acquisitions Editor: Andrew Allen
Project Manager: Agnes Hunt Byrne
Production Manager: Peter Faber
Illustration Specialist: Lisa Lambert
Book Designer: Karen O'Keefe Owens

FUNCTIONAL MOVEMENT DEVELOPMENT ACROSS THE LIFE SPAN

Permissions may be sought directly from Elsevier's Health Sciences Rights Department in Philadelphia, PA, USA: phone: (+1) 215 239 3804, fax: (+1) 215 239 3805, e-mail: healthpermissions@elsevier.com. You may also complete your request on-line via the Elsevier homepage (http://www.elsevier.com), by selecting 'Customer Support' and then 'Obtaining Permissions'.

ISBN-13: 978-0-7216-8122-1
ISBN-10: 0-7216-8122-0

Printed in the United States of America.

Last digit is the print number: 9   8   7   6   5   4   3

Contributors

Susan V. Duff, EdD, OTR/L, PT, CHT, BCP
Clinical Coordinator of the Upper Extremity and Limb Deformities Centers of Excellence, Shriners Hospital for Children, Philadelphia, Pennsylvania
Motor Learning and Motor Control; Prehension

Lori Quinn, EdD, PT
Associate Professor, New York Medical College, Physical Therapy Program, Valhalla, New York
Motor Learning and Motor Control

Patricia A. Wilder, PhD, PT
Associate Professor, Department of Physical Therapy, University of Wisconsin-LaCrosse, LaCrosse, Wisconsin
Muscle System Changes; Locomotion

Content Consultant

Jennifer M. Bottomley, PhD, MS, PT
Independent Geriatric Rehabilitation Consultant, Wayland, Massachusetts

Preface

We appreciate the feedback of our colleagues in response to the first edition of *Functional Movement Development Across the Life Span* and have endeavored to incorporate the suggestions in this second edition. Our text continues to be intended for students in physical therapy, occupational therapy, and other professions that address movement dysfunction. Development of functional movement and maintenance of functional skills throughout the life span are important to all individuals as well as being major goals for care and outcomes in today's health care market.

Movement is necessary for safety, survival, mobility, occupation, leisure, health, and fitness. Functional movement occurs throughout the span of everyone's life and contributes to our complete development. While motivation to move is innate, the ability to move changes across the life span. As biological organisms, we develop within a psychological and sociocultural environment. Birth and death are events we all share; what comes between these two events is unique to each of us.

This second edition continues to emphasize normal development and focuses on the definition of function, how it is attained, and how it is optimized across the life span. The basic premise of the text holds that students and therapists must have a solid grounding in normal development, including the cellular and systems changes that occur beginning in the embryo and continuing throughout life, in order to recognize, understand, and appropriately intervene in the presence of abnormal motor function. New and expanded text and more than 150 illustrations, of which 50 are new to this edition, help the reader achieve these goals more readily.

The book is carefully organized to provide the reader with the background and tools necessary to understand the components of functional movement. The context in Unit I has been revised to address the biophysical-psychological-sociocultural domains, significant research in the field, and the changes in rationales and steps for accurate assessment. The FIM™ and WeeFIM® tools, commonly used in the field today, are included. In addition, Chapters 3 and 4 have been completely revamped to bring students and clinicians the most current content on motor development, motor learning, motor control, and their complex interrelationships.

Building on this foundation, Unit II adds a more comprehensive review of how body systems develop and affect functional movement from the prenatal period through older adulthood. Specifically, the chapters dealing with the skeletal system, the cardiovascular and pulmonary systems, and the nervous system have been rewritten and are more comprehensively illustrated. New knowledge about the nervous system is included from a body of research that has increased exponentially in the last two years.

While the final unit continues to focus on age-related outcomes within the functional movement milieu, Chapter 11 offers a completely new perspective on vital functions. Chapter 12 has been significantly revised to include a more complete explanation of the relationship between posture and balance. Chapter 13 provides an expanded view of locomotion across the life span, including the components of gait. Chapter 14 presents the most recent research in the area of prehension.

Content related to development of specific age groups has been enhanced, with special attention to the ongoing development of the healthy older adult. Dr. Jennifer Bottomley's thoughtful consultation provides the basis for broader coverage of normal and problematic function after age 50.

In order to heighten awareness of wellness and prevention issues across the life span, we have provided a new feature in the systems and outcome chapters—Clinical Implications sidebars. We think these boxes greatly enhance the utility of the text by zeroing in on clinical application. This content works hand-in-hand with our continued focus on function and its importance to health and quality of life. In addition, we provide updated information about the World Health Organization's model of disablement and its relationship to the original Nagi model. Since this framework is shared with the *Guide to Physical Therapist Practice,* we also incorporate information from the *Guide* as appropriate to normal function.

Donna J. Cech, MS, PT, PCS
Downers Grove, Illinois

Suzanne "Tink" Martin, MACT, PT
Evansville, Indiana

Acknowledgments

We wish to thank the professional colleagues and many students who have provided feedback on our efforts and offered encouragement and support. A special thanks goes to coworkers at our respective universities for technical assistance and ongoing support. We especially thank Catherine McGraw, PhD, and Frank Underwood, PhD, PT, ECS, for reading and reviewing chapters. Jennifer Bottomley was invaluable to this project, helping us to better address issues related to older adulthood. We thank the contributors to the first edition, including Ann F. Vansant, PhD, PT, and those who have been a part of both editions, as well as Lori Quinn, who is new to our team.

We also want to thank our friends and family for their continued support and encouragement. Terry, Jim, and Alec, your patience and understanding is so important to us. We acknowledge our parents for instilling in us the confidence that helped us to pursue a project of this scope.

Lastly, thank you to the many people in the publishing world who have supported and worked with us over the course of this project. These include Andrew Allen, publishing director at W.B. Saunders, for patiently waiting for this second edition and believing in the book and Sue Bredensteiner, developmental editor, for her organization, insightful suggestions regarding text and artwork, and exceptional ability to keep us steadily moving toward completion. Our special regards go to Margaret Biblis for starting this entire process and her continued friendship and encouragement.

Donna J. Cech, MS, PT, PCS
Downers Grove, Illinois

Suzanne "Tink" Martin, MACT, PT
Evansville, Indiana

Contents

Unit

II   Body Systems Contributing to Functional Movement

Definition of Functional Movement

1 Functional Independence: A Lifelong Goal

OBJECTIVES

After studying this chapter, the reader will be able to:

1 Define function.
2 Appreciate the interrelationship of all domains of function in everyday life.
3 Discuss the relationship of functional abilities to health status.
4 Differentiate among functional independence, impairment, disability, and handicap.
5 Appreciate life-span issues related to functional abilities.
6 Identify the aspects of physical function that relate to quality of performance.

As humans, we learn to exist within our environment. Throughout our life span, we constantly develop or adapt our abilities and skills to live our lives in a satisfying and meaningful manner. The capacity to exist within the environment is influenced by our ability to function, and the quality of our functional ability is related to all aspects of development: physical, social, emotional, and mental. In this book, we approach development as an ongoing process and explore its influence on functional movement ability.

Improving our client's functional ability is frequently our goal as health care professionals. Various health care professionals strive to help their clients optimize different aspects of function to realize the most satisfying and meaningful life possible. To meet this goal most effectively, we must understand the meaning of the word *function* within our respective disciplines. For example, physicians and nurses may focus primarily on the attainment and maintenance of good health as related to function, whereas social workers concentrate on an individual's ability to function within his social system. Occupational therapists work to improve the ability to function in daily life and to perform occupational tasks, whereas physical therapists structure programs to enhance physical function and mobility. All of these aspects of function are, of course, interdependent, and when considered as a conceptual whole, they help to reflect a person's functional ability in our society and environment.

Function

Widely accepted definitions of the word *function* include such phrases as "normal, characteristic actions," "purpose," and "group of related actions." More generally, function is a natural, required, or expected activity. When related to the roles and activities of people, the term *function* can describe the action of an individual body part or the person as a whole. The heart functions to pump blood through the body, delivering nutrients to other organs and tissues. The legs function to support our body weight during standing and to propel us forward during walking. We gain mastery over the environment, functioning to complete roles and tasks important to everyday life.

FUNCTION AS RELATED TO HEALTH

Function is very closely related to health. As globally defined by the World Health Organization (WHO), *health* is a state of complete physical, mental, and social well-being, not merely the absence of disease and infirmity (WHO, 1958). This simple definition is difficult to use clinically because well-being is hard to measure and too broad a concept to accurately portray an individual's status. More specifically, health influences our ability to successfully complete the tasks expected by society. Without the necessary functional abilities, it is difficult to complete these tasks or to demonstrate a state of complete physical, mental, and social well-being. From another perspective, functional ability can be disrupted as a result of poor health. Disease, infirmity, and illness interfere with our capacity to perform socially expected roles. It therefore is not difficult to understand why health professionals endeavor to improve how an individual functions.

Client Assessment

To identify client needs and to develop interventions, health professionals must be able to measure an individual's health status. Health status can be measured by looking at three primary arenas: (1) physical manifestations, (2) client symptoms, and (3) functional status (Jette, 1985). *Physical manifestations* are those aspects of body function that can be measured or observed, such as muscle strength, body temperature, blood pressure, and the presence of edema. *Client symptoms* reflect the client's impression of his health. The client may report a painful knee, weakness, fatigue, or generally feeling good. *Functional status* reflects how well the client is able to perform day-to-day activities. Illness and injury, then, influence health status and can reduce one's ability to function. The impact of this reduction varies. Some people lose little ground in keeping up with their day-to-day tasks, whereas others may not be able to do the things they need to do. The terms *disability* and *handicap* are frequently used when daily tasks cannot be performed. In general, *disability* refers to an individual's diminished functional capacity (Jette, 1985). *Handicap* is a frame of reference defined by society; when an individual is no longer viewed as being able to perform the tasks expected by society, she is considered handicapped.

However, the loss of functional ability does not necessarily result in disability or handicap.

Health Status Models

Several models have been proposed to analyze the spectrum of status from functional independence to disability. This categorization is helpful in identifying appropriate services and in planning treatment programs. Historically, the two most popular models have been the International Classification of Impairments, Disabilities, and Handicaps (ICIDH) proposed by WHO (1980) and the model of health status proposed by sociologist Saad Nagi (1991). These two models are compared in Figure 1–1.

The ICIDH defines *impairment* as any limitation or abnormality in anatomical, physiological, or psychological processes. *Disability* refers to a deficit in the performance of daily activities. *Handicap* is related to an individual's inability to perform expected social roles, leading to a diminished quality of life. This model provides basic categories for classifying a client's functional outcome status. Not all clients fit easily and neatly into the categories. Some people can have impairments that do not automatically mean they are disabled in their performance of daily activities. Others may have the ability to perform a task such as dressing but choose not to perform this task independently if it takes too much time or is too exhausting. They may draw on the assistance of others, use assistive devices, or adjust the environment to make the task easier (Guccione, 1991; Haley et al, 1992). Do they then have a disability?

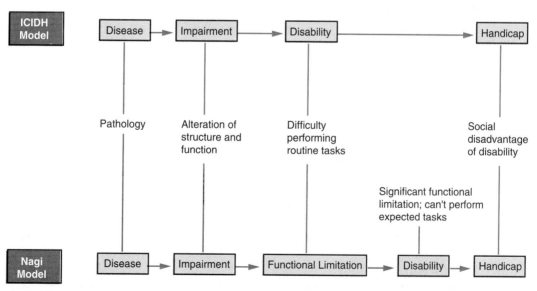

Figure 1–1

Comparison of International Classification of Impairments, Disabilities, and Handicaps (ICIDH) and Nagi classification systems of health status.

The model proposed by Nagi, although similar in its definition of impairment to the ICIDH, introduces another category into the classification scheme. The category of *functional limitation* describes deficits occurring because of an impairment and affecting the ability to perform usual activities. Within the Nagi model, the presence of disease and impairment does not necessarily result in functional limitations. Consider a client with an impairment of elbow range of motion who cannot fully extend the elbow. This impairment will cause more of a functional limitation for a baseball pitcher than it would for a pianist. The term *disability* is also used differently in the Nagi model. *Disability* refers to patterns of behavior that emerge when functional limitations are too great to allow successful completion of a task. The Nagi classification system supports the identification of limitations in functional tasks appropriate and important for the specific individual. Health care providers are aided in identifying the most appropriate focus for their interventions when they use this approach. The *Guide to Physical Therapist Practice* (American Physical Therapy Association, 2001) uses this model of disablement as a framework for the practice of physical therapy and to optimize client function.

In 1994, WHO launched an initiative to revise the ICIDH model. The new model is more similar to that proposed by Nagi than to the original ICIDH. The terminology used to relate functioning to disability has changed. The terms *body functions* and *body structures* now describe either the physiological or psychological function of the organs, limbs, and their components. Any problems with these body functions and structures that result in a deviation from the norm or a loss are referred to as *impairments*. The term *activity limitation* has replaced the term *disability* in the model and refers to difficulties in performance of activities by the individual. Finally, the term *participation restriction* has replaced the term *handicap*, referring to any problem the individual may have in participating in society. ICIDH-2 also considers possible roles of the environment and of personal factors such as health condition or status, fitness, age, and personality in an individual's ability to participate in society (Fig. 1–2). Overall, the new ICIDH-2 promises to describe human function and disability for all individuals, not only individuals with medical conditions (WHO, 2000).

In the assessment of the health status of individuals, health care providers need to understand and differentiate among the issues of impairment, functional limitation, and disability or activity limitation. Such assessment allows the provider to focus on the issues most important to the client and to consider whether interventions can effect change in an impairment, minimize a functional limitation, or diminish a disability or activity limitation.

In working with clients of different ages, it is also important to understand whether limitations reflect the presence of disability or normal development. Is the 3-year-old child who cannot tie his shoe disabled? Of course not. Developmentally, it is normal for a young child to require adult assistance with this task. By 8 years of age, the child usually has developed this skill and no longer needs adult assistance. If an older adult with severe arthritis cannot put on her shoe because of mobility limitations in hip flexion or finger mobil-

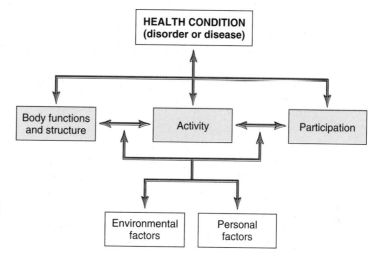

Figure 1–2

Classification system according to International Classification of Impairments, Disabilities, and Handicaps 2 (ICIDH-2).

ity, is she disabled? Again, not necessarily. If that adult uses a long-handled shoehorn, she may be quite good at completing the task. Developmental issues, social expectations, family attitudes, and adaptability of the environment are all issues that help determine whether limitations are present (Haley et al, 1992).

FUNCTIONAL SKILLS

Functional skills have been defined as the variety of skills that are frequently demanded in natural domestic, vocational, and community environments, allowing an individual to perform as independently as possible in all settings (Brown et al, 1979). Functional skills and activities not only support our biophysical and psychological well-being but also allow us to incorporate what we view as important into meaningful, everyday life. From early infancy to late adulthood, we must develop or adapt functional skills to best access the environment in which we live and to meet our own needs as independently as possible. The performance of functional activities not only depends on our physical abilities but also is affected by emotional status, cognitive ability, and sociocultural expectations. These factors together define an individual's functional performance (Fig. 1–3).

In general, certain categories of functional activities, such as eating, maintaining personal hygiene, dressing, ambulating, and grasping, are common to everyone. Other tasks related to our job or recreational activities vary from one person to the next. Within the health care model, personal care activities such as ambulating, feeding, bathing, dressing, grooming, maintaining continence, and toileting are referred to as *basic activities of daily living (BADL)*. Other important activities relate to how well we manage within the home setting and in the community. These activities are referred to as *instrumental activities of*

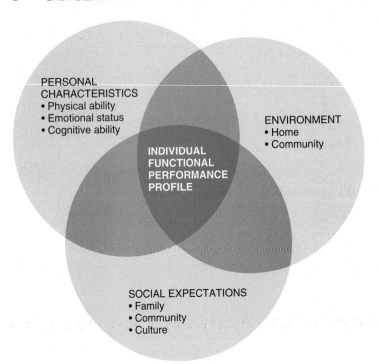

PERSONAL CHARACTERISTICS
• Physical ability
• Emotional status
• Cognitive ability

ENVIRONMENT
• Home
• Community

INDIVIDUAL FUNCTIONAL PERFORMANCE PROFILE

SOCIAL EXPECTATIONS
• Family
• Community
• Culture

Figure 1–3

Factors that define an individual's functional performance.

daily living (IADL) and include tasks such as cooking, cleaning, handling finances, shopping, working, and using personal or public transportation. The health care provider often assesses BADL and IADL to define client status and to develop appropriate intervention programs (see Chapter 5).

FUNCTION FROM A LIFE-SPAN PERSPECTIVE

Function defines mastery and competency over the environment. Throughout the life span, from conception until old age, we demonstrate varying abilities and levels of mastery over our environment. Initially, we are concerned with being able to survive and master a level of function concerned with the locus of self-need and control. Next, we learn to function well within the home environment, and finally we learn to function within the community (Fig. 1–4). For example, to ensure survival, the infant learns to cry for food or when experiencing discomfort. He can also turn his head to keep his airway clear and can coordinate important tasks such as breathing and swallowing. The toddler learns to function safely within his or her home: avoiding electrical outlets, climbing stairs, feeding herself, and using the toilet. The school-age child learns to safely cross the street on the way to school. These same levels of mastery are mirrored at all life stages, as functional expectations change. The adult masters the self-care tasks of eating by shopping and cooking or dining out and provides shelter for himself and keeps it clean and warm.

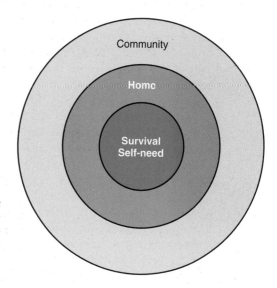

Figure 1–4

Acquisition of function. The concentric circles illustrate that acquisition of function begins with a focus on self, the locus of self-need and control, which evolves to increased levels of mastery over a broadening environment.

Finally, the adult masters functioning in a larger community, including the workplace.

From these examples, it is obvious that our functional ability is in part defined by age. As children become older, they are expected to gain independence in a wide variety of functional tasks and in an expanding environment. The 5-year-old child must meet the challenges of becoming competent within the new environment of school. Many 16-year-old youths assume the responsibilities of safely driving a car and functioning within their community. The functional expectations of adults expand as they have children and assume job responsibilities. Older adults may appear to be faced with fewer functional expectations as they retire and their children become independent. They may also be faced with challenges related to maintaining functional independence of even basic needs as they adapt to fixed incomes and declining physical abilities. It is clear that the definitions of function and functional independence change across the life span as our abilities change and the expectations of society vary.

Physical Growth and Function

In many ways, our functional abilities depend on physical abilities. Physical development not only influences the ability to perform physical activity but also affects our ability to interact with the environment. Movement has been related to cognitive development, social activity, and communication. Across the life span, the physical capacity of the individual changes and helps to define functional capacity.

During the embryonic development of a human, the first 7 to 8 weeks after conception are devoted to growth. Functional systems, although being formed, have not yet begun to work at their tasks. In the fetal period (8 weeks after conception until birth), the organ systems begin to function and the developing fetus becomes competent within the protective environment of the womb. After birth, the neonate must accommodate another environment, governed by the force of gravity. Infants attain functional skills in this new environment and systematically continue growing. The 1-year-old toddler may be very proud and excited about his ability to walk. Children who are 2 to 3 years old add important functional skills such as feeding and dressing themselves. Throughout childhood, physical growth occurs as the child becomes taller and stronger and demonstrates increasing endurance. The child actively explores his community on a bicycle or roller blades.

The balance between body growth and functional mastery continues until physical maturity is attained in young adulthood. Adults strive to attain and maintain functionally active lifestyles at home, in the workplace, and during leisure activities. The wear and tear that sometimes results from their functional activities can frequently be balanced by growth and the repair abilities of the body. By the time an adult reaches old age, growth and repair functions may be insufficient to maintain the optimal functional state of the body. Wide variations in functional ability are seen among older adults. Many older adults continue to live an active life, adapting as necessary to physical changes in their muscular and skeletal system. In other older adults, changes in strength, posture, or endurance may make efficient movement and physical function difficult. As the performance of functional skills becomes inefficient, the older adult may be less able to participate in activities that are important to him, diminishing his ability to function and maintain a level of mastery over his environment (Guccione, 2000; Sinclair and Dangerfield, 1998). The length of the average life span continues to extend, so many older adults can expect to live into their 70s, 80s, and 90s. A concomitant compression of the period of morbidity at the end of life has been demonstrated, most notably in older adults who have practiced good health behaviors (e.g., stress reduction, exercise, hydration, nutrition) throughout their life span (Blocker, 1992).

Relationship Between Development and Function

Each individual develops throughout the life span. Development occurs not only as a result of physical changes within the body but also because of environmental influences. As we interact within family, community, social, and cultural contexts, our development is shaped and functional roles or tasks are defined. From this perspective, development and function are intertwined throughout the life span, much like a piece of cloth is woven.

The *development of function* does not refer just to the growth process related to youth or to the decline often associated with aging. Similarly, it cannot necessarily be reflected linearly. Growth and development imply change, either positive or negative, which can be observed at any point within the life span. If the life span and functional development are considered two separate continuums, pleated onto one another to resemble the bellows of an accordion, their impact on each other is obvious (Fig. 1–5). As adolescents experience growth spurts, attaining new height, they also experience losses in flexibility

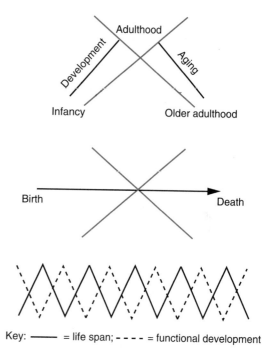

Figure 1–5

Interaction of life span and functional development.

because muscle growth does not keep up with bone growth. Adults may achieve new levels of productivity in the workplace but at a cost to family or social interactions. The life-span approach to development and function appreciates all of the changes seen in an individual's abilities at any point in the life cycle, whether the changes reflect progression, regression, or reorganization (VanSant, 1990).

DOMAINS OF FUNCTION

Functional activities with similar outcomes can be grouped together into categories or domains. We consider three domains of function here: biophysical domain, psychological domain, and sociocultural domain (Fig. 1–6). The *biophysical domain* includes the sensorimotor skills needed to perform activities of daily living, such as dressing, ambulating, maintaining hygiene, and cooking. The *psychological domain* is influenced by intellectual activities. Motivation, concentration, problem solving, and judgment are all factors that contribute to psychological function, as well as affective function, which allows a person to cope with everyday stresses. The psychological domain also influences how we perceive our ability to function. Factors such as anxiety, depression, emotional well-being, and self-esteem influence affective function (Guccione, 2000). The *sociocultural domain* relates to our ability to interact with other people and to successfully complete social roles and obligations. Cultural norms or expectations help define social function.

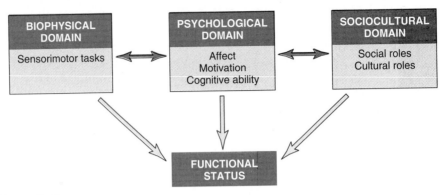

Figure 1-6

The three domains of function—biophysical, psychological, sociocultural—must operate independently as well as interdependently for human beings to achieve their best possible functional status.

These domains of function parallel domains of development discussed in Chapter 2, reinforcing the interrelationship of function and development. No one domain of function stands alone. All three are interrelated and interdependent in meeting everyday challenges. Many sociocultural functions depend on our mobility and ability to physically manipulate objects. Likewise, our physical level of function can be easily influenced by emotional status, intellectual ability, or motivation. Although all three domains of function are important, we are primarily concerned with the domain of physical function here.

Physical Function

Physical function can also be thought of as goal-directed movement. Function is the link between the physical actions we call *movement* and the environmental context in which they take place. For the act of reaching to be meaningful and therefore functional, it must take place when there is an object to reach for. Walking is functional because it is a means of moving from one place to another. People use movement every day as they interact with their environment. Goal-directed movement is important for an individual to survive, to adapt, and to learn within the environment. When our movement is inhibited, we may be less able to meet day-to-day needs. The young athlete with a broken leg suddenly must depend on crutches, making simple tasks such as walking to the bathroom or opening the door a challenge. As movement becomes less efficient, an individual may be faced with diminished functional independence. The individual with arthritis may not be able to quickly and efficiently button clothes. He may also have difficulty picking up coins when paying for purchases in a store. As physical function becomes impaired, we frequently turn to health professionals for assistance.

Physical and occupational therapy intervention is generally aimed at improving physical function. Improved physical functioning also may be a positive influence on psychological and sociocultural functioning. After the therapist identifies a client's basic functional difficulties, additional assessment of sensory, cardiopulmonary, neurological, or musculoskeletal systems may then identify impairments that interfere with overall function. Such impairments may include anatomical or physiological changes such as limited range of motion or diminished strength. Therapeutic programs can then be devised to improve function. The success of these programs is measured based on the functional change demonstrated by the client, not on isolated changes in range of motion or strength impairments.

It is important for therapists to understand how biophysical function changes over time, the relationship of physical function to other domains of function, and the components of physical function that contribute to the quality and efficiency of movement. With this knowledge, we, as therapists, can effectively create interventions that best meet individual needs.

DEVELOPMENT

How does physical function develop? What factors influence its development? Age, environment, and social expectations all contribute to a definition of normal biophysical function. Age not only defines size and biological capacity for movement but also reflects expectations about lifestyle.

During infancy and childhood, body size and the maturity of the body systems involved in movement limit and define functional abilities. For example, toddlers are able to walk, but because of their short legs, they have trouble keeping up with their parents. It is frequently more efficient and functional for them to be carried or pushed in a stroller. Young children may have trouble sitting at the table without fidgeting at a meal, perhaps because their feet do not reach the floor and they cannot easily sit in the large chair provided for them. Functional limitations in these examples are closely related to the immaturity of the child's skeletal system, but the neuromuscular and cardiopulmonary systems are also undergoing rapid development during this time frame and affect the child's physical abilities. Fundamental motor skills such as postural control, locomotion, and prehension develop rapidly during childhood.

Functional expectations of the infant and child also influence their development of functional skills. A young infant's abilities are basically survival oriented. He can lift and turn his head; coordinate suck, swallow, and breathing; cry to indicate needs; and socially interact with his caregivers. As the infant begins to control his movement, the major job or task is to explore the environment. Through play, an infant learns about the world around him; as the toddler and young child associate play with functional activities, such as eating and dressing, caregivers begin to have higher expectations for functional independence.

Through childhood and adolescence, social roles and expectations continue to undergo constant change. Body growth and maturation of the body systems also continue. Once maturity is attained in adolescence or young adulthood, the systems of the body that contribute to motor performance have completed their development. At this point, these body systems are ready to operate at peak efficiency. Practice and motivation to excel contribute to our ability to learn and refine new motor tasks. Skills are refined as we try to improve performance through recreational activities such as baseball, ballet, and gymnastics.

Societal roles and lifestyle changes that accompany adulthood again redefine physical function and may result in decreased physical activity levels. Commuting time, combined with a full day at work, may limit time available for physically active recreational pursuits. As activity levels decrease, so does our level of fitness. Cardiopulmonary functioning and muscle strength may not be supported to full capacity, resulting in decreased endurance and weakness. Refinement of skills associated with job pursuits continues through adulthood. As the body systems are continually used in day-to-day activities, wear and tear, as well as ongoing developmental changes related to adulthood, may decrease the efficiency of the body in physical functioning.

In the older adult, biophysical functional ability may decline further because of wear and tear on the body systems, normal development, and lifestyle changes. Retirement from a physically demanding job may result in a less active lifestyle. A common assumption made about older adults is that they have diminished ability to perform physical activities. It is important to remember that much variation exists in the abilities and activity levels demonstrated by older adults. Each older adult has her own unique history, experiences, and changes attributed to aging. When one considers the total population of older adults, the majority do not have significant functional limitations. They live independently and maintain a relatively active and satisfying lifestyle. Functional ability does decrease with age, but it is in the oldest populations (more than 85 years old) that physical disability is the greatest (Guccione, 2000). Numerous functional tasks are required of people who live independently, including BADL (self-care and mobility) and IADL (cooking, shopping, housekeeping, and transportation). Of these, housekeeping and transportation difficulties were reported most often by older adults (Jackson and Lang, 1989). Longitudinal studies of the functional status of adults older than 70 years report that many older adults remain functionally independent. In the study, difficulty in walking, doing heavy housework, and lower extremity function such as stooping were reported as the most difficult (Wolinsky et al, 1996).

COMPONENTS

"Efficient," "effective," "graceful," "fluid," and "smooth" are all adjectives frequently associated with movement. "Clumsy," "awkward," "disjointed," and "wasted" can also describe movement, but these words paint a very different picture. Sports science, physical education, and physical and occupational therapy professionals have tried to define the factors that contribute to efficient, effective movement. Flexibility, balance, coordination, power, and endurance are some dimensions that affect the quality of physical function.

Flexibility

Most simply, *flexibility* refers to the capacity to bend. Flexibility can be described for a specific joint, a series of joints, or a specific person. Within human movement, flexibility depends on two different components; the first is the flexibility of the muscles, connective tissue, and skin. These tissues must maintain an appropriate resting length and pliability to allow the joint mobility necessary for the completion of activities of daily living. The second component of flexibility refers to joint range of motion. The joint structure must be able to move through its entire range, completing the normal range of arthrokinematics and demonstrating adequate laxity of the joint capsule (Kisner and Colby, 1996; Zachazewski, 1989). When a person has good flexibility, the tissues more easily accommodate stress, which results in efficient, effective movement (Zachazewski, 1989).

Two types of flexibility can be assessed. *Static flexibility* refers to the range of motion available at a joint. *Dynamic flexibility* describes the resistance offered to active movement of the joint. As resistance increases, dynamic flexibility decreases. When optimal levels of resistance balance the motion around a joint, efficiency of movement is achieved. As flexibility increases, greater force can be exerted in a movement, and the speed of performance increases (Northrip et al, 1974).

Our flexibility is defined by the types of physical activities we pursue each day at work and in recreational activities. The flexibility of the baseball pitcher's throwing arm is certainly greater than that of a typist's arm. A gymnast is probably more flexible than a football player.

Developmentally, flexibility is fairly stable in boys from age 5 to 8 years and then decreases slightly until age 12 to 13 years. After that time, it again increases slightly until age 18. In girls, flexibility is stable from age 5 to 11 years and then increases until age 14. After that time, flexibility reaches a plateau. At all ages, females are more flexible than males (Malina and Bouchard, 1991). In older adults, flexibility may decrease because of cross-linkage of collagen fibers in connective tissue, inactivity, decreased muscle strength, and joint changes. Active older adults maintain greater levels of flexibility than do their more sedentary peers (Kaplan et al, 1993; Walker et al, 1984).

Balance

Balance is related to a state of equilibrium and is an important component of skilled movement. Balance is achieved when we can maintain our center of gravity over our base of support, thereby maintaining equilibrium. Several factors contribute to the ability to balance, including efficient function of the nervous system, musculoskeletal system, and sensory systems. Balance is necessary during static activities such as standing still (*static balance*) and during movement (*dynamic balance*).

Throughout childhood balance improves. Girls appear to perform better than boys in balance activities. In adolescence, both groups reach a plateau in balance skills; boys may perform slightly better than girls in this age group (Malina and Bouchard, 1991). In older adulthood, poor balance is frequently reported as a problem and may be related to developmental changes or impairments in the body systems that contribute to balance. Some of these changes include impaired reflex activity, vestibular dysfunction, posture changes, deconditioning from disuse, medications, and dehydration (Lord et al, 1991). Falling is also a problem related to balance issues in older adults. Falls within this population can lead to fractures, hospitalization, and loss of function.

Coordination

Coordination implies that various muscles are working together to produce a movement. Smooth, efficient movement results when the right muscles work at the right time with the right intensity (Kisner and Colby, 1996). Coordination is needed to successfully crawl, skip, run to catch a bus, make a bed, or put on a pair of pants in the morning. Another way of looking at coordination is to consider it as the function that constrains the body's limitless movement possibilities into one efficient, functional unit (Crutchfield et al, 1989).

Power

Power refers to the rate at which work is done. Related to movement, it is the rate at which a muscle can develop tension and produce a force, moving a body part through a range of motion (Mangine et al, 1989). Power is then related to both strength and speed. In childhood, power depends on size and maturity of the neurological and musculoskeletal systems. In older adults, as strength and speed decrease, power also decreases (Brown, 1987; Rogers and Evans, 1993).

Endurance

Endurance is related to the ability to continue to perform work over an extended period. Children, for example, can play actively for hours. We need endurance to perform repetitive activities of daily living, such as stirring food while cooking, using a blow dryer to dry our hair, or walking up steps. Recreational and job-related tasks also often require a high level of endurance.

Endurance can be affected by an individual muscle, a muscle group, or the total body. Total body endurance usually refers to cardiopulmonary endurance, reflecting the ability of the heart to deliver a steady supply of oxygen to working muscle. Muscle endurance is related to muscle strength. Developmentally, muscle endurance has been shown to increase linearly in boys between 5 and 13 years of age, after which a spurt is observed, whereas steady linear increase in muscle endurance is seen in girls (Malina and Bouchard, 1991).

Summary

Human function is an elusive entity. We discuss function from a life-span perspective as well as its relationship to the broader context of health. Models of health status help differentiate between function and dysfunction (disability or activity limitation). The interactions and interdependence of the biophysical, psychological, and sociocultural domains are what define our ability to function. The domain of biophysical function requires in-depth understanding because this is the area that we, as physical and occupational therapists, hope to improve when working with our clients. The components that make movement efficient, effective, and, most important, functional have been carefully reviewed. Using this knowledge base, we can assess how our clients are functioning and help them successfully meet their goals of improved function.

References

American Physical Therapy Association. *Guide to Physical Therapist Practice*, 2nd ed. Alexandria, VA: American Physical Therapy Association, 2001.

Blocker WP. Maintaining functional independence by mobilizing the aged. *Geriatrics* 47:42–56, 1992.

Brown L, Branston MB, Hamre-Mietupski S, et al. A strategy for developing chronological age appropriate and functional curricular content for severely handicapped adolescents and young adults. *J Spec Ed* 13:81–89, 1979.

Brown MA. Selected physical performance changes with aging. *Top Geriatr Rehabil* 2:68–76, 1987.

Crutchfield C, Shumway-Cook A, Horak F. Balance and coordination training. In Scully RM, Barnes MR (eds). *Physical Therapy*. Philadelphia: JB Lippincott, 1989, pp 825–843.

Guccione AA. Physical therapy diagnosis and the relationship between impairments and function. *Phys Ther* 71:499–504, 1991.

Guccione AA. *Geriatric Physical Therapy*, 2nd ed. St. Louis: Mosby, 2000.

Haley SM, Coster WJ, Ludlow LH, et al. *Pediatric Evaluation of Disability Inventory (PEDI)*. Boston: New England Medical Center Hospital, Inc, and PEDI Research Group, 1992.

Jackson OL, Lang RH. Comprehensive functional assessment of the elderly. In Jackson OL (ed). *Physical Therapy of the Geriatric Patient*, 2nd ed. New York: Churchill Livingstone, 1989, pp 239–277.

Jette AM. State of the art in functional status assessment. In Rothstein J (ed). *Measurement in Physical Therapy*. New York: Churchill Livingstone, 1985, pp 137–168.

Kaplan GA, Shawbridge WT, Camachs T, Cohen RD. Factors associated with change in physical functioning in the elderly. *J Aging Health* 5:140–153, 1993.

Kisner C, Colby LA. *Therapeutic Exercise: Foundations and Techniques*. Philadelphia: FA Davis, 1996.

Lord SR, Clark RD, Webster IW. Physiological factors associated with falls in an elderly population. *J Am Geriatr Soc* 39:1194–1200, 1991.

Malina RM, Bouchard C. *Growth, Maturation, and Physical Activity*. Springfield, IL: Human Kinetics Press, 1991.

Mangine R, Heckman TP, Eldridge VL. Improving strength, endurance and power. In Scully RM, Barnes MR (eds). *Physical Therapy*. Philadelphia: JB Lippincott, 1989, pp 739–762.

Nagi SZ. Disability concepts revisited: Implications for prevention. In Pope AM, Tarlov AR (eds). *Disability in America: Toward a National Agenda for Prevention*. Washington, DC: National Academy Press, 1991, pp 309–327.

Northrip JW, Logan GA, McKinney WC. *Introduction to Biomechanic Analysis of Sport*. Dubuque, IA: Wm C. Brown, 1974.

Rogers MA, Evans WJ. Changes in skeletal muscle with aging: Effects of exercise training. *Exerc Sport Sci Rev* 21:65–102, 1993.

Sinclair DC, Dangerfield P. *Human Growth After Birth*, 6th ed. New York: Oxford University Press, 1998.

VanSant AF. Life-span development in functional tasks. *Phys Ther* 70:788–798, 1990.

Walker JM, Sue D, Miles-Elkousy N. Active mobility of the extremities in older subjects. *Phys Ther* 64:919–923, 1984.

Wolinsky FD, Stump TE, Callahan CM. Consistency and change in functional status among older adults over time. *J Aging Health* 8:155–182, 1996.

World Health Organization. *The First Ten Years of the World Health Organization*. Geneva: World Health Organization, 1958.

World Health Organization. *International Classification of Impairments, Disabilities, and Handicaps*. Geneva: World Health Organization, 1980.

World Health Organization. *International Classification of Impairments, Disabilities, and Handicaps-2 (ICIDH-2)*. Available at: http://www.who.int./ICIDH. Accessed June 19, 2000.

Zachazewski JE: Improving flexibility. In Scully RM, Barnes MR (eds). *Physical Therapy*. Philadelphia: JB Lippincott, 1989, pp 698–738.

2 Theories Affecting Development

OBJECTIVES

After studying this chapter, the reader will be able to:

1 Define domains, periods, and concepts of development.

2 Define and give examples of growth, maturation, adaptation, and learning in all developmental domains.

3 Discuss representative biophysical, psychological, and sociocultural theories and theorists.

4 Discuss theories of life-span development, child development, and aging.

Development is a topic covered in many professional education curricula, including biology, education, psychology, and health sciences programs. Each program focuses on aspects of development unique to its profession, and vast amounts of information exist within these specialized areas. Our collective knowledge substantiates that an individual develops across the broad continuum of the life span, strongly influenced by three interrelated domains. Thus, normal human development is shaped by interaction among the biophysical, psychological, and sociocultural domains.

A general introduction to biophysical, psychological, and sociocultural theories describes how the different domains and disciplines are basic to our lives as well as the study of the development of human behavior. For example, a child in the United States learns to eat with a fork within the first or second year of life. This social skill cannot develop until physical coordination is sufficiently advanced to allow fine controlled movements of the arm and hand. The child must cognitively understand the relationship among food, the fork, hunger, and the action taken to satisfy that hunger. Social customs shape how the child performs the skill. In fact, an Asian child will be meeting the same functional need at about the same age but will be using chopsticks.

Human Development

Human development refers to changes that occur in our lives from conception to death. Change can occur on many levels—the cell, tissue, organ, and body systems. Change can be progressive, reorganizational, or regressive. In muscle, for example, where tissue increases during growth, fiber types differentiate or atrophy because of the use or loss of innervation and nutrition. Form and function change during the process of development, as occurs when a sapling grows into an oak tree or a caterpillar turns into a butterfly. The form a movement takes is shaped by its intended function. Because functional demands are different at different ages, the movement forms that emerge during development change as we age. Human behavior is the outward manifestation of development and changes through four processes: growth, maturation, adaptation, and learning. These processes occur simultaneously and concurrently in all domains of human development.

DOMAINS OF DEVELOPMENT

The processes of growth, maturation, adaptation, and learning operate at the same time in three different domains: biophysical, psychological, and sociocultural. Physical growth and development are accompanied by the acquisition of motor skills, intellectual development, and social-emotional development. For example, intellectually an infant may be unable to communicate or even understand his own physical actions. The parent supplies meaning to the gestures, looks, or early sound production. This shapes the infant's actions to his parents' expectations for motor performance or communication. Thus, we, as parents, may interpret a random swipe as a reach or the sound "ma" as recognition of mother.

We see the interrelationships of development in multiple domains when the infant develops perceptual awareness concurrently with motor control, beginning cognition, and attachment. A social smile is evident in most 2-month-old infants, although it usually takes 2 additional months before the infant demonstrates sufficient head control to focus attention on caregivers or objects and to be able to direct reaching. This process of human development is interactive, and each domain exerts a positive or negative impact on the other domains. The temperament of a baby can affect the quality of interaction with the caregiver or therapist and thereby affect the attachment process. The biophysical, psychological, and sociocultural selves interact to produce a unique individual. There are no two people who are exactly alike.

Each domain contributes to our understanding of motor behavior. We are biological organisms that develop within a psychological and sociocultural environment. This relationship is schematically represented in Figure 1–6. Even though our primary therapeutic emphasis is on our client's ability to move, as therapists, we must take into account his cognitive and psychosocial status as well as the familial, cultural, and societal movement and life expectations. Indeed, motor behavior will reflect age, ability, level of maturation, experience, and cultural bias.

PERIODS OF DEVELOPMENT

The life span is most often divided into age-related segments or periods (Table 2–1). The prenatal period averages 38 weeks in length, beginning with conception and culminating in birth. It is divided into three stages: the *germinal* period, the first 2 weeks of gestation; the *embryonic* period, when all major organ systems form (weeks 2 to 8); and the *fetal* period, when organ systems differentiate and rapid body growth occurs (weeks 9 to 38).

The lengthy postnatal period is usually broken down into the categories of infancy, childhood, adolescence, and adulthood. *Infancy* spans the first 2 years of life, from birth to the second birthday. *Childhood* begins at 2 years of age for both girls and boys but lasts longer for boys because of the time difference in the onset of puberty. *Adolescence* lasts 8 to 10 years, beginning at approximately 10 years of age for girls and 12 years of age for boys. It is divided into three stages: *prepubescence*, the 2 years before the onset of puberty; *pubescence*, the 4 years in which hormones produce secondary sexual characteristics; and *postpubescence*, the final 2 years of adolescence in which the final maturity of adulthood is reached.

Adulthood is concerned less with age than with role transition. Most of us are considered adult when we reach our 20s. Going to college, getting a job, and being able to vote have all been used as markers of adulthood, but no one task or age clearly defines this period. Adulthood can be divided loosely into young, middle, and older adulthood. Although transitions have been identified among the various divisions of adulthood, none appear to be as easily defined as the periods of child development.

Geriatrics and gerontology were established as fields of human service and research in the 1950s. Since that time, the field of gerontology has fostered an explosion of information on aging. Demographics document that the population continues to age. By 2050, almost 23% of the total population, or 68.5

TABLE 2–1

Periods of Development

	Period	Time Span
	Prenatal	Conception to birth
	• Germinal	• 1–2 weeks' gestation
	• Embryonic	• 2–8 weeks' gestation
	• Fetal	• 9–38 weeks' gestation
	Infancy	Birth to 2 years
	Childhood	2–10 years (female) 2–12 years (male)
	Adolescence	10–18 years (female) 12–20 years (male)
	Young adulthood	18–40 years
	Middle adulthood	40–65 years
	Older adulthood	65 years to death
	• Young-old	• 65–74 years
	• Middle-old	• 75–84 years
	• Old-old	• 85 years to death

million people, will be older than 65 years (Atchley, 1991). For purposes of research, gerontologists subdivide older adulthood into three stages: young-old, middle-old, and old-old (Atchley, 1991).

CONCEPTS OF DEVELOPMENT

Maturity

Development from birth to the attainment of biophysical, psychological, and sociocultural maturity constitutes the first part of the life span. *Maturation* is the process whereby an organism continues to grow, differentiate, and change from conception until achieving the mature state. Maturity is usually attained during adulthood between 25 and 30 years of age. Biological maturation is typically attributed to an individual's genetic makeup, whereas psychological and social-emotional maturity results from a combination of maturation and learning. Maturation is not considered the only determinant of development.

Senescence

Development continues throughout adulthood with structural and functional changes seen as a normal part of healthy aging. Therefore, aging can be viewed as a continuation of the developmental process. The term *senescence*, however, is appropriately used to describe later life because aging can refer to any time-related process. *Senescence* is the progressive physiological decline that results in our increasing vulnerability to stress and the progressing likelihood of death. Just like other phases of development, senescence is not a single process but rather many processes. Age-related changes produced in our organ systems and personal identity result from a lifetime of interactions among our internal environment, culture, and society.

Life Span

The concept of life-span development is not new. Baltes (1987) identified five characteristics to use when assessing a theory for its life-span perspective. These criteria ask that development be viewed as:

- Lifelong
- Multidimensional
- Plastic and flexible
- Contextual
- Embedded in history

Development within the biophysical, psychological, and sociocultural domains is enriched when viewed through a life-span perspective. Life-span development provides a holistic framework in which aging is a lifelong process of growing up and growing old. No one period of life can be understood without looking at its relationship to what came before and what lies ahead.

Life span is also defined as the maximum survival potential for a particular species (Atchley, 1991). Most gerontologists agree that our life span is species-specific and therefore intrinsically regulated (Cristofalo et al, 1999). Theoretically, the maximum length of life biologically possible for a human is 120 years, although documentation exists for one individual who lived to be 122. Numerous social and environmental factors, such as war, famine, radiation, and toxic chemicals, can negatively affect this figure. Although catastrophic disease is often thought to dramatically shorten our life spans, statistics reveal that if all major causes of death were eradicated, only 15 years would be added to our life expectancy (Hayflick, 2000).

Individual Differences

The development of human behavior is strongly influenced by both maturation and experience. Genetically, we are provided the physical base of our body that continually matures during our life span. Each of us builds a sense of identity and psychological wholeness within our mind, influenced by experiences within the social environment of our family, culture, and society. The interplay of maturation and experience is unique for each individual (Fig. 2–1).

Intelligence and personality can be influenced by the environment and heredity. Children exposed to enriched environments often improve their native intelligence. Conversely, environmental deprivation may contribute to a decrease in intellectual performance. Heredity can also influence the type of experiences an individual seeks, such as finding our niche in the world (Kail and Cavanaugh, 2000). Sociability has a genetic component that affects whether a child enjoys social interaction or prefers to observe the world from a distance. Shy children will tend to seek situations that allow peace and quiet, whereas extroverted children seek social contact.

Heredity accounts for about 35% of our longevity (Finch and Tanzi, 1997). In other words, one predictor of a longer life is to come from a family of long-lived people. The remaining 65% of our longevity is attributed to environmental influences: lifestyle as well as physical and social surroundings. Lifestyle factors considered to affect longevity include smoking, diet, stress, alcohol, and exercise. Living in a hostile physical or social environment also can be counterproductive to a long life.

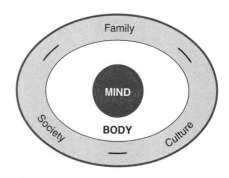

Figure 2–1

Depiction of the relationship of an individual's psychological (mind) and physical (body) self within the social environment of family, society, and culture.

PROCESSES OF DEVELOPMENT

Growth refers to the changes in physical dimensions of the body. Growth rates vary for specific body systems and tissues. Figure 2–2 provides a comparison of the general growth curve with that of specific systems and tissues. The general growth curve reflects rapid growth in infancy, slower growth in childhood, and again rapid growth in adolescence. Head circumference, height, and weight are all examples of dimensions that can be used to assess growth and can be plotted on growth charts. Changes in growth can be used to assess development by comparing the percentile growth achieved in these anthropometrical measures. Large variations among these measurements may signal a growth problem. Healthy children exhibit stable trends in growth throughout the developmental stages of life, although different body sections grow at proportionately different rates (Fig. 2–3).

Maturation contributes to development by producing physical changes that cause organs and body systems to reach their adult form and function. Changes that occur on a genetically controlled timetable can usually be attributed to the process of physical maturation. Maturation occurs in all body systems. One example from the skeletal system is the appearance of primary and secondary ossification centers in the bones (see Chapter 6). Reflexes and reactions emerge sequentially in response to maturation of the nervous system; myelination is one hallmark of nervous system maturation. Structures that are to function first are myelinated first, paralleling the development of function of those neuroanatomical structures (see Chapter 9). The integrity of nervous

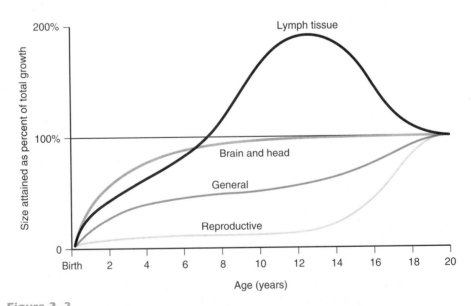

Figure 2–2

Differential rates of growth in three organ systems and tissues contrasted with the body's general growth curve.

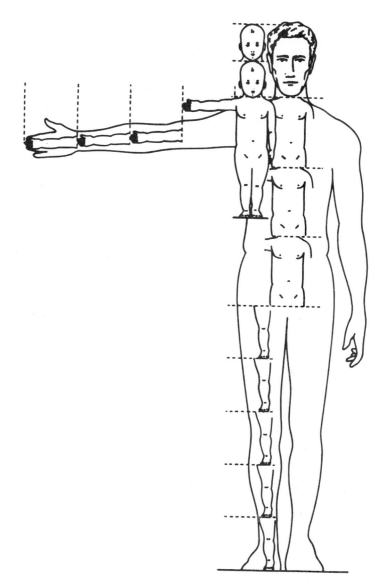

Figure 2-3

Proportional growth changes across the life span. While the whole body increases in length from birth to maturity, the length of the head increases about two times, the trunk increases about three times, the arms increase about four times, and the legs increase about five times. (From Valadian I, Porter D. *Physical Growth and Development: From Conception to Maturity*. Boston: Little, Brown, 1977, p 30.)

system development can be assessed by evaluating the presence of developmentally appropriate reflexes and reactions. The genetic substrate of behavior does not simply imprint its code on the environment; rather, the genetic base allows us to adapt to our environment. The environment also can influence maturation through adaptation and learning.

Adaptation and learning are sometimes difficult to separate from maturation. *Adaptation* is the body's accommodation to the immediate environment. Some structures and functions of organ systems are adaptations to exposure to the internal or external environment. Adaptation, like development, can produce positive or negative change. A positive change is exhibited by the production of antibodies after exposure to chicken pox. An example of a negative environmental effect was seen in the delayed motor behavior of understimulated, institutionalized infants in the 1940s. Exposure to some types of stimulus induces change, such as the development of joints in the embryo, which require primitive muscles to pull on bone to produce a joint cavity. If the muscles fail to produce movement, joint deformities occur in utero and result in *arthrogryposis*. Although each of us adapts differently, we all mature at varying rates in a similar manner.

Learning is a relatively permanent change in behavior resulting from practice and, as such, may be considered a form of adaptation. For example, rollerblading, or in-line skating, is an adaptation to having wheels on our shoes. To adapt to having wheels on our shoes, we must learn different ways to balance, start moving, and stop. Rollerblade takes practice. Many motor abilities, such as riding a bike, playing soccer, reading, writing, and speaking, are learned. We do not know if there is an optimal time for learning these tasks. We do know that experience plays a crucial role in mastering abilities that are not innate.

FACTORS AFFECTING DEVELOPMENT

The process of development is strongly influenced by four factors: genetics, maturation, environment, and culture. None of these influences alone can account for the many changes that occur throughout our life span. The interaction between maturation and experience within specific biophysical, psychological, and sociocultural environments may account for individual developmental differences. Two children grow up in the same neighborhood: one becomes a CEO for a Fortune 500 company and the other becomes a homeless drifter. What makes the difference? The values and life goals inherited from our family, society, and culture are just as real as our biological heritage.

Genetics and maturation contribute to and control our body's internal environment or milieu. The body's internal chemistry must be balanced to support growth, development, and functional activities such as movement. Hormones play a major role in controlling physical growth and initiating puberty, and they regulate the body's metabolism and ability to utilize chemical sources of energy for growth, maturation, adaptation, and learning.

Nutrition is part of the internal and external environment and contributes to the production of a healthy body. Adequate nutrition supplies fuel for efficient energy production and tissue development. For example, adequate nutrition is critical for the development and function of the nervous system, enabling the execution and control of movement. Fat must be present in the diet to produce myelin. Poor nutrition during pregnancy has been associated with intrauterine growth retardation, a significant cause of developmental disability in low-birth-weight infants (Lin and Evans, 1984). Effects of nutritional deprivation on brain development have been so thoroughly established that

U.S. manufacturers are considering adding supplements to baby formula to provide sufficient fatty acids for nervous system maturation. Infants who fail to thrive (i.e., do not gain weight at an appropriate rate) have poorer motor skills than do adequately nourished peers.

Our external environment or surroundings and culture contribute to the definition of personal nutrition. There is a vast nutritional difference between having rice and fish as dietary mainstays and having red meat and potatoes. These two different diets have been associated with Asian and Western cultures, respectively, and have been linked to differing incidences of illness such as heart disease and cancer (Helsing, 1984). Dietary differences may precipitate the earlier onset of puberty in Western societies because of a richer diet, whereas the effects of inadequate nutrition are painfully obvious in areas of the world that experience food shortages.

Culture helps us identify values and determine the task demands and roles that we play. There are similarities among cultural expectations as well as differences. Cultural expectations affect child-rearing practices and the attainment of adult status. Cultures vary in their focus on an individual or the group. Western cultures tend to focus on the individual, whereas Eastern cultures are collectivistic.

Theoretical Assumptions

The theoretical approach used to describe human development provides a framework for a discussion of the reasons for change and allows us to test our hypotheses regarding the ability of a theory to predict future development. The major assumptions about development center around the role of maturation and learning and the nature of developmental change over time. Theories and theorists differ in the way in which the origin of behavior is viewed. Is behavior innate, or is it the product of our experience? Maturationists argue that our genetic blueprint produces commonalities in our growth and development. Behaviorists take the stand that experience plays a strong role in our personal and social development.

The theorists discussed here have tried to explain the nature of developmental change over time (Table 2–2). All agree that orderly, sequential changes from simple to complex behavior occur in all domains of function. They differ on whether these changes occur in a smooth, continuous manner (continuity, or nonstage development) or with abrupt stops and starts (discontinuity, or stage development).

Continuity of development implies that later development is dependent on what came before. If development is viewed as continuous, earlier skills lead to the development of later skills. Continuity can be observed in psychological development (Gottlieb et al, 1998). In Erikson's theory (1968), successful resolution of each psychological dilemma is required to proceed to the next level. Development of cognition can be thought of as a continuous line from start to finish.

Stage theory provides another approach and can be thought of quantita-

TABLE 2-2

Theories of Human Development

Domain	Life Span	Child Development	Adulthood	Senescence
Biological/physical	Dynamic systems • Thelen • Schroots and Yates	Maturation • Gesell • McGraw		Programmed aging • Hayflick Stochastic changes Cross-linkage • Bjorksten Free radical • Harman Immune • Walford Neuroendocrine • Finch and Seeman
Psychological	Psychosocial stages • Erikson	Intelligence • Piaget Perception • Gibson and Gibson	Seasons of life • Levinson	Cognitive processing speed • Salthouse Selective optimization • Baltes
Sociocultural	Social learning • Bandura Motivation • Maslow Environmental • Bronfenbrenner	Behavioral • Skinner Social learning • Sears		Disengagement • Cumming and Henry Activity • Neugarten Continuity • Atchley

tively: A stair-step arrangement specifies different motor skills such as head control or sitting on each step. Stage theory also postulates that there are qualitative changes that occur throughout development. At each successively higher level of development, or next step, a new characteristic appears that was not previously present. In stage development, discontinuity is more prevalent than continuity in motor development (Gottlieb, 1983). For example, sitting and standing are sufficiently different to be considered stages in motor development.

Related to development is a third viewpoint—that of the child as a miniature adult. In some parts of the skeletal system, where miniature models of bones are first formed out of cartilage and then replaced by bone, it might appear that the theory is correct. Differential growth, however, occurs in the bones of the face during puberty, so that the adolescent looks much different from the child. Many body systems do not function on an adult level in the child. Because there are more instances in which this theory does not hold true, it is considered a false theory.

It is important to understand that theories provide the starting point from which to assess the complex process of human development. Regardless of the domain considered, theories attempt to explain why changes can and do occur over time. The time span covered by each developmental theory varies greatly. For example, Piaget's theory of intelligence begins at birth and ends in adolescence. Levinson's theory deals exclusively with adult development, a less well-understood phenomenon than either early or later development. Erikson's theory of personality development is the most easily recognized life-span approach because his theory accounts for changes that occur from birth to senescence.

Life-Span Theories of Development

BIOPHYSICAL DEVELOPMENT

Most theories of biophysical development focus on one age group. The only theoretical approach that remotely approximates a life-span perspective is the *dynamic systems theory*. Researchers from developmental psychology and gerontology have applied dynamic systems theory to development and aging (Lockman and Thelen, 1993; Schroots and Yates, 1999). Lockman and Thelen (1993) introduced the term *developmental biodynamics* to explain the organization of motor behavior based on interaction between perception and action. According to this theory, motor behavior emerges from that interaction rather than from nervous system maturation, as previously theorized. The application of dynamic systems theory to motor development is discussed in Chapter 3.

Dynamic systems theory grew out of *chaos theory*, which originated in mathematics and physical sciences to explain change over time in nonlinear systems. As a biological system, the human organism is an open system. It interacts with the internal and external environment. Open systems self-organize. "Dynamic systems theory hypothesizes that internal or external fluctuations of nonequilibrium systems can pass a critical point—the transformation point—and create order out of disorder through a process of self-organization" (Schroots and Yates, 1999, p 430). Energy is used in the development of a single cell into interacting organ systems. Living systems exhibit periods of stability or equilibrium and periods of disequilibrium during which significant change is possible. Energy is also used to keep the body going, make repairs, and preserve capacities in all systems. Living systems fluctuate and behave in complex ways.

Schroots and Yates (1999) applied dynamic systems theory to development and aging because they saw development and senescence as having similar features. These common features are change over time, with gradients and tapping of energy resources and the production of new structures and functions. Each new structure and function adds new dynamic constraints and information to the body through feedback to the genetic blueprint. Differences between development and senescence are the degree and rate of change that take place. During early development, the system is highly changeable; when maturity is reached, the system is more stable. The rate of change is faster early in development and slower during senescence. The first processes are negentrophic or anabolic and initially obscure the ongoing entropic or catabolic process of senescence. However, after maturity around the age of 30, the entropic processes dominate and lead to disorder (Yates and Benton, 1995). The more disordered the system, the more vulnerable it is to disease and degradation, and eventual cessation of activity.

PSYCHOLOGICAL DEVELOPMENT

Erikson (1968) transformed Freud's psychoanalytical theory into a psychosocial view of human development. Erikson's view combined biological needs with cultural expectations, producing the most broadly applicable theory of human psychological development for present-day society by replacing Freud's sexual focus with traits of social interaction. Erikson also addressed the entire life span in his eight stages of psychosocial development, as outlined in Table 2–3 and discussed in detail later. These stages incorporate more than one domain of function and are identified as necessary for an individual's growth. Each revolves around a psychosocial conflict that must be resolved to advance in the developmental process. Interestingly, as Erikson aged, his work increasingly dealt with adult stages and aging. He and his colleagues (1986) looked at generational differences and the role of expectations in aging.

Stage 1. The infant's first psychosocial conflict is whether to trust or mistrust the people within the world. Through physical contact and caregiving, the infant forms positive attachments that are mutually reinforcing. If this does not occur, negative attachments—mistrust of others, of the environment, and even of self—result. The basis of trust is seen in the establishment of positive contact with the environment and the people in it, including touch and the meeting of the infant's needs.

TABLE 2–3

Erikson's Eight Stages of Development

Life-Span Period	Stage	Characteristics
Infancy	Trust vs. mistrust	Self-trust, attachment
Late infancy	Autonomy vs. shame or doubt	Independence, self-control
Childhood (preschool)	Initiative vs. guilt	Initiates own activity
School age	Industry vs. inferiority	Works on projects for recognition
Adolescence	Identity vs. role confusion	Sense of self: physically, socially, sexually
Early adulthood	Intimacy vs. isolation	Relationship with significant other
Middle adulthood	Generativity vs. stagnation	Guiding the next generation
Late adulthood	Ego integrity vs. despair	Sense of wholeness, vitality, and wisdom

From Erikson EH. *Identity, Youth, and Crisis.* New York: WW Norton, 1986.

Stage 2. In toddlers, the basic trust learned in infancy is enhanced by resolving the next psychosocial conflict. The toddler expresses newfound independence, both motorically and socially, with the ever-popular statement, "Me do it." It is important during this stage that the toddler be allowed to be as independent as possible to prevent feelings of doubt concerning emerging abilities. Learning to control one's movements and those of people and objects within the environment is very important in early development. However, with the assertion of this newfound independence can come conflict between the child's wants and parental boundaries, as seen in the so-called terrible two's.

Stage 3. Self-regulation develops slowly in the third stage as the child learns the boundaries of appropriate social behavior. Just as an infant learns the rules of moving, the child experiments with social behavior. A growing sense of identity plus parental guidance allows for the development of self-regulation, whether that means becoming toilet trained, learning to share, or learning to take turns. Between 3 and 5 years, the preschooler has learned to master many tasks and feels free to initiate her own activities. By teaching the child which behaviors are acceptable under what circumstances, the parents encourage the child's confidence in her own planning without fear of a negative result or the burden of guilt. During this time, the parents' most important task is to encourage self-regulation of behavior. When a child begins to regulate her own behavior, she begins to rely on internalized value and reward systems.

Stage 4. The school-age child deals with the conflict between industry and inferiority. The initiative developed in the previous stage is applied to learning how to work hard on a project and to enjoy the satisfaction of a job well done. A positive self-image grows out of achievement. Without success, the child may learn to be helpless, which in turn can produce a negative self-image. The initial self-image formed between 2 and 3 years of age is expanded during middle childhood in the struggle with success or failure in school. As the student increases awareness of his values, goals, and strategies, he becomes more sensitive to the needs and expectations of others. It is during this time that tasks are often undertaken to gain the approval of a favorite teacher.

Stage 5. Adolescence produces one of the most trying psychosocial dilemmas: identity versus role confusion. An adolescent's identity is a unique blend of what she was in childhood and what she will become in adulthood. Identity formation is affected by social and sexual experiences, cognitive abilities, and self-knowledge. An adolescent must be capable of the highest level of cognition to ponder the philosophical question of "Who am I?" Anticipation of what she will do in a variety of situations causes her to enact every possible life scenario before it actually transpires. Self-knowledge is gleaned from past life experiences. This knowledge includes physical information gained from the five senses as well as knowledge of bodily functions. Emotionally, self-knowledge includes self-esteem and self-image.

The self is very important to the adolescent, so much so that self-centeredness or egocentrism engenders a feeling of performing on stage. Although emotions are part of adolescent development, they play only one role in the development of a stable identity: achievement of emotional independence from parents and other adults. Socially, the adolescent is expected to develop appropriate behavior toward her own and the opposite sex. Sexual identity is established along with a moral ideology to guide socially responsible behavior. The successful end result is a unique and stable view of self, a life philosophy, and a career path. The pursuit of a career or vocation allows the adolescent to move away from her previous egocentrism (Erikson, 1968).

The term *role confusion* describes the failure to form an identity during adolescence. Role confusion may result if adequate support systems are not available (Dennis and Hassol, 1983). The inability to form an identity leaves an adolescent confused about her role in society and makes it difficult to formulate a life philosophy, forge a career, or start a family.

Stage 6. Once an identity has been established, the young adult must deal with the conflict of intimacy versus isolation. Forming an intimate relationship with a significant other involves sharing the values, hopes, goals, and fears found during the search for identity. Schuster (1980) states that a person learns to share love in many different forms—parental love, spousal love, child love, friend love, and spiritual love. The negative result from losing the battle for intimacy is to become self-absorbed and unable to relate openly with other people. Social and emotional isolation may lead to an overly developed sense of righteousness and outward prejudice toward those with whom we disagree.

Stage 7. *Generativity* is an unconscious desire to guide and assist the next generation. The traditional way that this assistance is given is through parenting, but it can also be expressed through an occupation such as teaching or an avocation such as Big Brothers or Big Sisters. At the age of 80, Erikson (1986) wrote that making creative contributions to the world and caring for other people's children could substitute for having our own children. The common denominator in this stage is fostering another's well-being. To help others, we must be productive and creative. Stagnation is the alternative to generativity—the "Is that all there is?" attitude toward life.

Stage 8. The last hurdle of development is the conflict between integrity and despair—not ethical integrity, but ego integrity, a sense of wholeness of self related to the life already lived and the life yet to be experienced. There is a sense of vitality, expectation, and wisdom that comes from the life cycle being reflected back on itself (Erikson et al, 1986). If the older adult does not achieve ego integrity because inner resources from successful handling of previous psychosocial dilemmas have not been built up, despair replaces vitality.

Realistically, we understand that all determinants of late life satisfaction are not under our control. The body ages physically as well as psychologically. The physical self and the life situation, including socioeconomic status, activity level, and availability of transportation, have an impact on successful aging (Dennis and Hassol, 1983, p 268). There is a complex relationship between internal and external factors that shape the end result of a process that includes our past achievements and how we reacted to them. The task of coming to terms with how we led our life, the choices made, and the paths not taken is not easy. The challenge is best met with a strong sense of self-respect and a good sense of humor, remembering that "No one gets through this life alive."

SOCIOCULTURAL DEVELOPMENT

Social Learning

Bandura's (1986) social learning theory explains observational learning. As such, it may be more relevant to understanding the abstract learning that occurs from adolescence through adulthood. However, an essential process in Bandura's cognitive social learning theory is that of modeling. Modeling is described as a type of cognitive patterning. Some skills are taught directly by modeling the behavior being taught, such as having a child watch an adult sweep the floor. More complicated behaviors, such as learning values and developing problem-solving approaches, are transmitted more subtly. Adults are always amazed at what behaviors children pick up.

Social theory teaches us that experience is invaluable. We register personal experience with reference to our own level of biological and psychological maturity. A parent's raising her voice to a toddler may stop the child from an unwanted activity, but verbal warnings often go unnoticed by a teenager. Experience by itself is only an occurrence in time; experience paired with memory connotes learning. The pairing is possible because of the interaction among behavior, cognition, and the environment. Each area influences another; cognition can influence the environment and the environment can influence behavior. For example, teaching children not to play with matches does not preclude them from learning how to safely light a campfire.

Observational learning is used in the socialization process of becoming a professional. Expectations play a large role in structuring or motivating performance. The clinical instructor expects a certain level of performance from a student therapist, and that expectation motivates the student to perform. Thus, the reality that is observed in the clinic is more highly valued than a laboratory simulation. Learning is not the result of a single event but of many events within a context of interpersonal relationships.

Motivation

Maslow (1954) generated a theory to counteract the seemingly nonhumanistic approach of the psychoanalysts and the behaviorists. His theory of motivation is based on a needs hierarchy (Fig. 2–4) in which each life stage is seen from the perspective of fulfilling a certain need. We all have an innate drive to survive, grow, and find meaning to life. The sequence of needs progresses from the physiological needs related to survival and safety to the needs for love, self-esteem, and, ultimately, self-actualization. The last stage occurs when we have become all that it is possible for us to be, and it cannot be achieved unless all other needs have been met.

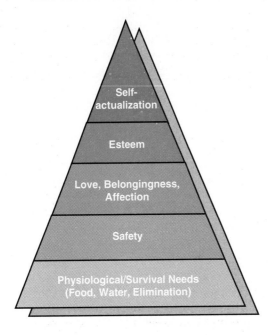

Figure 2–4

Maslow's hierarchy of needs.

Ecology

Bronfenbrenner's (1979) ecological systems approach is the application of the biological concept of studying organisms in their natural habitat or ecosystem to human development. For example, a biologist studies trout in a trout stream, not in a saltwater marsh. The model in Figure 2–5 represents Bronfenbrenner's perception of the family, community, and culture as interacting systems of society. Each system is named for its relationship to the child and encompasses an ever-widening sphere of influence. The child interacts with the members of the family, community, and culture, and they in turn act on the child. Research has focused on the effects of the varying levels of the system on developmental competence, child-rearing practices and developmental outcome, and parental attitudes within neighborhoods (Bronfenbrenner and Morris, 1998).

Theories of Child Development

BIOPHYSICAL DEVELOPMENT

Maturationists

The maturationist's view of motor development correlates all movement acquisition with the onset of changes in the nervous system relative to the onset and integration of reflexes/reactions, hierarchy of control, and a timetable of myelination. As biologists, maturationists might have considered the possibility

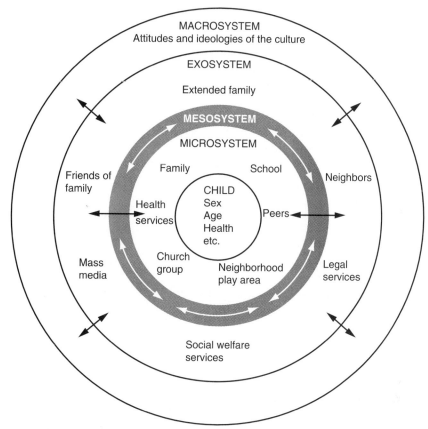

Figure 2–5

Bronfenbrenner's ecological model is one of the few comprehensive frameworks for understanding the role of the environment in the child's development. (*The Child: Development in a Social Context.* Kopp CB, Krakow JB. © 1982. Reprinted by permission of Pearson Education, Inc.)

that the maturation of other tissues, such as muscle or bone, could contribute to movement production.

.. Gesell and McGraw are the primary proponents of a biological maturation theory of development. The maturationists attributed developmental change to genetics and tended to ignore the role of experience. Gesell and associates (1974) studied motor development as a means to understand mental development, and in the process, Gesell became known as the "father of developmental testing." Gesell viewed motor development as the physical entity that allowed functional behavior. A believer in structure, he defined stages of motor development that he thought governed behavior during each age period. Gesell also recognized the role of individual differences in temperament as a variable during the development of stability and change in motor patterns.

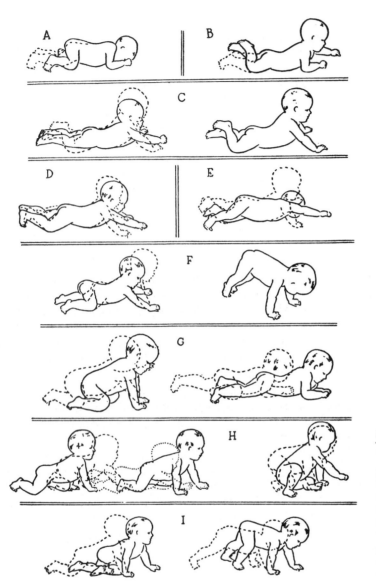

Figure 2–6

The nine phases (*A* to *I*) of the prone progression or assumption of an all-fours position including prone on elbows, prone on extended arms, and crawling to creeping. (From McGraw MB. *The Neuromuscular Maturation of the Human Infant.* New York: Columbia University Press, 1945.)

McGraw (1963) described in exquisite detail movement sequences in infants (Fig. 2–6). She also was interested in the relationship between structure and function in generating developmental change, and she related movement acquisition to biological maturation (Barnes et al, 1990). Like Gesell, she sought answers in the changing activity of the central nervous system. For example, she tried to correlate changes in an infant's patterns of movement in the prone position (prone progression) with central nervous system maturation.

TABLE 2–4

Piaget's Stages of Cognitive Development

Life-Span Period	Stage	Characteristics
Infancy	Sensorimotor	Pairing of sensory and motor reflexes leads to purposeful activity
Preschool	Preoperational	Unidimensional awareness of environment Begins use of symbols
School age	Concrete operational	Solves problems with real objects Classification, conservation
Pubescence	Formal operational	Solves abstract problems Induction, deduction

From Piaget J. *Origins of Intelligence.* New York: International Universities Press, 1952.

Dynamic Systems

Thelen and colleagues (1993 and 1994) applied a "dynamical systems" theory of motor control to early motor development. While studying reflexive lower extremity movements in infants, Thelen discovered a biomechanical explanation for the developmental change in motor behavior previously attributed to reflex integration. The cessation of infant stepping after 2 months of age was attributed to rapid changes in body weight and composition (Thelen and Fisher, 1982; Thelen et al, 1984). The recognition that nervous system maturation was not the only determinant of motor patterns had a significant effect on everyone's view of motor development and motor control. Movement patterns can change as a result of the weight of a limb, body orientation to gravity, and other biomechanical phenomena.

Thelen (1995) further questioned whether the separation between perception and action was real or imagined in developmental psychology. She proposed that perceptual development and motor development are tied together. The mover perceives the surroundings in order to move and moves in order to perceive. A child learns to adapt the original movement to the demands of the task and the environment in which the movement occurs. This premise is the basis of dynamic systems theory.

PSYCHOLOGICAL DEVELOPMENT

Intelligence

Piaget (1952), a well-known developmental psychologist, identified four stages of cognitive development in children: sensorimotor, preoperational, concrete operational, and formal operational. Each stage is characterized by different ways of interacting with the environment, as identified in Table 2–4 and described in detail later. His theory explained how humans acquire and process information and learn about the world. According to Flavell et al (1993), Piaget believed the individual's ultimate goal was to master the environment.

Piaget (1952) identified two basic functions of all organisms that make this mastery possible. The first is the individual's ability to organize, which he called *assimilation,* and the second is the ability to adapt, which he called *accommodation.* These two processes allow individuals to learn about and adapt to the world around them. *Assimilation* is the interpretation of external objects and events in terms of one's preferred way of thinking about them. *Accommodation* is a form of adaptation that involves noticing and taking into account the real properties and relationships of objects and events in the environment (i.e., collecting environmental data).

Sensorimotor Stage. The first 2 years of life mark the blending of sensory and motor experiences in which the infant uses sensory information or assimilation to cue movement and uses movement or accommodation to explore the environment. The child's sensorimotor system interacts with the environment and, by means of repeated interactions, undergoes developmental change and cognitive growth. Because the developmental therapist is concerned with the impact of maturation and experience on the motor development of infants and children with disabilities, a child's sensory and motor abilities are assessed, and treatment is designed to maximize potential.

Preoperational Stage. The next few years of life are dedicated to acquiring verbal expression as well as to using symbols, words, or objects to represent things that are not present. The child labels all forms of transportation as "ride" or all four-footed animals as "dog" or "cat," depending on his frame of reference. Behavior is self-centered, and reasoning is always in relation to the self. "To the right" means to her right. Objects are as alive as people, and they always have a purpose. Toward the end of this stage, most children begin to have some understanding of time, which eventually allows them to learn how to wait.

Concrete Operational Stage. During this period, children develop the ability to classify objects according to their characteristics. They can solve concrete problems—that is, those in which the objects are physically present, as in "Which cup is bigger?" or "Which string is longer?" Most of Piaget's famous conservation experiments were carried out to demonstrate a child's ability to transform objects from one set of circumstances to another while preserving the idea that the objects were unchanged. For example, two cups hold equal amounts of water. One cup (B) is poured into several other containers (A) and the child is asked whether the amount of water poured from cup B is the same as what is in A. If the child says yes, he demonstrates conservation.

Formal Operational Stage. Piaget and Inhelder (1967) described the highest level of cognitive development as formal operations in which early adolescents are able to deal with hypothetical as well as real situations. A person capable of abstract thought could grasp the experiments with the cups of water just described without having to physically see them. Being able to generate a hypothesis, engage in deductive reasoning, and check solutions are all characteristics of logical decision making. Not all adolescents and adults apply this type of thinking to all aspects of life. They may tend to selectively use this ability only in particular personal or professional situations.

By using biological terminology, Piaget introduced the concept of a cognitive system that develops in parallel with other bodily systems. Furthermore, Piaget used the model of assimilation and accommodation to describe cognition as another form of ontogenetic adaptation. *Ontogenetic adaptation* refers to the structural, physiological, or behavioral characteristics unique to an organism, in this case humans, that increase the survivability of the organism (Oppenheim, 1984).

Perception

Perception has been linked to cognition from the beginning of the field of psychology. Piaget linked sensation to movement as an initial step in the development of intelligence. With the advent of computers, information processing came into vogue as an explanation for the relationship of perception and cognition. The mind was viewed as a machine. Gibson's concept of environmental affordance highlights the ecological perspective of cognition.

Information Processing. Information processing theories are all predicated on the belief that thinking is information processing. The mind is described as working like a computer. When sensory information comes into the nervous system and is processed, that process is cognition. An information processing approach to development spans the biological and psychological domains and is concerned with memory, concept formation, and problem solving (Klar and MacWhinney, 1998). Information processing on a physiological level is an integral part of motor control and is discussed in more depth in Chapter 3.

Environmental Affordance. Gibson (1969, 1979, and 1982) viewed perceptual development from an ecological perspective. The environment affords a child the opportunity for interaction, and in that interaction the object and the child are somehow changed. A jungle gym may afford a seat for one child or a place to hang upside down for another child. Perception is the means by which the child comes in contact with the world and adapts to it. The ecological view of perceptual development does not require the child to construct actions with objects as did Piaget's model. Gibsonian research focuses on how perception guides action. Perceptual development is further explored in Chapter 10.

SOCIOCULTURAL DEVELOPMENT

Behaviorist

Probably the most famous behaviorist is B. F. Skinner (1938), the father of stimulus-response (S-R) psychology, whose experiments with rats and mazes clearly showed that certain behavior can be conditioned. He applied the principles of operant conditioning to the development of human behavior and believed that the environment was the most influential factor in determining

TABLE 2–5

Sears' Phases of Social Learning

Life-Span Period	Phase	Description
Infancy	I. Rudimentary behavior: initial behavioral learning	Basic need requirements met within intimate parental environment Positive reinforcement is primary socializing agent
Toddlerhood/preschool	II. Secondary motivational systems: family-centered learning	Socialization within larger family environment Negative reinforcement introduced as socializing agent
School age/adulthood	III. Secondary motivational systems: extrafamilial learning	Social penetration into neighborhood and beyond Controls universally defined and strictly enforced

From Sahler OJZ, McAnarney ER. *The Child from Three to Eighteen.* St. Louis: CV Mosby, 1981.

behavioral outcomes. Skinner was even able to condition a fear response in a child. Although the value of reinforcement is universally accepted and behavior modification is a legitimate form of therapeutic intervention, classic conditioning is not discussed as a formative aspect of development. Behaviorists do not represent a life-span view of human development because they focus on development in childhood and adolescence, but they do represent the opposing side to the nature-nurture debate. According to behaviorists, all behavior is learned by observation and imitation and can be conditioned or shaped through reinforcement.

Social Learning

Sears and colleagues (1965) attempted to explain the early behavior of the child according to observable social interactions—that is, overt behavior. Although Sears used the skinnerian S-R cycle, his theory became known as *social learning theory* and is predicated on identifying the common reinforcers used to produce social behavior. The theory states that behavioral development is learned with the parents as the first teachers, followed by the extended family, and then the social group (Table 2–5).

Theories of Adult Development

Biological development is considered complete by the time a person is considered to be an adult. Psychological and sociocultural development continues but has not been studied as rigorously as child development and aging. Therefore, less has been written about adult development. Instead, specific phenomena associated with adulthood, such as midlife crisis, social roles, and family systems, have been examined. For more information, the student is referred to psychology texts on adult development.

If a phenomenon occurs often enough, it will become the subject of study, as is the case of the so-called midlife crisis. The initial findings from the study of men aged 35 to 45 years led to a new view of adult development that extended Erikson's original work by identifying four eras: preadulthood, early adulthood, middle adulthood, and late adulthood (Levinson, 1986). These are frequently referred to as the "seasons of a man's life."

The theory includes the elements of a life course and life cycle, individual life structure, and a conception of adult development. Life structure, as defined by Levinson, is a pattern of relationships between the self and the world. This relationship includes psychological aspects such as feelings and outer social aspects such as ways of relating to people. He further identified periods during the adult years in which structure building is most prevalent and other periods when structure changing is more prevalent. The structure-changing periods are seen as transitions between the more stable structure-building periods. His research supports the notion that the character of living changes considerably between early and middle adulthood and is associated with age-related periods (Levinson, 1986).

Theories of Aging

DEVELOPMENT IN THE OLDER ADULT

In contrast to adulthood, there are literally hundreds of theories on aging. Theorists observing the later aspect of the life span hypothesize that aging occurs because of biological or physical changes in the human body. Aging can be defined as the sum of all the changes that normally occur in an organism with the passage of time (Matteson, 1997). Aging also can be described as a process that transforms healthy adults into frail ones (Miller, 1994). Biological aging results in diminished reserves in most physiological systems and an increasing vulnerability to most diseases and death (Hayflick, 1998).

BIOPHYSICAL THEORIES

The biological theories of aging are usually subdivided into genetic and nongenetic investigation. Genetic research is based on the premise that aging is programmed in the cell nucleus. This process of cellular aging is considered a *purposeful event* (Cavanaugh, 1999). Nongenetic research is related to environmental factors outside the cell nucleus. Here, aging is viewed as part of the same continuum as the process of development—genetically controlled and probably programmed but subject to environmental influence.

Genetic Research

Programmed Aging. The best known block of genetic research, the programmed aging theories, grew out of biological investigation in the 1960s. Hayflick and Moorehead (1961) made a profound observation while studying human tumor viruses. When growing human cells in tissue culture, they observed a waxing and waning of cellular proliferation, followed by senescence and eventual death of the cultures. Before this time, tissue cultures had been reported to be immortal (Carrel, 1912). Hayflick and Moorehead interpreted their findings to mean that aging was a cellular as well as an organismic phenomenon, and dramatically changed the way we view aging and aging research (Hayflick, 1965).

Hayflick (1965) subsequently described, in the *Hayflick limit theory*, the number of cell replications (population-doubling potential) possible in the life span to be about 50. Martin and colleagues (1970) later linked the replicative life span of specific tissue types in culture to the age of their donor cells. The younger the donor cells, the greater was their life span; the older the donor cells, the shorter their life span. Röhme (1981) proved that this holds true for the species from which the cells are derived. In individuals with premature aging, called progeria, the donor cells show a lower Hayflick limit (Fries and Crapo, 1981).

Programmed Cell Death. Many biogerontologists think that aging is determined by a biological clock that turns on death genes or causes certain hormones to be secreted. Programmed cell death, called *apoptosis*, is apparent during early development when unwanted or unused cells are destroyed. Research has shown that cells do eventually cease dividing; when DNA is replicated, the ends of the chromosome, called telomeres, shorten with each successive replication until they are so short that replication stops. Theoretically, this shortening could act as a replication clock to time cell death.

The theory of *programmed aging* is not as popular as it was in the 1960s, in part because from an evolutionary standpoint, it would mean that the species has selected for aging in order for it to occur. "The expression of age changes is not essential for the survival of the species. Humans have survived, and sometimes flourished, with a life expectancy at birth of 20 or 30 . . ." (Hayflick, 2000, p 365). Hayflick points out that we confuse the aging process with age-related disease and end up investigating diseases rather than biological processes.

Nongenetic Research

Nongenetic research assumes that aging changes occur because of influences outside of the cell nucleus and involve some maladaptive response to cell, tissue, or system damage. The damage may be from external, environmental sources or from internal sources. These events eventually reach a level that is no longer compatible with life. If the events occur randomly and represent environmental insults to the human body, they are called *stochastic changes*.

The major stochastic theories include the cross-linkage theory, free radical theory, immune system theory, and the neuroendocrine theory. All of these theories could be considered developmental because they represent change over time and focus on wear and tear on the body. The idea that the body wears out as a result of a lifetime of use is very attractive, especially because other objects in our world have an estimated time to failure. Although there is evidence of wear in joints in the form of osteoarthritis and the accumulated affects of free radicals, the damage from wear and tear does not explain why these things occur with age.

Cross-Linkage. Bjorksten (1976) first related the idea of cross-linkage of protein molecules to aging in the 1940s. According to the *cross-linkage theory*, a cross-linking agent attaches itself to two large molecules as a result of a chemical reaction. If the cross-link attaches to only one strand of DNA, it can be repaired. However, if two strands of DNA are cross-linked, the strands are unable to part normally. With aging, the body's ability to repair cross-linkages is thought to decline, causing an increase in cell death related to incomplete division. In looking at collagen, elastin, and DNA molecules, Bjorksten (1976) recognized that the occurrence of cross-linkages between compounds might be responsible for the secondary and tertiary signs of aging. One obvious example is seen in the skin. Tanning of the skin produces cross-linkages between collagen and elastin, which leads to a loss of tissue elasticity. Over time, these cross-linking compounds build up and interfere with cell function by impeding cell-to-cell transport. Although age-related changes in collagen such as loss of flexibility have been well documented (Hayflick, 1994), the negative relationship between flexibility and age can be partially compensated for by diet and exercise (Lee and Paffenbarger, 2000; Leslie and Frekaney, 1975).

Free Radical. Harman (1956) originally described the *free radical theory of aging*. Free radicals are highly charged ions with an orbiting unpaired electron. The separated electron with its high energy level is thought to attack neighboring molecules. The radicals have an affinity for lipid molecules, which are found in abundance in mitochondrial and microsomal membranes. The free radicals then damage cell membranes in a chemical process called lipid peroxidation, which leads to structural changes and malfunctions in the cell. One of the results of the oxidative reactions within the cells is the deposition of lipofuscin, an aging pigment (Cavanaugh, 1999). Lipofuscin accumulates in many organs with aging, particularly in postmitotic organs such as the heart, skeletal muscle, and central nervous system that are no longer dividing. In general, the presence of lipofuscin is an aging characteristic of some cells such as neurons.

In addition to forming age pigments, free radicals produce cross-links in some cells that can damage DNA. They also play a role in formation of neuritic plaques, a structural hallmark of Alzheimer's disease. The accumulation of reactive oxygen species in the form of free radicals increases with age, and the body's ability to produce antioxidants to counteract their effects declines. Hayflick (1994) has reported that the administration of antioxidants delays the appearance of free radical–related diseases such as cancer and cardiovascular disease and the age-related decline in the immune system.

Immune System. The immune system consists of the bone marrow, thymus gland, spleen, and lymph nodes. The first two are primary organs of immunity; the latter two are considered peripherally or secondarily responsible for developing immunity. The bone marrow and thymus are the two organs most affected by the aging process. The thymus gets smaller with age. By age 50, it is 5% to 10% of its peak mass (Whitbourne, 1999). After young adulthood, the thymus loses its ability to produce the differentiated T cells needed for cell-mediated immune response declines. As the bone marrow becomes less efficient, the rate of infections, autoimmunity, and cancer rises (Aldwin and Gilmer, 1999; Dickson, 1999). Walford (1969) first postulated the *immunity theory* based on these facts. Hayflick (1994) questioned whether another process, such as the neuroendocrine system or degradation of proteins, might not be responsible for the age-related decline in the immune system. Moderate exercise and endurance training have been shown to increase immune function (Nieman, 1997; Venjatraman and Fernandes, 1997).

Neuroendocrine. Genetic and nongenetic theories are not mutually exclusive. Aging may result from purposeful programmed events, random events, or the interaction of the two types of events. The decline in neuroendocrine function may be preprogrammed or a result of accumulated effects of stress, and as such is an example of such interaction.

Several theories on aging implicate the endocrine system as the culprit in the aging process. The maintenance of a stable internal environment is the purview of the endocrine system and the sympathetic division of the autonomic nervous system. As we age, the hormones produced by the endocrine system appear to be intact and potent, although their effective interaction with target body cells is decreased. Put another way, the body's tissues are less responsive. The hypothalamic-pituitary-adrenal (HPA) interconnections act as a system to control the body functions of growth, reproduction, and metabolism. This HPA axis has been postulated as the master time-keeper for the body because the pituitary gland controls the thyroid gland, which controls the metabolic rate of the body through the secretion of thyroxin. A major question related to aging is whether the body slows down the rate at which it burns calories as we age.

Finch and Seeman (1999) postulated a *stress theory of aging* that targets age-related changes in the ability of the HPA axis to respond to challenges. These authors link the changes in resiliency to cumulative exposure to glucocorticoids, which predispose the individual to increased risk for certain types of illness. Although hormonal changes do occur in many systems of the body, they do so differentially based on gender, with women living on average 7 years longer than men (Cavanaugh, 1999).

PSYCHOLOGICAL THEORIES

The study of cognitive development in adulthood is referred to as *cognitive aging* (Dixon and Hultsch, 1999). After peaking in early adulthood, intelligence

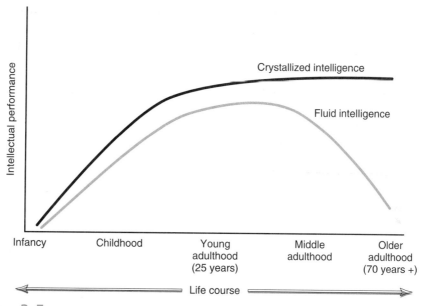

Figure 2–7

Comparison of age-related changes in fluid and crystallized intelligence.

declines through late adulthood. There are individual differences and multiple causes for change. Schaie (1996) studied the age at which cognitive decline actually begins, as part of the Seattle longitudinal study. He found that intellectual decline in all dimensions is not observed on average until the late 60s. Cognitive processing theories have been proposed to explain the decline and selective optimization to compensate for the decline.

Horn and Cattell (1966) described two dimensions of intelligence: fluid and crystallized. *Fluid intelligence* refers to learning reflective of induction, deduction, and abstract thinking, whereas *crystallized intelligence* is related to knowledge of life experiences and education or cultural knowledge. Fluid intelligence declines at some point in adulthood, whereas crystallized intelligence is maintained or may even increase during the adult years (Fig. 2–7). Fluid intelligence is more dependent on physiological functioning, especially the neurological system, both of which decline with advancing age (Medina, 1996).

Cognitive Processing

Information-processing theories of cognition have been used to assess the age-related differences seen in attention, reaction time, and working memory. The *processing-speed theory* states that a decrease in the speed of processing operations leads to impairment in cognitive functioning (Salthouse, 1996). Older adults are slower to respond, with increased reaction time being well documented (Kail and Salthouse, 1994). The degree to which the response time slows is dependent on the difficulty of the task being performed. Attending to tasks of increasing complexity is more difficult for older than for younger adults (Stine-Morrow and Soederberg Miller, 1999). Salthouse (1994) has shown that 40% to 80% of the age-related variance in associative learning can be explained by speed measures. Slower processing appears to produce a less durable memory trace in older adults. In comparing performances on free recall, a paper-folding task, inductive reasoning, and associative learning, Salthouse demonstrated pronounced age trends. On many variables, there was as much as a 1.5 standard deviation difference between the performances of the average 25- and 75-year-old adults (Salthouse, 1999). The processing-speed theory is a persuasive construct to explain age-related changes in fluid cognition.

Selective Optimization With Compensation

Although the data are very persuasive in regard to cognitive decline for fluid intelligence, crystallized intelligence remains and in some instances may increase with increasing age. *Selective optimization* is a popular theory that attempts to explain why some individuals compensate for age-related declines. Successful aging is viewed as optimizing gains while minimizing losses. For example, the pianist Arthur Rubinstein, at age 80, practiced fewer pieces (selection) more frequently (optimalization), compensating for his slower speed by purposively slowing down before rapid sequences to increase the contrast in movement speed (Baltes et al, 1998).

SOCIOCULTURAL THEORIES

Age may be the only thing a group of older adults have in common. Life histories and experiences are only a few of the variables present in our life course. Two divergent social theories emerged since the 1960s: the activity-disengagement debate viewed what happened as we aged in very different ways.

Disengagement

Cumming and Henry (1961) proposed the *disengagement theory*, suggesting that aging adults turned inward as a means of withdrawal from family and society. This served to ease the eventual loss of the older adult on the family. Researchers originally thought that this was normal, but after considerable investigation, they found that it was neither normal nor natural for this disengagement to occur, at least not totally (Atchley, 1991). Disengagement may occur partially or completely, but it is usually because of circumstances beyond our control, such as placement in a nursing home some distance from the remaining family, a terminal illness, or Alzheimer's disease.

Activity

In sharp contrast to the disengagement theory, the *activity theory*, postulated by Neugarten and associates (1968), suggested that staying actively involved with friends, family, and society was necessary for successful aging. Activity was positively correlated with happiness in old age. Being active allowed for adaptation, which has always been part of life and becomes an even more important part of aging. Depending on life circumstances, we may need to adjust to less income, increased dependency, loss or change of a job role, or an inability to participate in leisure activities. Those who adapt and remain active are most successful in aging.

Continuity

Continuity theory has replaced the debate between the activity and disengagement viewpoints (Kail and Cavanuagh, 2000). Atchley (1989) described this widely accepted theory as one in which the individual seeks continuity by linking things in the past with changes in the future. For example, applying a study strategy used in college to taking on a new task at work is combining prior knowledge for future change. Continuity can be internal or external. Internal continuity is lost in a patient with Alzheimer's who loses awareness of himself, but external continuity allows adaptation to changing environmental demands.

The range of sociocultural theories is vast and multilayered. Aging is viewed within the context of our relationship with the larger society and culture. Our relationships can be defined in terms of sociocultural roles, as in continuity theory, or as a linkage to the larger group, as seen in the activity or disengagement models.

Summary

Development, as a process of change, reflects the transactional nature of our interaction with the environment and encompasses our need to survive, organize, and adapt to our surroundings. The child changes, and so do the people and things with which the child interacts. Each experience is different. The variables within the physical, psychological, and social environments need to be considered in the development of functional skills. We should not envision this interaction as a robot-like series of actions but as one in which variation occurs to produce an adaptive response. The environment includes people, places, and things. We develop a sense of identity through psychological interaction with our environment. Motor learning also occurs as a function of the interactions between our physical body and environmental task demands. Although it may be true that "Just because your father was a concert pianist, it doesn't mean you will inherit his musical talent," our genetic makeup will predispose us to certain traits. The physical, psychological, and social environments in which we develop, however, can have an equally potent affect.

Theories of development evolve over time and are modified to reflect what we currently know about development and to provide a basis for our clinical decision making. If the development of functional movement is based solely on neuromaturation, our therapeutic intervention must follow the developmental sequence. If we believe that the environment and task also help shape the development of functional movement, we also will consider these factors in designing interventions. If motor learning is necessary during motor development, our therapeutic intervention must incorporate knowledge of results and practice at solving movement problems. We must remember that theories are changeable; none are totally correct. As theorists of human development and clinicians seek to integrate the changes in all domains of function across the life span, the process of the development of functional movement will become clearer.

References

Aldwin CM, Gilmer DF. Immunity, disease processes, and optimal aging. In Cavanaugh JC, Whitbourne SK (eds). *Gerontology: An Interdisciplinary Perspective*. New York: Oxford University Press, 1999, pp 123–154.

Atchley RC. A continuity theory of normal aging. *Gerontologist* 29:183–190, 1989.

Atchley RC. *Social Forces and Aging*, 6th ed. Belmont, CA: Wadsworth, 1991.

Baltes PB. Theoretical propositions of life-span developmental psychology: On the dynamics between growth and decline. *Dev Psychol* 23:611–626, 1987.

Baltes PB, Lindenberger U, Staudinger UM. Life-span theory in developmental psychology. In Damon W, Lerner RM (eds). *Handbook of Child Psychology*, 5th ed. New York: John Wiley & Sons, 1998, pp 1029–1144.

Bandura A. *Social Foundations of Thought and Action: A Social Cognitive Theory*. Englewood Cliffs, NJ: Prentice-Hall, 1986.

Barnes MR, Crutchfield CA, Heriza CB, et al. *Reflex and Vestibular Aspects of Motor Control, Motor Development and Motor Learning*. Atlanta: Stokesville Publishers, 1990.

Bjorksten J. The crosslinkage theory of aging: Clinical implications. *Compr Ther* 2:65, 1976.

Bronfenbrenner U. *The Ecology of Human Development. Experiments by Nature and Design*. Cambridge, MA: Harvard University Press, 1979.

Bronfenbrenner U, Morris PA. The ecology of developmental processes. In Damon W, Lerner RM (eds). *Handbook of Child Psychology*, 5th ed. New York: John Wiley & Sons, 1998, pp 993–1028.

Carrel A. On the permanent life of tissues outside the organism. *J Exp Med* 15:516–528, 1912.

Cavanaugh JC. Theories of aging in the biological, behavioral, and social sciences. In Cavanaugh JC, Whitbourne SK (eds). *Gerontology: An Interdisciplinary Perspective*. New York: Oxford University Press, 1999, pp 1–32.

Cristofalo VJ, Tresini M, Francis MK, Volker C. Biological theories of senescence. In Bengtson VL, Schaie KW (eds). *Handbook of Theories of Aging*. New York: Springer, 1999, pp 98–112.

Cumming E, Henry WE. *Growing Old: The Process of Disengagement*. New York: Basic Books, 1961.

Dennis LB, Hassol J. *Introduction to Human Development and Health Issues*. Philadelphia: WB Saunders, 1983.

Dickson G. The aging immune system. In Kaufman TL (ed). *Geriatric Rehabilitation Manual*. New York: Churchill Livingstone, 1999, pp 53–57.

Dixon RA, Hultsch DF. Intelligence and cognitive potential in late life. In Cavanaugh JC, Whitbourne SK (eds). *Gerontology: An Interdisciplinary Perspective*. New York: Oxford University Press, 1999, pp 213–237.

Erikson EH. *Identity, Youth, and Crisis*. New York: WW Norton, 1968.

Erikson EH, Erikson JM, Kivnick HQ. *Vital Involvement in Old Age*. New York: WW Norton, 1986.

Finch CE, Seeman TE. Stress theories of aging. In Bengtson VL, Schaie KW (eds). *Handbook of Theories of Aging*. New York: Springer, 1999, pp 81–97.

Finch CE, Tanzi RE. Genetics of aging. *Science* 278:407–411, 1997.

Flavell JH, Miller PH, Miller SA. *Cognitive Development*, 3rd ed. Englewood Cliffs, NJ: Prentice Hall, 1993.

Fries I, Crapo L. *Vitality and Aging*. San Francisco: WH Freeman, 1981.

Gesell A, Ilg FL, Ames LB, et al. *Infant and Child in the Culture of Today*, revised. New York: Harper & Row, 1974.

Gibson EJ. *Principles of Perceptual Learning and Development*. New York: Appleton-Century-Crofts, 1969.

Gibson EJ. *The Ecological Approach to Visual Perception*. Boston: Houghton Mifflin, 1979.

Gibson EJ. The concept of affordance in development: The renaissance of functionalism. In Collins WA (ed). *Minnesota Symposium on Child Psychology*, vol 15. Hillsdale, NJ: Erlbaum, 1982.

Gottlieb G. The psychobiological approach to developmental issues. In Haith MM, Campos JJ (eds). *Infancy and Developmental Psychobiology*, vol 2. New York: John Wiley & Sons, 1983, pp 1–26.

Gottlieb G, Wahlsten D, Lickliter R. The significance of biology for human development: A developmental psychobiological systems view. In Damon W, Eisenberg N (eds). *Handbook of Child Psychology*, 5th ed. New York: John Wiley & Sons, 1998, pp 233–273.

Harman D. A theory based on free radical and radiation chemistry. *J Gerontol* 11:298–300, 1956.

Hayflick L. The limited in vitro lifetime of human diploid cell strains. *Exp Cell Res* 37:614–636, 1965.

Hayflick L. *How and Why We Age*. New York: Ballantine Books, 1994.

Hayflick L. How and why we age. *Exp Gerontol* 33:639–653, 1998.

Hayflick L. New approaches to old age. *Nature* 403:365, 2000.

Hayflick L, Moorehead PS. The serial cultivation of human diploid cell strains. *Exp Cell Res* 25:585–621, 1961.

Helsing E. *Malnutrition in an Affluent Society*. Geneva: World Health Organization, October 1984, pp 14–15.

Horn JL, Cattell RB. Refinement and test of a theory of fluid and crystallized intelligence. *J Educ Psychol* 57:253–270, 1966.

Kail KM, Cavanaugh JC (eds). *Human Development: A Lifespan View*, 2nd ed. Belmont, CA: Wadsworth, 2000.

Kail KM, Salthouse TA. Processing speed as a mental capacity. *Acta Psychol* 86:199–225, 1994.

Klar D, MacWhinney B. Information processing. In Damon W, Kuhn D, Siegler RS (eds). *Handbook of Child Psychology*, 5th ed. New York: John Wiley & Sons, 1998, pp 631–678.

Lee IM, Paffenbarger RS Jr. Association of light, moderate, and vigorous intensity physical activity with longevity. The Harvard Alumni Health Study. *Am J Epidemiol* 151:293–299, 2000.

Leslie D, Frekaney G. Effects of an exercise program on selected flexibility measurements of senior citizens. *Gerontologist* 15:182, 1975.

Levinson DJ. A conception of adult development. *Am Psychol* 41:3–13, 1986.

Lin CC, Evans MI. *Intrauterine Growth Retardation: Pathophysiology and Clinical Management*. New York: McGraw Hill, 1984.

Lockman JJ, Thelen E. Developmental biodynamics: Brain, body, behavioral connections. *Child Dev* 64:953–959, 1993.

Martin GM, Spargue CA, Epstein CJ. Replication lifespan of cultivated human cells: Effects of damage, tissue, and genotype. *Lab Invest* 23:86–92, 1970.

Maslow A. *Motivation and Personality*. New York: Harper & Row, 1954.

Matteson MA. Biological theories of aging. In Matteson MA, McConnel ES, Linton AD. *Gerontological Nursing: Concepts and Practice*, 2nd ed. Philadelphia: WB Saunders, 1997, pp 158–173.

McGraw MB. *The Neuromuscular Maturation of the Human Infant*. New York: Halfner, 1963.

Medina JJ. *The Clock of Ages*. Cambridge: Cambridge University Press, 1996.

Miller RA. The biology of aging and longevity. In Hazard WR, Bierman EL, Blass JP, et al (eds). *Principles of Geriatric Medicine and Gerontology*, 3rd ed. New York: McGraw-Hill, 1994, pp 3–18.

Neugarten BL, Havinghurst RJ, Tobin SS. Personality and patterns of aging. In Neugarten BL (ed). *Middle Age and Aging*. Chicago: University of Chicago Press, 1968, pp 173–177.

Nieman DC. Exercise immunology: Practical applications. *Int J Sports Med* 18(suppl 1):S91–S100, 1997.

Oppenheim RW. Ontogenetic adaptation in neural development: Toward a more "ecological" developmental psychobiology. In Prechtl HFR (ed). *Continuity of Neural Functions From Prenatal to Postnatal Life*. Philadelphia: JB Lippincott, 1984, pp 16–30.

Piaget J. *Origins of Intelligence*. New York: International Universities Press, 1952.

Piaget J, Inhelder B. *The Child's Concept of Space*. New York: WW Norton, 1967.

Röhme, D. Evidence for a relationship between longevity of mammalian species and lifespan of normal fibroblasts in vitro and erythrocytes in vivo. *Proc Natl Acad Sci USA* 78:3584–3588, 1981.

Salthouse TA. The nature of the influence of speed on adult age differences in cognition. *Dev Psychol* 30:240–259, 1994.

Salthouse TA. The processing-speed theory of adult age differences in cognition. *Psychol Rev* 103:403–428, 1996.

Salthouse TA. Theories of cognition. In Bengtson VL, Schaie KW (eds). *Handbook of Theories of Aging*. New York: Springer, 1999, pp 196–208.

Schaie KW. *Intellectual Development in Adulthood: The Seattle Longitudinal Study*. Cambridge, UK: Cambridge University Press, 1996.

Schroots JJF, Yates FE. On the dynamics of development and aging. In Bengtson VL, Schaie KW (eds). *Handbook of Theories of Aging*. New York: Springer, 1999, pp 417–433.

Schuster CS. Study of the human life span. In Schuster CS, Asburn SS (eds). *The Process of Human Development: A Holistic Approach*, 2nd ed. Boston: Little, Brown, 1986.

Sears RR, Rau L, Alpert R. *Identification and Child Rearing*. Stanford, CA: Stanford University Press, 1965.

Skinner BF. *The Behavior of Organisms: An Experimental Analysis*. New York: Appleton-Century-Crofts, 1938.

Stine-Morrow EAL, Soederberg Miller LM. Basic cognitive processes. In Cavanaugh JC, Whitbourne SK (eds). *Gerontology: An Interdisciplinary Perspective*. New York: Oxford University Press, 1999, pp 186–212.

Thelen E. Timing and developmental dynamics in the acquisition of early motor skills. In Turkewitz G, Devenny D (eds). *Timing as an Initial Condition of Development*. Hillsdale, NJ: Erlbaum, 1993, pp 85–104.

Thelen E. Motor Development: A new synthesis. *Am Psychol* 50:79–95, 1995.

Thelen E, Fisher DM. Newborn stepping: An explanation for a "disappearing reflex." *Dev Psych* 18:760–775, 1982.

Thelen E, Fisher DM, Ridley-Johnson R. The relationship between physical growth and a newborn reflex. *Infant Behav Dev* 7:479–493, 1984.

Thelen E, Smith LB. *A Dynamic Systems Approach to the Development of Cognition and Action*. Cambridge, MA: MIT Press, 1994.

Venjatraman JT, Fernandes G. Exercise, immunity and aging. *Aging (Milano)* 9:42–56, 1997.

Walford RL. *The Immunological Theory of Aging*. Baltimore: Williams & Wilkins, 1969.

Whitbourne SK. Physical changes. In Cavanaugh JC, Whitbourne SK (eds). *Gerontology: An Interdisciplinary Perspective*. New York: Oxford University Press, 1999, pp 91–122.

Yates FE, Benton LA. Rejoinder to Rosen's comments on biological senescence: Loss of integration and resilience. *Can J Aging* 14:125–130, 1995.

3 Motor Development and Motor Control

Development results from the interrelated processes of maturation, physical growth, and learning and may be observed in genetic and environmental adaptation. *Maturation* guides development genetically in the physical changes that occur during organ differentiation in the embryo, myelination of nerve fibers, and the appearance of primary and secondary ossification centers. *Growth* is the process whereby changes in physical size and shape take place, as witnessed during adolescence when dramatic changes in facial and body growth occur. *Adaptation*, on the other hand, is the body's response to environmental stimuli. A muscle increases bulk with strength training, the immune system produces antibodies when exposed to a pathogen, bones heal after a fracture—all of these processes illustrate adaptation.

Motor Development

Motor development is the change in motor behavior experienced over the life span. The process and the product of motor development are related to age, and its study has roots in psychology. Typically, researchers in motor development study individuals of different ages performing the same task, describe age differences in terms of performance, and suggest age-appropriate standards for judging the motor performance of infants, children, teenagers, adults, and older adults. Motor development studies are less likely to be concerned with changing one's performance than with documenting naturally occurring age-related change.

Motor behavior changes occur to meet our needs across the life span. Observable changes are the result of the interaction between biological and environmental factors. Biological factors are not stable over time and are evidenced by differences in rate of growth, magnitude of growth, sensory processing, flexibility, strength, and speed of response (VanSant, 1989). Maturation and learning depend on each other because learning does not occur unless the system is ready to learn. The rate of maturation is affected by the amount and type of learning experiences, and the type of learning experiences is affected by the sociocultural environment (Higgins, 1985). Environmentally, the variables are infinite and include physical surroundings, family structure, access to motor learning experiences, and culture. Needs are related to survival, safety, motivation, psychological development, and societal and cultural expectations. Together, all of these factors produce change or adaptation in the motor behaviors of the individual.

Changes in growth are used as markers for development. Children can be classified as an early, an average, or a late maturer according to the relationship between physiological growth parameters and chronological age. Although we routinely use age as the yardstick of motor development, we should think more about relating body size to motor skill achievement. Think of a small 3-year-old child being assessed on how he ascends a standard set of stairs. Does he use the railing because of poor motor skills or because the steps are too tall for his short legs? The effects of physical size and body proportion on motor skill acquisition or movement proficiency have been examined in adolescence but are just beginning to be explored in younger age groups. Does the changing weight and proportion of the limb segments constrain the production of movement? Thelen and Fisher's (1982) research supports the possibility that infants cease reflex stepping because the limbs get too heavy, not because of any change in the nervous system.

Other factors that affect how a person develops movement are genetic coding and culture. Group differences are reflected in gender and in the culture in which children are raised. Males have an innate ability to develop more muscle and greater strength (Malina and Bouchard, 1991). A child's experience gleaned from various child-rearing practices (including physical handling), sensory and motor feedback, and sensorimotor integration combine with a genetic predisposition to produce movement skills. Why does one person become a triathlete and another a prima ballerina, whereas others have difficulty riding a bike, water skiing, or hitting a ball? Culture and child rearing practices influence movement skill acquisition by rewarding some motor behaviors and avoiding others.

MOTOR DEVELOPMENT CONCEPTS

Many conceptual themes have been used to describe the acquisition and production of movement across the life span. One major concept related to movement skill acquisition is that it is sequential. Another framework that appears to influence movement outcomes seen across the life span is the direction in which growth and development, and hence change, occur. Movement, by its nature, also requires a point of mobility and a point of stability. Last, sensation plays a very important role in the acquisition and refinement of movement skill acquisition.

Developmental Sequence

One of the most important concepts about movement, and possibly the most universal concept, is that movement skill development is sequential. Movement development in the broadest sense is based on what came before. Each movement learned is used again in a slightly different way to achieve something else. Although the rate of development may vary normally from individual to individual and is referred to by the term *individual differences*, the sequence is the same for similar populations and cultures. In Western cultures, infants master sitting before creeping, standing, or walking.

Directional Concepts

Cephalocaudal

Traditionally, development is said to progress *cephalocaudally*, that is, from the head to the foot. Head control develops before trunk control. Control of arm movements for reaching develops before control of leg movements for creeping. The first part of the body to develop is the neck. In utero, the neural tube closes first at the level of the fourth cervical vertebra and continues to close in two directions, toward the head (cephalo) and toward the feet (caudal). From this perspective, development is said to proceed from the neck cervicocephalocaudally.

Proximal-Distal

The second concept of directional development is that development occurs from proximal to distal. In this case, *proximal* refers not only to the proximal parts of the extremities, such as the shoulder or pelvic girdles, but also to the midline of the neck and the midline of the trunk. The infant controls the midline of the neck, the midline of the trunk, the shoulders, and the pelvis before controlling arms, legs, hands, and feet.

Proximal and distal structures are inseparable because the body is a system of linked structures. Movement in one area affects the relationship of the structures not only in the moving part but also in the other parts. Although the infant has not developed sufficient trunk control to sit alone, the infant can reach for and hold objects. Control of the midline of the trunk occurs before shoulder and pelvic girdle control is established.

Mobility and Stability

Controlled movement occurs within the framework of mobility and stability, or movement and posture. The relationship between *stability* (holding a posture) and *mobility* (moving) is called *postural control*. Mobility is present before stability. Once a stable posture is established, movement control within that posture develops.

Infants are very mobile and initially demonstrate random movements such as kicking in the supine position. These random leg movements occur within the available range of motion. Some postures are assumed briefly, such as head lifting in the prone position. Next, the infant learns to hold postures such as propping on elbows in prone (prone on elbows). Stable postures provide a base from which movement can occur. Infants and children are able to maintain a posture such as sitting before they are able to attain the posture independently, move in and out of the posture, or demonstrate the ability to preserve the posture if balance is disturbed.

Some postures are inherently stable and require little or no muscular effort. A prime example is W-sitting, in which the legs are internally rotated, the pelvis in anteriorly tilted, and the knees are flexed. It is as if a peg (the trunk) has been placed in a puzzle hole (the pelvis). Biomechanically, the child is locked in place with no need for active trunk control and is free to use the hands for play rather than support. The child is exhibiting *positional stability*, the stability that comes from the mechanics of the position, not from muscular control of the trunk. *Dynamic stability* is the use of muscular control to maintain a position. Frequently, infants use mechanical stability before sufficient muscular control has developed. For example, an infant elevates the shoulders to assist in maintaining the head in a midline position, when first supported up in an unstable sitting position.

Dynamic stability is necessary for the child to develop skilled movements such as walking, running, and climbing. A child must be able to move into and out of postures, make subtle corrections to maintain balance, and control movement over a stable base for these functional movement patterns to emerge. Dynamic postural control is necessary to move safely from one posture to another and involves both dynamic stability and controlled mobility.

Sensation

Sensory information plays an important role in movement skill acquisition. The first movements experienced by the newborn are reflexively cued by sensation. Before vision, touch cues help the newborn find food. "Sensation is an ever-present cue for motor behavior in the seemingly reflex-dominated infant" (Martin and Kessler, 2000, p 29). Voluntary movement emerges as the nervous system and body mature. Sensory information from visual, somatosensory, and vestibular systems cue automatic postural responses in a reactive manner as postural control is acquired. Sensation from weight bearing reinforces postures such as quadruped, kneeling, and standing. Sensory information is used by the infant, toddler, or child to entice, direct, or guide interaction with objects and navigate the environment. Later, sensory information is used to cue postural readiness, such as when a person sees a bulging grocery sack and he needs to recruit a few more muscles before lifting it.

MOTOR DEVELOPMENT THEORIES

Motor development scholars describe changes in motor behavior that are related to age. There are three theoretical views that have been most prevalent in motor skill acquisition: the maturation perspective, the perceptual-cognitive perspective, and the dynamic systems perspective. The maturationists Gesell and colleagues (1974) and McGraw (1945) predicated motor development and emerging motor behaviors on the neuromaturation of the cerebral cortex. The perceptual-cognitive perspective came from researchers in the field of motor learning and motor control (Clark et al, 1990). They viewed information processing/perceptual development as a foundation for movement. In the dynamic systems perspective, multiple systems of the body interact and in that interaction, movement emerges (Thelen and Smith, 1998).

Maturation Theories

From the maturationist's point of view, central nervous system maturation is one of the primary determinants of early motor behavior. In the infant's nervous system, there is a vertical hierarchy of control, with the infant exhibiting spinal cord reflexes in response to touch or pain. As the nervous system matures, reflexes and reactions that are mediated by the brain stem and midbrain emerge. Finally, voluntary control from the cortex is seen with purposeful movements such as reaching and walking. There also is a horizontal hierarchy of increasingly complex connectivity within the nervous system. Synaptic connections increase between areas of the cortex, allowing exchange of information. These horizontal connections monitor the timing and execution of motor commands as well as storing movement and perceptual information. Although central nervous system maturation is only one part of the explanation for motor development, Gesell's theory has provided an invaluable concept about movement skill acquisition that is still important. That concept is reciprocal interweaving.

Gesell's Reciprocal Interweaving

Gesell (1974) coined the term *reciprocal interweaving* to describe the spiral-like development that alternates between periods of equilibrium and disequilibrium. Periods of equilibrium are marked by stable behavior, whereas periods of disequilibrium are marked by instability. The cycles occur frequently in the first year and decrease in frequency with increasing maturity. Gesell applied this concept to all types of behavior—motor, adaptive, linguistic, and personal-social.

The application of reciprocal interweaving can be seen by looking at the pattern of development of head control. Head control in a newborn is relatively good. The newborn is able to hold the head in the midline if he is held upright and is able to lift the head when held at one's shoulder or in the prone position. At 2 months, the head appears to be more wobbly; but at 4 months, control is again excellent in upright and in prone positions. A cycle of stability, instability, and renewed stability is evident in this development of head control.

The development of balance in children is another example of this concept. Shumway-Cook and Woollacott's (1985) study of the growth of stability in standing also reinforces Gesell's concept of reciprocal interweaving. They found that the immature pattern of postural response, the hip strategy, was replaced by the adult pattern, the ankle strategy. *Strategies* are patterns of muscle activation observed when the supporting surface is moved. Between the two extremes was an intervening period in which highly variable postural responses were seen. This sequence of immature, transitional, and mature motor patterns can be documented throughout development, in fact, throughout the life span.

McGraw's Longitudinal Perspective

Myrtle McGraw was a developmental psychologist whose work chronicled the development of motor skills longitudinally, identifying phases in the development of skills such as rolling and crawling. Figure 2–6 illustrates her nine phases of the prone progression. Along with Gesell, she emphasized the role of nervous system maturation as the guiding force behind motor development. In reviews of her work, Bergenn and associates (1992) and Campbell (2000a) recognized that McGraw's theory of motor development possessed some recognizable similarities to the preeminent motor control theory, the *dynamic systems theory* (DST). These commonalities included that movement is important for its own sake (i.e., movement acts as an incentive to move) and that movements come and go along with periods of stability and instability. McGraw believed in sensitive periods when development could be disrupted and the outcome (motor behavior) could be affected.

Perceptual-Cognitive Theory

The perceptual-cognitive perspective champions the importance of sensory processing and the effect that intellectual abilities related to that processing have on the acquisition and performance of motor skills. The role of sensation in movement changes over the life span. First, sensation is paired with movement in the form of reflexes. The sensory input cues a phasic motor response. Next, sensation is used as feedback to refine volitional movement and as a stimulus for postural responses. Eventually, sensation is fed forward in anticipation of a motor action and is used less in feedback of familiar actions. When learning a new movement, sensation is still used for reinforcement or refinement.

Gibson (1987) reviewed the research findings related to infant perception in an attempt to shed some light on the theories involved in human perceptual performance. She discussed eight conclusions that provide a view of the perceptual-cognitive perspective, as indicative of the relationships between perception and movement:

1. Perception is an active and exploratory process.
2. Perception is externally directed toward distal sources of stimulation.
3. Perception not only uses but depends on information given in motion.
4. Perception is of a three-dimensional world.
5. Perceptual constancy for various object properties such as size and shape exists before reaching, grasping, and handling objects become manifest.

6. Perception is coherent, that is, makes sense.
7. Perception is coordinated between different sensory modalities.
8. Perceptually guided actions are organized and flexible, not reflexive or mechanical stimulus-response sequences.

These conclusions point out the sophistication present in the perceptual abilities of the infant. Movement plays an important role in affording perception. The concept of affordance was introduced in Chapter 2. A 4-month-old infant can distinguish an object's movement from his or her own movement (Kellman et al, 1987). Perceptual information reinforces posture, as when visual information is used to stabilize head posture at 2 months (Butterworth and Pope, 1982, cited in Gibson, 1987) and to stabilize the trunk at 6 months (Butterworth and Hicks, 1977). Just as movement appears to organize behavior, perception may be the ability to detect order and structure in the world, not merely the means to organize sensory information.

The goal of perception is action (Gibson, 1979). Perception of the surrounding environment, which includes objects and people, serves the functional purpose of bringing about contact and interaction. The objects afford the opportunity to act, and in acting, the object and the action are changed. Perception affords adaptation of the individual and the environment. Infants who creep recognize action-specific properties of surfaces and use visual information to guide locomotion (Adolph et al, 1993; Gibson et al, 1987).

The speed of processing information can significantly affect motor performance. Information processing improves rapidly in the first 2 years of life (Coren et al, 1999). Positive changes continue to be seen in childhood with the rate of change slowing in adulthood. Around age 40, declines in sensory processing begin. Movement time provides information about sensorimotor processing. *Fitts' law* (1954) is a mathematical calculation that describes the relationship among speed, accuracy, and distance in motor performance. It describes the speed-accuracy trade-off. The faster a person responds, the less accurate are the responses. Fitts' law also establishes a relationship between movement time and an index of difficulty for aiming movements. The relationship is linear; the greater the index of difficulty, the greater is the movement time. Children perform in a fashion similar to that of adults but at a lower absolute level of performance. Older adults perform even more slowly and are disproportionately affected by the index of difficulty (Fig. 3–1).

With advanced age, the speed of processing sensory information declines. The decline makes it more difficult for someone to learn a new motor skill, such as playing the guitar or piano, later in life. As seen in Figure 3–1, the slowing of movement time is not constant but increases with advanced age, such that the older person takes much longer to perform a difficult movement. There is an interaction between cognition and sensation in learning that also applies to motor skills.

Dynamic Systems Theory

A third perspective on motor development comes again from developmental psychology. Thelen and Smith (1994 and 1998) proposed a functional view of

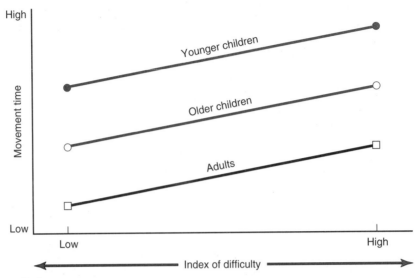

Figure 3–1

General relationship between movement time and index of difficulty for different age groups. (Adapted from Keogh J, Sugden D. *Movement Skill Development*. New York: Macmillan, 1985, p 355.)

the process of motor development. In this perspective, movement is described as emerging from the interaction of multiple body systems. The DST incorporates developmental biomechanical aspects of the mover, along with the developmental status of the mover's nervous system and the environmental context in which the movement occurs. Movement abilities associated with the developmental sequence are the result of motor control, which organizes movements into motor programs. The DST is discussed in greater detail later in the chapter.

COMPARISON OF MOTOR DEVELOPMENT, MOTOR CONTROL, AND MOTOR LEARNING ON MOTOR BEHAVIOR

The studies of motor development, motor control, and motor learning all uniquely contribute to our understanding of functional motor behavior. It is important to appreciate the similarities and differences in these three areas to have a full understanding of how functional movement is produced and controlled.

Motor control theory was influenced by a developmental model of neural function: one that grew from a view of how the nervous system evolved. Similarly, motor development scholars were strongly influenced by studies of reflexes (Peiper, 1963; Wyke, 1975), which have long been considered a fundamental unit of motor control. Motor learning and motor control theory share common themes such as the use of feedback (Rosenbaum, 1991), and researchers in these areas share ideas that mutually influence each other's work

(Brooks, 1986; Schmidt and Lee, 1999). An understanding of the differences between these areas helps one to appreciate the unique contributions of each to our knowledge of motor behavior.

Time Frames

One way to distinguish between motor development, motor control, and motor learning is to focus on the time base that is used to study motor behavior within each area (VanSant, 1991) (Fig. 3–2). Motor development processes transpire across intervals typically referred to as "age." Commonly, age is measured in years. Motor control processes occur within very small intervals, typically, fractions of seconds. Motor learning is a process that occurs across hours, days, and weeks and is discussed in Chapter 4.

Maturation of Systems

The development of motor control begins with the control of self-movements and proceeds to the control of movements in relationship to changing conditions. Control of self-movement is largely due to the development of the neuromotor systems. As the nervous and muscular systems mature, movement emerges. Motor control allows the nervous system to direct which muscles should be used and in what order and how quickly to solve a movement problem. The infant's first movement problem relates to overcoming the effect of gravity. A second but related problem is how to move a proportionately

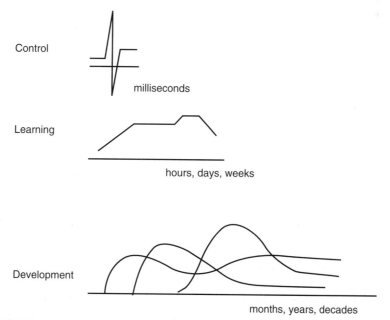

Figure 3–2

Time scales of interest from a motor control, motor learning, and motor development perspective.

larger head in relation to a smaller body to establish head control. Later, movement problems are related to controlling the interaction between stability and mobility of the head, trunk, and limbs. Control of task-specific movements such as stringing beads or riding a tricycle is dependent on cognitive and perceptual abilities. The task to be carried out by the person within the environment dictates the type of movement solution that is going to be needed.

Because the motor abilities of a person change over time, the motor solutions to a given motor problem also may change. The motivation of the individual to move may also change over time and affect the intricacy of the movement solution. An infant encountering a set of stairs, sees a toy on the top stair. She creeps up the stairs but then has to figure out how to get down. She can cry for help, bump down on her buttocks, creep down backwards, or even attempt to creep down forward. A toddler faced with the same dilemma may walk up the same set of stairs one step at a time holding onto a railing and descend in sitting, holding the toy, or she may be able to hold the toy with one hand and the railing with the other and descend the same way she came up. The child will go up and down stairs without holding on, and an even older child may run up those same stairs. The relationship among the task, the individual, and the environment is depicted graphically in Figure 3–3. All three components must be considered when thinking about motor development, motor control, and motor learning.

Motor Control Dependency on Maturation

The degree of maturation of the body's systems affects motor control because motor control occurs on a physiological level. Physiological maturation occurs in all body systems involved in movement production: muscular, skeletal, nervous, cardiovascular, and pulmonary. For example, if maturation of the contractile properties of muscle is incomplete, certain types of movements may not be possible. Weakness can impair movement. If synaptic connections are not complete, movement quality could be affected. Inability to perceive a threat visually will prevent a person from making a protective movement. Muscle strength, posture, and perceptual abilities exhibit maturation and can affect the rate of motor development by affecting the process of motor control.

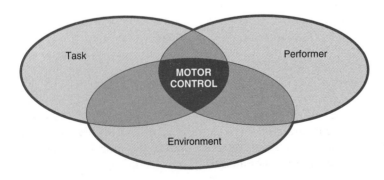

Figure 3–3

Motor control relationship among the task, the individual as performer, and the environment.

Motor Control

Motor control is the ability to organize and control functional movement. The field of motor control grew primarily from the specialized study of neurophysiology in an attempt to explain how functional movement is produced and regulated in humans. From a historical perspective, several different theories and models have been proposed. Some models approach motor control from a physiological perspective, and others have a psychological perspective. Regardless, it is important to realize that these theories are ever changing and evolving based on contemporary thought and the current research. When the explanations of an existing theory are no longer sufficient to interpret the research data, new theories are developed.

During the 20th century, scholars attempted to explain the mechanisms of motor control. Initially, it was thought that the brain organized movement through a hierarchical model. Later models were developed that described feedback and programming within the nervous system. A systems perspective has been described. Motor control is the set of processes that organize and coordinate functional movements physiologically and psychologically. The blending of physiological and psychological perspectives has greatly enriched the study of how movements are governed. Each of these models is discussed in turn.

HIERARCHICAL MODELS

Hierarchical models of motor control are characterized by three main concepts: (1) the role of reflexes in movement production, (2) hierarchical levels of control within the nervous system, and (3) the role of volitional movement. The reflex or reaction is seen as the basic unit of movement in this model of motor control. Reflexes are stereotypical responses to specific sensory stimuli. In the hierarchical model of motor control, specific reflexes or reactions are associated with a specific neuroanatomical level (Fig. 3–4). Reflexes mediated in the spinal cord are deemed *phasic* because they are typically of short duration. The monosynaptic stretch reflex and the flexor withdrawal are examples of phasic reflexes. Spinal reflexes are characterized by patterns of reciprocal innervation. Reflexes mediated at the brain stem level are characterized as *tonic* because of their long duration. Tonic reflexes such as the asymmetrical tonic neck and tonic labyrinthine produce changes in tone and posture. Co-contraction of agonist and antagonist muscles enables primitive forms of posture. The positive support reflex, brought about by pressure on the ball of the foot, turns the lower limb into a pillar of support.

The second characteristic of the hierarchical model is that there are levels of control within the nervous system: spinal cord, brain stem, midbrain, and cortex. These levels traditionally constitute reflex responses as indicated earlier, with the highest-level reflexive responses exerting dominance over lower-level reflexive responses. The brain stem reflexes inhibit the phasic spinal cord reflexes and so on up the chain of command.

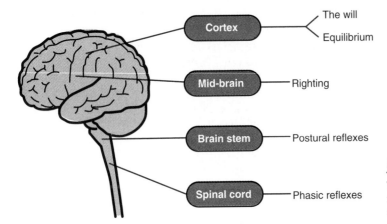

Figure 3–4

The classic reflex hierarchy with reflexes or reactions assigned to specific neuroanatomical levels.

The motor behaviors of the midbrain are complex behaviors that align the body with respect to gravity. This function is termed *righting*. The righting function is composed of a series of movements that bring the body from recumbency to standing. Righting behaviors believed to be mediated at the midbrain level are brought about by complex sensory signals arising from a variety of sources, including the eyes, the labyrinths of the ears, and the cutaneous and proprioceptive sensory receptors of the body. The stimulus for these reactions is any complex set of sensory signals that indicate discomfort or misalignment of the head or segments of the body. Righting behaviors are quite variable in their form and, as a result, were termed "reactions" rather than reflexes. The term *reaction* emphasizes their variability compared with stereotypical reflex responses (see Chapter 12 for a description of various righting reactions).

The highest level of the motor control hierarchy is the cortical level. Two functions are attributed to this level. First, equilibrium or balance reactions are thought to be mediated at this level. The use of the term *reaction* is also quite appropriate to describe these balance activities, because they also vary considerably in form and, like righting reactions, arise from a complex set of sensory signals. Equilibrium reactions are more fully described in Chapter 12. In addition to balance reactions, the cortex is the site of the will, or volitional functions that inhibit and control reflexes and initiate purposeful action.

Neurologists have explained motor behavior exhibited by patients with brain injury using this traditional hierarchy (Denny-Brown, 1950; Seyffarth and Denny-Brown, 1948; Twitchell, 1951). According to classic theory, disease or damage to the brain causes "dissolution" of brain function. *Dissolution* means that neural function regresses to a primitive level characteristic of an earlier phase of nervous system development. After the patient performs a clinical test of reflexes, the behavior of the patient is interpreted to represent a particular level of function. For example, if the patient's behavior is dominated by tonic reflex responses, the behavior is interpreted as representing brain stem—

level function. Classic treatment theories for individuals with brain damage were founded on this view of motor control.

The last characteristic of the hierarchical model is the view of volitional movement. Volitional movement is thought to replace reflexive movement. As stated earlier, when an individual is able to exert cortical control over his actions, he is displaying volitional control of movement. The ability of the cortex to use feedback related to the performance of motor tasks contributes to the volitional control of movement. Feedback is an important factor in both motor control and motor learning (see Chapter 4). A variety of motor control models further examine the concept of feedback.

FEEDBACK AND PROGRAMMING MODELS

Feedback is a very crucial feature of motor control. *Feedback* is defined as sensory or perceptual information received as a result of movement. This is intrinsic feedback, or feedback produced by the movement. Sensory feedback can be used to detect errors in movement. Feedback and error signals are important for two reasons. First, feedback provides a means to understand the process of self-control. Reflexes are initiated and controlled by sensory stimuli from the environment surrounding the individual. Motor behavior generated from feedback is initiated as a result of an error signal produced by a process within the individual. Many motor hierarchies have included at the highest level a volitional, or self-control, function, but there has been very little explanation of how self-control operates.

Feedback also provides the fundamental process for learning new motor skills. For this reason, feedback is a common element in motor control and motor learning theories. Although the kinds of feedback of concern may vary between these two fields, the common interest in feedback mechanisms is apparent.

Open- and Closed-Loop Feedback

Open-loop and *closed-loop* are used to designate two different types of motor control. Closed-loop processes are based on feedback. If one were to draw a model of the feedback process (Fig. 3–5*A*), one would say that information regarding a motor action is fed back into the nervous system to assist in planning the next action. A loop between sensory information and motor actions is created; this is a closed loop. An example of a closed-loop action can be seen in many computer games that require guiding a figure or object across a screen. No one can learn without feedback. Whether one relies on a teacher or coach to provide the feedback or on one's capacity to gather information about performance, feedback is necessary to correct faulty actions. Movements that have already been learned can proceed without feedback.

Open-loop movements are driven by either a central structure (Schmidt and Lee, 1999) or sensory information from the periphery without benefit of feedback (Fig. 3–5*B*). This is particularly true for very fast actions termed *ballistic movements*. For example, when a baseball pitcher fires off his favorite

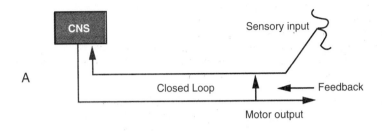

A

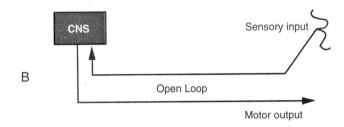

B

Figure 3–5

Models of the feedback process. *A*, Closed loop. *B*, Open loop. CNS, central nervous system.

pitch, the movement occurs so fast that it is completed before feedback loops can provide information that would alter the action.

Program Models

As a result of a debate over the role of sensory information in motor actions, another concept of importance to current control and learning theories arose (Lashley, 1951). That concept is the motor program. A *motor program* is a memory structure that provides instructions for the control of actions. A program is a plan that has been stored for future use. The concept of a motor program is useful because it provides a means by which the nervous system can avoid having to create each action from scratch and thus can save time when initiating actions. There has been much debate over what is contained in a motor program. Different researchers have proposed a variety of programs. We discuss a contemporary theory of motor control that uses the motor program concept extensively.

Brooks' Model

Brooks, a well-known motor physiologist, proposed a hierarchy of motor control that parallels the functions of the traditional motor control hierarchy (Brooks, 1986). Reflexes are predominantly the function of the lowest level of the spinal cord, and volitional, or intended, movements depend on the sensorimotor cortex. The levels are also composed of functional elements termed *plans*, *programs*, and *subprograms*. Brooks views motor plans and programs as communication systems within the nervous system that are based on previous experiences and contribute to the creation of intended actions. Plans, programs, and subprograms are learned. Plans are made up of several programs, which in turn are made up of several subprograms. Reflexes, mediated at the lower level of the hierarchy, unlike plans and programs, are innate rather than learned functional elements.

The nervous system creates and controls motor actions through two fundamental divisions of the nervous system: the sensorimotor system and the limbic system (Brooks, 1986). The sensorimotor system is concerned with sensations, perceptions, and motor actions. The limbic system is involved in the control and regulation of emotions and drives related to feeding, reproduction, and other activities that are vital for the preservation of the species. In addition, the limbic system is involved in the process of learning. The relationship between the limbic system and the sensorimotor system is important because it assists in understanding how goal-directed behavior is initiated. Drives arising through the limbic system are formatted into motor goals through cortical processes carried out in the sensorimotor system. The two systems are described by Brooks as "essential and inseparable partners" (Brooks, 1986, p 22) that function together to produce motor behavior. Figure 3–6 illustrates the command hierarchy beginning at the level of the limbic system, which is superimposed on the sensorimotor hierarchy of plans, programs, and subprograms used in the execution of motor behavior.

Despite an emphasis on plans, programs, and subroutines, all of Brooks' control levels receive feedback and therefore represent a potential for closed-

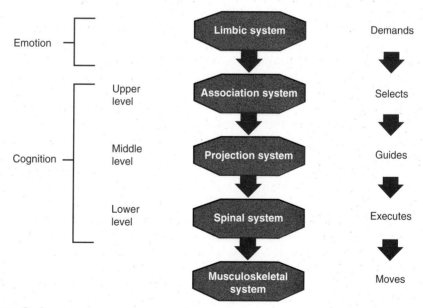

Figure 3–6

Brooks' hierarchical control model.

loop motor control and motor learning. However, they also suggest that learned movements can be carried out without the benefit of feedback through programs and subroutines that have been stored in memory.

LEARNING-BASED MODELS

There are two theories of motor learning that have generated a great deal of study about how we control and acquire motor skills. Both theories use programs to explain how movements are controlled and learned; they are Adams' closed-loop theory of motor learning (Adams, 1971) and Schmidt's schema theory (Schmidt, 1975). The two theories differ in the amount of emphasis placed on open-loop processes that can occur without the benefit of ongoing feedback (Schmidt and Lee, 1999). Schmidt incorporated many of Adams' original ideas when formulating his schema theory in an attempt to explain the acquisition of both slow and fast movements.

Adams' Closed-Loop Theory

The name of Adams' theory emphasizes the crucial role of feedback. The concept of a closed loop of motor control is one in which sensory information is funneled back to the central nervous system for processing and control of motor behavior.

The basic premise of Adams' theory is that movements are performed by comparing the ongoing movement with an internal reference of correctness that is developed during practice. This internal reference is termed a *perceptual trace,* which represents the feedback one would receive if the task were performed correctly. Through ongoing comparison of the feedback with the perceptual trace, a limb may be brought into the desired position. The quality of performance is directly related to the quality of the perceptual trace. A perceptual trace, formed as the learner repeatedly performs an action, is made up of a set of intrinsic feedback signals that arise from the learner. Intrinsic feedback here means the sensory information that is generated through performance: for example, the kinesthetic feel of the movement. The perceptual trace becomes stronger with repetition and more accurately represents correct performance as a result of external feedback provided by a teacher or therapist.

In the closed-loop theory, there are two types of feedback: intrinsic feedback arising from the learner, and extrinsic feedback arising from the teacher or therapist. Extrinsic feedback in motor learning is referred to as "knowledge of results" (KR). Rather than just viewing KR as a means of reinforcing correct performance, Adams emphasized the role KR plays in providing information to help the learner solve a motor problem. KR does not produce learning; rather, it helps the learner accomplish the process of learning.

Adams' theory no longer reflects our knowledge of motor learning (Schmidt and Lee, 1999). A specific limitation of the theory may be its development as an explanation of *slow positioning movements,* such as those used to track slowly moving targets. Adams' theory did not explain how fast movements were controlled and learned, nor did it address the presence of central pattern generators that produce rhythmic movements without feedback. Central pattern generators are groups of neurons that when activated produce rhythmic movements such as those that occur in walking.

Schmidt's Schema Theory

Schmidt's schema theory was developed in direct response to Adams' closed-loop theory and its limitations. Schema theory is concerned with how movements that can be carried out without feedback are learned, and it relies on an open-loop control element—specifically, the motor program.

Schema refers to an abstract memory that represents a rule, or generalization, about skilled actions. According to schema theory, when an individual produces a movement, four kinds of information are stored for a brief period:

1. The initial conditions under which the performance took place (e.g., the position of the body, the kind of surface on which the individual carried out the action, or the shapes and weights of any objects that were used to carry out the task)
2. The parameters assigned to the motor program (e.g., the force or speed that was specified at the time of initiation of the program)
3. The outcome of the performance, or KR
4. The sensory consequences of the movement (e.g., how it felt to perform the movement, the sounds that were made as a result of the action, or the visual effect of the performance)

These four kinds of information are analyzed to gain insight into the relationships among them and to form two types of schema.

The *recall schema* is an abstract representation of the relationship among the initial conditions surrounding performance, parameters that were specified within the motor program, and the outcome of the performance (KR). The learner, through the analysis of parameters that were specified in the motor program and the outcome, begins to understand the relationship between these two factors. For example, the learner may come to understand how far a wheelchair travels when varying amounts of force are generated to push the chair on a gravel pathway. The learner stores this schema and uses it the next time the wheelchair is moved on a gravel path.

The *recognition schema* represents the relationship among the initial conditions, the outcome of performance (KR), and the sensory consequences that are perceived by the learner. Because it is formed in a manner similar to that of the recall schema, once established, the recognition schema is used to produce an estimate of the sensory consequences of the action that will be used to adjust and evaluate motor performance given a motor program. However, the formation of the motor program is not explained. This model emphasizes the role of practice in developing motor skill (see Chapter 4).

SYSTEMS MODELS

A systems view of motor control assumes that motor control is distributed throughout the nervous system and proposes that movement emerges as a result of an interaction among many subsystems (Campbell, 2000a; Shumway-Cook and Woollacott, 1995; Thelen and Smith, 1998). The nervous system and its subsystems are composed of a set of structural-functional units. A systems model differs from traditional control models in that the units participate collectively in the process of control. Also, other systems, such as the muscular and skeletal systems, are incorporated into movement decisions. Through co-operative and interactive processes among the structural-functional units, the individual is capable of self-regulation and can construct and control motor behavior.

Four features can be used to distinguish a systems model of control from a traditional hierarchy (Davis, 1976).

1. In a hierarchy, information typically flows in one direction: from the top downward. This is not the case in a system. Rather, there is a reciprocal flow of information among units of the system.
2. In a hierarchy, functions are attributed to specific levels. For example, in the classic hierarchy described earlier in this chapter, phasic reflexes were specifically related to the spinal level of the nervous system, and tonic reflexes were controlled at the brain stem level. In contrast, in a system, a function is a property of the system as a whole. Thus, functions are shared or distributed among the units of the system.
3. Properties of a hierarchy are the properties of each unit within the hierarchy. In contrast, properties of the system emerge though interaction among the elements of the system. For example, a rhythmic repetitive movement may arise through a circular arrangement of neural elements rather than being the property of one neuron.
4. In a hierarchy, the command function is typically the province of the highest level. In a systems model, command is usually an emergent property arising from the cooperation, collaboration, and sharing of information among units of the system.

In contemporary systems models, units other than the central nervous system are given a role in motor control (Forssberg, 1999; Penn and Shatz, 1999). Other biological systems, such as the musculoskeletal, cardiovascular, and pulmonary systems, as well as the biophysical, psychological, and sociocultural environments in which we function, also contribute to motor control.

Bernstein (1967), a physiologist, looked at the body in a new way and helped spawn the systems approach to motor control. The body is seen as a mechanical system of levers, joints, and muscles. The nervous system task in directing movement is to control the muscles to work together. Each joint has many possible movements, with these movements representing the degrees of freedom of the joints. If the nervous system could constrain groups of muscles to work together in synergies, the degrees of freedom problem presented by the body's multilinked segments could be controlled. Biomechanical properties of the body's muscular and skeletal system became recognized as contributing to motor control.

One of the advantages of a systems model of control is its flexibility. The system can vary its coordinative arrangements depending on the context or situation in which the individual must operate. Actions are organized to meet specific goals. The process of motor control can be envisioned as a process of solving a problem. Depending on the goal, a variety of structural-functional units have the potential to assume control. Which unit is in command is a function of the specific situation in which the goal must be attained. An example of a motor control/motor development theory that reflects the systems model is the DST.

Dynamic Systems Theory

The DST is the imminent motor control perspective. A dynamic system is any system that demonstrates change over time (Heriza, 1991). Thelen and Smith (1998, p 563) identify two themes relative to DST:

1. Development can only be understood as the multiple, mutual, and continuous interaction of all the levels of the developing system, from the molecular to the cultural.
2. Development can only be understood as nested processes that unfold over many time scales, from milliseconds to years.

Embryogenesis is an example of the DST on a molecular, cellular level, and motor development is an example on a systems level. The theory has evolved during the past several years and provides a framework for an integrated account of motor development and motor control. Thelen and associates (1990) proposed four fundamental assumptions of the DST.

The first assumption holds that every action, such as walking, requires the cooperation of numerous systems, including neuromuscular, sensory, perceptual, cardiovascular, and pulmonary. Motor behavior emerges from cooperation among the many subsystems within a task-specific context. Originally, the theory identified the nervous system as just one of many components that interact to produce motor behavior. It was not necessarily viewed as more or less important than other salient components. This was probably done in an effort to distance itself from the long-held view that nervous system maturation explained motor behavior. However, the role of the nervous system has been elevated by the statement that the neurological basis of the dynamic systems model of development is neuronal group selection (Thelen and Smith, 1998).

Neuronal group selection (Sporns and Edelman, 1993) proposes that motor skills result from the interaction of developing body dynamics and the structure/functions of the brain. The brain's structures are changed by how the body is used (moved). The brain's nascent neural networks are sculpted to match efficient movement solutions. Three requirements must be met for neuronal selection to be effective in a motor system: the presence of a basic repertoire of movement, the availability of sensory information to identify and select adaptive forms of movement, and the means to strengthen the preferred movement responses.

The infant is genetically endowed with spontaneously generated motor behaviors. Figure 3–7 illustrates rudimentary neural networks that subserve

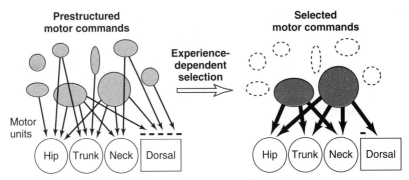

Figure 3-7

A developmental process according to the neuronal group selection theory is exemplified by the development of postural muscle activation patterns in sitting infants. Prior to independent sitting, the infant exhibits a large variation of muscle activation patterns in response to external perturbations, including a backward body sway. Various postural muscles on the ventral side of the body are contracted in different combinations, sometimes together with inhibition of the dorsal muscles. Among the large repertoire of response patterns are the patterns later used by adults. With increasing age, the variability decreases and fewer patterns are elicited. Finally, only the complete adult muscle activation patterns remain. If balance is trained during the process, the selection is accelerated. (Redrawn from Forssberg H. Neural control of human motor development. *Curr Opin Neurobiol* 9:676–682, 1999.)

initial motor behaviors. This example involves activation of postural muscles in sitting infants. As the infant's multiple sensory systems provide perception, the strength of synaptic connections between brain circuits is varied with selection of some networks that predispose one action over another. Environmental and task demands can become part of the neural ensemble for producing movements. Spatial maps are formed and mature neural networks emerge as a product of use and sensory feedback. The maps that are developed by use connect large amounts of the nervous system and provide an interconnected organization of perception, cognition, emotion, and movement (Campbell, 2000b).

The theory of neuronal group selection supports the DST of motor control/motor development. According to neuronal group selection, the brain and nervous system are guided in development by a genetic blueprint and activity within rudimentary neuronal circuits. The use of certain circuits over others reinforces synaptic efficacy and strengthens those circuits. Last, maps are developed that provide the organization of spontaneous movement in response to mover and task demands. Other body systems, such as the skeletal, muscular, cardiovascular, and pulmonary systems, develop and interact with the nervous system so that the most efficient movement pattern for the mover is chosen. There are no motor programs, and the brain should not be thought of as a computer or as hard wired. This theory supports the idea that neural plasticity may be a constant feature across the life span.

Order parameters are expressions of complex relationships within a motor behavior. They represent observable collective variables involved in temporal and spatial phasing between limbs. According to neuronal selection theory of motor control, the most appropriate neuronal group would be selected based on the task requirements, the environmental conditions, and the state of the body systems. Movement variability has always been considered a hallmark of normal movement. This integration of multiple systems allows for a variety of movement strategies to be available to perform a functional task; think of how many different ways it is possible to move across a room.

The second assumption posits that there are "self-organizing properties" inherent in developing systems and that movement patterns arise from an interaction of these component parts. In the DST, recurrent interactions among sensory, perceptual, and neuromusculoskeletal activities give rise to coordinative patterns of reaching, walking, and talking (Thelen and Smith, 1994). Self-organization is the unifying theme that establishes a single theory of development by integrating diverse viewpoints and multiple facets of development (Lewis, 2000).

Four principles of self-organization illustrate an integrated view of development (Lewis, 2000). First, self-organizing systems permit true novelty, the structure of movement is emergent. For example, the stages seen in the developmental sequence represent periods of stability that emerge from the self-organization of multiple body systems. Second, self-organizing systems become more complex. The complexity serves the purpose of adapting to varying functional needs. Third, the system is able to reorganize and transition to new patterns of movement after or during a period of instability. Phase transitions are points of instability and turbulence that occur when old patterns break down and new ones appear. For example, stereotypical rhythmic movements described by Thelen (1979) (Fig. 3–8) appear to represent transitional behaviors that emerge as the child is gaining control over a new posture. Last, self-organizing systems are both sensitive to change and inherently stable. The system recognizes aspects of the environment via feedback. However, the repetition of a pattern of movement such as walking increases the likelihood of that pattern of coordinative movement continuing.

The third assumption notes that component structures and skill processes develop in an asynchronous, nonlinear manner. For example, the number of motor skills and the rate of acquisition of those skills are markedly different during the first year of life and the subsequent 2 years. Maturation of component systems such as the skeletal and muscular systems does not occur at the same rate. The rate-limiting nature of select components may mask or facilitate the expression of select elements at any given time. Campbell (2000a) identified strength, posture, and perceptual analysis as possible rate-limiting factors in motor development.

The fourth assumption states that shifts from one behavioral mode to another are discontinuous. At varying periods of development, different subsystems act as control parameters.

Control parameters are those variables that act as catalysts for change in motor behavior. Changes in motor behavior are being attributed to parameters that previously went unnoticed, such as the weight of a limb. In their now

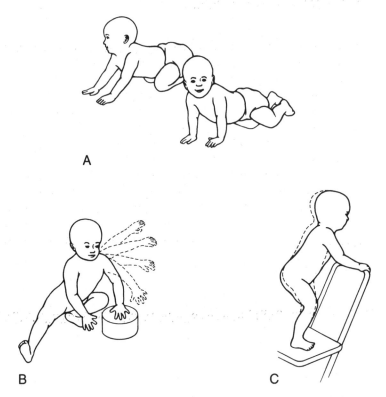

Figure 3-8

Stereotypical rhythmic movements. *A*, Hands-and-knees rocking. *B*, Arm-banging against a surface. *C*, Stand-bouncing. (Modified from Thelen E. Rhythmical stereotypies in infants. *Anim Behav* 27[3]: 704, 706, 1979.)

classic experiment, Thelen and Fisher (1982) demonstrated that the cessation of infant stepping movements is due to the increased weight of the legs, not to reflex inhibition. When the weight of the limbs was discounted, the stepping movement reappeared (Thelen et al, 1984).

The DST holds a great deal of promise for advancing our understanding of the changing form of movements that we observe in our clients.

Relationship to Other Models

We need to recognize that the three major theoretical perspectives on motor development and motor control parallel each other. The maturationist view of development can be supported by the hierarchical view of motor control, whereas the perceptual-cognitive perspective of motor development seems in line with the learning-based view of motor control (see Chapter 4). The greatest overlap between motor development theory and motor control theory is demonstrated in the dynamic systems perspective, which is a theory of both motor development and motor control.

For physical therapists, the hierarchical theory is classic and has been fundamental to our basic understanding of motor control as intervention models have evolved. Reflexes fulfill a basic role in hierarchical theories as the fundamental unit of behavior. In the hierarchical theories, hierarchies are composed of levels closely related to anatomical structures. Volitional movements, which are complex and variable in form, are hypothesized to be carried out by the higher levels, whereas more simple, reflexive behaviors are characteristic of lower levels of a motor hierarchy. In light of today's understanding of motor control, a hierarchy may exist, but the traditional assumption of higher levels of the hierarchy controlling lower centers is more questionable. Can it be that lower hierarchical levels influence the higher centers?

Functional Implications

The functional implications of motor development, motor control, and motor learning are that movement abilities change over time, or across the life span. Each individual develops functional movement in a similar sequence, but the rate of acquisition shows variation. The ages noted in the following discussion are approximations.

LIFE SPAN CHANGES

Infancy

An infant's movements are intimately associated with reflexes for the first 3 months of life. Although a typically developing infant is not limited to reflex motor behavior, reflexes do play a role in pairing sensory and motor action. Reflexes are stereotypical responses to sensory stimuli. Reflexes occur early in developmental time, with some appearing during gestation or shortly after birth, and are integrated by 4 to 6 months of age. A list of primitive, or early occurring, reflexes is found in Table 3–1.

Motor skill development progresses sequentially over the first year of life, with the infant able to roll, sit, creep, pull to stand, and walk by 1 year. Reaching and prehension change from swiping at objects at 5 months to discrete movement of the thumb and index finger by 10 months. The motor milestones and the ages at which these skills can be expected to occur can be found in Tables 3–2 and 3–3.

Head control is achieved by 4 months of age and is evidenced by the infant's ability to keep the head in line with the body (ear in line with the acromion) when pulled to sit from a supine position (Fig. 3–9). The infant also develops from the ability to lift the head momentarily at 1 month to 90 degrees from the support surface while in a prone position (Fig. 3–10A and B). Segmental rolling is possible around 6 to 8 months and replaces the earlier log rolling in which the infant's trunk moved as a single unit without segmentation. *Independent sitting* is defined as sitting alone when placed. The infant's back is straight and no hand support is needed; this milestone is achieved by 8

TABLE 3–1

Primitive Reflexes

Reflex	Age at Onset	Age at Integration
Suck-swallow	28 weeks' gestation	2–5 months
Rooting	28 weeks' gestation	3 months
Flexor withdrawal	28 weeks' gestation	1–2 months
Crossed extension	28 weeks' gestation	1–2 months
Moro	28 weeks' gestation	4–6 months
Plantar grasp	28 weeks' gestation	9 months
Positive support	35 weeks' gestation	1–2 months
Asymmetrical tonic neck	Birth	4–6 months
Palmar grasp	Birth	9 months
Symmetrical tonic neck	4–6 months	8–12 months

Data from Barnes MR. Crutchfield CA, Heriza CB. *The Neurophysiological Basis of Patient Treatment*, vol 2. Atlanta: Stokesville Publishing, 1982.

months of age. To achieve the milestone, the child does not have to attain sitting but does need to exhibit head or trunk rotation while in the position. These abilities are important for dynamic balance while interacting with the environment, such as when playing with toys.

As the infant learns the rules of moving, he learns postural control. Sensory information is used as feedback to refine movement accuracy. The infant needs to know how much force to generate and when and in what direction to do so. Feedback allows refinement of movement parameters and assists the infant in organizing movement against gravity. The vestibular system processes sensory information related to gravitational orientation. Increased weight bearing through both upper and lower extremity joints provides proprioceptive information, as does movement itself. By 7 to 9 months of age, most infants are pulling to stand and beginning to cruise or walk sideways

TABLE 3–2

Gross Motor Milestones

Milestone	Age
Head control	4 months
Rolling	6–8 months
Sitting	8 months
Creeping	9 months
Cruising	10 months
Walking	12 months

From Martin ST, Kessler M. *Neurologic Intervention for Physical Therapist Assistants*. Philadelphia: WB Saunders, 2000, p 57.

TABLE 3–3

Fine Motor Milestones

Milestone	Age
Palmar grasp reflex	Birth
Raking	5 months
Voluntary palmar grasp	6 months
Radial palmar grasp	7 months
Radial digital grasp	9 months
Inferior pincer grasp	9–12 months
Superior pincer grasp	12 months
Three-jaw chuck	12 months

From Martin ST, Kessler M. *Neurologic Intervention for Physical Therapist Assistants.* Philadelphia: WB Saunders, 2000, p 57.

around low objects such as the coffee table. Independent walking is achieved anywhere from 9 to 15 months of age.

The prone progression includes the infant's ability to progressively move up against gravity, beginning with head lifting, assumption of prone on elbows, prone on extended arms, and, finally, four point or quadruped. Positions identified as part of the prone progression are shown (Fig. 3–10*A* to *C*). Creeping is a means of mobility is used by a majority of infants before mastering upright walking.

Most infants attempt forward locomotion by 1 year of age and then are referred to as toddlers. Typical first attempts at independent ambulation are

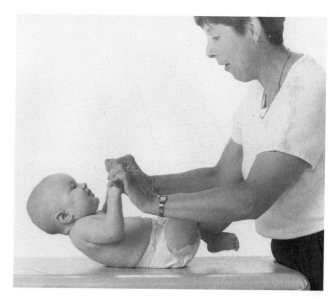

Figure 3–9

Head in line with the body when pulled to sit is a hallmark of head control typically seen at 4 months of age. (From Martin ST, Kessler M. *Neurologic Intervention for Physical Therapist Assistants.* Philadelphia: WB Saunders, 2000, p 58.)

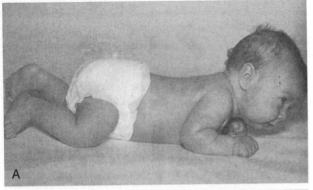

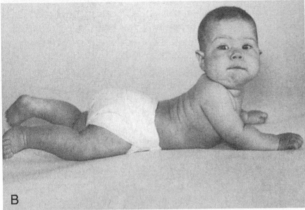

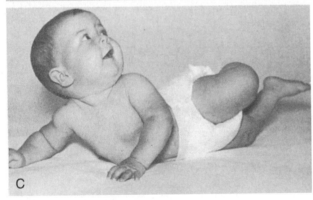

Figure 3–10

Prone progression of head control. *A*, Head lifting in prone. Infant momentarily lifts head at 1 month. *B*, Prone on elbows. A 4-month-old infant lifts and maintains head past 90 degrees. *C*, Prone on extended arms. A 6-month-old infant lifts head, chest, and upper abdomen and can bear weight on extended arm and hands. (From Wong DL, Perry SE. *Maternal Child Nursing Care.* St. Louis: CV Mosby, 1998, p 940.)

characterized by a wide base of support with arms held in high guard (scapula adducted, shoulders externally rotated and abducted, elbows flexed, and wrist and fingers extended). The upper trunk extension afforded by this arm posture compensates for the toddler's lack of hip extension. As the trunk is more easily maintained against gravity, the arms will be lowered to midguard, low guard, and no guard.

The beginning walker keeps hips and knees slightly flexed to bring the center of mass closer to the ground. Weight is shifted from side to side as the toddler moves forward, with each flexed limb moving as a unit with the hips remaining externally rotated during the gait cycle. Toddlers take many small steps and walk slowly. They exhibit minimal ankle movements, and the foot is pronated when the entire foot makes contact with the ground. The instability of their gait is seen in the short amount of time they spend in single-limb stance (Martin, 1989). As trunk stability improves, the legs are brought more under the pelvis. As the hips and knees become more extended, the feet develop the plantar flexion needed for push off.

By 17 months, the toddler is so at ease with walking that a toy can be carried or pulled at the same time. With help, the toddler goes up and down stairs, one step at a time. Without help, the toddler creeps up the stairs and may creep or scoot down on the buttocks. Most children will be able to walk sideways and backwards at this age if they began walking at 12 months or earlier. The typically developing toddler will come to stand from a supine position by rolling to prone, pushing up on hands and knees or hands and feet, assuming a squat, and rising to standing (Fig. 3–11A to F).

Most toddlers exhibit a reciprocal arm swing and heel strike by 18 months of age, with other adult gait characteristics being manifested later in life. Toddlers walk well and exhibit a running-like walk. The toddler may still occasionally fall or trip over objects because eye-foot coordination is not completely developed. Fewer falls seem to be the result of improvement in standing balance reactions and the ability to monitor trunk and lower extremity movements kinesthetically and visually. The first signs of jumping appear as a stepping off jump from the bottom step of a set of stairs. Children are ready for this after being able to walk down stairs holding the hand of an adult (Wickstrom, 1983). Momentary one-foot balance is also possible.

Childhood

A 2-year-old child can go up and down stairs one step at a time, jump off a step with a 2-foot takeoff, stand on one foot for 1 to 3 seconds, kick a large ball, and throw a small ball. Stair climbing and kicking are indicative of improved stability while shifting body weight from one leg to another (Conner et al, 1978). Stepping over low objects encountered in the environment is part of the child's movement abilities. True running emerges in the second year and is characterized by a flight phase when both feet are off the ground at the same time. Despite the running, quick starts and stops remain difficult, with directional changes requiring a large area to make a turn. Jumping off the ground with both feet is eventually mastered. Beginning attempts result in only one foot leaving the ground, followed by the second foot as if the child were stepping in air.

Fundamental motor patterns such as hopping, galloping, and skipping develop from 3 to 6 years of age. Wickstrom (1983) also includes running, jumping, throwing, catching, and striking in this category. Other reciprocal actions mastered by age 3 are pedaling a tricycle and climbing a jungle gym or

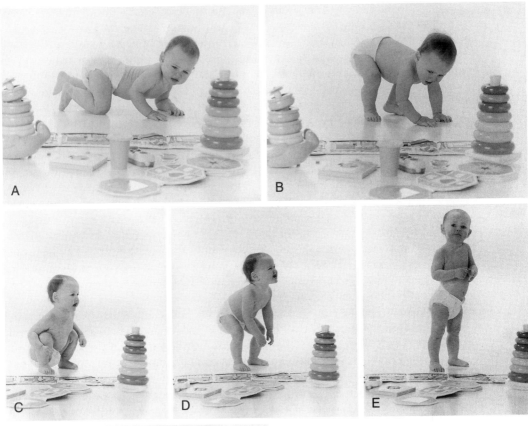

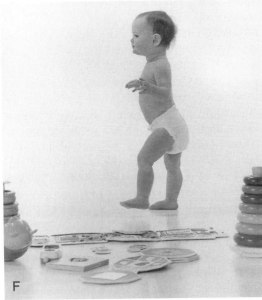

Figure 3–11

Progression of rising to standing to independent walking. *A*, Assuming four point. *B*, Assuming plantigrade. *C*, Squatting. *D*, Rising from a squat. *E*, Standing. *F*, Walking independently. (From Martin ST, Kessler M. *Neurologic Intervention for Physical Therapist Assistants*. Philadelphia: WB Saunders, 2000, pp 72–73.)

ladder. Locomotion can be started and stopped based on the demands from the environment or from a task such as playing dodge ball on a crowded playground. A 3-year-old child can make sharp turns while running and can balance on toes and heels in standing. Standing with one foot in front of the other, known as tandem standing, is possible, as is standing on one foot for at least 3 seconds. A reciprocal gait is now used to ascend stairs with the child placing one foot on each step in alternating fashion but marking time (one step at a time) when descending.

Hopping on one foot is a special type of jump requiring balance on one foot and the ability to push off the loaded foot. It does not require a maximum effort. "Repeated vertical jumps from 2 feet can be done before true hopping can occur" (Wickstrom, 1983, p 70). Neither type of jump is seen at an early age. Hopping one or two times on the preferred foot may also be accomplished by age 3½. A 4-year-old child should be able to hop on one foot four to six times. Improved hopping ability is seen when the child learns to use the nonstance leg to help propel the body forward. Before that time, all the work is done by pushing off with the support foot. A similar pattern is seen in arm use; at first, the arms are inactive, and later they are used opposite the action of the moving leg.

Sexual differences for hopping are documented in the literature, with girls performing better than boys (Wickstrom, 1983). This may be related to the fact that girls appear to have better balance than do boys in childhood. Rhythmic relaxed galloping is possible for a 4-year-old child. Galloping consists of a walk on the lead leg followed by a running step on the rear leg. Galloping is an asymmetrical gait. A good way to visualize galloping is to think of a child riding a stick horse. Toddlers have been documented to gallop as early as 20 months after learning to walk (Whithall, 1989), but the movement is stiff with arms held in high guard as in beginning walking.

At 5 years of age, a child can stand on either foot for 8 to 10 seconds, walk forward on a balance beam, hop 8 to 10 times on one foot, make a 2- to 3-foot standing broad jump, and skip on alternating feet. Skipping requires bilateral coordination. A 6-year-old child is well coordinated and can stand on one foot for more than 10 seconds, with eyes open or eyes closed. This ability is important to note because it indicates that vision can be ignored and balance maintained. The 6-year-old child can walk on a balance beam in all directions without stepping off. The child also uses alternate forms of locomotion, such as riding a bicycle or roller skating.

Fundamental game-playing skills are learned in early childhood (3 to 6 years). All children typically develop the ability to run, jump, throw, and catch. These patterns of movement form the basis for later sports skills. Between 6 and 10 years of age, a child masters the adult forms of running, throwing, and catching (Porter, 1989). Throughout the process of changing motor activities and skills, the nervous, muscular, and skeletal systems are maturing, and the body is growing in height and weight. Power develops slowly in children, because strength and speed within a specific movement are required (Bernhardt-Bainbridge, 2000).

Adolescence

The onset of puberty can have a short-term positive effect on motor perform-ance of boys, which is related to an increase in adrenergic hormones. Boys who mature early demonstrate greater strength and endurance than do boys who have not yet matured. The growth spurt seen in adolescent males is marked by rapid gain in strength. Motor performance peaks during late ado-lescence, which for males occurs around 17 to 18 years of age.

The onset of puberty occurs 2 years earlier in girls than in boys. Static strength increases in females during adolescence, but gains do not show a spurt as they do in males. Although strength changes are related to skeletal maturity, such as peak height velocity (rate of fastest growth), motor perform-ance is not (Malina and Bouchard, 1991). Although females demonstrate an increase in motor performance to around 14 years of age (Bailey et al, 1986), performance on tasks is highly variable during the remainder of adolescence. The variability is probably due to a complex interaction of strength, peak height velocity, and the onset of menses. Motivation, interest, and attitudes toward physical activity may also be factors.

The adolescent may continue to gain prowess in motor skills with practice. Parameters of performance such as power, speed, accuracy, form, and endur-ance can be changed. The amount of change is highly variable and depends on practice and innate ability. The maximum degree of skill possible on most tasks is related to the individual's satisfaction with his or her performance within the limits of cognitive, structural (physical), or sociocultural factors (Higgins, 1991). In other words, working with the resources at hand, the movement is as efficient as possible given the raw materials of the individual within the environment. Some improvement in motor performance in most sports has been thought to occur relatively early.

Spirduso (1995) examined the effect of age on sport-specific abilities. Gen-erally, peak performance of sports requiring explosive bursts of power or speed over time occurred in the person's early 20s. However, because older athletes (30s) put in record-breaking performances in the 1990s, she thinks the concept of age at peak performance may need to be reevaluated. Years of training and a competitive edge may allow an over-30 athlete to triumph over a more physiologically robust 20-year-old in some sports. The physical de-mands of the task, such as power, speed, or endurance, must be taken into consideration.

Age-Related Differences in Movement Patterns Beyond Childhood

Many developmentalists have chosen to look only at the earliest ages of life when motor abilities and skills are being acquired. The belief that mature motor behavior is achieved by childhood led researchers to overlook the possi-bility that movement might change as a result of factors other than nervous system maturation. Although the nervous system is generally thought to ma-ture by the age of 10, changes in movement patterns do occur in adolescence and adulthood.

VanSant (1988a and 1988b) and Sabourin (1989) studied the movement patterns used by people of different ages to accomplish a simple motor task. VanSant and others studied the task of rising from supine to standing by describing the movement components for different regions of the body. Although an explanation of the method used in the many studies is beyond the scope of this text, a summary of the results is most appropriate.

Research shows a developmental order of movement patterns across childhood and adolescence with trends toward increasing symmetry with increasing age (VanSant, 1988a). VanSant (1988b) identified three common ways in which adults move from supine to standing (Fig. 3–12*A* to *C*). The most common

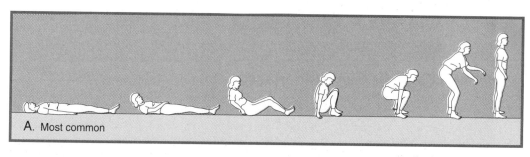

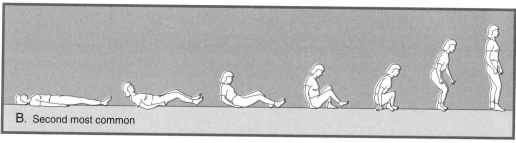

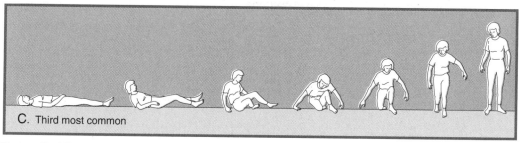

Figure 3–12

Common forms of rising to a standing position. *A*, Most common using upper extremity component, symmetrical push; axial component, symmetrical; lower extremity component, symmetrical squat. *B*, Second most common using upper extremity component, symmetrical push; axial component, symmetrical; lower extremity component, asymmetrical squat. *C*, Third most common using upper extremity component, asymmetrical push and reach; axial component, partial rotation; lower extremity component, half-kneel. (Adapted and reprinted from VanSant AF. Rising from a supine position to erect stance: Description of adult movement and a developmental hypothesis. *Phys Ther* 68:185–192, 1988, with permission of the American Physical Therapy Association.)

pattern was to use upper extremity reach; symmetrical push; forward head, neck, and trunk flexion; and a symmetrical squat. The second most common pattern was identical to the first pattern up to an asymmetrical squat. The third most common pattern involved an asymmetrical push and reach followed by a half-kneel. In a separate study of adults in their 20s through 40s, there was trend toward increasing asymmetry with age (Ford-Smith and Van-Sant, 1993). Adults in their 40s were more likely to demonstrate the asymmetrical patterns of movement seen in young children (VanSant, 1991). The asymmetry of movement in 40-year-old adults may reflect less trunk rotation due to stiffening of joints or lessening of muscle strength, making it more difficult to come straight forward to sitting from a supine position.

Thomas and colleagues (1998) studied movement from a supine position to standing in older adults using VanSant's descriptive approach. In a group of community dwelling older adults with a mean age of 74.6 years, the 70- and 80-year-old adults were more likely to use asymmetrical patterns of movement in the upper extremity and trunk regions, whereas those younger than 70 demonstrated more symmetrical patterns in the same body regions. Furthermore, the researchers found shorter time to rise was related to lower age, greater knee extension strength, and greater hip and ankle range of motion (flexion and dorsiflexion, respectively). However, older adults who maintain their strength and flexibility rise to standing faster and more symmetrically than do those who are less strong and flexible (Thomas et al, 1998).

Although the structures of the body are mature at the end of puberty, changes in movement patterns continue throughout a person's life. Mature movement patterns have always been associated with efficiency and symmetry. Early in motor development, patterns of movement appear to be more homogeneous and follow a fairly prescribed developmental sequence. As a person matures, movement patterns become more symmetrical. With aging, movement patterns again become more asymmetrical. In general, more mature patterns of movement are symmetrical. Because an older adult may exhibit different ways of moving from supine to standing than a younger person, treatment interventions should be taught that match the individual's usual patterns of movement.

Summary

Motor development includes the change in motor behavior over the life span and the sequential, continuous, age-related process of change. It is determined by the merging of our genetic blueprint for movement and our experiences. The mover and the environment are both changed in the process. Motor control is the physiological process whereby motor development occurs, and motor learning allows motor development to occur systematically, resulting in a permanent change in motor behavior due to experience. The contents in this chapter and Chapter 4 seek to relate motor control to both motor development and motor learning.

In 1989, Roberton proposed that the DST of motor control be applied to life span motor development research. Thelen and Smith (1994 and 1998) have done so with great effect. The DST and its underlying premise, neuronal selection theory, are being hailed as the unifying theme for viewing motor development (Lewis, 2000). If motor development is viewed as the study of change in motor behavior across a lifetime, age becomes a marker variable and may not be the cause of change. Altering the way in which we think about age may allow therapists and researchers to discover new information about why individuals move the way they do at different times in their lives. Knowledge of motor development across the life span is critical for therapists to ascertain the most appropriate therapeutic strategies for people to function optimally regardless of age or occupation.

References

Adams JA. A closed-loop theory of motor learning. *J Mot Behav* 3:110–150, 1971.

Adolph KE, Eppler MA, Gibson EJ. Crawling versus walking infants' perception of affordances for locomotion over sloping surfaces. *Child Dev* 64:1158–1174, 1993.

Bailey DA, Malina RM, Mirwald RL. Physical activity and growth of the child. In Falkner FT, Tanner JM (eds). *Human Growth: A Comprehensive Treatise*, vol 2, 2nd ed. New York: Plenum, 1986, pp 147–170.

Bergenn VW, Dalton TC, Lipsitt LP, Myrtle B. McGraw: A growth scientist. *Dev Psychol* 28:381–395, 1992.

Bernhardt-Bainbridge D. Sports injuries in children. In Campbell SK, Vander Linden DW, Palisano RJ (eds). *Physical Therapy for Children*, 2nd ed. Philadelphia: WB Saunders, 2000, pp 429–467.

Bernstein N. *The Coordination and Regulation of Movements*. London: Pergamon, 1967.

Brooks VB. *The Neural Basis of Motor Control*. New York: Oxford University Press, 1986.

Butterworth G, Hicks L. Visual proprioception and postural stability in infancy: A developmental study. *Perception* 6:255–262, 1977.

Campbell SK. The child's development of functional movement. In Campbell SK, Vander Linden DW, Palisano RJ (eds). *Physical Therapy for Children*, 2nd ed. Philadelphia: WB Saunders, 2000a, pp 3–44.

Campbell SK. Revolution in progress: A conceptual framework for examination and intervention. Part II. *Neurol Report* 24:42–46, 2000b.

Clark JE, Truly TL, Phillips SJ. Dynamical systems approach to understanding the development of lower limb coordination in locomotion. In Block H, Bertenhal BI (eds). *Sensorimotor Organization and Development in Infancy and Early Childhood*. Dordrecht: Kluwer Publishing, 1990, pp 363–378.

Conner FP, Williamson GG, Siepp JM. *Program Guide for Infants and Toddlers with Neuromotor and Other Developmental Disabilities*. New York: Teacher's College Press, 1978.

Coren S, Ward LM, Enns JT (eds). *Sensation and Perception*, 5th ed. Fort Worth, TX: Harcourt Brace College Publishers, 1999.

Davis WJ. Organizational concepts in the central motor networks of invertebrates. In Herman RL, Grillner S, Stein PSG, et al (eds). *Advances in Behavioral Biology: Neural Control of Locomotion*. New York: Plenum Publishing, 1976, pp 265–292.

Denny-Brown D. Disintegration of motor function resulting from cerebral lesion. *J Nerv Ment Dis* 112:1–45, 1950.

Fitts PM. The information capacity of the human motor system in controlling the amplitude of movement. *J Exp Psychol* 47:381–391, 1954.

Ford-Smith CD, VanSant AF. Age differences in movement patterns used to rise from a bed in the third through fifth decades of age. *Phys Ther* 73:300–307, 1993.

Forssberg H. Neural control of human motor development. *Curr Opin Neurobiol* 9:676–682, 1999.

Gesell A, Ilg FL, Ames LB, et al. *Infant and Child in the Culture of Today*, 2nd ed. New York: Harper and Row, 1974.

Gibson EJ. Introductory essay: What does infant perception tell us about theories of perception? *J Exp Psychol Hum Percept Perform* 13:515–523, 1987.

Gibson EJ, Riccio G, Schmuckler MA, et al. Detection of the traversibility of surfaces by crawling and walking infants. *J Exp Psychol Hum Percept Perform* 13:533–544, 1987.

Gibson JJ. *The Ecological Approach to Visual Perception.* Boston: Houghton Mifflin, 1979.

Heriza C. Motor development: Traditional and contemporary theories. In Lister M (ed). *Contemporary Management of Motor Control Problems. Proceedings of the II Step Conference.* Alexandria, VA: Foundation for Physical Therapy, 1991, pp 99–126.

Higgins S. Movement as an emergent form: Its structural limits. *Hum Mov Sci* 4:119–148, 1985.

Higgins S. Motor skill acquisition. *Phys Ther* 71:123–139, 1991.

Kellman PJ, Gleitman H, Spelke ES. Object and observer motion in the perception of objects by infants. *J Exp Psychol Hum Percept Perform* 13:586–593, 1987.

Lashley KS. The problem of serial order in behavior. In Jeffress LA (ed). *Cerebral Mechanisms in Behavior.* New York: John Wiley and Sons, 1951, pp 112–136.

Lewis MD. The promise of dynamic systems approaches for an integrated account of human development. *Child Dev* 71:36–43, 2000.

Malina RM, Bouchard C. *Growth, Maturation and Physical Activity.* Champaign, IL: Human Kinetics, 1991.

Martin S, Kessler M. *Neurologic Intervention for Physical Therapist Assistants.* Philadelphia: WB Saunders, 2000.

Martin T. Normal development of movement and function: Neonate, infant, and toddler. In Scully RM, Barnes MR (eds). *Physical Therapy.* Philadelphia: JB Lippincott, 1989, pp 63–82.

McGraw M. *The Neuromuscular Maturation of the Human Infant.* New York: Hafner Publishing, 1945.

Peiper A. *Cerebral Function in Infancy and Childhood.* New York: Consultants Bureau, 1963.

Penn AA, Shatz CJ. Brain waves and brain wiring: The role of endogenous and sensory-driven neural activity in development. *Pediatr Res* 45:447–458, 1999.

Porter RE. Normal development of movement and function: Child and adolescent. In Scully RM, Barnes MR (eds). *Physical Therapy.* Philadelphia: JB Lippincott, 1989, pp 83–98.

Roberton MA. Motor development: Recognizing our roots, charting our future. *Quest* 41:213–223, 1989.

Rosenbaum DA. *Human Motor Control.* San Diego: Academic Press, 1991.

Sabourin P. *Rising from Supine to Standing: A Study of Adolescents.* Unpublished master's thesis, Virginia Commonwealth University, 1989.

Schmidt RA. A schema theory of discrete motor skill learning. *Psychol Rev* 82:225–260, 1975.

Schmidt RA, Lee TD. *Motor Control and Learning: A Behavioral Emphasis,* 3rd ed. Champaign, IL: Human Kinetics, 1999.

Seyffarth H, Denny-Brown D. The grasp reflex and the instinctive grasp reaction. *Brain* 71:109, 1948.

Shumway-Cook A, Woollacott MH. Growth of stability: Postural control from a developmental perspective. *J Motor Behav* 17:131–147, 1985.

Shumway-Cook A, Woollacott MH. *Motor Control: Theory and Practical Applications.* Philadelphia: Williams & Wilkins, 1995.

Spirduso WW. *Physical Dimensions of Aging.* Champaign, IL: Human Kinetics, 1995.

Sporns O, Edelman GM. Solving Bernstein's problem: A proposal for the development of coordinated movement by selection. *Child Dev* 64:960–981, 1993.

Thelen E. Rhythmical sterotypies in infants. *Anim Behav* 27:699–715, 1979.

Thelen E, Fisher DM. Newborn stepping: An explanation for a disappearing reflex. *Dev Psychol* 18: 760–775, 1982.

Thelen E, Fisher DM, Ridley-Johnson R. The relationship between physical growth and a newborn reflex. *Infant Behav Dev* 7:479–493, 1984.

Thelen E, Smith LB. *A Dynamic Systems Approach to the Development of Cognition and Action.* Cambridge, MA: MIT Press, 1994.

Thelen E, Smith LB. Dynamic systems. In Damon W (ed). *Handbook of Child Psychology,* 5th ed. New York: John Wiley and Sons, 1998, pp 563–634.

Thelen E, Ulrich BD, Jensen JL. The developmental origins of locomotion. In Woollacott MH, Shumway-Cook A (eds). *Development of Posture and Gait Across the Life Span*. Columbia, SC: University of South Carolina Press, 1990, pp 25–47.

Thomas RL, Williams AK, Lundy-Ekman L. Supine to stand in elderly persons: Relationship to age, activity level, strength, and range of motion. *Issues Aging* 21:9–18, 1998.

Twitchell TE. The restoration of motor function following hemiplegia in man. *Brain* 74:443 480, 1951.

VanSant AF. Age differences in movement patterns used by children to rise from a supine position to erect stance. *Phys Ther* 68:1130–1138, 1988a.

VanSant AF. Rising from a supine position to erect stance: Description of adult movement and a developmental hypothesis. *Phys Ther* 68:185–192, 1988b.

VanSant AF. A life span concept of motor development. *Quest* 41:224–234, 1989.

VanSant AF. Life-span motor development. In Lister M (ed). *Contemporary Management of Motor Control Problems. Proceedings of the II Step Conference*. Alexandria, VA: Foundation for Physical Therapy, 1991, pp 77–83.

Whithall, J. A developmental study of the inter-limb coordination in running and galloping. *J Mot Behav* 21:409–428, 1989.

Wickstrom RL. *Fundamental Movement Patterns*, 3rd ed. Philadelphia: Lea & Febiger, 1983.

Wyke B. The neurological basis for movement: A developmental review. *Clin Dev Med* 55:19–33, 1975.

Susan V. Duff
Lori Quinn

Chapter

4 Motor Learning and Motor Control

OBJECTIVES

After studying this chapter, the reader will be able to:

1 Explain key concepts related to a systems view of motor control.

2 Describe mechanisms contributing to neural plasticity.

3 Describe stages of learning and the difference between implicit and explicit processes related to motor learning.

4 Identify key variables used to measure motor learning.

5 Describe effective strategies that can be used to promote motor learning across the life span.

How do infants learn to crawl and walk? How do children and adults learn to accurately throw a baseball at a target or safely traverse a steep incline on skis? These tasks are initially attempted with an abundance of determination and physical aptitude, and with practice, the necessary motor skill is gained. *Motor skills* are defined as voluntary body or limb movements used to accomplish action or task goals (Magill, 1993). As we move toward proficiency in a particular action or task, performance becomes more consistent and efficient yet flexible enough to be executed in a variety of contexts (Higgins, 1991).

Attaining motor skills involves a process of motor learning (Newell, 1991). *Motor learning principles* integrate information from psychology, neurology, physical education, and rehabilitation research. An infant learning to navigate across the floor uses the perceptions she has of her own body and skill to move within a particular environment successfully. As an older adult accommodates to strength and sensory changes that occur with aging, she often must modify how she performs tasks such as walking or manipulating objects. An individual with a neurological deficit, orthopedic problem, or even cardiopulmonary disease, may need to *relearn* previously acquired motor skills, but an altered number and quality of resources are available to her. For instance, after an individual has sustained a stroke, he may need to relearn how to get dressed or to get up and down from a chair despite limitations in strength or cognition. When we, as researchers and clinicians, gain insight into this multifaceted process, theories about how humans learn and relearn motor skills continue to be modified.

What we learn, as we engage in motor learning of select skills, is associated *motor control* processes tailored to an environmental context. The *neural mechanisms* related to plasticity of the central nervous system (CNS) provide a substrate for skill learning and relearning. The evolving perspectives and concepts related to both motor control processes and neural plasticity provide the foundation for an understanding of the stages of learning and strategies that may be used to promote skill acquisition (see Chapter 3).

Motor Control Concepts Associated with Learning

Perspectives or theories in motor control are based on models of the nervous system and represent the paradigm shifts that have taken place throughout history. When existing theories begin to limit the way movement and behavior are interpreted, new paradigms are developed (Kuhn, 1970). Because motor control theories are used to analyze and understand the changes that occur with motor learning, they provide a framework for interpreting movement and behavior.

HISTORICAL VIEW

This section provides a brief overview of motor control models. A systems model is the most contemporary model, at this time, and we use it as a basis for our clinical applications throughout this chapter. A more detailed discussion of all motor control models can be found in Chapter 3.

Reflex Model and Hierarchical View

Early perspectives of motor control date back to the late 1800s, when two similar views were proposed that pointed to a hierarchical organization. In separate research, the authors claimed that sensory input was necessary for the control of motor output. James (1890) suggested that a successive chain of muscular contractions inherent in an habitual motor act were triggered in sequence by associated sensations, or *chaining*. By the turn of the century, Sherrington (1906) proposed his *reflex model* wherein a sequence of reflexes formed the building blocks of complex motor behavior. Unfortunately, these two related theories did not explain movement that occurs without a sensory stimulus, nor did they explain how actions are modified depending on the context in which they occur (e.g., varying speed, novel conditions).

Motor Program Model

During the 1900s, different perspectives have emerged in an attempt to demonstrate that movement could be generated from within the nervous system, not just following a sensory stimulus, and that motor control may be distributed throughout the nervous system. *Motor program theory* was developed to directly challenge the notion that all movement was generated through chaining or reflexes, because even slow movements occur too fast for sensory input to influence them (Gordon, 1987). Motor programs are associated with a set of muscle commands specified at the time of action production, which do not require sensory input (Wing et al, 1996, p 504). Schmidt (1988) expanded motor program theory to include the notion of a generalized motor program or an abstract *neural representation* of an action, distributed among different systems.

Systems Model

A *systems model* disputes the assumption that motor control is hierarchically organized and instead argues that it is distributed throughout the nervous system (Shumway-Cook and Woollacott, 2001) (see Chapter 3). Although the CNS is organized in a hierarchical fashion to a certain degree, the direction of control is not simply from the top down (Gordon, 1987; Horak, 1991). For example, lower levels of the nervous system can assume control over higher levels depending on the goals and constraints of the task.

The brain undergoes anatomical growth during development, which includes cell proliferation, migration, and differentiation (Nowakowski, 1993), as well as functional and organizational changes in response to environmental and task demands. Because the nervous system has the ability to self-organize, it is feasible that several systems are engaged in resolving movement problems; therefore, solutions typically are unique to the context and goal of the task at hand (Carr and Shepherd, 1998; Thelen, 1995). The advantage of the systems model is that it can account for the flexibility and adaptability of motor behavior in a variety of environmental conditions. Functional goals as well as environmental and task constraints are thought to play a major role in determining movement (Horak, 1991). This frame of reference provides a foundation for developing intervention strategies based on task goals that are aimed at improving motor skills.

One theory that developed out of the systems model is the *dynamic systems theory* (DST) (Thelan and Ulrich, 1991). DST is supported by the *theory of neuronal group selection*, which emphasizes the dynamic variability of neural circuitry (Edelman, 1993; Sporns and Edelman, 1993) (see Chapter 3). Specifically, DST proposes that in contrast to behavior unfolding in a set ontogenetic sequence, motor patterns are softly assembled (Thelen, 1995). *Softly assembled* means that although there is some level of neural organization that determines motor behavior, particular motor patterns are not simply preprogrammed but instead have some flexibility based on characteristics of the performer and the specifics of the task and environment.

Motor control theories continue to be developed, and although the associated assumptions may differ, most current models have incorporated a systems view of distributed control of the nervous system. One assumption that remains controversial is whether a central neural representation of movement exists. Bernstein (1967) suggested that the *outcome* of a movement is represented in a motor plan (e.g., aiming a ball toward a target) and distributed at different levels of the CNS. Many theorists have adopted this concept. *Early motor program theory* suggested that some form of neural storage of motor plans took place (Keele, 1968). It is questionable whether the CNS has the capacity to store motor plans, or whether the motor plan is a hypothetical concept (Morris et al, 1994). Conversely, DST proposes that nothing is stored; instead, motor learning is an emergent property (Thelen and Ulrich, 1991). Although the specific organization of motor plans is not known, flexible neural representations of the dynamic and distributed processes through which the nervous system can solve motor problems seem to exist (Gordon, 1994; Weiss et al, 2000). We advocate that learning does evolve from an interaction and strengthening among multiple systems and that there may be strong neural connections between related systems that can be crudely viewed as representations.

APPLICATION OF MOTOR CONTROL CONCEPTS WITHIN SYSTEMS THEORY

Three key concepts are pertinent to the application of the systems theory of motor control to skill acquisition:

1. How we resolve the *degrees of freedom* problem inherent in movement
2. How we *optimize* our movements
3. How we *use sensory information*

Degrees of Freedom

There are multiple levels of redundancy within the CNS. Bernstein (1967) suggested that a key function of the CNS is to control this redundancy by minimizing the degrees of freedom or the number of independent movement elements that are used. For example, muscles can fire in different ways to control particular movement patterns or joint motions. In addition, many different kinematic or movement patterns can be executed to accomplish one specific outcome or action. During the early stages of learning novel tasks, the body may produce very simple movements, often linking together two or more degrees of freedom (Gordon, 1987, p 12), and limiting the amount of joint motion by holding some joints stiffly via muscle co-contraction. As an action or task is learned, we first hold our joints stiffly through muscle coactivation and then, as we learn the task, we decrease coactivation and allow the joint to move freely. This increases the degrees of freedom around the joint (Vereijken et al, 1992). With improved skill, greater fluidity may be observed, reflecting the ability of the CNS to use multiple motor resources to accomplish select tasks. This is exemplified when learning a task such as downhill skiing, in which a skier's body initially is held stiff and rigid. As the skier becomes more proficient, the movement becomes smoother and the skier can express multiple degrees of joint motion, which are required to adapt to environmental changes such as icy surfaces and a range of inclines.

Certainly, an increase in joint stiffness used to minimize degrees of freedom at the early stages of skill acquisition may not hold true for all types of tasks. In fact, different skills require different patterns of muscle activation. For example, Spencer and Thelen (1997) reported that muscle coactivity increases with learning of a fast vertical reaching movement. They proposed that high-velocity movements actually result in the need for muscle coactivity to counteract unwanted rotational forces. However, during the execution of complex multijoint tasks, such as walking and rising from sitting to standing, muscle coactivation is clearly undesirable and may in fact negatively affect the smoothness and efficiency of the movements. The resolution of the degrees of freedom problem varies depending on the characteristics of the learner as well as on the components of the task and environment. Despite the various interpretations of Bernstein's original hypothesis (1967), the resolution of the degrees of freedom problem continues to form the underlying basis for a systems theory of motor control.

Optimization Principles

Optimization theory suggests that movements are specified to optimize a select cost function (Cruse et al, 1990; Nelson, 1983; Wolpert et al, 1995). Cost functions are those kinematic (spatial) or dynamic (force) factors that influence movement at an expense to the system. Motor skill development or relearning is aimed at achieving select objectives while minimizing cost to the system. Reducing such cost while meeting task demands and accommodating to task constraints theoretically solves the degrees of freedom problem and enhances movement efficiency.

Flash and Hogan (1985) theorized that the cost function being reduced during point-to-point reaching movements is *jerk* (rate of change in acceleration). This results in a straighter hand path, as exemplified in a 1997 study by Konczak and Dichgans (Fig. 4–1). These authors found that the distance the hand traveled during reaching movements in young infants was initially prolonged with a noticeable curvature in the sagittal hand path or paths. However, with practice, the distance the hand traveled was reduced, the hand path became straighter, and the overall movement was smoother. Hypothetically, optimization principles drive the nervous system toward greater efficiency within the confines of task demands, environmental constraints, and performer limitations.

As children and adults struggle to achieve functional gains during development or during recovery from neural injury, they may appear to use inefficient movement strategies, at least from an outside view. In actuality, they may be expressing the most efficient movements available to them given their current resources. For example, a child with hemiplegic cerebral palsy may have the physical constraints of shoulder or wrist weakness and reduced finger fractionation (isolation). In an effort to reduce cost to the system while meeting tasks demands, he may use a "flexion synergy," in which elbow flexion is used in combination with shoulder elevation and lateral trunk flexion to reach for objects placed at shoulder height. This flexion synergy is a strategy that seems to reduce the number of movement elements yet allows for successful attain-

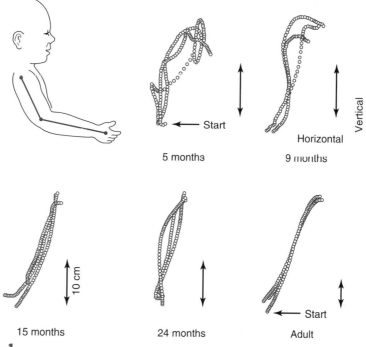

Figure 4–1

Progressive smoothing of sagittal hand paths during reaching from infancy to adulthood. (Redrawn from Konczak J, Dichgans J. The development toward stereotypic arm kinematics during reaching in the first 3 years of life. *Exp Brain Res* 117:348, 1997.)

ment of the target object. Although this strategy may be useful in a specific situation, it may become habitual and may not be effective in performing a wide range of tasks. Furthermore, persistent use of a specific movement pattern may lead to related musculoskeletal impairments.

Once strengths and weaknesses are known, coaches, therapists, and educators can guide individuals toward successful motor function by structuring tasks to work on overcoming weaknesses. For example, to encourage reaching and grasping in the aforementioned child with hemiplegia, the task could be altered to require a reach toward large objects positioned at knee versus shoulder level (in sitting). This new movement strategy may reduce the demands on select muscle groups, such as shoulder and elbow musculature, while encouraging the full use of the upper limb, including the long finger flexors and wrist extensors needed for gross grasp. Alternatively, the environment can be arranged so those habitual patterns are no longer effective, thus forcing different ones to emerge. For instance, an individual who tends to circumduct the leg to clear the floor when walking may be forced to use an alternate gait pattern if presented with obstacles in the path, necessitating some hip and knee flexion. The movement patterns selected by the performer become habitual (not necessarily efficient) unless alternate patterns are demanded and practiced more.

Utilization of Sensory Information

Sensory information most pertinent to motor control comes from three key sources: somatosensory (proprioceptive and tactile), visual, and vestibular processes. Patla (1995) introduced a model for examining the use of sensory information to maintain equilibrium during locomotion that incorporates two control processes: proactive and reactive control (Fig. 4–2). *Proactive (anticipatory* or *feedforward) control* refers to the use of previous sensory information for planning before movement execution. *Reactive control* refers to the use of sensory information to adjust and adapt movement responses after an unexpected event (Patla, 1995). In addition to locomotion, this model is useful to understand how we use sensory information during other motor tasks.

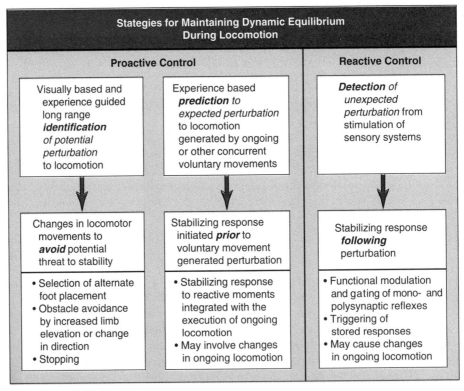

Figure 4–2

Proactive and reactive control. Example of maintaining dynamic equilibrium during locomotion. (From Patla AE. A framework for understanding mobility problems in the elderly. In Craik RL, Oatis CA [eds]. *Gait Analysis: Theory and Application.* St. Louis: Mosby, 1995, p 439.)

Proactive Control

The following scenario clearly exemplifies proactive control.

> A young college student walks across a busy street, carrying several books in one hand and a cup of coffee in the other. On reaching the other side, she marvels at the fact that she arrived safely at her destination without being injured by the onslaught of traffic, while her books and coffee remain intact.

As she made her way across the street, she probably made use of previous experiences and sensory information to *predict* and *respond* in advance of upcoming events. These events included steering herself around an oncoming car, avoiding a pothole in the street, and coordinating her movements to minimize jerkiness, which might have caused her to drop the books or spill the coffee she was holding. For proactive control to be effective, regulatory conditions in the environment that do not change or vary, such as the road surface and the distance to cross the street (Gentile, 1987), combined with previous sensory information are held in memory and are used to scale muscle forces in advance (Ghez et al, 1990; Johansson, 1996). After completion of the task, revisions can be made to the internal representation (sensorimotor memories) based on sensory feedback and are used in the planning of future movements.

According to Patla's model (1995), proactive control also encompasses prediction to expected perturbations generated by ongoing movements. In preparation for destabilizing forces, such as propulsive forces or slippery contact surfaces, anticipatory muscle responses are activated in a timely manner. Learning to predict the impact external forces and environmental characteristics have on a particular movement is a difficult but important process in proactive motor control. Essentially, a person must initially stabilize responses before an expected perturbation (destabilizing force) to minimize the effects of that perturbation. For instance, without proactive control, we may exert too much or too little force during object manipulation, crushing fragile objects or letting them slip from our grasp. Proactive control, particularly during locomotion, involves changes in movement strategy to avoid potential threat to stability. In many voluntary movements, such as raising the arm, muscle activity begins in proximal postural musculature close to the base of support (paraspinal musculature) even before the onset of the prime mover (anterior deltoid) (Nashner, 1977). The early activation of postural musculature is termed *anticipatory postural adjustments*. Anticipatory postural adjustments prevent a loss of balance due to displacement of the body's center of mass and minimize the effects of perturbations induced by the movement itself (see Chapter 12). The specificity and intensity of these anticipatory postural adjustments seem to be dependent on many factors, including initial body position and postural support, speed and amplitude of the movement, and the context in which all are taking place (Bouisset and Zattara, 1987; Cordo and Nashner, 1982).

Reactive Control

Sensory information has an important role in adjusting and adapting our movement responses after an unexpected event. *Reactive control* uses sensory feedback to detect and stabilize the body after unexpected perturbations (Patla, 1995). Examples of perturbations include tripping on an unexpected obstacle while walking, losing one's balance while standing on a bus that stops suddenly, or the unexpected slipping of an object between the fingertips. For example, the student crossing the street makes use of reactive control to counteract a fall if she slips on slick pavement. Although avoidance of these events is the best preventative measure for ensuring stability, it is not always possible. Therefore, we must be able to quickly and appropriately react to unexpected external events. Fortunately, with practice, muscle responses to unexpected perturbations become more efficient and effective (Horak et al, 1989).

Neural Plasticity

The capacity of the brain to modify its structure or function in response to learning or brain damage is termed *plasticity* (Lebeer, 1998). As concepts of neural plasticity have gained acceptance, the functional changes seen during learning and after recovery from brain damage are being interpreted within a systems theory framework. The plasticity associated with motor learning may be attributed to changes at the chemical, synaptic, and structural levels (axonal and dendritic branching) of the nervous system (Coulson and Klein, 1997). Although we lose neurons with age, the number of synapses per neuron increases (Buell and Coleman, 1981) and may support new learning or relearning in older adults. In addition to synaptic transmission of information, evidence supports the notion of *nonsynaptic diffusion neurotransmission*, which is the diffusion of neurotransmitters and other substances through extracellular fluid and may play a role in brain plasticity (Bach-y-Rita, 1995).

In infancy and early childhood, there is a high degree of neuroplasticity. However, there are critical or sensitive periods during which a child's brain may be most adaptable to certain experiences (Acredolo and Goodwin, 2000). As we age, we lose a certain degree of adaptability. Evidence does suggest, however, that reorganization is also present in adults (Goldman and Plum, 1997; Lebeer, 1998).

Early in the 1900s, various theories were postulated to explain why there was a lack of CNS regeneration in adult mammals ranging from the lack of catalytic elements or a conductor for regrowth to the existence of mechanical blocks. Evidence supports the brain's capacity (animal and human) to regenerate and reorganize throughout life as a result of functional use, strength training, immobilization, and related cellular processes (Classen et al, 1998; Enoka, 1995; Nudo et al, 1996). Neural mechanisms that take place at synapses and on the cell membrane away from synapses (nonsynaptic diffusion neurotransmission) may play a significant role during the recovery of function after brain damage (Bach-y-Rita, 1990). Interestingly, Hallet and colleagues have found that transcranial magnetic stimulation influences the plasticity of particular brain areas and may be useful in recovery during select periods after brain injury (Corthout et al, 1999 and 2000; Hallet, 2000).

An attempt by the brain to recover from injury may initially involve resolution from shock as noted by a reduction in edema. The majority of recovery, however, is due to neural reorganization. Key hypotheses regarding mechanisms for adaptive and maladaptive reorganization after injury, which are not mutually exclusive, include the following:

- Unmasking or strengthening of silent synapses or those from subthreshold connections (Calford and Tweedale, 1991; Jenkins et al, 1990; Merzenich and Sameshima, 1993; Pascual-Leone and Torres, 1993; Recanzone et al, 1992s)
- Development of extrasynaptic receptors on the membrane of surviving cells via diffusion (Bach-y-Rita and Illis, 1993)
- Reactive synaptogenesis (Cotman and Nieto-Sampedro, 1985) or sprouting and the construction of new functional pathways (Berman and Sterling, 1976; Jones, 2000; Wainer et al, 1997)
- Migration of cells into the deafferentated region (Allard et al, 1993; Mogiler et al, 1993; Ramachandran et al, 1992)
- Subcortical reorganization projected to the cortex (Pons et al, 1991)

The extensive research on plasticity provides strong justification to enhance motor learning and relearning across all ages and skill levels. We continue with a description of the behavioral aspects of motor learning related to neural plasticity and the key concepts inherent in a systems view of motor control.

Stages of Motor Learning

FITTS' CATEGORIES

A behavioral analysis of motor skill learning often begins with three overlapping stages first described by Fitts (1964). The first stage is identified as the *cognitive phase* because it requires a high degree of conscious involvement. Initially, the learner must understand the goal of the task to be performed and recognize the regulatory features of the environment to which the movement must conform (Gentile, 1987). In a task such as walking across a crowded room, the surface of the floor and the location and size of people within the room are considered regulatory features. If the floor is slippery, a person's walking pattern probably is different than if the floor is carpeted. Although nonregulatory or background features, such as lighting or noise, are not critical to shaping the movements, they may affect task performance.

During this initial cognitive stage of learning, an individual naturally tries a variety of strategies to achieve the action-goal, often exhibiting a great deal of movement variability (Gentile, 1987 and 1998). With practice, the learner often develops appropriate and effective strategies for accomplishing the goal, while simultaneously discarding ineffective ones. The performance gains that occur in the cognitive stage are usually dramatic, although most of the improvements involve learning what to do rather than learning the specific motor patterns involved (Schmidt, 1988). When a child learns to bat a baseball, the focus in this initial stage of learning is on successfully hitting the ball rather than exhibiting of a particular movement pattern, such as a level swing of the bat.

At the next stage of learning, the *associative phase*, the learner presumably has picked the best strategy to use for a specific task and has begun to refine it. Performance is less variable, and more subtle adjustments take place as she makes use of error information to correct subsequent movements. The learner can persist in this phase while producing small changes in movement patterns, which ultimately allow for more effective and efficient performance. During this phase, the focus of the learner switches from "what to do" to "how to do the movement" (Schmidt, 1988). The child learning to bat a baseball might begin to shift her focus of attention toward a certain movement form and style that may result in greater efficiency and consistency, such as choking up on the bat to allow greater control.

In the final stage of learning, the *autonomous stage*, the skill becomes more "automatic" because the learner does not need to focus all of her attention on the motor skill. Therefore, she is able to attend to other components of the task, such as scanning for subtle environmental obstacles. Research supports this reduction in mental effort in planning skilled actions with evidence of decreased movement-related brain potentials after long-term practice of a motor skill (Fattapposta et al, 1996). The autonomous stage allows the learner to fine-tune her performance, working toward consistent and efficient achievement of the movement and task goals. At this phase, the learner is better able to adapt to changes in regulatory and nonregulatory features in the environment. The child, in our example, will be relatively successful at hitting the ball when using different bats (regulatory feature) or if a crowd is present (non-regulatory feature).

EXPLICIT AND IMPLICIT PROCESSES

New theories have begun to emerge that provide more in-depth analysis of the stages of motor skill learning described by Fitts (1964). Gentile (1998) suggested that motor skill learning involves two parallel yet distinct learning processes: *explicit* and *implicit*. Although these two processes change at different rates and appear to take place in different stages, they probably overlap during skill learning. Explicit learning has traditionally been linked with declarative memory (conscious recall of information), however, it appears that there is little relationship between motor learning ability and declarative memory ability (Sullivan, 1998). Instead explicit learning may be reflected by a conscious focus on attainment of the action-goal, as in the initial stage of learning. In an attempt at early success, the performer develops a map between his body structure and the conditions within the environment. Thus, he remains consciously aware of changes in the movement's shape or structure and its relationship to external conditions and demands as he attempts to problem solve through a task. For example, a boy who is learning to throw a basketball into a net must learn about the size and texture of the ball and how he can manipulate it with his hands and must obtain a general representation of the distance and size of the net. Whenever movement patterns can be consciously adapted by the performer, they are considered to be regulated by *explicit* processes (Gentile, 2000).

With prolonged practice in the later stages of learning, we begin to refine motor control strategies, indicating the predominance of *implicit* processes. Traditionally, *implicit learning* has been defined as "the learning of complex information in an incidental manner, without awareness of what has been learned" (Segar, 1994, p 163). Implicit learning of motor skills typically occurs over a gradual period of time as we learn to unconsciously merge successive movements, couple simultaneous components, and regulate intersegmental force dynamics inherent in specific tasks (Gentile, 1998). Intersegmental force dynamics incorporate active forces produced through muscle contraction and passive forces such as motion-dependent torques (joint movement obtained without muscle contraction) that occur naturally in the environment or as a result of movement. The variability typically observed in young children and novel performers as they learn particular motor skills allows them to develop a range of force production patterns (Gentile, 1998).

We learn how to exploit passive forces, thus minimizing the energy we need to expend for active forces or muscle contraction with internal and external feedback. For example, execution of an efficient basketball throw involves the use of gravity (pulling the ball downward toward the target) and exploitation of motion-dependent torques (reactive forces that result from links to other joints) to reduce the active muscle force required to push off from a slightly crouched position and throw the ball with ease. Gentile (1998) suggested that implicit learning occurs only through active, task-specific practice. Skill is visible as learners work on achieving the most efficient and optimal outcome to the task, at a minimal cost to their system.

When a child learns to throw a basketball into a net, we can envision the balance that occurs between explicit and implicit processes. Initially, all his resources must attend to his movements or arm position and the regulatory conditions in the environment, in this case ball size and net height, to ensure he hits the net. Such concentration places greater emphasis on explicit learning. Implicit learning is used when the focus is on controlling the dynamics of the movements, such as the force expended to propel the ball through the air. Once physical ability develops, the explicit processes are less involved in basic movement planning and organization. Now implicit learning begins to dominate, allowing him to attend to many different things at once, including other children trying to steal away the ball. After considerable practice, the learner begins to demonstrate the ability to exploit the force dynamics with minimal awareness of the movement process. For instance, he may be able to throw a ball while his attention is diverted toward the yelling crowd during a game and still accurately hit the net.

Motor Learning

KEY FEATURES

Motor skills are discrete acts that involve the use of our hands or body to accomplish a specific goal. Gross motor skills are characterized by movements that involve large proximal musculature and include such activities as walking, jumping, climbing, and ball throwing. Fine motor skills require control of the small distal muscles and incorporate such activities as buttoning, picking up small objects, and turning a key in a door.

Although specific movement patterns are typically associated with highly skilled performance, it is critical to have flexibility and a range of available movement patterns. We often adopt movement patterns that conform to our own body type and resources. Therefore, rather than being concerned with a perfect or normal quality of movement, it is more important that movement patterns are efficient given the individual's available resources, yet flexible enough to be used in a variety of contexts.

Although movement variability is evident in adults learning novel tasks (McDonald et al, 1989; Moore and Marteniuk, 1986), it is even greater in young children, aging adults, and clinical populations (Van Thiel et al, 2000). Young children show high degrees of intertrial variability when trying to maintain their balance in response to platform perturbations (Shumway-Cook and Woollacott, 1985) or attempting to clear their toes when stepping over obstacles (Law et al, 1996). Older adults demonstrate high degrees of both intrasubject and intersubject variability in motor performance (Light and Spirduso, 1990). In general, movement variability is high if resources or experiences are limited and usually decreases with practice, except in select clinical populations. This variability and subsequent reduction that occur with practice must be considered when designing and implementing intervention programs. Variability in motor performance, not stereotypy, is a natural part of motor skill learning. Coaches, therapists, and educators may actually promote variability in early learning by encouraging a learner to explore a wide variety of movement strategies. Later in learning, consistent movement patterns may become more apparent, as the learner begins to focus on the most optimal strategy given her resources, the environmental context, and demands of the task.

CLASSIFICATION

Although gross and fine motor skills are useful broad classifications, a more detailed view of motor skill is necessary to optimally assess and promote acquisition. Two useful classification systems for motor skills are (1) defining the beginning and end points and (2) defining the stability of the environment in which the task is being performed.

Within the beginning and end points classification system, three separate types of motor skills are identified: discrete, serial, and continuous. *Discrete* motor skills are movements that have a clear beginning and end, as seen when we throw a ball at a target. *Serial* motor skills can be put together in a series,

TABLE 4–1

Classification of Movement Tasks Based on Beginning and End Points

Classification	Task Examples
Discrete	Reaching, flipping a light switch, sit to stand
Serial	Getting dressed, driving a car, brushing teeth
Continuous	Walking, running, swimming

where the sum of the parts equals the whole, as seen in the process of dressing. The variability experienced in walking provides a good illustration of the more arbitrary beginning and end points that are defined by the performer using *continuous* motor skills (Table 4–1).

Another way of classifying motor tasks is by describing the environment as being either closed or open (Gentile, 1987). An environment is considered *closed* if the features remain constant and objects, people, or supporting surfaces are stationary. In closed tasks, regulatory features in the environment remain consistent and predictable such as when an individual walks alone in his own home. In such an environment, the individual does not have to account for variability or unexpected occurrences when planning movement strategies. This contrasts with *open* environments, in which objects, people, or supporting surfaces within it are in motion or vary. Open tasks require a greater amount of information processing and advanced planning. When a person walks across the street, she must consider and predict the speed of oncoming traffic, the moving path of pedestrians passing by, and alterations in the walking surface. A closed versus open task classification can be incorporated into a more complex taxonomy for analyzing functional activities and creating intervention programs (Gentile, 1987).

MEASUREMENT

In behavioral research, motor learning is measured by analyzing performance at three distinct levels: acquisition, retention, and transfer of skills (Magill, 1993). *Acquisition* is the initial practice or performance of a novel skill, or new control aspect of a motor skill. *Retention* is the ability to demonstrate attainment of the skill or improvement in some aspect, following a short or long time delay in which the task is not practiced. *Transfer* requires the performance of a task similar in movement yet different than the original task practiced in the acquisition phase, such as altered force or timing. Although we may demonstrate acceptable performance of a motor skill within a single session or series of sessions, it is not considered truly learned until retention or transfer of that particular skill is established.

Consider a young child who is just learning to sit up on the floor. Among other variables, his skill might be measured in the amount of time that he can maintain the sitting position independently. This ability could be evaluated from all three levels of motor learning: acquisition, documenting sitting time over multiple trials when he is learning to sit and is actively engaged in practice; retention, determining whether he can maintain sitting after a period of not doing so, possibly the next day; and transfer, determining whether he can perform a similar skill, such as sitting on a grassy surface versus a wooden floor.

Three measures of skill learning—consistency, flexibility, and efficiency— provide another framework for establishing criteria for skilled motor performance. Although the specifics clearly differ depending on the task, virtually all motor tasks incorporate all three components when skilled performance is considered. Table 4–2 provides examples of how these three aspects of skill can be measured.

Consistency refers to the repeatability of performance. Returning to the young child: can he perform the task consistently over a period of trials conducted over a number of sessions? For example, can he sit for a sustained time period, repeatedly? *Flexibility*, or transferability, refers to the ability to adapt and to modify task performance based on changing environments or conditions. For instance, can he sit on various surfaces successfully? Flexibility, in essence, represents transfer of the skill. *Efficiency* typically pertains to the capabilities of the cardiovascular and musculoskeletal systems. *Cardiovascular efficiency* refers to an ability to preserve or minimize energy expenditure during task performance as documented through physiological variables such as heart and respiratory rate. *Musculoskeletal efficiency* refers to optimal movement coor-

TABLE 4–2

Assessment of Functional Skills

Skill Component	Definition	Objective Measurements
Flexibility	Ability to perform a skill under a variety of environmental conditions	• Height, surface, or position of equipment or objects • Environment (e.g., open versus closed) • Ability to do two tasks at once
Efficiency	Ability to perform a skill within a certain level of both cardiovascular and musculoskeletal efficiency	• Time to complete task • Distance • Speed of movement • Reaction time • Kinematics, electromyographic patterns • Heart rate, respiratory rate, or blood pressure changes
Consistency	Ability to successfully perform a skill repeatedly over multiple trials or days	• Errors (number, percent) • Number of successful trials • Number of days or weeks able to perform

dination with respect to kinematics (spatial or temporal factors) or kinetics (force dynamics). For example, is the child able to reach for toys in front of him using a relatively straight hand path without excessively listing his trunk to one side?

PROMOTION

Individuals of all ages can learn most motor skills with little or no intervention. Young children learn to sit up, crawl, pull-to-stand, and walk without anyone teaching them to do so. Children, who are delayed in learning early mobility skills, or older children, adolescents, and adults who wish to learn particular skills for recreational or occupational endeavors may benefit from intervention. In addition, individuals who have sustained musculoskeletal or neurological damage often must relearn certain basic skills previously taken for granted, such as brushing their teeth or getting out of bed. Therefore, information on how to enhance motor skills may be beneficial to coaches and educators as well as therapists.

Promoting skill acquisition across the life span requires consideration of the critical interactions out of which movement emerges: the *task,* the *environment,* and the *performer* (see Fig. 3–3). Once task goals and the level of the learner are determined, intervention can occur at one or all three levels of interaction (see Clinical Implications—Task-Based Intervention to Enhance Skill Learning). Incorporated within this task-oriented approach to clinical intervention are methods to address underlying impairments and motor control strategies that optimize motor performance (Carr and Shepherd, 1998; Shumway-Cook and Woollacott, 2001).

Motor skill promotion can occur at the task level by structuring practice, at the environmental level by structuring the environment, and at the performer level through modeling, mental practice, and feedback.

Structuring Practice

Structuring practice of a task is one of the most important aspects of motor learning. The amount and schedule of the practice must be considered as well as transferability of the task.

Amount of Practice

It is well supported that the best way to improve at any skill is to practice, practice, practice. However, what amount of practice leads to the best improvement in motor performance?

Early intensive training or rehabilitation is optimal to take advantage of neural plasticity. Young children who learn motor skills such as ice skating or golf at an early age often have a better chance of becoming highly skilled than do individuals who learn these skills later in life. This can be due to many factors. The young child simply has devoted more time on task—practice time is related to skilled performance—than the older adult. Also, as discussed

The steps describe the components to consider before task practice is initiated. Practice itself can incorporate methods to structure practice, set up the environment, or provide augmentative input to the learner before, during, and after performance of the task.

Step 1: *Determine the goal and define the task to be learned.*

- Consider type of task: serial, discrete, or continuous.
- Analyze environmental conditions by identifying regulatory features of the environment and recognizing the task as closed or open.

Step 2: *Determine level of skill learning.*

- Cognitive, associative, or automatic stage of learning
- Explicit versus implicit processes

Step 3: *Choose method of intervention based on task, environment, and performer characteristics.*

Task Level–Structuring Practice

- Task-specific practice
- Amount of practice
- Schedule of practice
  - Massed versus distributed practice
  - Contextual interference–random versus blocked practice
- Transfer of training
  - Whole versus part practice

Environment Level–Structuring the Environment

- Closed versus open environment
- Consider affordances

Performer Level–Before, During, and After Performance

- Before task performance
  - Demonstration and modeling
  - Mental practice and imagery
- During task performance–concurrent feedback
  - Manual assistance and manual guidance (manual facilitation, physical assistance, braces, assistive devices)
  - Verbal information
- After task performance–terminal feedback
  - Knowledge of results (KR)
  - Knowledge of performance (KP)

earlier, the brain of a young child exhibits a high degree of neural plasticity and may be more amenable to specific experiences than adults.

The early practice of activities in an individual recovering from neurological damage can significantly affect learning and may positively affect neural recovery (Bassile and Bock, 1995; Malouin et al, 1992). Nudo and colleagues (1996) studied the effects of intense rehabilitation in adult squirrel monkeys that were given an insult to motor areas of the cortex. These authors reported that recovery of function and prevention of loss of function in the monkeys were dependent on the intensity of practice, in some cases up to 8 hours per day. Cortical remapping was documented and indicated that the animals still had an extensive region responsible for movement of the arms and fingers.

Scheduling Practice

The often-quoted adage, "Use it or lose it," can be translated into the maintenance and relearning of motor skills. After extended disuse of an impaired limb, a condition termed *learned nonuse* or *learned helplessness* can develop, where an individual does not use the affected limb because it is easier and faster to use the unaffected limb (Peterson et al, 1995; Taub, 1980). Suppression of active movement may stem from sensory impairments, pain, or inefficient sensorimotor control in the involved limb. Children and adults with hemiplegia typically favor the noninvolved hand during prehensile tasks due to the limited grasp and manipulation patterns and poor sensorimotor control (among other factors) in the involved hand. Without task demands to engage the involved extremity, problem-solving skills and motor learning capabilities may be affected, which can perpetuate the motor dysfunction in the involved limb.

Massed Versus Distributed Practice. *Massed practice* incorporates greater practice time than rest time. Under *distributed practice* conditions, practice is spread out to allow greater rest time. Constraint-induced therapy can be considered a modified form of massed practice in which learned nonuse is overcome by shaping or reinforcement (Taub et al, 1993). In an individual with hemiplegia, the uninvolved arm or hand is constrained, thereby forcing use of the involved arm or hand in functional tasks. Ogden and Franz (1917) introduced this concept when they reported significant recovery of function from experimentally induced hemiplegia in monkeys via forced use of the impaired upper limb. This type of therapy has been reintroduced not only as a means to force practice of the involved limb but also to prevent learned nonuse or helplessness. Human studies have begun to examine the effectiveness of this technique as a mode of promoting recovery of function, particularly after unilateral brain damage (Blanton and Wolf, 1999; Charles et al, 2001; Taub and Wolf, 1997). Focal transcranial magnetic stimulation has provided evidence of neural reorganization corresponding to improved motor performance in the involved limb after 12 days of constraint-induced movement therapy in individuals after a stroke (Liepert et al, 2000). In general, the results of constraint-induced therapy are promising.

aaaaaaaaa *bbbbbbbbb* *ccccccccc*	*acbcbacab* *cbacabacb* *bcacabaca*
Blocked	Random

Figure 4–3

Sample practice schedules for reach to grasp activity illustrate blocked and random practice: a, reach and grasp for a paper cup; b, reach and grasp for a coffee mug; c, reach and grasp for a glass.

Random versus Blocked Practice. *Random practice* order refers to the practice of different tasks or task variations in a varying sequence on successive trials rather than the practice of multiple repetitions of any one task. In contrast, a *blocked practice* schedule assumes that multiple trials are completed on one task or task variation before moving onto a different one (Fig. 4–3). Random practice has a greater degree of contextual interference than blocked practice. The literature supports a *contextual interference effect* among healthy adults (Battig, 1966 and 1979; Magill and Hall 1990; Shea and Morgan 1979) and

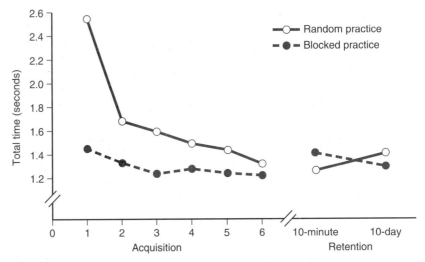

Figure 4–4

Effect of blocked versus random practice on acquisition and retention of a motor skill. Although blocked practice led to better performance during acquisition, random practice led to greater learning as measured by retention tests. (Adapted with permission from Shea JB, Morgan RL. Contextual interference effects on the acquisition, retention, and transfer of a motor skill. *J Exp Psychol* 5[2]:183, 1979.)

adults after a stroke (Hanlon, 1996; Winstein et al, 1999). This effect is graphically illustrated in Figure 4–4. Although blocked practice leads to better performance during acquisition, adults perform better during retention and transfer of motor skills following a random practice order.

The cognitive processes involved in the contextual interference effect may be argued from either an elaboration hypothesis (Battig, 1979) or a reconstructionist view (Lee and Magill, 1983). The *elaboration hypothesis* (Battig, 1979) claims that elaborate and distinct memory representations are developed during random practice based on comparison of the multiple strategies used by the learner. The *reconstructionist view* (Lee and Magill, 1983) asserts that because previously encoded information is at least partially forgotten during random trials, the learner must continually reconstruct the action plan for each response. This leads to a stronger representation and better retention of the skill.

Unlike adults, typically developing children, low-skilled performers, and children from clinical populations may learn best under a blocked or mixed schedule (blocked before random practice) (Edwards et al, 1986; Herbert et al, 1996). Del Rey and colleagues (1983) had typically developing children (approximately 8 years old) practice an anticipation timing task at different speeds in either a blocked or random order and then tested them on a transfer test with new coordination pattern. The researchers found that blocked practice led to better performance on the transfer task than did random practice. Pinto-Zipp and Gentile (1995) studied the effects of contextual interference on unskilled (novice) adults and children learning to throw a Frisbee to a target. Accuracy was determined by measuring the distance from the target and documented by the root-mean-square error. On retention, accuracy improved in adults following random practice, whereas in the children, it was enhanced following blocked practice. Similar results were reported in other studies (Jarus and Goverover, 1999; Pigott and Shapiro, 1984).

Although most of the literature on children supports a blocked or mixed schedule for learning whole body tasks, some researchers have found that typically developing children may learn best following a random practice order (Edwards et al, 1986; Pollack and Lee, 1997). The discrepancy in findings may stem from a difference between learning tasks incorporating whole body movements versus simple manipulative tasks (Gentile, 2000).

An effective practice schedule depends on the task being learned and the characteristics of the learner, such as age. The best practice design not only promotes immediate performance effects but, more important, also promotes long-term learning. Blocked practice may help the learner of any age "get into the ballpark" of a movement or task. In addition, it may be effective when the performer's cognitive or memory function, as seen in individuals with mental retardation or Alzheimer's disease, or need to generalize their movements is compromised, as demonstrated by a person living in a very controlled environment such as a nursing home. Conversely, a random practice schedule may be best for highly skilled learners, because it allows them to derive a range of solutions to the task that can be used at a later time. A mixed practice schedule incorporates both random and blocked practice and may be a useful combination for some learners.

Transfer of Training

By definition, *transfer of training* is the benefit obtained from having had previous training or experience in acquiring a new skill or in adapting an old skill to a new situation. Although practice is the key ingredient to motor skill learning, how much does practice on one type of task transfer to other types of tasks?

Whole Versus Part Practice. A task can be practiced as a complete action (whole) or broken up into its component parts. For the task of walking, *whole task practice* involves the entire action of walking, whereas *part practice* could entail stepping back and forth. For continuous tasks such as walking, running, or stair climbing, whole task practice is preferred over part practice. Winstein and associates (1989) found that practicing a weight-shifting task (part practice) resulted in improvements in weight-shifting abilities in standing but did not transfer to improvements in walking in adults after a stroke any better than did other interventions. Continuous and discrete tasks are not well suited for part practice. Artificially breaking down a task into parts may not benefit motor learning and may even be detrimental.

Serial tasks are more naturally divisible into distinct parts; they are usually more amenable to part practice. Thus, if a whole task is overwhelming, breaking it into its components may help make it more manageable. For example, upper body dressing could be broken down into separate components, such as donning the sleeves and buttoning the buttons. Ultimately, after practicing a task in its component parts, the whole task should be practiced in sequence.

Task-Specific Practice

Select clinical studies indicate that there is limited transferability of certain tasks (Richards et al, 1993; Winstein et al, 1989) and that task-specific or task-related practice is more beneficial (Dean and Shepherd, 1997). For example, Richards and colleagues (1993) found that gait velocity, in adults after a stroke, was strongly correlated with time dedicated to gait training in therapy. However, total time spent in therapy correlated poorly with gait velocity, suggesting that task-specific gait training, not total therapy time, improved gait velocity. Dean and Shepherd (1997) studied individuals at least 1 year after a stroke in a task-related program of progressive reaching beyond arms' length in sitting and compared them with a control group. They found that those who participated in the reaching task not only could reach further and faster but also demonstrated improved sitting balance and increased the load taken through the affected leg. In essence, due to the difficulty ensuring transfer of training, it may be best to focus on task-specific or task-related practice.

Despite its benefits, task-specific practice is not always possible. For instance, an individual may not be capable of practicing the task due to weakness or endurance limitations. Furthermore, practicing the task by itself may prove to be frustrating and even boring for the learner. Worse yet, practice of the same movement pattern over and over again, although useful for learning, may lead to musculoskeletal injuries or may actually reinforce an ineffective habitual pattern if not structured correctly. Practicing different tasks may augment performance of the initial skill, but this often depends on the similarities of the two tasks. For example, bicycle riding, stair climbing, and treadmill training may help improve walking performance in individuals with neurological and other conditions (Guiliani, 1994; Hesse et al, 1994 and 1995; Richards et al, 1993). The key to success is to incorporate essential components of a skill within the tasks that are practiced. Addressing impairments such as weakness and range-of-motion deficits may also improve task performance (Shumway-Cook and Woollacott, 2001).

Structuring the Environment

Tasks cannot be separated from the environment and the context in which they are performed. For closed tasks, the environment is stable, and therefore the performance is constrained only by the spatial organization of the movement (Gentile, 2000). In contrast, open tasks that incorporate timing constraints and thus demand that an individual predicts the speed and location of moving objects, people, or supporting surfaces require heightened proactive control.

Structuring and creating environments that provide appropriate affordances for movement is one important aspect of environmental intervention. An *affordance* is the reciprocal relationship or fit between a performer and the environment needed to perform functional tasks (Gibson, 1979). The age and level of the learner must be considered when setting up the environment for this purpose. For infants and toddlers, an environment that provides the perception of affordances may include couches that can be pulled up onto instead of sat upon or mats that can be crawled on instead of walked on (Gibson et al, 1987). A room full of enticing toys placed on low furniture that is perceived by an infant as "easy to pull up onto" may motivate her to explore and facilitate learning the task of pulling to stand.

The positive effect of environmental stimulation on brain reorganization is referred to as *ecological plasticity* (Lebeer, 1998; Walsh, 1981). As demonstrated in animal studies, enriched environments significantly contribute to physiological and behavioral changes (Held et al, 1985; Rosenzweig et al, 1973). In consideration of this, the typical hospital rehabilitation setting may need considerable reshaping. An environment limited to smooth shiny floors, adjustable-height mat tables with smooth firm surfaces, and specific areas dedicated for walking does not provide an enriching and challenging environmental context. Structuring the rehabilitation environment to create variability, and even more open environments that demand higher levels of adaptation, may enhance recovery and help individuals to transfer their skills to the real world. Something as simple as changing the height of a mat table or altering the chair from which someone has to stand up forces a change in movement strategy and kinematics, not to mention changing force production and flexibility requirements.

Performer Reinforcement

Characteristics of the performer can have a significant impact on motor skill learning. It is important to consider individual differences such as age, height, and weight. Furthermore, underlying impairments such as weakness or difficulties with motor control strategies, including poor advanced planning, must be identified. Such performer characteristics affect learning and how practice is structured. In addition, various methods specifically aimed at the learner or performer have been found to affect motor skill learning; these reinforcements include modeling, mental practice, and feedback.

Modeling

Modeling "refers to the process of reproducing actions that have been executed by another individual" (McCullagh et al, 1989, p 475). These demonstrations are powerful sources of information given before task performance. Studies indicate that the learner readily adopts the demonstrated strategies for use to perform a motor skill, whether effective or ineffective (Martens et al, 1976; McCullagh, 1987).

The type of model used has been found to influence motivation and therefore subsequent learning. Although mastery or expert models provide important strategies for the learner, a less-skilled demonstration can provide more information on error detection and correction made by the model. Coaches, therapists, and educators are often considered *expert* models, whereas older siblings or individuals with higher, yet imperfect, skill may be thought of as *coping* models. *Peer* models are those who have similar characteristics. For example, for a poststroke older adult, a peer model might be another person close to his age who has also had a stroke. Schunk and colleagues (1987) examined the effect of peer mastery and coping models among children learning mathematical skills and found a peer coping model to be an effective motivational tool. Another study examined the acquisition of swimming skills in children (mean age of 6.2 years) identified as fearful of the water using a peer mastery or coping model (Weiss et al, 1998). The authors found that peer modeling (mastery or coping) combined with swimming lessons affected behavior more than did swimming lessons alone (i.e., without a model). Peer versus adult models have also been found to be most effective in promoting early gross motor skill acquisition (Little and McCullagh, 1989).

Modeling can be used to augment therapeutic intervention for children, older adults, and persons with musculoskeletal or neurological impairments. It can take place within small group-related tasks, thereby fostering interaction among peer groups, which also allows greater opportunity for demonstrations by coping models. As skill improves, the mastery or expert model may help the learner focus on key strategies that may lead to greater success.

Mental Practice

Mental practice involves cognitive rehearsal and visualization of an action in the absence of overt movement (Magill, 1993). Due to its effect on the psychomotor aspects of motor skill learning, it is similar in many respects to actual physical practice of the task. Evidence supports the notion that neural processes involved in imagining movements are very similar to those required for its performance (Jeannerod, 1994; Pascual-Leone et al, 1995; Roland et al, 1980; Roth 1996). Furthermore, magnetic resonance imaging studies have confirmed that in addition to the primary motor cortex being engaged during motor imagery, the supplementary motor area, premotor cortex, and parietal areas may also be activated (Roland et al, 1980; Roth, 1996; Stephan et al, 1995). In addition to neural findings, kinematics may improve, as exemplified by Yaguez and colleagues (1998) in their study of writing. Specifically, they found improvements in the movement synchrony and a shift in the peak velocity after mental practice of the writing task.

The ability to perform mental imagery may be task dependent. Certain types of tasks may be easier to mentally carry out than others. In one study, Porretta and Surburg (1995) randomly assigned a group of adolescents with mild mental retardation to strike a bat at a string when the last light on a runway was illuminated. In comparison to this group with physical practice only, a similar group was asked to imagine the task before physically practicing it. The imagery plus practice group performed with significantly less error and variability over a five-session period. Although the effectiveness of mental imagery and mental practice varies (Warner and McNeill, 1988), their application may prove beneficial in enhancing motor skills.

Feedback

Information given during task performance is known as *concurrent feedback*. Coaches, therapists, and educators often use concurrent feedback by altering sensory input, providing manual cues, or giving verbal information to facilitate specific movement patterns. Concurrent feedback has several purposes: to help guide the learner so she can feel the desired movement pattern, to enhance execution of a certain pattern of movement by encouraging activation of specific musculature, and to assist the individual in successfully accomplishing a goal. Similar to other types of augmented information, when concurrent feedback is used too frequently, it may actually impede learning because the learner may become dependent on it. Furthermore, the person providing the feedback becomes a part of the performer's environment. Thus, the performer still needs to learn how to move effectively when the feedback is removed.

Studies in healthy populations suggest that individuals retain skills more effectively when feedback is provided less frequently. This is not to say that no feedback should be provided. Coaches, therapists, and educators, however, must consider that individuals naturally become dependent on feedback when it is provided. The more frequently feedback is provided, the less capable the performer is at performing those skills without it. Wulf and Toole (1999) investigated learning in subjects engaging in a ski-simulation task. They found that subjects who had control over whether they used assistance (i.e., using a pole to support themselves) had better retention of the task than did individuals who had no influence over whether assistance was provided. Allowing the performer to have some control and decision-making influence over when and what type of assistance is provided during task practice may enhance learning.

Studer and Yeager (1994) discussed the concept of direct versus indirect verbal cueing in a clinical setting. They suggest that rather than providing direct cues, coaches, therapists, and educators should start by providing indirect cues to learners. They propose that integration of cognitive and motor skills is essential to enhance problem-solving capabilities and resultant independence. For example, with an older adult who is learning to get out of a wheelchair, a therapist may say, "Is there something you need to do before you stand up?" Similar information can also be provided in the form of manual cueing, in which the therapist might tap the brakes as a hint to lock the brakes or tap the performer's leg to cue him to produce a certain movement pattern. This type of cueing forces the learner to arrive at a solution, rather than simply having the therapist or a caregiver provide the answers.

Winstein and colleagues (1996) reported differences in the performance and learning of a partial weight-bearing task by healthy adults based on the type of feedback provided. Subjects who practiced the task while receiving concurrent feedback were more accurate as indicated by the lower percent of absolute error during practice sessions compared with those given terminal feedback after completion of the task (KR-1, KR-5) (Fig. 4–5). During retention, however, the concurrent feedback group was less accurate. This suggests that while during initial learning performance on the task improved, ultimately the concurrent feedback was detrimental to long-term learning. Furthermore, post-response feedback led to better learning as measured by retention. In essence, although direct cues or concurrent feedback can be useful in the early stages of learning, individuals may achieve greater success if given indirect cues and encouraged to solve problems independently.

Terminal Feedback

Information given after task performance is considered *terminal feedback* and typically can be categorized in two forms: knowledge of results and knowledge of performance (Table 4–3). *Knowledge of results* is information related to the outcome, whether successful or not, and typically is inherent in most tasks that we perform. We know whether we have been successful in picking up a cup or walking across the room. *Knowledge of performance* pertains to information received regarding execution of the task and typically relates to the type or quality of the movement. Although knowledge of results is useful at any time during the learning process, knowledge of performance should be used selectively. Individuals are involved in highly cognitive processing as they attempt to understand the demands of task during the early stages of learning. Providing detailed information of movement patterns at this stage can be confusing and may be detrimental to long-term learning. Whether using

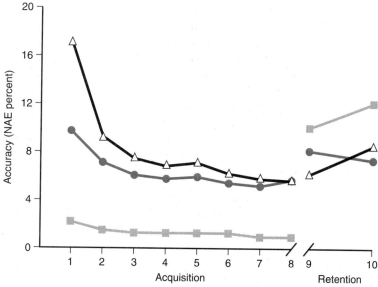

Figure 4–5

Effect of feedback on accuracy of performance. Subjects received either concurrent feedback (CF/■) or postresponse feedback (KR-1/● or KR-5/△) during training on a weight-bearing task. Data points represent group block means for normalized absolute error (NAE) percent. Performance was best during training when subjects received concurrent feedback. Postresponse feedback led to better learning as measured by retention. (Adapted Winstein C, Pohl PS, Cardinale C, et al. Learning a partial-weight-bearing skill: Effectiveness of two forms of feedback. *Phys Ther* 76:990, 1996.)

knowledge of results or knowledge of performance, the frequency at which feedback is provided is an important consideration. Therapists and coaches can provide intermittent feedback (less than 100% frequency), faded feedback (frequency is greater in early stages of learning), and summary feedback (feedback is summarized over several trials). These feedback schedules decrease a performer's reliance on external feedback and may untimately enhance learning of a motor skill (Winstein et al, 1994).

TABLE 4–3

Examples of Feedback Given After Task Performance

Knowledge of Results	Knowledge of Performance
Outcome of success or failure	Task execution
"You walked across the room!"	"You did not keep your elbow straight."
"That task took you 1 minute 30 seconds to complete."	"You are not bearing as much weight on your right side when you walk."
"You scored 5 points out of 8!"	"You were looking at your feet."

The key concepts related to providing concurrent or terminal feedback for any population include (1) use of feedback that is specific to the task and the performer's needs, (2) minimizing use of excessive feedback, and (3) encouragement of active problem solving that allows time to self-assess, rather than rely on feedback. An individual's ability to learn is limited not only by age and developmental level but also by the ability to solve motor problems. A learner with cognitive deficits can still demonstrate motor learning or learn to perform motor skills. The context or environment in which he can execute the task, however, may limit him, or he may be dependent to some degree on others for guidance or feedback.

Summary

Motor learning is a life-long process. The best indicators of skill learning are retention and transfer testing, yet the consistency, flexibility, and efficiency of select movements and behaviors clearly measure the depth of learning for a particular task. Because infants and children discover the capabilities of their bodies and how they can successfully interact with the environment, they display a great deal of motor skill variability. The movements of adolescents and adults become more consistent, efficient, and flexible as they refine and modify skills to fit the context. As they learn novel tasks, variability may again be evident. Older adults must often adjust to changes in their neuromuscular system, resulting again in greater movement variability. To adequately promote motor skills, we must be aware of the characteristics of the performer and how he interacts within particular tasks and environments.

Practice is strongly associated with skill acquisition. How practice is structured can have tremendous influence on the learning of particular motor skills. A low-skilled performer may require different practice conditions—before, during, and after performance—than does someone who is fine-tuning specific movement components as he perfects his ability. For example, although adults may learn best following a random order of practice, children or low-skilled performers may learn best following a blocked or mixed practice schedule. The effect of various practice schedules on motor skill acquisition is being examined more closely in various clinical populations and may affect service delivery in the future.

Research that examines current assumptions about how motor skills are controlled and learned may begin to validate the concepts put forth in this chapter. We hope that as research advances, our ability to extract information from the literature and apply it in education and clinical practice also increases.

ACKNOWLEDGMENTS

We would like to thank James Gordon, PT, EdD, Clare Bassile, PT, EdD, and Michael Majsak, PT, EdD, for their insight and thoughtful reviews of this manuscript. We would also like to extend our appreciation to Ann Gentile,

PhD, for sharing her expertise and views on motor learning with her students at Teachers College, Columbia University.

References

Acredolo L, Goodwyn S. *Baby Minds*. Toronto: Bantam Books, 2000.

Allard T, Clark SA, Jenkins WM, Merzenich MM. Reorganization of somatosensory area 3b representations in adult owl monkeys after digital syndactyly. *J Neurophysiol* 66:1048–1058, 1991.

Bach-y-Rita P. Brain plasticity as a basis for recovery of function in humans. *Neuropsychologia* 28: 547–554, 1990.

Bach-y-Rita P. *Nonsynaptic Diffusion Neurotransmission and Late Brain Reorganization*. New York: Demos, 1995.

Bach-y-Rita P, Illis LS. Spinal shock: Possible role of receptor plasticity and non-synaptic transmission. *Paraplegia* 31:82–87, 1993.

Bassile CC, Bock C. Gait Training. In Craik R, Oatis C (eds). *Gait Analysis*. Mosby: St. Louis, 1995, pp 420–435.

Battig WF. Facilitation and interference. In Bilodeau ED (ed). *Acquisition of Skill*. New York: Academic Press, 1966, pp 215–244.

Battig WF. The flexibility of human memory. In Cermak LS, Craik FIM (eds). *Levels of Processing in Human Memory*. Hillsdale, NJ: Erlbaum, 1979, pp 23–44.

Berman N, Sterling P. Cortical suppression of the ritino-collicular pathway in the monocularly deprived cat. *J Physiol* 255:263–273, 1976.

Bernstein N. *The Coordination and Regulation of Movements*. Oxford, UK: Pergamon, 1967.

Blanton S, Wolf S. An application of upper extremity constraint-induced movement therapy in a patient with subacute stroke. *Phys Ther* 79:847–853, 1999.

Bouisset S, Zattara M. Biomechanical study of the programming of anticipatory postural adjustments associated with voluntary movements. *J Biomech* 20:735–742, 1987.

Buell SJ, Coleman DP. Dendritic growth in aged human brain and failure of growth in senile dementia. *Science* 206:854–856, 1981.

Calford MB, Tweedale T. Immediate expansion of receptive fields of neurons in area 3b of macaque monkeys after digit denervation. *Somatosens Mot Res* 8:249–260, 1991.

Carr J, Shepherd R. *Neurological Rehabilitation: Optimizing Motor Performance*. Oxford: Butterworth Heinemann, 1998, pp 3–22.

Charles J, Lavinder G, Gordon AM. Effects of constraint-induced therapy on hand function in children with hemiplegic cerebral palsy. *Pediatr Phys Ther*, 13:68–76, 2001.

Classen J, Liepert J, Wise SP, et al. Rapid plasticity of human cortical movement representation induced by practice. *J Neurophysiol* 79:1117–1123, 1998.

Cordo P, Nashner L. Properties of postural adjustments associated with rapid arm movements. *J Neurophysiol* 47:287–302, 1982.

Corthout E, Uttl B, Walsh V, et al. Plasticity revealed by transcranial magnetic stimulation of early visual cortex. *Neuroreport* 11:1565–1569, 2000.

Corthout E, Uttl B, Ziemann U, et al. Two periods of processing in the (circum)striate visual cortex as revealed by transcranial magnetic stimulation. *Neuropsychologia* 37:137–145, 1999.

Cotman CW, Nieto-Sampedro M. Progress in facilitating the recovery of function after central nervous system trauma. *Ann N Y Acad Sci* 457:83–104, 1985.

Coulson RL, Klein M. Rapid development of synaptic connections and plasticity between sensory neurons and motor neurons of Aplysia in cell culture: Implications for learning and regulation of synaptic strength. *J Neurophysiol* 77:2316–2327, 1997.

Cruse H, Wischmeyer M, Bruwer P, et al. On the cost functions for the control of the human arm movement. *Biol Cybern* 62:519–528, 1990.

Dean CM, Shepherd RB. Task-related training improves performance of seated reaching tasks after stroke. *Stroke* 28:722–728, 1997.

Del Rey P, Whitehurst M, Wughalter E, Barnwell J. Contextual interference and experience in acquisition and transfer. *Percept Mot Skills* 57:241–242, 1983.

Edelman GM. Neural darwinism: Selection and reentrant signaling in higher brain function. *Neuron* 10:115–125, 1993.

Edwards JM, Elliot D, Lee TD. Contextual interference effects during skill acquisition and transfer in Down's Syndrome adolescents. *Adapt Phys Activity Q* 3:250–258, 1986.

Enoka RM. Neural adaptations with chronic physical activity. *Proceedings of XVth Congress of ISB.* Jyvaskyla, Finland, 1995, pp 20–21.

Fattapposta F, Amabile G, Cordischi MV, et al. Long-term practice effects on a new skilled motor learning: An electrophysiological study. *Electroencephalogr Clin Neurophysiol* 99:495–507, 1996.

Fitts PM. Categories of human learning. In Melton AW (ed). *Perceptual-Motor Skills Learning*. New York: Academic Press, 1964, pp 243–285.

Flash T, Hogan N. The coordination of arm movements: An experimentally confirmed mathematical model. *J Neurosci* 5:1688–1703, 1985.

Gentile AM. Implicit and explicit processes during acquisition of functional skills. *Scand J Occup Ther* 5:7–16, 1998.

Gentile AM. Skill acquisition: Action, movement, and neuromotor processes. In Carr JA, Shepherd RB (eds). *Movement Science: Foundations for Physical Therapy in Rehabilitation*. Rockville, MD: Aspen Publishers, Inc, 1987, pp 93–154.

Gentile AM. Skill acquisition: Action, movement, and neuromotor processes. In Carr JA, Shephard RB (eds). *Movement Science: Foundations for Physical Therapy in Rehabilitation*, 2nd ed. Rockville, MD: Aspen Publishers, Inc, 2000, pp 111–187.

Ghez C, Gordon J, Ghilardi MF, et al. Roles of proprioceptive input in the programming of arm trajectories. *Cold Spring Harbor Symp Quant Biol* 55:837–847, 1990.

Gibson JJ. *The Ecological Approach to Visual Perception*. Boston: Houghton Mifflin, 1979.

Gibson EJ, Riccio G, Schmuckler MA, et al. Detection of the transversability of surfaces by crawling and walking infants. *J Exp Psycho Hum Percept Perform.* 13:533–544, 1987.

Goldman S, Plum F. Compensatory regeneration of the damaged adult human brain neuroplasticity in a clinical perspective. *Adv Neurol* 73:99–107, 1997.

Gordon J. Assumptions underlying physical therapy intervention. In Carr JA, Shephard RB (eds). *Movement Science: Foundations for Physical Therapy in Rehabilitation*. Rockville, MD: Aspen Publishers, Inc, 1987, pp 1–30.

Gordon J. Current status of the motor program—invited commentary. *Phys Ther* 74:748–751, 1994.

Guiliani CA. Strength training in neurologic patients. *Neurol Rep* 1994.

Hallet M. Transcranial magnetic stimulation and the human brain. *Nature* 406:147–150, 2000.

Hanlon RE. Motor learning following unilateral stroke. *Arch Phys Med Rehabil* 77:811–815, 1996.

Held JM, Gordon J, Gentile AM. Environmental influences on locomotor recovery following cortical lesions in rats. *Behav Neurosci* 99:678–690, 1985.

Herbert EP, Landin D, Solmon MA. Practice schedule effects on the performance and learning of low-and high-skilled students: An applied study. *Res Q Exerc Sport* 67:52–58, 1996.

Hesse S, Bertelt C, Jahnke T, et al. Treadmill training with partial body weight support compared with physiotherapy in nonambulatory hemiparetic patients. *Stroke* 26:976–981, 1995.

Hesse S, Bertelt C, Schaffrin A, et al. Restoration of gait in nonambulatory hemiparetic patients by treadmill training with partial body-weight support. *Arch Phys Med Rehabil* 75:1087–1093, 1994.

Higgins S. Motor skill acquisition. *Phys Ther* 71:123–139, 1991.

Horak B. Assumptions underlying motor control for neurologic rehabilitation. In Lister M (ed). *Contemporary Management of Motor Control Problems: Proceedings of the II STEP Conference*. Alexandria, VA: Foundation for Physical Therapy, 1991.

Horak FB, Diener HC, Nashner LM. Influence of central set on human postural responses. *J Neurophysiol* 62:841–853, 1989.

James W. Habit. 1890. Reprinted in Shoben EJ, Ruch F (eds). *Perspectives in Psychology*. Fairlawn, NJ: Scott, Foresman & Co, 1963.

Jarus T, Goverover Y. Effects of contextual interference and age on acquisition, retention, and transfer of motor skill. *Percept Mot Skills* 88:437–447, 1999.

Jeannerod M. The representing brain: Neural correlates of motor intention and imagery. *Behav Brain Sci* 17:187–245, 1994.

Jenkins WM, Merzenich MM, Recanzone G. Neocortical representational dynamics in adult primates. *Neuropsychologia* 28:573–584, 1990.

Johansson RS. Sensory control of dexterous manipulation in humans. In Wing AM, Haggard P, Flanagan J (eds). *Hand and Brain: The Neurophysiology and Psychology of Hand Movements*. New York: Academic Press, 1996, pp 381–414.

Jones EG. Cortical and subcortical contributions to activity dependent plasticity in primate somato sensory cortex. *Annu Rev Neurosci* 23:1–37, 2000.

Konczak J, Dichgans J. The development toward stereotypic arm kinematics during reaching in the first 3 years of life. *Exp Brain Res* 117:346–354, 1997.

Kuhn TS. *The Structure of Scientific Revolutions,* 2nd ed. Chicago: University of Chicago Press, 1970.

Law S-H, Gentile AM, Bassile CC. Gait adaptations of children and adults while stepping over an obstacles. *Soc Neurosci Abstr* 22:2038, 1996.

Lebeer J. How much brain does a mind need? Scientific, clinical, and educational implications of ecological plasticity. *Dev Med Child Neurol* 40:352–357, 1998.

Lee TD, Magill RA. The locus of contextual interference in motor-skill acquisition. *J Exp Psychol Learning Memory Cogn* 9:730–746, 1983.

Liepert J, Bauder H, Wolfgang HR, et al. Treatment-induced cortical reorganization after stroke in humans. *Stroke* 31:1210–1216, 2000.

Light KE, Spirduso WW. Effects of adult aging on the movement complexity factor of response programming. *J Gerontol* 45:107–109, 1990.

Little WS, McCullagh P. Motivation orientation and modeled instruction strategies: The effects on form and accuracy. *J Sport Exerc Psychol* 11:41–53, 1989.

Magill RA. *Motor Learning: Concepts and Applications*, 4th ed. Madison, WI: Brown and Benchmark, 1993.

Magill RA, Hall KG. A review of the contextual interference effect in motor skill acquisition. *Hum Move Sci* 9:241–289, 1990.

Malouin F, Potvin M, Prevost J, et al. Use of intensive task-oriented gait training program in a series of patients with acute cerebrovascular accidents. *Phys Ther* 72:781–793, 1992.

Martens R, Burwitz L, Zuckerman J. Modeling effects on motor performance. *Res Q* 47:277–191, 1976.

McCullagh P. Model similarity effects on motor performance. *J Sports Psychol* 9:249–260, 1987.

McCullagh P, Weiss MR, Ross D. Modeling considerations in motor skill acquisition and performance: An integrated approach. *Exerc Sport Sci Rev* 17:475–513, 1989.

McDonald PV, Vanemmerik REA, Newell KM. Effect of task constraints on limb kinematics in a throwing task. *J Mot Behav* 21:245–264, 1989.

Merzenich MM, Sameshima K. Cortical plasticity and memory. *Curr Opin Neurobiol* 3:187–196, 1993.

Mogiler A, Grossman JA, Ribary U, et al. Somatosensory cortical plasticity in adult humans revealed by magnetoencephalography. *Proc Natl Acad Sci USA* 90:3593–3597, 1993.

Moore SP, Marteniuk RG. Kinematic and electromyographic changes that occur as a function of learning a time-constrained aiming task. *J Mot Behav* 4:397–426, 1986.

Morris ME, Summers JJ, Matyas TA, Iansek R. Current status of the motor program. *Phys Ther* 74: 738–748, 1994.

Nashner LM. Fixed patterns of rapid postural responses among leg muscles during stance. *Exp Brain Res* 30:13–24, 1977.

Nelson WL. Physical principles for economics of skilled movements. *Biol Cybern* 46:135–147, 1983.

Newell KM. Motor skill acquisition. *Annu Rev Psychol* 42:213–237, 1991.

Nowakowski RS. Basic concepts of CNS development. In Johnson MH. (ed). *Brain Development and Cognition*. Cambridge, MA: Blackwell, 1993, pp 54–92.

Nudo RJ, Milliken GW, Jenkins WM, Merzenich MM. Use-dependent alterations of movement representations in primary motor cortex of adult squirrel monkeys. *J Neurosci* 16:785–807, 1996.

Ogden R, Franz SI. On cerebral motor control: The recovery from experimentally produced hemiplegia. *Psychobiology* 1:33–50, 1917.

Pascual-Leone A, Nguyet D, Cohen LG, et al. Modulation of muscle responses evoked by transcranial magnetic stimulation during the acquisition of new fine motor skills. *J Neurophysiol* 74: 1037–1045, 1995.

Pascual-Leone A, Torres F. Plasticity of the sensorimotor cortex representation of the reading finger in Braille readers. *Brain* 116:39–52, 1993.

Patla AE. A framework for understanding mobility problems in the elderly. In Craik RL, Oatis CA (eds). *Gait Analysis: Theory and Application.* St. Louis: Mosby, 1995, pp 436–449.

Peterson C, Maier S, Seligman M. *Learned Helplessness: A Theory for the Age of Personal Control.* New York City, NY: Oxford University Press, Inc, 1995.

Pigott RE, Shapiro DC. Motor schema: The structure of the variability session. *Res Q Exerc Sport* 61: 169–177, 1984.

Pinto-Zipp G, Gentile AM. Practice schedules in motor learning: Children vs. adults. *Soc Neurosci Abstr* 21:1620, 1995.

Pollock BJ, Lee TD. Dissociated contextual interference in children and adults. *Percept Mot Skills* 84: 851–858, 1997.

Pons TP, Garraghty PE, Ommaya AK, et al. Massive cortical reorganization after sensory deafferentation in adult macaques. *Science* 252:1857–1860, 1991.

Porretta DL, Surburg PR. Imagery and physical practice in the acquisition of gross motor timing of coincidence by adolescents with mild mental retardation. *Percept Mot Skills* 80:1171–1183, 1995.

Recanzone GH, Merzenich MM, Jenkins WM, et al. Topographic reorganization of the hand representation in cortical area 3b owl monkeys trained in a frequency-discrimination task. *J Neurophysiol* 67:1031–1056, 1992.

Ramachandran VS, Rogers-Ramachandran D, Stewart M. Perceptual correlates of massive cortical reorganization. *Science* 258:1159–1160, 1992.

Richards CL, Malouin F, Wood-Dauphinee S, et al. Task-specific physical therapy for optimization of gait recovery in acute stroke patients. *Arch Phys Med Rehabil* 74:612–619, 1993.

Roland PE, Larsen B, Lassen NA, Skinhoj E. Supplementary motor area and other cortical areas in organization of voluntary movements in man. *J Neurophysiol* 43:118–136, 1980.

Roth M, Decety J, Raybaudi M, et al. Possible involvement of primary motor cortex in mentally simulated movement: A functional magnetic resonance imaging study. *Neuroreport* 7:1280–1284, 1996.

Rosenzweig MR, Bennet EL. Diamond M. Effects of differential experience on dendritic spine counts in rat cerebral cortex. *J Comp Physiol Psychol* 82:175–181, 1973.

Schmidt R. *Motor Control and Learning.* Champaign, IL: Human Kinetics Publishers, 1988.

Schunk DH, Hanson AR, Cox CD. Peer model attributes and children's achievement behaviors. *J Educ Psychol* 79:54–61, 1987.

Segar CA. Implicit learning. *Psychol Bull* 115:163–196, 1994.

Sherrington CS. *The Integrative Action of the Nervous System.* New York: Cambridge University Press, 1906.

Shea JB, Morgan RL. Contextual interference effects on the acquisition, retention, and transfer of a motor skill. *J Exp Psychol* 5:179–187, 1979.

Shumway-Cook A, Woollacott M. The growth of stability: Postural control from a developmental perspective. *J Mot Behav* 17:131–147, 1985.

Shumway-Cook A, Woollacott M. *Motor Control: Theory and Practical Applications,* 2nd ed. Baltimore, MD: Williams & Wilkins, 2001.

Spencer JP, Thelen E. A multimuscle state analysis of adult motor learning. *Exp Brain Res* 128:505–516, 1997.

Sporns O, Edelman GM. Solving Bernstein's problem: A proposal for the development of coordinated movement by selection. *Child Dev* 64:960–981, 1993.

Stephan KM, Fink GR, Passingham RE, et al. Functional anatomy of the mental representation of upper extremity movements in healthy subjects. *J Neurophysiol* 73:373–386, 1995.

Studer M, Yeager KK. The cognitive and the motor: Inseparable. A transdisciplinary approach. *PT Magazine* June:52–56, 1994.

Sullivan KJ. Functionally distinct learning systems of the brain: Implications for brain injury rehabilitation. *Neurology Report* 22:126–131, 1998.

Taub E. Somatosensory deafferentation research with monkeys: Implications for rehabilitation medicine. In Ince LP (ed). *Behavioral Psychology in Rehabilitation Medicine: Clinical Implications.* Baltimore, MD: Williams & Wilkins, 1980, pp 371–401.

Taub E, Miller NE, Novack TA, et al. Technique to improve chronic motor deficit after stroke. *Arch Phys Med Rehabil* 74:347–354, 1993.

Taub E, Wolf SL. Constraint-induction/forced use techniques to facilitate upper extremity use in stroke patients. *Top Stroke Rehabil* 3:38–61, 1997.

Thelen E. Motor development: A new synthesis. *Am Psychol* 50:79–95, 1995.

Thelen E, Ulrich BD. Hidden skills: A dynamic systems analysis of treadmill stepping during the first year. *Monogr Soc Res Child Dev* 56:1–98, 1991.

Van Thiel E, Meulenbroek RG, Hulstijn W, Steenbergen B. Kinematics of fast hemiparetic aiming movements toward stationary and moving targets. *Exp Brain Res* 132:230–242, 2000.

Vereijken B, van Emmerik REA, Whiting HTA, Newell KM. Free(z)ing degrees of freedom in skill acquisition. *J Motor Behav* 24:133–142, 1992.

Wainer BH, Kwon J, Eves EM, et al. Neural plasticity as studied in neuronal cell lines. *Adv Neurol* 72:133–142, 1997.

Walsh RN. Effects of environmental complexity and deprivation on brain anatomy and histology: A review. *Int J Neurosci* 12:33–51, 1981.

Warner L, McNeil ME. Mental imagery and its potential for physical therapy. *Phys Ther* 68:516–521, 1988.

Weiss MR, McCullagh P, Smith AL, Berlant AR. Observational learning and the fearful child: Influence of peer models on swimming skill performance and psychological responses. *Res Q Exerc Sport* 69:380–394, 1998.

Weiss PH, Jeannerod M, Paulignan Y, Freund H. Is the organization of goal-directed action modality specific? *Neuropsychologia* 38:1136–1147, 2000.

Wing AM, Haggard P, Flanagan J. *Hand and Brain: The Neurophysiology and Psychology of Hand Movements.* New York: Academic Press, 1996.

Winstein CJ, Gardner ER, McNeal DR, et al. Standing balance training: Effect on balance and locomotion in hemiparetic adults. *Arch Phys Med Rehabil* 70:755–762, 1989.

Winstein CJ, Merians AS, Sullivan KJ. Motor learning after unilateral brain damage. *Neuropsychologia* 37:975–987, 1999.

Winstein CJ, Pohl PS, Cardinale C, et al. Learning a partial-weight-bearing skill: Effectiveness of two forms of feedback. *Phys Ther* 76:985–993, 1996.

Winstein CJ, Pohl PS, Lewthwaite R. Effects of physical guidance and knowledge of results on motor learning: Support for the guidance hypothesis. *Res Q Exerc Sport* 65(4):316–323, 1994.

Wolpert DM, Ghahramani Z, Jordan MI. Are arm trajectories planned in kinematic or dynamic coordinates? An adaptation study. *Exp Brain Res* 103:460–470, 1995.

Wulf G, Toole T. Physical assistance devices in complex motor skill learning: Benefits of a self-controlled practice schedule. *Res Q Exerc Sport* 70:265–272, 1999.

Yaguez L, Nagel D, Hoffman H, et al. A mental route to motor learning: Improving trajectorial kinematics through imagery training. *Behav Brain Res* 90:95–106, 1998.

5 Evaluation of Function

OBJECTIVES

After reading this chapter, the reader will be able to:

1 Discuss the importance of evaluating a client's functional performance.

2 Identify well-developed, standardized functional assessment instruments.

3 Discuss reliability and validity issues of functional assessment measurement tools.

4 Compare and contrast commonly used functional assessment instruments.

As discussed in Chapter 1, our success at meeting the challenges of everyday life reflects our functional independence. Is a small child capable of shopping for groceries, cooking, and managing finances? What about the older adult? Can an adult successfully balance the demands of work, home, family, and self? The answer to the first question is, of course, no. Within our society, we care for children until they are capable of these activities. Children do, however, develop skills in mobility, dressing, and hygiene that allow them some degree of functional independence. We hope that the answer to the latter two questions is yes. Adults and older adults want to live their lives as successfully and independently as possible. Occasionally, illness or injury may limit our ability to physically function as independently as we would wish. At this point, we may turn to the health care community for support and assistance in regaining a self-sufficient lifestyle.

The primary task of health care professionals is to improve the health and functional independence of the client. In medical, surgical, psychosocial, and rehabilitation intervention, professionals strive to maintain or restore function. Health professionals in these areas of intervention hope to improve a person's functional capacity (Liang and Jette, 1981).

For the physical or occupational therapist, the focus of intervention is on physical functioning. The area of physical function includes a person's ability to move through the environment, perform self-care activities, successfully complete job tasks, and enjoy recreational pursuits (Guccione, 2000). How well can the client move from place to place? Is she able to successfully perform the tasks related to a profession or job? Can she take care of basic daily tasks such as bathing, dressing, and eating? How about more difficult tasks, such as shopping, taking a bus, or cleaning the house? Can the client enjoy leisure and recreational activities? By focusing intervention at these areas, the physical and occupational therapist can improve a client's ability to live as independently as possible and can improve her quality of life.

For health care professionals to best serve their clients, they must be able to clearly, efficiently, and reliably identify what activities are meaningful and necessary to them. They must then determine at what level they are able to perform these important everyday tasks. Functional evaluation can be used to identify a client's strengths and needs, develop appropriate treatment plans, and evaluate the effectiveness of that treatment over time.

To evaluate a client's function, the therapist must observe the performance of functional activities as well as consider the underlying impairments. Range of motion or muscle strength offers some degree of quantitative information that can be used to document a need for services or how well the client has progressed in treatment. But do these measures in and of themselves reflect how the client is functioning? If it is demonstrated that someone's range of motion in shoulder flexion has improved 5 degrees, progress has been made in range of motion, but it is unclear whether that 5 degrees makes the difference in being able to put on a shirt or reach into the kitchen cabinets. To measure the success of intervention in these functional tasks, assessment must focus on function. Goniometry and muscle strength testing do not provide information on how function has changed. Instead, they may provide information on impairments, which ultimately affect function.

Comprehensive evaluation of function allows health care providers to develop meaningful treatment programs that will improve the quality of life for their clients (Haley et al, 1991). When appropriate assessment instruments are used as a basis for intervention, therapists can measure success in achieving the primary goal of therapy—improvement of the functional independence of their clients.

Characteristics

An evaluation of functional performance can take many different forms and be implemented in many ways. We bring a unique set of functional tasks to our day, based on self-care, work, and leisure activities. All of these activities relate to how well we can complete the necessary tasks of everyday life and should be included when function is evaluated. Self-care activities such as dressing, washing, eating, and ambulating are referred to as *basic activities of daily living* (BADL). More advanced activities that allow us to live independently in our communities, such as shopping, using transportation, cooking, and cleaning, are referred to as *instrumental activities of daily living* (IADL). Functional assessment needs to look at both of these categories of activities, as well as at abilities in job-related tasks and recreation. By addressing all areas of our life, the evaluation reflects important aspects of how successfully we can independently care for ourselves.

In evaluating function, the health care provider must be sure that the entire spectrum of activities performed during the client's day is represented.

The evaluation must address issues related to emotional, social, and environmental issues, not just physical functioning. How does a person interact with the environment? Can he easily commute to the workplace or get to the grocery store when necessary? Is it easy to move from place to place within the home regardless of whether the floor is carpeted or tiled? It must be clear that the goal of the assessment is to identify how the individual is functioning in everyday life, not to document the issues specific to such medical problems such as weakness, depression, or confusion. It is important to understand how the client reacts to his medical problems and how medical issues interfere with successfully meeting the demands of daily life. All in all, a functional assessment must try to assess an individual's maximal functional potential, encompassing all domains of function.

STANDARDIZED VERSUS NONSTANDARDIZED FORMAT

Functional evaluations can include standardized or nonstandardized formats. *Standardized* assessment uses a formal functional assessment tool; the assessment is administered in the same way to everyone, every time it is used. The items included in a standardized assessment are carefully selected and very clearly defined. *Nonstandardized* evaluation is more informal and includes a review of activities the evaluator considers important for an individual client.

Whenever a therapist works with a client and evaluates how well that person can get out of bed, walk to the bathroom, or get dressed, the therapist is evaluating function. When using this nonstandardized format, it is difficult to ensure that the evaluation is complete. Have all of the important aspects of the client's daily routine been included, or just the activities important to the therapist? When it is time to reevaluate, can the initial evaluation be replicated? If not, how can the therapist accurately note client progress? Use of nonstandardized evaluation makes it difficult to effectively communicate client status among health care professionals or to compare the functional status of clients with similar disabilities. Standardized assessment procedures can effectively minimize some of these problems. When standardized functional assessment instruments are developed, care is taken to include information on all tasks that are important in defining a client's functional status. Data obtained from the assessment are easy to communicate to other professionals familiar with the assessment instrument. Because standardized assessments are performed in the same way on repeated assessments, it is also easier to report on client change.

Comprehensive functional evaluation should contain both standardized and nonstandardized components. The use of a formal standardized assessment provides the therapist with a body of reliable, valid information for all clients. Alone, this assessment strategy may not represent all activities that the client feels are important and meaningful in her everyday life. By also including a more individualized, nonstandardized component within the functional evaluation, the therapist identifies important information unique to the client (Guccione, 2000).

CONSIDERATION IN SELECTING STANDARDIZED FUNCTIONAL ASSESSMENTS

Focus

Several standardized functional assessment instruments are available today. As clinicians, we must choose an instrument that best meets the needs of each individual client. For some clients, disease-specific factors may interfere with function, such as the pain of arthritis. Young children certainly participate in a different set of functional activities than do adults. Other individuals may perform functional tasks quite well only when using an assistive device or may require the assistance of a caregiver. We need to consider all of these issues when selecting a functional assessment instrument.

Many of the formal functional assessment instruments in use were developed to meet the needs of specific client populations. For example, the Arthritis Impact Measurement Scale (AIMS) was developed to assess the status of adults with rheumatoid arthritis and includes items related to ability to complete functional tasks as well as information on pain (Meenan et al, 1980). As originally developed, it is not optimal for use with children, older adults, or individuals with other medical problems. A functional assessment tool for children with juvenile rheumatoid arthritis is the Juvenile Arthritis Functional Assessment Scale (Lovell et al, 1989). The GERI-AIMS (an adaptation of the AIMS) was designed for use with older individuals with osteoarthritis or rheumatoid arthritis. It also assesses functional impairments related to other common medical problems of older adults, independent of the arthritis-specific functional impairment (Hughes et al, 1991). Other types of instruments are available for individuals who demonstrate neurological involvement. The Gross Motor Function measure was developed specifically for use with children with cerebral palsy (Russell et al, 1989). General functional assessments, such as the Functional Status Index, consider a wide variety of BADL and IADL (Table 5–1) and are useful for clients with chronic disabilities.

Care must be taken to choose the appropriate assessment instrument. Instruments that are developed for specific client populations can specifically focus on issues particular to a disease process that limits function, such as the pain of the arthritic client. These instruments, however, are not necessarily appropriate for use with other client populations, because they may not be sensitive enough to other problem areas of his performance. Also, instruments developed for use with a specific age group may not address issues important for older or younger individuals. In general, functional assessment instruments may not be valid for use in client populations other than those for which they were developed.

Design

Once we, as clinicians, decide which assessment instrument best assesses a specific client's functional skills and limitations, we must also decide which type of assessment can best be used with the client. The three basic types of functional assessment designs are interview assessments, self-administered assessments, and performance-based assessments (Guccione, 2000).

TABLE 5–1

Categories of the Functional Status Index

Gross mobility	Personal care
• Walking inside	• Washing all parts of your body
• Stair climbing	• Putting on pants
• Chair transfers	• Putting on a shirt
Hand activities	• Buttoning a shirt
• Opening containers	**Home chores**
• Writing	• Doing laundry
• Dialing a telephone	• Reaching into a low cupboard
Interpersonal activities	• Doing yardwork
• Driving a car	• Vacuuming a rug
• Visiting family or friends	
• Attending meetings	
• Performing your job	

From Jette AM. Functional Status Index: Reliability of a chronic disease evaluation instrument. *Arch Phys Med Rehabil* 61:395–401, 1980.

The *interview assessment* is completed by a trained interviewer who asks the client a set of standard questions and records the answers in a standardized format. The information gleaned from this type of assessment is most useful when the interviewer has had training in how to administer and score the assessment. It is important that the interviewer not expand on questions or prompt answers to avoid influencing the client.

Self-administered assessments are generally presented as questionnaires. The directions for completion of the questionnaire and questions themselves must be clearly written, so that the client can understand what is being asked. It is also important to ensure that the way questions are asked or focused does not bias the answers. The accuracy of these types of assessments depends on the quality of the instrument itself and the person's ability to complete the questionnaire.

Both interview and self-administered assessments are based on a client's self-report of his functional status. Studies that compare the validity of self-report with direct observation assessments have shown that agreement between the client's report and the direct observation is good to excellent in BADL. Research has shown that skill in IADL was slightly underreported in client self-reports (Harris et al, 1986). The validity of self-report measures makes them attractive for use in health care settings, especially because they are easy and relatively inexpensive to administer.

Performance-based assessments are those in which an evaluator observes the client's performance in functional tasks. This type of assessment does report someone's ability to complete BADL but is not as easily applied to the evaluation of IADL. Because the assessment is completed in a structured test environment, performance in the home environment may not be reflected. Direct observation assessment is also time consuming and therefore an expensive process. The type of information gathered from this type of assessment may be most useful for developing and evaluating the success of therapeutic intervention programs.

Rating Performance

Functional assessments vary in how they rate an individual's performance. In the simplest rating format, a skill is noted as being present or absent, thereby documenting whether something can be done. Checklist-type assessments favor this type of rating format but do not address the quality of that performance. It cannot be determined whether the skill is accomplished efficiently, consistently, or to the degree necessary for functional independence within a wide variety of environments. For example, if the client can walk 20 to 30 feet with a cane and ascend the stairs in the therapy department, he would certainly pass a checklist assessment that includes these tasks. What happens if the individual then goes home and encounters thick, plush carpeting or a steeper flight of stairs with higher steps than those in the therapy department? His ability to get into his apartment and to walk from room to room may be very different from the performance seen in the therapy department. From another perspective, if while an individual walks with a cane the other arm becomes stiff and the hand clenches, the quality of ambulation may not be sufficient for her to perform daily tasks such as carrying a plate to the table or bringing in the newspaper.

Another type of rating system uses a visual analog scale. A client is asked to rate her performance on a linear scale, on which one end of the line reflects one extreme and the other end the other extreme of performance. She responds by placing a mark on the line at the point she feels best represents her performance. This system allows her to express a level of skill in a functional task at some point between being fully dependent and fully independent. An example of this type of scale is given in Figure 5–1.

Other scales use a summative rating system, in which different items are weighted so that independent completion of all tasks represented in the assessment results in a total score of 100. In the development of this type of scale, weighting of items is generally based on professional judgment. Therefore, this scale reflects the developer's values about the importance of different functional skills, not necessarily how important certain skills are to a client's life. The performance of each task is evaluated and scored to reflect total or partial

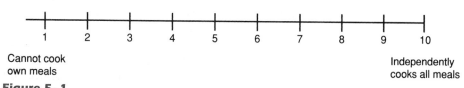

Figure 5–1

Linear rating scale for ability to prepare meals.

completion of the task independently. Scores for all tasks are added and compared with a perfect total score of 100. A score of 100 does not necessarily reflect normal performance, just as a score of 85 does not mean that someone is functioning within 15% of normal. Another confusing aspect of summative scale formats is that scores can be compared mathematically. When an individual achieves a score of 10 on the initial assessment and a score of 50 on a subsequent assessment, it is not necessarily true that he is performing five times better than initially. We must remember that the score can be compared only within the context of the assessment instrument. This type of rating scale is good for measuring whether change has occurred over time or with intervention.

Another approach to rating performance is to rate the quality of performance of a skill. This approach is especially useful when using performance-based assessment strategies. For instance, it is possible to measure the efficiency with which a task is performed by measuring a person's heart rate before and after an activity. An evaluator can also use time tests to see how long it takes someone to walk 30 feet. This is important information when assessing a client's ability to efficiently cross a street or to get from one high school class to another.

When choosing an assessment instrument, a therapist must consider all of the factors we discussed. For what client population is the assessment appropriate? What type of assessment best and most accurately measures a person's functional skills? How does the assessment rate the performance? What type of assessment and rating system provides the best information to identify clients who require services, to develop treatment plans, or to assess the effectiveness of intervention? Even after answering all of these questions, the therapist must consider additional aspects of assessment instruments that contribute to their effectiveness as measurement tools and affect the interpretation of the data they provide. These aspects include the reliability and validity of the instrument.

MEASUREMENT ISSUES FOR STANDARDIZED INSTRUMENTS

Several characteristics of assessment instruments affect their ability to accurately measure functional skills. Well-developed assessment strategies incorporate the principles of measurement science into their format. Measurement science involves the use of specific rules to evaluate a situation. By adhering to rules in the evaluation process, several important properties of measurement science are supported, including (1) reliability, (2) validity, (3) responsiveness, and (4) precision. Information regarding the reliability and validity of published functional assessments should be reported in assessment manuals or research reports. The health care professional should use the reported information to determine whether the tool has been proved to be reliable and valid.

Reliability refers to the ability of the test instrument to report findings in a consistent and repeatable fashion. The assessment should yield very similar results when administered to the same client by two different therapists (*inter-*

rater reliability) or when administered by the same therapist on two separate occasions within a short time frame *(intrarater reliability)*. Consistency between two administrations of the same test within a short period is also called *test-retest reliability.*

Validity implies that the assessment is achieving its intended function and truly measuring what it is supposed to measure. Four issues have been identified that may diminish the validity of functional assessment instruments (Kaufert, 1983):

1. Effect of the use of aids, adaptations, or helpers to achieve a functional task
2. Situational variation (i.e., between home and hospital settings) and individual motivation
3. Professional perspective of the rater
4. Role expectations of the client

For example, an individual may not be able to walk independently to the bathroom unless she uses a cane. If the assessment does not allow this person to use an assistive device, she will be rated inaccurately as unable to perform a basic functional task. On the other hand, someone who can independently use the bathroom in the hospital that is furnished with grab bars or an elevated toilet seat may not be as independent in his home environment without similar environmental modifications. Motivation also plays a role. If someone feels good about the prospect of going home or living independently, he may perform much differently than another individual who is depressed about the need to live in a long-term care facility. With regard to role expectation, if an assessment measures an individual's ability to cook or clean and this is not part of that person's social responsibility, he is not as likely to perform independently in these tasks. The professional perspective of the rater is another issue that affects validity. If the rater is a physical therapist, his impressions of functional independence in certain tasks may be very different from the impressions of a social worker.

Precision and specificity of an instrument are also considerations if therapists anticipate that the use of a standardized functional assessment will allow them to document changes in a client's status over time, as a result of either therapy or progression of disease or secondary to development. *Precision* refers to the ability to detect appropriate levels of change (Liang and Jette, 1981). For example, consider the client with poor endurance who has a spinal cord injury and must learn to walk with bilateral lower extremity orthotics and crutches. If an assessment tool contains only one item to assess walking that requires the client to walk 50 yards independently, this client will not be able to pass the item for a very long time. A more precise test for this client may have several items related to the ability to walk (i.e., for 10 feet, 10 yards, 25 yards, and so on). *Responsiveness* to change refers to a test's ability to measure an aspect of performance that is anticipated to change as a result of therapy. For example, consider a client who has had an injury that makes it impossible to use his right hand in functional activities. In therapy, you are working with the client to help him learn to use his left hand to feed himself and to write. A responsive assessment tool will measure his ability to perform these activities with his left hand. An unresponsive tool will measure the return of function of the right hand.

Survey of Measurement Instruments

In this section, we review a sample of standardized functional assessment instruments; only a small number of the assessments tools available to clinicians are discussed. These specific instruments were chosen because they are assessment instruments appropriate for individuals of different ages or because they are commonly used in clinical practice.

PEDIATRIC FUNCTIONAL ASSESSMENT INSTRUMENTS

Pediatric Evaluation of Disability Index

The Pediatric Evaluation of Disability Index (PEDI) assesses the capability and performance of functional skills by children between the ages of 6 months and 7.5 years in the areas of self-care, mobility, and social function (Table 5–2). The index is meant to be used to detect functional deficits of individual

TABLE 5–2

Types of Activities Assessed in Pediatric Evaluation of Disability Index

Self-care
- Eating—types of food, use of utensils, use of drinking containers
- Hygiene—toothbrushing, hair brushing, nose care, hand washing
- Dressing—pullovers, fasteners, pants, shoes/socks
- Toileting tasks

Mobility
- Transfers—toilet, tub, chair, car, bed
- Indoor locomotion
- Outdoor locomotion
- Stairs

Social function
- Comprehension of language
- Functional use of communication
- Problem resolution
- Peer interaction
- Play
- Orientation to self, time
- Household chores
- Function in community

children with disabilities, to monitor the child's progress in rehabilitation, and to assist in program evaluation. The PEDI can be administered in a structured interview format with the child's parents (which is reported to take 45 to 60 minutes) or by recording the judgment of therapists and teachers about the child's abilities (which is reported to take 20 to 30 minutes). Three different aspects of the child's functional performance are assessed: (1) the child's functional skill level, (2) the need for modification or adaptive equipment to achieve the task, and (3) the amount of physical assistance the child requires (Feldman et al, 1990; Haley et al, 1992).

The PEDI was used to assess 412 nondisabled children from New England. This normative sample represented all age groups for whom the test is appropriate and attempted to reflect demographics of the U.S. Census in 1980 (Haley et al, 1992). Results from this study have provided some information on the development of functional skills in children and permit comparisons between children with and without disabilities. The normative scores also allow the nominal data recorded in the PEDI to be converted to ratio scales that reflect item difficulty.

Good reliability and validity of the PEDI have been demonstrated. High internal consistency has been reported. Using a structured interview administration format, researchers have documented good interrater reliability. Nichols and Case-Smith (1996) suggested that reliability is increased when both the parents and primary therapist complete the PEDI. Concurrent validity of 0.70 to 0.73 between the PEDI and Batelle Developmental Inventory Screening Test (BDIST) has been demonstrated, implying that the two tests address similar but not identical issues. Good concurrent validity among the PEDI, BDIST, and Functional Independence Measure for Children (WeeFIM®) instrument has also been demonstrated with a population of children with severe disabilities. The PEDI demonstrated the ability to correctly discriminate between disabled and normal populations and to detect change over time with intervention. Construct validity is achieved because the PEDI supports the assumptions that functional behaviors change with age and that attainment of a functional skill precedes independence in that skill. The latter assumption implies that the degree of caregiver assistance is an important changeable dimension to monitor in a functional assessment framework (Feldman et al, 1990; Haley et al, 1992).

School Function Assessment

The School Function Assessment (SFA) is intended to assess how well an elementary school student with disabilities, who attends kindergarten through sixth grade, can meet the functional demands of the school setting. The SFA is administered as a judgment-based questionnaire, documenting a student's typical behavior compared with same-age or -class peers. Criterion-referenced scoring represents the student's interaction within the school context, and criterion-referenced cutoff scores compare the student's performance with grade-level expectations (Coster et al, 1998).

The SFA consists of three separately scored sections, including (1) social

TABLE 5–3

Types of Activities Assessed in the School Function Assessment

Social Participation in School Activities	Activity Performance in School-Related Function	
	Physical	*Cognitive or Behavioral*
Classroom	Travel	Communication
Recess or playground	Maintain or change position	Computer or equipment use
Transportation	Set up or clean up	Behavior regulation
Bathroom or toileting	Hygiene	Memory or understanding
Transition to or from class	Clothing management	
Mealtime or snack time	Stairs	

participation in school activities, (2) task supports necessary to participate in activities, and (3) activity performance in school-related functional activities (Table 5–3). Raw scores from each of the three sections are converted into criterion scores using a Rasch analysis statistical model. Tables of criterion scores and standard error of measurement are provided in the test manual. The authors suggest that the Participation and Task Support scales can be used as a screening device to identify students who demonstrate functional limitations in the school setting. Selective scales can also be assessed individually to address specific areas of concern for intervention. In addition, the SFA can be used to support Individualized Education Plan development and document progress or effects of intervention.

In development of the SFA, a standardization sample of 363 students with disabilities was used. The criterion cutoff scores reflect the performance of 318 nondisabled peers. The test manual also reports good internal reliability of each item (0.92 to 0.98) and test reliability (0.82 to 0.98 in a study with 23 participants; 0.80 to 0.99 in a study with 29 participants). Content validity is also supported by expert review during the development and piloting of the SFA.

Functional Independence Measure for Children

The WeeFIM® instrument is an adaptation of the Functional Independence Measure (FIM™* instrument) designed to measure the acquisition of functional skills in children with disability from 6 months through 7 years of age (Fig. 5–2). The WeeFIM® instrument measures the severity of the child's disability and evaluates outcomes of pediatric rehabilitation. It can be used in both inpatient and outpatient settings, and it can be administered by a variety of health and education professionals to measure the child's actual performance of functional tasks.

---

*FIM™ is a trademark of the Uniform Data System for Medical Rehabilitation, a division of U B Foundation Activities, Inc.

WeeFIM® instrument

L E V E L S	7 Complete Independence (Timely, Safely) 6 Modified Independence (Device)	**No Assistance**
	Modified Dependence 5 Supervision (Subject = 100%) 4 Minimal Assist (Subject = 75%+) 3 Moderate Assist (Subject = 50%+) **Complete Dependence** 2 Maximal Assist (Subject =25%+) 1 Total Assist (Subject = less than 25%)	**Assistance**

ASSESSMENT   GOAL

Self-Care
1. Eating
2. Grooming
3. Bathing
4. Dressing - Upper
5. Dressing - Lower
6. Toileting
7. Bladder
8. Bowel
   Self-Care Total   *Quotient*

Mobility
9. Chair, Wheelchair
10. Toilet
11. Tub, Shower
12. Walk/Wheelchair   W Walk / C wheelChair / L crawL / B comBination
13. Stairs
    Mobility Total   *Quotient*

Cognition
14. Comprehension   A Auditory / V Visual / B Both
15. Expression   V Vocal / N Nonvocal / B Both
16. Social Interaction
17. Problem Solving
18. Memory
    Cognitive Total   *Quotient*

    WeeFIM Total   *Quotient*

NOTE: Leave no blanks. Enter 1 if patient not testable due to risk

Figure 5–2

WeeFIM® instrument. (*WeeFIM Systems^SM Clinical Guide: Version 5.01.* Buffalo, NY: Center for Functional Assessment Research and UDSMR, State University of New York at Buffalo, 2000.)

Like the FIM™ instrument, the WeeFIM® instrument focuses on BADL with six domains: self-care, sphincter control, mobility, locomotion, communication, and social cognition. A seven-point ordinal scale is used to reflect level of independence in these tasks. A score of 7 indicates ability to perform a task independently, and a score of 1 indicates a need for total assistance. Scores of 1 to 5 are used when caregiver assistance is necessary, and a score of 6 indicates modified independence (i.e., need for assistive device) (Msall et al, 1993).

The WeeFIM® instrument has demonstrated good reliability whether administered via direct observation or structured interview (Ottenbacher et al, 1996; Sperle et al, 1997). Instrument validity was originally determined for children in the United States but has also been accepted for Japanese children (Liu et al, 1998). Reported limitations for the WeeFIM® instrument concern its use of an ordinal scoring scale and the sensitivity of the scale (Deutsch et al, 1996).

Gross Motor Function Measure

The Gross Motor Function Measure is a criterion-referenced assessment designed to be used with children with cerebral palsy. It evaluates the child's ability to complete motor functions such as rolling, crawling, sitting, standing, walking, running, stair use, and jumping. A four-point ordinal scale of measurement is used to assess each item. A score of 0 indicates the task cannot be done, 1 indicates the task can be initiated (<10% completion), 2 indicates partial completion of the task (10% to <100% completion), and 3 indicates the task can be completed. Summary scores can also be calculated, resulting in ratio data. Interrater and test-retest reliability are reported to be excellent (>0.80). Content and construct validity are also reported to be good. GMFM construct validity for children with diplegic cerebral palsy during a 12- to 24-month period also has been demonstrated (Bjornson et al, 1998). The measure is considered to be sensitive to changes in performance in functional tasks, making it an effective tool for documenting change in the motor performance of children with cerebral palsy (Russell et al, 1989).

ADULT FUNCTIONAL ASSESSMENT INSTRUMENTS

Katz Index of Activities of Daily Living

This instrument was originally designed to measure how independently clients in institutional settings could perform BADL, including bathing, dressing, toileting, continence, feeding, and transfer skills (Katz et al, 1963). Ambulation, or client mobility, was not measured, limiting the usefulness of this tool. The original instrument has been adapted for use with community-based clients, with the addition of two functional categories (ambulation and grooming) and the deletion of continence (Branch et al, 1984). Reliability studies judge the instrument as fair to good. Agreement scores of 0.68 to 0.98 between raters have been demonstrated. Test-retest reliability coefficients range from 0.61 to

0.78 (Liang and Jette, 1981). The predictive validity of some of the Katz items has also been demonstrated with an older adult population living in senior housing or at home (Reuben et al, 1992).

Clients are rated on whether they can complete tasks in the six functional areas independently, with some assistance, or totally dependently. Both client self-report and direct observation are used to score the assessment. A letter score of A, B, C, D, E, F, or G is assigned, according to which of the six basic activities the client performs independently. For example, if the client is independent in all six tasks, she receives a score of A. If she is independent in all except bathing and one additional function, she receives a score of C.

Functional Status Index

The Functional Status Index was derived from the Katz Index for use with individuals with arthritis. BADL and IADL are assessed, making this an appropriate tool for use with community-dwelling, chronically disabled populations (see Table 5–1). Not only is the degree of dependence in achieving the task measured, but also the amount of pain experienced with each activity and the client's perceived difficulty in completing the task are rated.

Either the interviewer- or self-administered format can be used. Reliability studies have indicated fair interrater and test-retest reliability coefficients, ranging from 0.61 to 0.81. Construct validity also has been supported (Jette, 1980; Jette and Deniston, 1978; Liang and Jette, 1981).

Barthel Index

The Barthel Index was developed to measure improvement in clients with chronic disability who were participating in rehabilitation (Table 5–4). BADL are assessed, including toileting, bathing, eating, dressing, continence, transfers, and ambulation. Clients receive numerical scores based on whether they require physical assistance to perform the task or can complete it independently. Items are weighted according to the professional judgment of the developers. A client scoring 0 points would be dependent in all assessed activities of daily living, whereas a score of 100 would reflect independence in these activities (Mahoney and Barthel, 1965).

Specific reliability and validity studies have not been reported, but Barthel Index scores of adult clients who have had a stroke or have severe disabilities correlate with clinical outcomes and functional status (Granger et al, 1979a and b). Specific, detailed instructions are provided, supporting standardized use of the measure (Jette, 1985).

The Barthel Index was one of the earliest standardized functional assessments. The FIM™ instrument was developed to be a more comprehensive tool. Research shows a relationship between the two instruments, because a Barthel Index score can be derived from FIM™ instrument motor item scores (Nyein et al, 1999). The Barthel Index, total FIM™ instrument score, and motor FIM™ instrument score all demonstrate similar responsiveness in the evaluation of inpatient rehabilitation clients with multiple sclerosis and stroke (van der Putten et al, 1999).

TABLE 5–4

Barthel Index: A Functional Evaluation Tool to Assess a Client's Level of Independent Activity

Activity	Independent Function	Dependent Function
Feeding	Independent = **10.** The client can feed himself a meal from a tray or table when someone puts the food within his reach. He must put on an assistive device if this is needed, cut up the food, use salt and pepper, spread butter, etc. He must accomplish this in a reasonable time.	Some help is necessary (with cutting up food, etc.) = **5.**
Moving from wheelchair to bed and return	Independent in all phases of this activity = **15.** Client can safely approach the bed in his wheelchair, lock brakes, lift footrests, move safely to bed, lie down, come to a sitting position on the side of the bed, change the position of the wheelchair (if necessary) to transfer back into it safely, and return to the wheelchair.	Either some minimal help is needed in some step of this activity or the client needs to be reminded or supervised for safety of one or more parts of this activity = **10.** Client can come to a sitting position without the help of a second person but needs to be lifted out of bed, or she transfers with a great deal of help = **5.**
Doing personal toilet	Client can wash hands and face, comb hair, clean teeth, and shave = **5.** The client may use any kind of razor but must put in blade or plug in razor without help as well as get it from drawer or cabinet. Female clients must put on own makeup, if used, but need not braid or style hair.	With help = **0.**
Getting on and off toilet	Client is able to get on and off toilet, fasten and unfasten clothes, prevent soiling of clothes, and use toilet paper without help = **10.** He may use a wall bar or other stable object for support if needed. If it is necessary to use a bed pan instead of a toilet, he must be able to place it on a chair, empty it, and clean it.	Client needs help because of imbalance or in handling clothes or in using toilet paper = **5.**
Bathing	Client may use a bath tub or a shower or take a complete sponge bath = **5.** He must be able to do all the steps involved in whichever method is used without another person being present.	With help = **0.**

Continued

TABLE 5–4 Continued

Barthel Index: A Functional Evaluation Tool to Assess a Client's Level of Independent Activity

Activity	Independent Function	Dependent Function
Walking on a level surface	Client can walk at least 50 yards without help or supervision = **15.** He may wear braces or prosthesis and use crutches, canes, or a walkerette, but not a rolling walker. He must be able to lock and unlock braces if used, assume the standing position and sit down, get the necessary mechanical aides into position for use, and dispose of them when he sits.	Client needs help or supervision in any of the above but can walk at least 50 yards with a little help = **10.**
Propelling a wheelchair	If a client cannot ambulate, but can propel a wheelchair independently = **5*.** He must be able to go around corners, turn around, maneuver the chair to a table, bed, toilet, etc. He must be able to push a chair at least 50 yards. * Do not score this item if the client gets score for walking.	With help = **0*.**
Ascending and descending stairs	Client is able to go up and down a flight of stairs safely without help or supervision = **10.** He may and should use handrails, canes, or crutches when needed. He must be able to carry canes or crutches as he ascends or descends stairs.	Client needs help with or supervision of any one of the above items = **5.**
Dressing and undressing	Client is able to put on and remove and fasten all clothing, and tie shoe laces (unless it is necessary to use adaptations for this) = **10.** The activity includes putting on and removing and fastening corset or braces when these are prescribed. Such special clothing as suspenders, loafer shoes, or dresses that open down the front may be used when necessary.	Client needs help in putting on and removing or fastening any clothing = **5.** He must do at least half the work himself. He must accomplish this in a reasonable time.
Continence of bowels	Client is able to control his bowels and have no accidents = **10.**	Client needs help in using a suppository or taking an enema or has occasional accidents = **5.**
Controlling bladder	Client is able to control his bladder day and night = **10.** Clients who wear an external device must be able to care for it independently.	Client has occasional accidents or cannot wait for the bed pan or get to the toilet in time or needs help with an external device = **5.**

The best possible score is 100. A score of 0 indicates that the client cannot meet the criteria as defined for each function.
Adapted from Mahoney FI, Barthel DQ. Functional evaluation: The Barthel Index. *Md State Med J* 14:61–65, 1965.

Functional Independence Measure

The FIM™ instrument was developed as part of the Uniform Data System for Medical Rehabilitation at the State University of New York at Buffalo (1990), and Version 5.1 of the FIM System™ was published in 1997 (*Guide for Uniform Data Set for Medical Rehabilitation*, 1997). The FIM™ instrument assesses the functional skills of individuals over 7 years of age (Fig. 5–3). This data set has been used widely in the United States and internationally; it consists of more than 1 million records (Deutsch et al, 1996). It is used in inpatient rehabilitation settings, as well as in long-term care, subacute rehabilitation, and home care environments.

The FIM™ instrument is meant to reflect an individual's usual performance rather than his best performance. The assessment can be completed by direct client observation or interview. Six domains of function are evaluated: self-care, sphincter control, transfers, locomotion, communication, and social cognition. Self-care activities include dressing, eating, grooming, and bathing. Transfers from the bed to chair, to the toilet, and to the tub or shower are included in the mobility section. Locomotion includes walking, managing stairs, and propelling a wheelchair. Items are scored on a 7-point ordinal scale, with 7 reflecting complete independence and 1 reflecting total dependence. Scores of 1 to 5 indicate a need for caregiver assistance. Scores in all domains are added to obtain a total FIM™ instrument score; motor and cognitive scores can be calculated separately.

Reliability and validity of the FIM™ instrument are reported to be good, with very good interrater reliability to the total score (0.96), motor score (0.96), and cognitive score (0.91). Some individual subtest interrater reliability scores are weaker, such as the memory subtest, which depends on the training of the examiner (0.53, untrained; 0.69, trained) (Hamilton et al, 1994). Concurrent validity with the Barthel Index has been reported (Kidd et al, 1995). Construct validity research summarized by Deutsch and colleagues (1996) and a study with clients with multiple sclerosis (Brosseau, 1994) indicate good FIM™ instrument construct validity. Functional independence is a multidimensional entity and may be better reflected by the subscores (Ravaud et al, 1999). The responsiveness of the FIM™ instrument also has been reported to be good; scores can differentiate client populations and improve over the course of rehabilitation (Deutsch et al, 1996).

Summary

The desire for positive outcomes is directly related to the importance of evaluating a client's functional ability in clinical practice. The primary goal of physical and occupational therapy intervention is to improve the functional skills of the clients served. Functional outcome measures can easily be developed into functional goals for the client. By emphasizing functional outcomes, intervention focuses on the client's independence, rather than on attainment of normality (Haley et al, 1991).

FIM™ instrument

LEVELS		NO HELPER
	7 Complete Independence (Timely, Safely) 6 Modified Independence (Device)	**NO HELPER**
	Modified Dependence 5 Supervision (Subject = 100%+) 4 Minimal Assist (Subject = 75%+) 3 Moderate Assist (Subject = 50%+) **Complete Dependence** 2 Maximal Assist (Subject =25%+) 1 Total Assist (Subject = less than 25%)	**HELPER**

	ADMISSION	DISCHARGE	FOLLOW-UP
Self-Care A. Eating B Grooming C. Bathing D. Dressing - Upper Body E. Dressing - Lower Body F. Toileting			
Sphincter Control G. Bladder Management H. Bowel Management			
Transfers I. Bed, Chair, Wheelchair J. Toilet K. Tub, Shower			
Locomotion L. Walk/Wheelchair M. Stairs	W Walk C Wheelchair B Both	W Walk C Wheelchair B Both	W Walk C Wheelchair B Both
Motor Subtotal Score			
Communication N. Comprehension O. Expression	A Auditory V Visual B Both V Vocal N Nonvocal B Both	A Auditory V Visual B Both V Vocal N Nonvocal B Both	A Auditory V Visual B Both V Vocal N Nonvocal B Both
Social Cognition P. Social Interaction Q. Problem Solving R. Memory			
Cognitive Subtotal Score			
TOTAL FIM Score			

NOTE: Leave no blanks. Enter 1 if patient not testable due to risk

FIM™ Instrument. Copyright©1997 Uniform Data System for Medical Rehabilitation, a divison of U B Foundation Activities, Inc. Reprinted with the permission of UDSMR, University at Buffalo, 232 Parker Hall, 3435 Main Street, Buffalo, NY 14214.

Figure 5–3

FIM™ instrument. (*Guide for the Uniform Data Set for Medical Rehabilitation [including the FIM™ instrument], Version 5.1.* Buffalo, NY: Center for Functional Assessment Research and UDSMR, State University of New York at Buffalo, 1997.)

Evaluation of a client's functional abilities can include both standardized and nonstandardized components. A functional assessment should encompass activities that are important throughout a client's day as well as consider social, emotional, environmental, and cognitive issues relevant to that client. The spectrum of tasks assessed must reflect those necessary for the client to function in his environment. For example, the School Function Assessment will better assess how a first grader is functioning in school than the Pediatric Evaluation of Disability Index. Likewise, the Katz or Barthel Index may adequately reflect the functional ability of a client in a long-term care facility but will not address the IADL necessary for that client's discharge to a home setting.

Use of standardized assessment instruments increases the reliability and validity of the evaluation, assists in objectively documenting outcomes, and improves communication between professional caregivers. The mode of administration, scoring format, and measurement characteristics of reliability and validity are important, as noted in the descriptions of the instruments reviewed in this chapter.

Establishing a client's level of function is the first step to designing interventions that address that person's individual needs. The clinician must decide what domains of function are involved and which components of function are limiting performance based on an evaluation of functional skills. Strength, endurance, balance, mobility, or coordination may be the factor that limits physical performance. Specific therapeutic programs can be designed to address any of those factors.

We, as therapists, must have a working knowledge of the human body to thoroughly understand physical function and the factors that influence it. The next unit of this book explores the role of each body system involved in movement and discusses the effect of life-span development on these systems.

References

Bjornson KF, Graubert CS, Buford VL, McLaughlin JF. Validity of the Gross Motor Function Measure. *Pediatr Phys Ther* 10:43–47, 1998.

Branch LG, Katz S, Kneipmann K, Papsidero JA. A prospective study of functional status among community elders. *Am J Public Health* 74:266–268, 1984.

Brosseau L. The inter-rater reliability and construct validity of the Functional Independence Measure for multiple sclerosis subjects. *Clin Rehabil* 8:107–115, 1994.

Coster W, Deeney T, Haltiwanger J, Haley S. *The School Function Assessment*. San Antonio, TX: Therapy Skill Builders, 1998.

Deutsch A, Braun S, Granger C. The Functional Independence Measure (FIM™ Instrument) and the Functional Independence Measure for Children (WeeFIM® Instrument): Ten years of development. *Crit Rev Phys Rehabil Med* 8:267–281, 1996.

Feldman AB, Haley SM, Coryell J. Concurrent and construct validity of the pediatric evaluation of disability inventory. *Phys Ther* 70:602–610, 1990.

Granger CV, Albrecht GL, Hamilton BB. Outcome of comprehensive medical rehabilitation: Measurement by PULSES Profile and Barthel Index. *Arch Phys Med Rehabil* 60:145–154, 1979a.

Granger CV, Dewis LS, Peters NC, et al. Stroke rehabilitation: Analyses of repeated Barthel Index measures. *Arch Phys Med Rehabil* 60:14–17, 1979b.

Guccione AA. *Geriatric Physical Therapy*, 2nd ed. St. Louis: Mosby, 2000.

Guide for the Uniform Data Set for Medical Rehabilitation (Including the FIM™ Instrument), Version 5.1. Buffalo, NY 14214: State University of New York at Buffalo, 1997.

Haley SM, Coster WJ, Ludlow LH. Pediatric functional outcome measures. *Phys Med Rehabil Clin North Am* 2:689–723, 1991.

Haley SM, Coster WJ, Ludlow LH, et al. *Pediatric Evaluation of Disability Inventory (PEDI).* Boston: New England Medical Center Hospital and PEDI Research Group, 1992.

Hamilton BB, Laughlin JA, Fiedler RC, Granger CV. Interrater reliability of the 7 level functional independence measure (FIM). *Scand J Rehabil Med* 26930:115–119, 1994.

Harris BA, Jette AM, Campion EW, Cleary PD. Validity of self-report measures of functional disability. *Top Geriatr Rehabil* 1:31–41, 1986.

Hughes SL, Edelman P, Chang RW, et al. The GERI-AIMS: Reliability and validity of the arthritis impact measurement scales adapted for elderly respondents. *Arthritis Rheum* 34:856–865, 1991.

Jette AM. State of the art in functional status assessment. In Rothestein J (ed). *Measurement in Physical Therapy.* New York: Churchill Livingstone, 1985, pp 137–168.

Jette AM. Functional Status Index: Reliability of a chronic disease evaluation instrument. *Arch Phys Med Rehabil* 61:395–401, 1980.

Jette AM, Deniston OL. Inter-observer reliability of a functional status assessment instrument. *J Chronic Dis* 31:573–580, 1978.

Katz S, Ford AB, Moskowitz RW, et al. Studies of illness in the aged—The Index of ADL: A standardized measure of biological and psychosocial function. *JAMA* 185:914–919, 1963.

Kaufert JM. Functional ability indices: Measurement problems in assessing their validity. *Arch Phys Med Rehabil* 64:260–267, 1983.

Kidd D, Stewart G, Baldry J, et al. The Functional Independence Measure: A comparative validity and reliability study. *Disabil Rehabil* 17:10–14, 1995.

Liang MH, Jette AM. Measuring functional ability in chronic arthritis: A critical review. *Arthritis Rheum* 24:80–86, 1981.

Liu M, Toikawa H, Seki M, et al. Functional Independence Measure for Children (WeeFIM): A preliminary study in nondisabled Japanese children. *Am J Phys Med Rehabil* 77:36–44, 1998.

Lovell DJ, Howe S, Shear E, et al. Development of a disability measurement tool for juvenile rheumatoid arthritis: The Juvenile Arthritis Functional Assessment Scale. *Arthritis Rheum* 32:1390–1395, 1989.

Mahoney FI, Barthel DW. Functional evaluation: Barthel Index. *Md State Med J* 14:61–65, 1965.

Meenan RF, Gertman PM, Mason JH. Measuring health in arthritis: The Arthritis Impact Measurement Scale. *Arthritis Rheum* 23:146–152, 1980.

Msall ME, DiGaudio KM, Duffy LC. Use of functional assessment in children with developmental disabilities. *Phys Med Rehabil Clin North Am* 4:517–527, 1993.

Nichols DS, Case-Smith J. Reliability and validity of the Pediatric Evaluation of Disability Inventory. *Pediatr Phys Ther* 8:15–24, 1996.

Nyein K, McMichael L, Turner-Stokes L. Can a Barthel score be derived from the FIM? *Clin Rehabil* 13:56–63, 1999.

Ottenbacher KJ, Taylor ET, Msall ME, et al. The stability and equivalence reliability of the Functional Independence Measure for Children (WeeFIM®). *Dev Med Child Neurol* 38:907–916, 1996.

Ravaud JF, Delcey M, Yelnik A. Construct validity of the Functional Independence Measure (FIM): Questioning the unidimensionality of the scale and the "value" of FIM scores. *Scand J Rehabil Med* 31:31–41, 1999.

Reuben DB, Sui AL, Sokkun K. The predictive validity of self-report and performance-based measures of function and health. *J Gerontol* 47:M106–M110, 1992.

Russell DJ, Rosenbaum PL, Cadman DT, et al. The gross motor function measure: A means to evaluate the effects of physical therapy. *Dev Med Child Neurol* 31:341–352, 1989.

Sperle FA, Qttenbacher KJ, Braun SL, et al. Equivalence reliability of the Functional Independence Measure for Children (WeeFIM®) administration methods. *Am J Occup Ther* 51:35–41, 1997.

van der Putten JJ, Hobart JC, Freeman JA, Thompson AJ. Measuring change in disability after inpatient rehabilitation: Comparison of the responsiveness of the Barthel Index and the Functional Independence Measure. *J Neurol Neurosurg Psychiatry* 66:480–484, 1999.

WeeFIM System™ Clinical Guide: Version 5.01. Buffalo, NY 14214: University at Buffalo, 1998, 2000.

Body Systems Contributing to Functional Movement

6 Skeletal System Changes

OBJECTIVES

After studying this chapter, the reader will be able to:

1 Describe the structure of the components of the skeletal system.

2 Identify the function of bone and cartilage in supporting posture and movement.

3 Discuss unique structural and functional characteristics of the skeletal system in the developing fetus, infant, child, adolescent, adult, and older adult.

4 Relate the age-related characteristics of the skeletal system to functional movement abilities and risk factors.

5 Incorporate issues of life-span development of the skeletal system into patient assessment and treatment planning.

The ability to walk, run, lift, and manipulate objects is influenced by the strength and resilience of the skeletal system. A young infant cannot walk, climb stairs, push a stroller, or tie shoes. Not only do infants lack the experience and practice necessary for these tasks, their immature skeleton does not provide a structural framework on which these movements can take place. Older adults may not have the spring in their step, power in their tennis serve, or manual dexterity they enjoyed when they were younger. The changes in the skeletal system that occur with aging may contribute to decreased efficiency of movement. Across the life span, the skeletal system evolves and influences our ability for unrestricted movement.

The skeletal system, as discussed in this chapter, consists of the bony skeleton and cartilage. The skeleton provides a structure on which muscles can work. The size and shape of the bones and location of muscular attachments form an efficient system of levers and struts. Joints allow bones to articulate with each other, and the shape of the joint contributes to efficiency of movement. Cartilage acts as a shock absorber and protects joint surfaces from wear and tear. We better appreciate the contribution of the skeletal system to functional movement when we understand the role of its components and their changing properties throughout development.

Components of the Skeletal System

CARTILAGE

Cartilage, a type of connective tissue, can tolerate mechanical stress and acts as a supporting structure in the body. It provides a mechanism for shock absorption, acts as a sliding surface for the joints, and plays a role in the development and growth of bone. During fetal development, a cartilage model is laid down from which the long bones of the body will develop. The ends of immature long bones as well as some sites of muscular attachment also contain cartilage plates, which are sites of bone growth.

Three types of cartilage exist, each meeting different functional needs (Fig. 6–1). *Hyaline cartilage* is the most abundant and rigid. It is found at the articular surfaces of joints and the walls of respiratory passages such as the trachea and bronchi. Hyaline cartilage also makes up the fetal model of the future long bones and can be found at the epiphyseal growth plates of immature bone. *Fibrocartilage* is found at the acetabulum, intervertebral disks, menisci, and tendinous insertions. It is more pliable than hyaline cartilage but still provides strength and support to the skeletal system. Fibrocartilage fibers are arranged parallel to the stress forces that the tissue experiences. *Elastic cartilage* is the most pliable cartilage and can be found at the larynx, ear, and epiglottis, where it provides support with flexibility.

Hyaline cartilage covers the ends of the bones that make up synovial joints, and in this capacity, it is called *articular cartilage*. It is responsible for facilitating motion at the joints and can tolerate a variety of loading forces. Synovial fluid and the compression of fluids from within the surface of the articular cartilage contribute to lubrication of the joint. Articular cartilage provides a low friction surface and allows joints to move freely and easily for 80 or even 100 years (Gradisar and Porterfield, 1989). Years of microtrauma, isolated instances of more severe joint trauma, and aging of the cartilaginous tissue eventually result in a breakdown of articular cartilage, which contributes to the development of *osteoarthritis*.

Properties

Cartilage consists of water, collagen fibers, cartilage cells (*chondrocytes*), and a ground substance in which the collagen fibers are embedded. Elastic cartilage also contains elastin fibers. The fibers and ground substance make up the extracellular matrix surrounding the chondrocytes. Differences in the extracellular matrix and amount of water in the tissue help to differentiate the three types of cartilage. For example, the water content of articular cartilage is 80% but that of fibrocartilage is only 50% (Gradisar and Porterfield, 1989).

Cartilage has no nerve supply and no vascular supply of its own. Oxygen and nutrients must be obtained from surrounding tissues. Most cartilage is covered by a layer of dense connective tissue called the *perichondrium*. The perichondrium is vascularized and supplies nutrients to the cartilage via diffusion. Articular cartilage is not covered with perichondrium and depends on

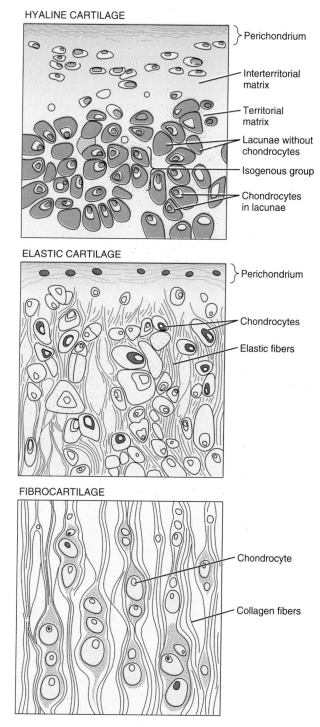

Figure 6-1

Diagram of the types of cartilage. (From Gartner LP, Hiatt JL. *Color Textbook of Histology*, 2nd ed. Philadelphia: WB Saunders, 2001, p 130.)

diffusion of nutrients from synovial fluid. In articular cartilage, periods of compression and decompression facilitate the exchange of fluids: during decompression, osmotic forces allow nutrients to diffuse into the cartilage, and during compression, fluids and waste products can be squeezed out (Gradisar and Porterfield, 1989; Pickles, 1989). Both processes are necessary to maintain adequate nutrition of the cartilage. Compressive forces also promote production of hyaluronic acid, which lubricates the tissues (Ryan, 1994).

Formation

Cartilage is derived from embryonic mesoderm, as is other connective tissue. Cartilage growth occurs through two different processes: interstitial growth and appositional growth. Interstitial growth occurs within the cartilage through mitotic division of the existing chondrocytes. It occurs in the early phases of cartilage development to increase tissue mass, at the epiphyseal plates of long bones, and at articular surfaces. In appositional growth, new cartilage is laid down at the surface of the perichondrium. In this process, chondroblasts of the perichondrium, which are precursors to chondrocytes, form an extracellular matrix and develop into mature chondrocytes. Nonarticular cartilage loses the capacity for interstitial growth early and then undergoes only appositional growth.

In the formation of articular cartilage, collagen fibers of the extracellular matrix weave together and form a loop parallel to the joint surface. These collagen fibers are embedded in the subchondral bone or deep cartilage tissue. This structural arrangement helps the cartilage to retain water and to maintain its shape (Gradisar and Porterfield, 1989; Pickles, 1989).

Mechanical loading, including compression, is necessary to maintain healthy articular cartilage. In the absence of mechanical loading, atrophy of the articular tissue may be seen.

Constant compression, however, leads to a thinning of cartilage, and excessive compression contributes to degeneration of the cartilage (LeVeau and Bernhardt, 1984). With use, cells of the articular surface are worn away, the cartilage thins, and eventually the surface changes. Cartilage repair depends on interstitial growth and the ability of chondrocytes to synthesize and maintain the extracellular matrix. Articular cartilage has the ability to repair itself, undergo limited mitosis, metabolize nutrients, and maintain its matrix even during aging, although less so than younger cartilage because of decreased ability to synthesize new extracellular matrix (Guccione, 2000; Kauffman, 1999). For example, with rest, a young individual with chondromalacia is able to recover from articular cartilage damage. In the older individual, similar cartilage degeneration cannot be repaired, and osteoarthritis results. Others report that articular cartilage has poor ability for repair, except in infancy (Gradisar and Porterfield, 1989). They suggest that damaged articular cartilage is replaced by scar tissue or fibrocartilage, whose mechanical properties are not optimal for providing low friction joint motion under high mechanical loads. Most authors do agree that wear and tear over time result in a worn, less efficient articular surface.

Aging

The composition of cartilage changes with age as a result of dehydration, poor nutrition, an imbalance between rest and weight bearing over the life span, and basic wear and tear from life-long stresses. Water content of cartilage decreases from 80% to 90% in the fetus to 70% in the adult (VanderWeil, 1983). Increased cross-linkage of collagen and elastin fibers causes the extracellular matrix to become more rigid and eventually calcify, making diffusion of nutrients more difficult. If cartilage nutrition cannot be maintained, chondrocytes die.

Whitbourne (1985) and Pickles (1989) suggest that thinning of articular cartilage occurs with age. Decreased numbers of cells are seen throughout the cartilage, especially at weight-bearing surfaces. Repeated exposure to mechanical loading wears away the cartilage and compromises its ability to protect the articulating bony surfaces. The extracellular matrix of the articular cartilage becomes hard and brittle, resulting in decreased resiliency, strength, and efficiency. Friction increases during joint movement with the thinning, fraying, and cracking of articular cartilage.

BONE

The bony skeleton accounts for 14% of adult weight and for 97% to 98% of total height (Sinclair and Dangerfield, 1998). Intervertebral disks contribute to the remaining height. In humans, bone has several functions, including (1) protection of vital organs, (2) support of body weight, (3) storage for minerals, (4) structural leverage for movement, and (5) bone marrow storage.

Bony protection of the central nervous system is provided by the skull, which forms a vault around the brain, and by the vertebral column, which encases the spinal cord. The rib cage protects the lungs and heart. The bones of the vertebral column, shoulder girdle, pelvic girdle, upper extremities, and lower extremities are arranged to effectively support the body weight in upright postures. Joints functionally connect the bones, enhancing their support functions or fostering efficient articulations. Muscles are strategically attached to this bony framework, allowing efficient movement to occur with muscular contraction.

In addition to providing protection and support, bone is a storage site for materials used by the body. Bone marrow, which is important in the formation of blood cells, is stored in bone. Calcium, phosphate, and other ions are stored in bone as crystalline salts. These salts contribute to the strength of the bone and its ability to withstand the compressive forces of weight bearing. The stored minerals are also used to maintain blood mineral levels when changes in diet or metabolic demand occur. If the blood levels of calcium and phosphate drop, these minerals are accessed from the bone. Likewise, after a meal, calcium is deposited in bone or excreted rather than increased in blood levels (Guyton and Hall, 1997; Lanyon, 1989).

The structure of bone, as well as its stiffness and strength, allows it to meet the functional demands of everyday activities. Throughout development, bone must be produced and maintained in sufficient quantity to withstand a lifetime of weight bearing, movement, and functional activity.

General Structure and Form

Bone is a connective tissue composed of bone cells and bone matrix. These elements are held together by a ground substance. The bone matrix is a hard, calcified substance made up of collagen fibers and mineral salts. It surrounds the primary bone cell, the *osteocyte*, which functions to maintain the nutrition and mineral content of the bone matrix. Two other types of bone cells are the *osteoblast*, which is active in the formation of new bone, and the *osteoclast*, which is associated with resorption of bone. Osteoblasts are found on the surface of bone and synthesize new bone matrix. As they are encased in sufficient bone matrix, they become osteocytes. Osteoclasts are found in areas of bone resorption, where they break down the bone matrix and release minerals into the circulation (Malina and Bouchard, 1991).

The external surface of bone, except at articular surfaces, is covered with periosteum. The periosteum is made up of collagen fibers and bone-forming cells, which provide a source of osteoblasts. The internal surface of bone, the *endosteum*, is thinner than the periosteum but also supplies osteoblasts for bone growth and repair. Both surfaces are vascularized and play a role in nutrition of bone.

All bones are made up of two types of bone tissue: *compact bone* and *cancellous bone*, also called *trabecular bone* (Fig. 6–2). Compact bone, which is hard and dense, represents the majority of bone in the human skeleton. It makes up the shaft of long bones and provides a thin outer covering for areas of cancellous bone. Compact bone is formed when thin plates of bone (*lamellae*) are arranged concentrically around a channel containing blood vessels and nerves (*haversian canals*). This vascular channel is formed when new bone matrix surrounds existing blood vessels. Four to 20 lamellae surround a haversian canal, making up an osteon (*haversian system*). Osteons provide a mechanism to maintain nutrition of the bone. They are continuously being destroyed and rebuilt throughout the life span. Cancellous bone, made up of loosely woven strands of bone tissue (*trabeculae*), represents only about 20% of bone in the human skeleton. It is found at the ends of the long bones and surrounds the inner bone marrow cavity of the shaft. The open spaces of the cancellous bone house the bone marrow and vessels that nourish the bone. Figure 6–2 shows compact bone surrounding a portion of cancellous bone. Bones of the spine, wrist, and hip are made up of a high proportion of cancellous bone. As we age, loss of cancellous bone occurs earlier than that of cortical bone. It is not surprising, then, that the wrist, spine, and hip are frequent sites of fracture in older adults with osteoporosis.

The general form of each bone, its muscular attachments, and its anatomic relationships are all genetically determined. Heredity and the mechanical stresses placed on developing bone dictate the shape, size, and structure of the mature bone. Bone mass, girth, cortical thickness, curvature, density, and ar-

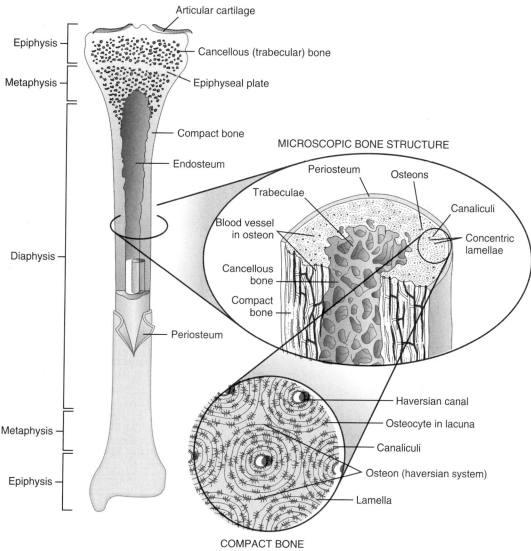

Figure 6-2

The structural components of a long bone with cross sections depicting the microscopic structure and enlarged view of compact bone with haversian system.

rangement of trabeculae are influenced by the mechanical stresses produced during functional activities. Heredity also appears to influence bone mass as evidenced by the greater skeletal weight and bone mineral content of black children compared with white children (Parfitt, 1997). Weight bearing and the pull of muscular attachments on bone during activities direct the arrangement of collagen fibers within bone trabeculae in the same direction as the stress forces (Smith, 1981). In the absence of functional loading of the bone, deficiencies in bone architecture and structure will result (Lanyon, 1989). The relationship between bone structure and the mechanical loads it experiences was identified by J. Wolff in 1892. According to Wolff's law of bone transformation, the structure of bone will change in response to the mechanical loads placed on it, according to certain mathematical laws (LeVeau and Bernhardt, 1984; Martin and Brown, 1989).

Nutrition and hormones are important factors in the growth and development process of bone. People who do not have sufficient protein, calcium, vitamin D, and vitamin C in their diet experience abnormal bone growth. Without adequate dietary protein, insufficient collagen is produced by the osteoblasts, leading to poor calcification of the bone matrix. In vitamin C deficiency, the cartilage formed for bone growth also lacks collagen. In severe vitamin C deficiency (*scurvy*), decreased rate of growth at the cartilage growth plates of the long bones results in deficient bone formation. Vitamin D deficiency in children causes rickets. In this disorder, growth in the region of the cartilage growth plate is distorted because calcification of the cartilage is deficient (Smith, 1981). Vitamin D is also important in the absorption of calcium in the gastrointestinal tract. The role of hormones in bone development is evidenced by the influence of growth hormone on growing bone. A rapid growth period accompanies the hormonal changes of adolescence. Low levels of estrogen are needed for the pubertal growth spurt of bone in both boys and girls (Cutler, 1997). In contrast, accelerated loss of bone mineral content occurs immediately after menopause, again related to hormonal changes in the body.

Development

In embryologic development, bone forms from the mesoderm. Fetal bone is made of primary or woven bone tissue. Woven bone consists of an irregular array of collagen fibers and is less mineralized than mature bone. As osteons form, mineralization of the bony matrix increases and mature bone tissue replaces woven bone. A similar process can be seen throughout development as new, woven bone is laid down and other bone tissue is resorbed. Therefore, woven bone, mature bone, and areas of bone resorption are all found in adult bone tissue.

Bone develops through one of two different processes: intramembranous ossification or endochondral ossification. *Intramembranous ossification* takes place directly within mesenchyme tissue, beginning near the end of the embryonic period and proceeding rapidly. Mesenchymal cells produce an organic matrix called *osteoid*, which is composed of collagen fibers. Calcium phosphate crystals accumulate on the collagen fibers, resulting in ossification (Gould, 1990). In this process, numerous ossification centers are formed, which fuse into cancellous bone tissue. With time, some of this cancellous bone will become compact bone. The skull, carpals, tarsals, and part of the clavicle are formed by intramembranous ossification.

In *endochondral ossification*, a hyaline cartilage model of the bone is laid down first and then replaced by bone in an orderly fashion. Endochondral bone growth is seen in the long bones of the body and is the method by which bones increase in length (see Fig. 6–2). The parts of the long bone are defined as the following:

- Diaphysis—the shaft of the long bone; the portion of bone formed by the primary center of ossification
- Epiphysis—the ends of the long bone; the portions formed by secondary centers of ossification
- Epiphyseal plate—the bone's growth zone, which is composed of hyaline cartilage
- Metaphysis—the wider part of the shaft of the long bone, adjacent to the epiphyseal plate, that consists of cancellous bone during development; in adulthood, it is continuous with the epiphysis

Endochondral bone development is illustrated in Figure 6–3. Primary centers of ossification form at the center of the diaphysis. First, a bony collar is laid down around the center of the diaphysis via intramembranous ossification of the perichondrium. Cartilage cells in the central diaphysis then become hypertrophied and are destroyed. As the remaining cartilage matrix becomes calcified, the area is infiltrated by osteoblasts and capillaries. The osteoblasts lay down ossified bone matrix. Ossification proceeds toward the ends of the diaphysis. Secondary ossification centers form in the epiphysis. Ossification radiates in all directions from the secondary ossification center. Endochondral ossification is also seen in the vertebrae, as depicted in Figure 6–4.

A growth (epiphyseal) plate, composed of hyaline cartilage, is formed between the diaphyses and epiphyses. This is the site of longitudinal bone growth. Interstitial growth of the hyaline cartilage continues at the surface of the epiphysis. The new cartilage undergoes endochondral ossification in the metaphysis. As the bone approaches its adult length, chondrocyte formation slows while endochondral ossification at the metaphysis continues. The epiphyseal plate narrows and eventually closes.

Mechanical loading of the epiphyseal plate affects longitudinal bone growth. The growth plate is usually aligned perpendicular to the load that crosses it (LeVeau and Bernhardt, 1984), and formation of new bone is stimulated as tension or compression forces are applied. If the compression or tension forces are too great, they may interfere with bone growth. Unequal forces along the epiphyseal plate may stimulate a change of direction of bone growth, whereas torsional forces at the growth plate may result in rotational changes. The changes in angle of inclination between the femoral neck and shaft from approximately 135 to 145 degrees in infancy to 125 degrees in the adult and 120 degrees in the older adult provide an example of directional change in normal bone development (Bernhardt, 1988) (Fig. 6–5). The torsional changes in the femur, from retroversion prenatally to 25 to 30 degrees of anteversion at birth and 10 to 15 degrees of anteversion in the adult (Norkin and Levangie, 1992), are also illustrated in Figure 6–5. Table 6–1 summarizes some of these changes in lower extremity structure. It should also be noted that shearing forces applied across the epiphyseal plate may contribute to

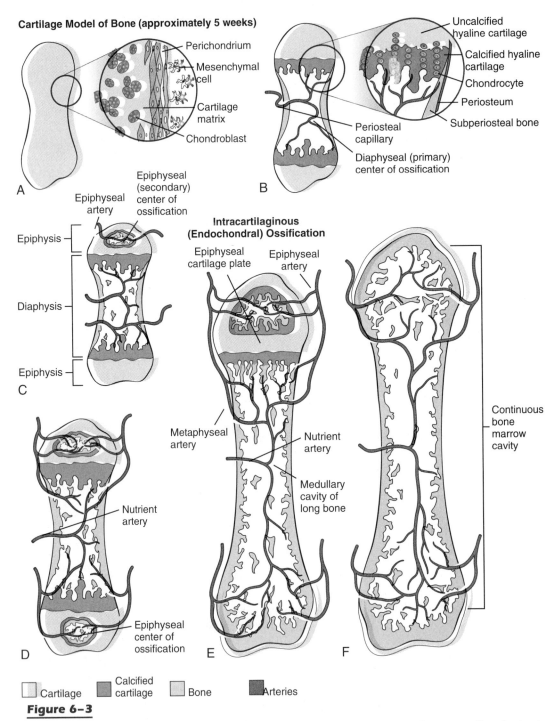

Cartilage Model of Bone (approximately 5 weeks)

Perichondrium

Mesenchymal cell

Cartilage matrix

Chondroblast

A

Uncalcified hyaline cartilage

Calcified hyaline cartilage

Chondrocyte

Periosteum

Subperiosteal bone

Periosteal capillary

Diaphyseal (primary) center of ossification

B

Epiphyseal artery

Epiphyseal (secondary) center of ossification

Epiphysis

Diaphysis

Epiphysis

C

Intracartilaginous (Endochondral) Ossification

Epiphyseal cartilage plate

Epiphyseal artery

Metaphyseal artery

Nutrient artery

Medullary cavity of long bone

Nutrient artery

Epiphyseal center of ossification

D

E

Continuous bone marrow cavity

F

Cartilage   Calcified cartilage   Bone   Arteries

Figure 6–3

Stages in endochondral ossification of a long bone. *A*, Cartilage model. *B*, Periosteal stage; cartilage begins to calcify. *C*, Vascular mesenchyme enters the calcified cartilage matrix and divides the cartilage matrix into two zones of ossification; blood vessels and mesenchyme enter the upper epiphyseal cartilage. *D*, The epiphyseal ossification center develops in the cartilage. A similar ossification center develops in the lower epiphyseal cartilage. *E*, Intracartilaginous ossification; the lower epiphyseal plate disappears. *F*, Next, the upper epiphyseal plate disappears, forming a continuous bone marrow cavity.

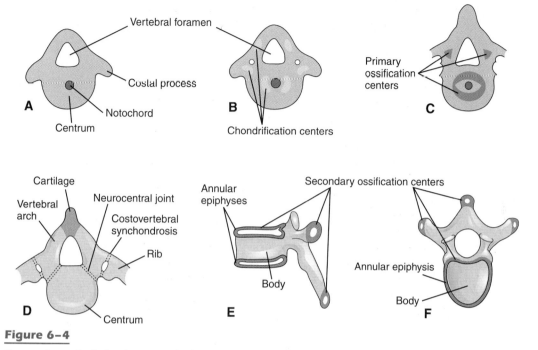

Figure 6–4

Stages of vertebral development. *A,* Precartilaginous vertebra at 5 weeks. *B,* Chondrification centers in a mesenchymal vertebra at 6 weeks. *C,* Primary ossification centers in a cartilaginous vertebra at 7 weeks. *D,* A thoracic vertebra at birth, consisting of three bony parts. Note the cartilage between the halves of the vertebral neural arch and between the arch and the centrum. *E* and *F,* Two views of a typical thoracic vertebra at puberty showing the location of the secondary centers of ossification. (From Moore KL, Persaud TVN. *The Developing Human,* 6th ed. Philadelphia: WB Saunders, 1998, p 413.)

displacement of the growth plate. Therapeutically, this is an important consideration when working with individuals whose skeleton has not reached maturity, because displacement of the epiphyseal plate interferes with normal growth.

Cartilaginous growth plates are found not only at the ends of long bones but also at points of muscular attachment, where they are called *traction epiphyses,* or *apophyses.* Muscle contraction places a traction force on the bone and stimulates bone growth. This is demonstrated at the proximal femur. Figure 6–6 reflects the effects of muscle pull on the greater trochanter and lesser trochanter of the femur. The greater trochanter has broad muscular attachments, whereas the lesser trochanter has only one muscular attachment. The traction force exerted by the muscular activity stimulates varying degrees of bone growth at these locations, helping shape the developing bone into its mature form. Muscle weakness can affect bone growth, as demonstrated in Figure 6–6, as well as bone length, which is exemplified by a 5% to 10% decrease in bone length in the affected limbs of a person with hemiplegia (Smith, 1981).

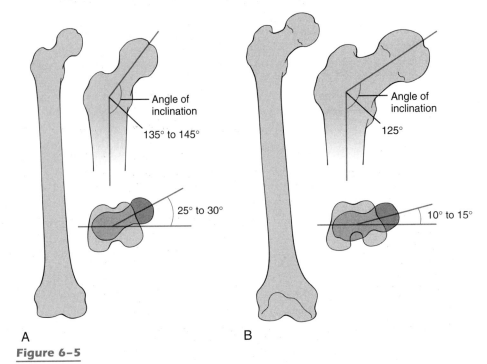

A   B

Figure 6–5

Comparison of the newborn *(A)* and adult *(B)* femoral angle of inclination *(top)* and femoral angle of torsion *(bottom)*. The enlarged views of the femoral angle or torsion show a superior perspective, looking down from the head/neck of femur to the femoral condyles.

TABLE 6–1

Developmental Changes in Lower Extremity Alignment

	Birth	**3 Years**	**Adult**
Acetabular roof	7 degrees from vertical	17 degrees from vertical	
Femur			
Angle of inclination	135–145 degrees		125%
Angle of torsion	25- to 30-degree anteversion		10- to 15-degree anteversion
Tibial torsion	5- to 10-degree internal tibial torsion		20- to 25-degree external tibial torsion
Calcaneus	22-degree varus		0- to 3-degree varus

Data from Bernhardt DB. Prenatal and postnatal growth and development of the foot and ankle. *Phys Ther* 68:1831–1839, 1988.

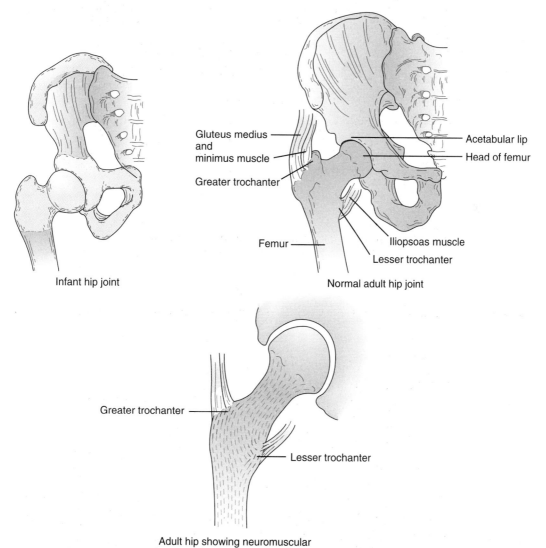

Gluteus medius
and
minimus muscle

Greater trochanter

Acetabular lip

Head of femur

Femur

Iliopsoas muscle

Lesser trochanter

Infant hip joint

Normal adult hip joint

Greater trochanter

Lesser trochanter

Adult hip showing neuromuscular
weakness and underdeveloped trochanters

Figure 6–6

The muscular attachments to an immature bone help to shape bone growth. Compared with the hip joint of a normal adult, an infant's hip joint shows neuromuscular weakness and an underdeveloped trochanter.

Bones grow not only in length but also in diameter. New bone is laid down on the outer surface of the bone and is absorbed from the inner surface, determining the thickness of bone and size of the marrow cavity within the bone. This process is called *appositional growth* and continues throughout life, but the proportion of bone formation to resorption varies. In childhood and adolescence, formation is greater than resorption, increasing bone diameter and

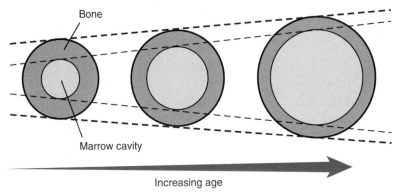

Figure 6-7

Schematic approximates the effect of appositional bone growth over time, which leads to an increase in the diameter of bone. Bone thickness decreases and the width of the marrow cavity increases because resorption is greater than production.

thickness. Throughout early and middle adulthood, equilibrium between the two processes maintains bone size. In later adult life, resorption exceeds formation, resulting in loss of bone mass. Because resorption occurs at the inner surface of the bone, the marrow cavity becomes larger and the bony shell surrounding it becomes thinner (Fig. 6-7). Muscle weakness can also affect appositional bone growth.

The ongoing reconstruction of bone tissue via resorption in some areas and subsequent formation of new bone in other areas is called *bone remodeling*. Through this process, bone achieves adult form, adapts its architecture to accommodate changes in mechanical loading, and renews its structure. Remodeling of bone improves its mechanical resilience and structural alignment. Mechanical strain, especially compression, is an important force in the bone remodeling process because it provides the stimulus for bone growth. Fibers within the bone tissue are aligned in response to mechanical stress, allowing the bone to withstand functional load bearing (Lanyon, 1989). Sufficient bone mass with optimal internal architecture is necessary to meet the demands of everyday life.

Because bone serves as the storage site for calcium, serum calcium levels will also affect bone remodeling. As the concentration of calcium in the blood changes, calcium in the bone is accessed through one of two processes. In the first process, calcium is quickly transferred into or out of younger, less-calcified lamellae, adjusting to food intake or functional demands of the body. The second process is slower and depends on stimulation of calcium-regulating hormones. Parathyroid hormone is released when blood calcium levels drop. This hormone activates osteoclasts to begin resorption of bone matrix, which releases the calcium stores in well-established bone matrix. Calcitonin, another thyroid hormone, is released as blood calcium levels increase, inhibiting resorption.

Bone is an adaptable tissue, responding to hormonal demands and the mechanical stresses placed on it. To maintain bone mass and architecture, a balance must be achieved between these two processes. Good nutrition and exercise are important throughout the life span to build and maintain maximal bone mass and structural competence of the skeleton. Although research findings have been conflicting, many studies of the effect of exercise on bone mass suggest that increased functional loading results in increased bone mass, whereas decreased functional loading results in bone loss (Bouxsein and Marcus, 1994; Lanyon, 1989, 1996; Welten et al, 1994).

Aging

As discussed, adaptation of bone through remodeling continues throughout life. Skeletal maturity, however, as measured by closure of the epiphyseal plate, occurs within the first two decades of life. *Maximal bone mass*, which is the total bone growth in length and thickness, is obtained during the late 20s or early 30s (Anderson, 1996; Duncan and Parfitt, 1984; Welten et al, 1994). Between the ages of 35 and 40 years, bone resorption can begin to exceed bone formation (Thibodeau and Patton, 1999). Bone loss appears to vary between racial groups and with gender. Although such loss appears to be less severe in black adults than it is in white adults, this may be reflective of the greater bone mass attained during the bone growth of blacks (Parfitt, 1997). Women also appear to begin losing bone mass earlier than do men (Duncan and Parfitt, 1984). A decrease in mass eventually results in a more fragile bone, which is less able to withstand mechanical forces such as compression and bending.

Other changes involved in the aging of bone include cross-linkage, architectural rearrangement of collagen fibers, and excessive mineralization of trabecular bone. Fibrils are arranged more longitudinally. Osteons become shorter and narrower as the haversian canals become wider. Excessive mineralization of bone occurs as bone matrix deteriorates, because as the bone becomes more porous, more sites for mineral deposition are provided (Klein and Rajan, 1984). These changes increase the brittleness of bone and compromise its ability to withstand mechanical loads.

Throughout life, the body must maintain the necessary serum calcium level. Intestinal absorption of calcium declines with age, increasing the amount of calcium that must be retrieved from bone to meet the needs of the body. As a result, bone mass is gradually lost because bone resorption frequently occurs faster than new bone can be formed. The loss of bone tissue during remodeling leaves the bone thinner and more susceptible to injury. The increased brittleness due to internal changes in bone structure also increases the risk of fracture.

JOINTS

The joints provide the functional connection between bones. The primary purpose of most joints is to enable a wide range of movement. Within the joint,

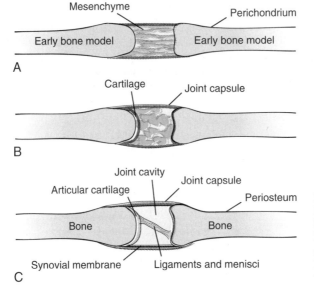

Figure 6–8

Development of synovial joints. *A*, Mesenchyme collects in the space between early bone models. *B*, Differentiation of mesenchyme into cartilage and joint capsule. Beginning of cavitation. *C*, Formation of joint cavity and structure.

bones can be connected by ligaments, tendons, muscles, other connective tissue structures, and the joint capsule. Two types of joints are found in the mature skeletal system: synarthroses and diarthroses.

Synarthrosis joints allow minimal to no movement and provide areas of stability to the skeleton. The sutures of the skull and tibular-fibular joint are examples of this type of joint. The articulation between the bones consists of connective tissue, which may be replaced by bone during aging.

Diarthrosis joints allow movement. The joint capsule functionally connects two adjoining bones to form a cavity that is filled with synovial fluid, which bathes the joint surfaces with nutrition and provides a cushion between the bones (Fig. 6–8). Diarthrodial joints are found in several shapes and sizes; their shape and form help define the type of movement that can be produced at the joint. For example, hinge joints, such as the elbow, allow movement in one axis only, whereas a ball-and-socket type of joint, such as the hip, allows a wide range of motion in multiple axes.

Skeletal System Development

Skeletal system development follows a pattern of maturation that begins before birth and continues through the last decades of life.

PRENATAL PERIOD

As discussed earlier, bone and cartilage are differentiated from the mesoderm layer early in the gestational period. Development of bone, via either intramembranous or endochondral ossification, begins in the embryonic period (third to eighth gestational weeks). By the fifth week of gestation, mesenchymal models of bones appear in the extremities, with upper extremity development preceding lower extremity development. In the sixth week, mesenchymal cells have differentiated into chondroblasts, which form the cartilage model of the long bones. Primary centers of ossification appear as early as the seventh to eighth week (Fig. 6–9); by the 12th week of gestation, they have appeared in almost all bones of the extremities (Moore and Persaud, 1998). The diaphyses are fairly well ossified by birth, but the epiphyses remain cartilaginous. A few secondary ossification centers begin to appear late in fetal development (Figs. 6–9 and 6–10).

Vertebral development also begins in the embryonic period. Cartilage models of the vertebrae are formed from mesenchymal cells located around the notochord. By the seventh to eighth gestational week, three ossification centers have formed in the vertebrae model. These bony parts remain connected by cartilage at birth (Moore and Persaud, 1998) (see Fig. 6–4).

After the early models of bone are present, joint formation occurs, and by the early fetal period, most joints have been formed. In articular joints, mesenchyme differentiates into the joint capsule, ligaments, tendons, and menisci. Depressions then begin to form in the mesenchyme, resulting in formation of the joint cavity and bursae (see Figs. 6–8 and 6–9). Once the joint is formed, intrauterine movement is important for ongoing joint development.

The confined intrauterine environment in the later weeks of gestation limits the positioning options of the fetus and applies forces to the fetal skeletal system. Intrauterine molding of the developing skeletal system can occur and results in deformities such as congenital hip dislocation, tibial bowing, metatarsus adductus, calcaneus varus, and extreme ankle dorsiflexion. Some of these deformities will spontaneously improve in the first few years of life. Others, such as congenital hip dislocation, require early orthopedic management, applying corrective mechanical forces to the skeleton during infancy (Hensinger and Jones, 1982).

Functionally, early intramembranous ossification of the skull serves to protect the developing brain. The bones of the skull are not fused, as evidenced by the "soft spots," called *fontanelles*. Expansion and molding of the cranium accommodate brain growth. The lack of fusion of the bones of the skull also allows adaptation of the cranium to the intrauterine environment and passage through the birth canal.

INFANCY AND CHILDHOOD

Infancy and childhood are times of bone growth, modeling, and remodeling. Bone mineral content increases more before puberty than at any other time in life. Children attain 50% of their peak bone mass by 10 years of age and an additional 40% by age 20 (Anderson, 1996). As mentioned, the diaphyses of the long bones are fairly well ossified at birth. Secondary ossification centers in the epiphyses continue to appear through adolescence (see Fig. 6–9). Through-

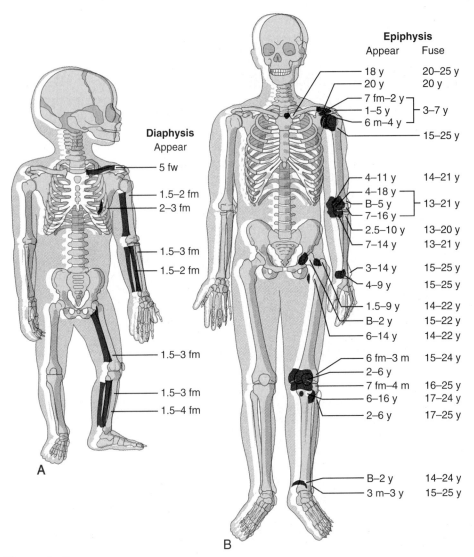

Figure 6-9

Appearance of primary and secondary ossification centers. *A*, Appearance of diaphyses. *B*, Appearance and fusion of epiphyses. fw, fetal weeks; fm, fetal months; m, postnatal months; y, years; B, birth. (Modified from Anson B. *Morris Human Anatomy*, 12th ed. New York: McGraw-Hill, 1966.)

out infancy and early childhood, bone growth occurs rapidly. Factors such as genetic makeup, nutrition, general health, and hormonal levels affect the rate of bone growth and time of appearance of the secondary ossification centers (Hensinger and Jones, 1981). Physical activity has also been demonstrated to increase bone mineral content and bone mineral density in prepubertal children (Bradney et al, 1998; Cooper et al, 1995; Courteix et al, 1998).

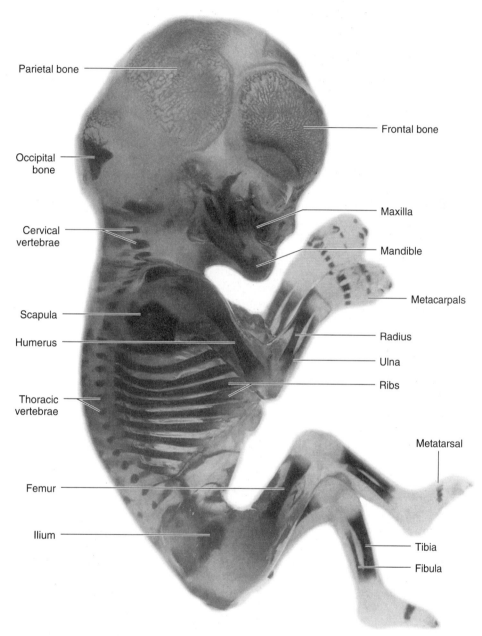

Figure 6–10

Electron micrograph of 12-week human fetus shows the progression of ossification from the primary centers that are endochondral in the appendicular and axial parts of the skeleton except for most of the cranial bones. (From Moore KL, Persaud TVN. *Before We Are Born: Essentials of Embryology and Birth Defects*, 5th ed. Philadelphia: WB Saunders, 1998, p 395. [Courtesy of Dr. Gary Geddes, Lake Oswego, Oregon])

Dynamic Bone Growth

The dynamic quality of bone growth contributes to the spontaneous correction of skeletal abnormalities and the responsiveness to orthopedic treatment seen in children. The infant born with congenital bony deformities, such as metatarsus adductus or club foot, may benefit greatly from early orthopedic intervention. Corrective forces can be applied with casting or taping procedures to correct bony alignment. Bleck (1982) reports that all except 5% to 15% of childhood lower extremity deformities resolve spontaneously. Abnormal skeletal development also occurs if unbalanced muscle action around a joint is present, as in cerebral palsy or spina bifida. For example, bone growth will proceed in response to the strong adduction and internal rotation forces exerted by muscles at the hip of the child with cerebral palsy. This abnormal force interferes with normal development of the acetabulum, femoral torsion, and the femoral neck/shaft angle. The hip can become unstable, and the risk for dislocation is increased.

The epiphysis is an active site for new bone formation and plays an important role in early skeletal development. During periods of rapid growth, forces acting on the epiphysis can have dramatic effects. Injury or infection to the epiphysis can result in abnormal bone growth and limb length deficiencies (Hensinger and Jones, 1982). The newborn infant is especially susceptible to infection of the epiphysis because the epiphyseal plate is very thin at this age and does not provide a significant barrier between the metaphysis and the epiphysis. Blood vessels easily cross the growth plate, allowing infection to be spread from the metaphysis to the epiphysis. As the epiphyseal plate becomes thicker, the blood vessels can no longer cross it, eliminating the possibility for transmission of infection. Fractures of the epiphyseal plate will interfere with bone growth patterns, resulting in asymmetric bone growth or the cessation of growth.

Structural differences between growing and adult bone make children more susceptible to injuries such as plastic deformation of the bone, greenstick fractures, and apophyseal avulsion (avulsion of muscle tendon from its insertion) (Wojtys, 1987). In general, growing bone is less dense and more porous than adult bone. As a result, it is more sensitive to both compressive and tensile stress. The cortex of the metaphysis is also thinner than that of the diaphysis, making it less resistant to compressive forces. The periosteum, however, is thicker than in adult bone and less readily torn, resulting in less displaced fractures.

Areas of Bone Growth

The head and trunk of the newborn infant make up a proportionately larger part of the total skeleton than in the adult. During childhood, the growth of the axial skeleton does not contribute as much to a child's increasing height as does the growth of the lower extremities.

The lower extremities and pelvis undergo angular, rotational, and length changes as the infant learns to move. At birth, the ilia and sacrum are more upright than they are in the adult. Once the infant starts walking, the curvature of the sacrum increases, the ilia thicken, and the acetabular depth increases (Sinclair and Dangerfield, 1998). The acetabular roof rotates from a relatively vertical position to one of more forward inclination (Bernhardt, 1988). Bernhardt describes changes throughout the developing lower extremity (see Table 6–1). The femoral angle of inclination decreases (see Fig. 6–5), creating a better lever arm for force production of the hip abductors. The femoral angle of torsion also changes (see Fig. 6–5), decreasing the amount of anteversion from birth to adulthood. Different rates of growth in the three epiphyseal zones of the proximal femur contribute to the angular and rotational changes of the bone (Bernhardt, 1988). By 8 years of age, the proximal femur has attained its adult form (Ogden, 1983).

Angular and torsional changes also take place in the tibia and ankle/foot complex. External tibial torsion increases from the newborn period to adulthood. The relationship between the femur and tibia changes from a position of bow legs (genu varum) in infancy to one of knock knees (genu valgus) by 3 years of age. The degree of valgus then decreases to normal adult values. The newborn's foot also is in a position of varus at the calcaneus and forefoot, which slowly decreases until adult values are reached. Slight forefoot varus may persist until 2 years of age. Weight bearing and the torsional forces of muscles actively contracting during creeping (four-point), standing, and walking contribute to these changes.

Not only does the lower extremity skeleton undergo transformation as the infant develops functional movement skills, but also changes are seen in the spine. In the newborn, the anteroposterior spinal curve is relatively concave. The cervical lordosis is present at birth, possibly because of early ossification of the occipital bone, but it becomes more evident by 3 months of age, when the infant has developed head control. The lumbar lordosis develops as the infant learns to sit. Iliopsoas tightness from fetal positioning combined with antigravity work in prone, four-point, and kneeling positions may contribute to development of the lumbar lordosis (LeVeau and Bernhardt, 1984; Walker, 1991). Orthopedic management of spinal deformities, such as scoliosis and kyphosis, can be achieved by bracing the immature skeleton.

ADOLESCENCE

During adolescence, bone continues to grow and remodel in response to mechanical loading stresses. Physical activity and body weight have been shown to increase bone mineral density and to influence peak bone mass in adolescence (Welten et al, 1994). Adequate caloric and calcium intake contributes to the growth of bone, formation of bone matrix, and bone mineralization (Barr and McKay, 1998). The adolescent experiences sudden increases in height and weight, with growth of the trunk exceeding the lower extremities. The adolescent growth spurt of girls begins at an average of 12 to 13 years of age, preceding that of boys by approximately 2 years. A growth spurt in bone width is seen through adolescence in boys and up to age 14 in girls. The width of the bone cortex increases in both boys and girls, but boys also demonstrate an increase in width of the central marrow cavity (Malina and Bouchard, 1991). Rapid bone growth frequently outpaces increases in muscle length, resulting in decreased flexibility. Injuries can result if adolescents do not modify their activities to accommodate these changes in flexibility.

Vulnerability of the Skeletal System

Skeletal system problems such as scoliosis often become obvious and may progress rapidly during adolescence. Mild scoliosis of 5 degrees or less is seen in 10% of children during puberty; boys and girls are equally represented. Only a small percentage of scoliotic curves progress to greater than 15 degrees (Staheli, 1983).

The rapid growth spurt seen during adolescence increases the vulnerability of the open epiphysis. The epiphysis is less stable than the joints, making epiphyseal injury likely when the joint area is involved. Apparent joint sprains in this age group should be critically evaluated to rule out involvement of the epiphysis.

Stress fractures and apophyseal avulsion fractures are also seen, especially in the adolescent athlete when activity or training level changes. These injuries are related to overuse and stress on the system beyond the ability for self-repair. Common sites for stress fracture in the adolescent are the lumbar spine, tibia, and fibula. Gymnasts or individuals performing repetitive activities that place an axial load on an extended spine are at risk for lumbar spondylolysis, a stress fracture of the pars interarticularis (Smith, 1988). Long distance runners frequently present with fractures at the tibia or fibula (Wojtys, 1987).

Apophyseal avulsion fractures occur when traction forces are applied at the apophysis and it is pulled away from the bone. Common sites for avulsion fractures are the anterior superior iliac spine, anterior inferior iliac spine, lesser trochanter, and ischium (Smith, 1988). Osgood-Schlatter disease may also be associated with avulsion of the apophysis at the tibial tuberosity after a traction injury. The definite cause of this disease is unknown, but it affects adolescent boys (10 to 15 years of age) and girls (8 to 13 years of age) (Wojtys, 1987). Physical conditioning programs, thorough preseason screening examinations, and appropriate supervision during athletic activities are important to prevent these stress-related injuries.

Cartilage injury can also be seen in adolescence. Chondromalacia of the patella, with softening and fibrillation of the cartilage, results from stress on the kneecap. Rotational or angular malalignment of the patella is usually seen. Restriction of overactivity allows the cartilage to repair itself.

Attainment of Skeletal Maturity

Skeletal maturity is attained when the epiphyseal plates close. Epiphyseal closure begins in childhood and is usually complete by 25 years of age (see Fig. 6–9). Fusion of the vertebral arches is seen in the cervical spine in the first year of life and in the lumbar spine by 6 years of life. Fusion of the vertebral arch and centrum occurs between 5 and 8 years of age. Secondary centers of ossification in the vertebrae do not unite until the 25th year (Moore and Persaud, 1998). Fusion of the epiphyses occurs earlier in girls than in boys and has been linked to the fact that estrogen levels are higher in girls than in boys (Cutler, 1997).

ADULTHOOD

After the epiphyses have closed, the bones no longer lengthen. Throughout adulthood, only bone remodeling occurs. Weight bearing and muscle contraction continue to stimulate bone remodeling and to increase bone density (Whitbourne, 1985). Adequate nutritional and calcium intake also supports appropriate mineralization of the remodeled bone. Both men and women attain their maximal bone mass by their late 20s or early 30s; the last 10% of peak bone mass is attained in early adulthood (Anderson, 1996). Bone formation and resorption remain balanced until 35 to 40 years of age (LeVeau and Bernhardt, 1984; Martin and Brown, 1989). After that time, bone loss is greater than bone replacement. In the adult skeleton, cortical bone loss has been reported to begin in the fourth decade and cancellous bone loss to begin in the third decade of life (Borner et al, 1988).

Several different estimates of the amount of bone loss with aging are reported in the literature. Raab and Smith (1985) estimate that women lose 1% of bone mass per year before menopause. For the 4 to 5 years after menopause, 2% to 4% of bone mass per year is lost. After this time, the rate of loss returns to 1% per year. Men are reported to lose 0.5% of bone mass per year. This loss translates into a decline in bone strength, which increases the risk for spontaneous fractures and functional motor deficits.

Fibrous cartilage changes also become apparent in adulthood as the intervertebral disk loses water. The nucleus pulposus is primarily affected; most water content is lost in the second to fourth decades of life. Water loss continues slowly in older adulthood, during which the annulus fibrosus also undergoes fibrotic changes. The intervertebral disk becomes flattened and less resilient. Considering the early changes in the disk, it is not surprising that the highest incidence of back pain is reported between the ages of 30 and 50 years (Koeller et al, 1986; Lewis and Bottomley, 1996).

OLDER ADULTHOOD

With aging, the skeletal system becomes progressively more compromised. Loss of bone mass continues in older adulthood and can be related to osteopenia, osteomalacia, or osteoporosis. *Osteopenia* occurs when either organic or inorganic components of bone fail to develop. *Osteomalacia* refers to abnormal mineralization of the bone matrix due to calcium and phosphate deficiencies. It affects both recently formed and well-established bone, decreasing the amount of mineral per unit of bone matrix. *Osteoporosis* refers a reduction in bone mass due to decreased formation of new bone or increased resorption while bone chemistry is normal. Age-related bone loss may be related to hormonal

TABLE 6–2

Age-Related Skeletal System Concerns Related to Physical Activity

Age Period	Skeletal System Concern
Prenatal	Intrauterine molding late in gestation
Newborn	Epiphyseal infection
Childhood	Epiphyseal injury
	Apophyseal avulsion
	Greenstick fracture
Adolescence	Scoliosis
	Epiphyseal injury
	Apophyseal avulsion
	Stress fracture
Adulthood	Back pain secondary to disk changes
Older adulthood	Osteoporosis
	Osteoarthritis

changes, dietary changes, and the decreased activity level of older adults, which limits both the mechanical loading of bone and circulation. Decreased estrogen levels decrease both bone production and the intestinal absorption of calcium. Vitamin D metabolism is also affected by decreased levels of calcitonin. In addition, the diet may contain lower amounts of calcium, vitamins, and minerals (Spirduso, 1995). Borner and colleagues (1988), Bouxsein and Marcus (1994), MacKinnon (1988), and Pickles (1989) examined studies that reported the effects of continued weight-bearing activities on bone density and conclude that physical activity can help to maintain bone density. Continued functional loading of the skeletal system appears to help balance bone formation and resorption. Site-specific increases in bone mineral density have been demonstrated in older adults participating in exercise programs (Bravo et al, 1996; Prior et al, 1996).

Functional Implications of Skeletal System Changes

Changes in the skeletal system affect its effectiveness at all age levels, requiring special concern with relation to functional activities (Table 6–2). Osteoporosis and osteoarthritis are common problems for older adults. When we, as therapists, understand the processes underlying these two disorders, we can develop individualized prevention programs that will help limit the functional losses experienced by older adults (see Clinical Implications: Osteoporosis Prevention—A Lifelong Process).

OSTEOPOROSIS

Osteoporosis due to the progressive loss of bone mass with aging is referred to as *senile*, or *involutional*, *osteoporosis*. Pathologic conditions such as poor nutri-

CLINICAL IMPLICATIONS
Osteoporosis Prevention—A Lifelong Process

Osteoporosis is a common, costly condition of older adults that results in bone fracture, pain, and disability. The best way to prevent or minimize risk for osteoporosis is to maximize the amount of bone tissue present in adulthood. Peak bone mass is attained in young adulthood and can be enhanced by several factors throughout childhood. These factors include dietary intake of adequate amounts of calories, calcium, and vitamin D; physical activities that provide weight bearing and mechanical strain stimuli to the bone and muscle; and maintenance of appropriate body weight. Research has shown that the effects of increased physical activity and calcium supplementation in increasing bone mineral concentration and bone mineral density are greatest in prepubertal children (Anderson, 1996; Barr and McCay, 1998; Copper et al, 1995; Courteix et al, 1998; Snow, 1996; Welten et al, 1994). For this reason, it is important to begin preventative measures for osteoporosis early. Such programs should continue across the life span. Health care providers can guide their patients of all ages to the most effective methods that will optimize bone growth and minimize the risk of osteoporosis.

Osteoporosis prevention strategies for individuals of all ages include the following:

- Participation in a variety of diverse movement activities that provide different patterns of mechanical strain; high-strain activities have been associated with the greatest gains in bone density (Lanyon, 1996)
- Participation in weight-bearing exercise
- Regular, ongoing physical activity that begins in childhood and continues throughout adulthood; daily participation is best for skeletal health, but positive effects have been seen with participation several times per week
- Exercise that increases strength, flexibility, and coordination; muscle strength gains positively influence bone density (Snow, 1996), and improved flexibility and coordination also decrease the likelihood of falls in older adults
- Eating a well-balanced diet to support the energy demands of the growing body and to provide appropriate vitamins and minerals for bone growth and maintenance
- Intake of appropriate levels of calcium from the diet to enhance mineralization of the developing bone and to maintain appropriate levels of blood calcium
- Maintaining optimal body weight; increased body weight, especially of lean muscle mass has been associated with increased bone mass (Snow, 1996)
- Ensuring optimal hormonal function; periods of amenorrhea should be avoided and delayed puberty should be managed medically; appropriate levels of estrogen are necessary to trigger the adolescent growth spurt and to optimize bone growth; in postmenopausal women, hormonal replacement therapy may be recommended to minimize the amount of bone lost when estrogen levels diminish in the body
- Avoiding periods of immobilization when bone density is rapidly lost

tion, metabolic disorders, neoplasm, and hormonal influences can also be related to the development of osteoporosis. Physical inactivity related to aging, long periods of bedrest, and exposure to weightless environments have been identified as factors that contribute to osteoporosis. The individual most at risk for the development of osteoporosis is the slightly built, sedentary white woman.

The clinical features of osteoporosis are pain, loss of height, kyphosis, and decreased function, because bone is unable to withstand the compression forces of weight bearing. MacKinnon (1988) reports that 40% of normal bone strength should be adequate to withstand normal mechanical loading. When the amount of bone mass is no longer sufficient to support the body during activity, spontaneous fracture may result (Fig. 6–11). The most frequent sites for spontaneous fracture secondary to osteoporosis are the spine, proximal femur, and wrist. Anterior compression fractures of the vertebrae result in wedge-shaped vertebrae and lead to kyphotic posturing. Central collapse of adjacent vertebra lead to fish-shaped vertebrae, decreasing the disk space and skeletal height. In general, the microfractures related to osteoporosis cause pain and lead to a flexed posture. No specific criteria exist for the diagnosis of osteoporosis. Generally, when bone mass content falls below 2 standard deviations of the mean bone mass content for young normal adults, osteoporosis is present (Borner et al, 1988).

Two categories of involutional osteoporosis exist. One category, related to decreased intestinal absorption of calcium, occurs in both men and women and affects both cortical and cancellous bone. For these individuals, clinical management with dietary calcium is reportedly beneficial (Kauffman, 1987). However, Borner and colleagues (1988) review other studies that question the effectiveness of calcium supplementation. The second category of involutional osteoporosis is associated with menopause and affects primarily cancellous

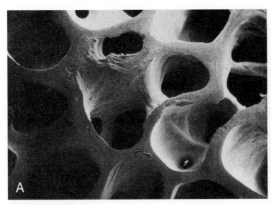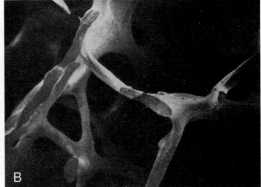

Figure 6–11

Electron micrograph of normal (A) and osteoporotic (B) bone. (Dempster DW, Shane E, Horbert W, Lindsay R. A simple method for corrective light and scanning electron microscopy of human iliac crest bone biopsies. Reproduced from *J Bone Miner Res* 1:16–21, 1986, with permission of the American Society of Bone and Mineral Research.)

bone. When estrogen secretion decreases with menopause, the bone is thought to become more sensitive to parathyroid hormone, increasing the rate of bone resorption (MacKinnon, 1988). Calcium and fluoride supplements combined with estrogen therapy are of some value for women with this type of osteoporosis (Borner et al, 1988).

Good nutrition and a lifelong commitment to exercise may influence the maximal bone mass attained in early adulthood and maintenance of that bone mass. Exercise programs may effectively slow or prevent the bone loss associated with aging or even increase the bone mass (Borner et al, 1988; Bouxsein and Marcus, 1994; Bravo et al, 1996; MacKinnon, 1988; Martin and Brown, 1989; Prior et al, 1996). In the planning of exercise programs, weight-bearing and strengthening activities should be included. Weight-bearing activities such as walking and running provide mechanical loading to the bones of the lower extremities and spine. Twisting, explosive, and staccato movements should be avoided because of the forces they place on bone tissue. Spinal extension exercises should be emphasized because flexion exercises may be problematic, contributing to anterior wedging and compression fractures of the vertebrae (MacKinnon, 1988). Although previous studies emphasized the need for weight-bearing activities, one study reported increased vertebral and radial bone density in male swimmers compared with their peers who did not exercise. No differences were noted between female swimmers and nonexercisers (Orwoll et al, 1989).

OSTEOARTHRITIS

Osteoarthritis refers to the degeneration of articular cartilage with age. It affects 70% of people at some point in their life and most adults older than 70 years (Gradisar and Porterfield, 1989). The cartilage thins, and clefts and cracks form, leaving the surface uneven and unable to efficiently provide frictionless joint motion. Underlying bone, which is innervated, becomes exposed to mechanical stress, resulting in pain. Bony spurs or outgrowths covered with hyaline cartilage may also develop in the joint. The individual with osteoarthritis experiences pain with movement and limited range of motion.

Treatment for osteoarthritis is limited to the protection of affected joints from undue stress, minimization of joint range-of-motion limitations, and relief of pain. Anti-inflammatory medications offer some relief. Weight loss in overweight individuals will also help decrease pain by lessening the loading of the joint. Individuals with osteoarthritis benefit from participation in exercise programs that emphasize balanced loading of the joint surface. The exercises should address improvement in muscle strength, preservation of joint range of motion, and improved efficiency when performing everyday tasks so that loading forces on the cartilage are equalized (Kauffman, 1989). Prolonged jogging or impact exercises should be avoided, because they put high loads on the cartilage and may increase tissue destruction. When conservative treatment approaches do not relieve symptoms, surgical débridement of the joint surface or joint replacement is considered.

Summary

Cartilage, bones, and joints are the essential components of the skeletal system that develop over a lifetime and have the capacity to increase or limit physical ability to function. Together, these elements provide a structural base on which movement can take place. Optimal, healthy development of the skeletal system depends not only on genetics and nutrition but also on an active lifestyle. The mechanical stresses of everyday functional activities and exercise help the system achieve its most efficient form and maintain its stability. Lifelong commitment to good nutrition and exercise helps the attainment of maximal bone mass and maintenance of a strong skeletal system well into older adulthood.

References

Anderson J. Calcium, phosphorus, and human bone development. *J Nutr* 126:1153S–1158S, 1996.

Barr SI, McKay HA. Nutrition, exercise and bone status in youth. *Int J Sports Nutr* 8:124–142, 1998.

Bernhardt DB. Prenatal and postnatal growth and development of the foot and ankle. *Phys Ther* 68: 1831–1839, 1988.

Bleck EE. Developmental orthopedics, III: Toddlers. *Dev Med Child Neurol* 24:533–555, 1982.

Borner JA, Dillworth BB, Sullivan KM. Exercise and osteoporosis: A critique of the literature. *Physiother Can* 40:146–155, 1988.

Bouxsein MS, Marcus R. Overview of exercise and bone mass. *Rheum Dis Clin North Am* 20:787–802, 1994.

Bradney M, Pearce G, Naughton G, et al. Moderate exercise during growth in prepubertal boys: Changes in bone mass, size, volumetric density and bone strength—A controlled prospective study. *J Bone Miner Res* 13:1814–1821, 1998.

Bravo G, Gauthier P, Roy PM, et al. Impact of a 12-month exercise program on the physical and psychological health of osteopenic women. *J Am Geriar Soc* 44:756–762, 1996.

Cooper C, Cawley M, Bhalla A, et al. Childhood growth, physical activity and peak bone mass in women. *J Bone Miner Res* 10:940–947, 1995.

Courteix D, Lespessailles E, Peres SL, et al. Effect of physical training on bone mineral density in prepubertal girls: A comparative study between impact-loading and nonimpact-loading sports. *Osteoporosis Int* 8:152–158, 1998.

Cutler GB. The role of estrogen in bone growth and maturation during childhood and adolescence. *J Steroid Biochem Mol Biol* 61(3–6):141–147, 1997.

Duncan H, Parfitt AM. The biology of aging bone. In Nelson CL, Dwyer AP (eds). *The Aging Musculoskeletal System-Physiologic and Pathological Problems.* Lexington, MA: DC Heath, 1984.

Gould JA III. *Orthopedic and Sport Physical Therapy,* 2nd ed. St. Louis: Mosby, 1990.

Gradisar IA, Porterfield JA. Articular cartilage: Structure and function. *Top Geriatr Rehabil* 4:1–9, 1989.

Guccione AA. *Geriatric Physical Therapy,* 2nd ed. St. Louis: Mosby, 2000.

Guyton AC, Hall JE. *Human Physiology and Mechanisms of Disease,* 6th ed. Philadelphia: WB Saunders, 1997.

Hensinger RN, Jones ET. *Neonatal Orthopedics.* New York: Grune & Stratton, 1981.

Hensinger RN, Jones ET. Developmental orthopedics, I: The lower limb. *Dev Med Child Neurol* 24: 95–116, 1982.

Kauffman T. Posture and age. *Top Geriatr Rehabil* 2:13–28, 1987.

Kauffman TE. *Geriatric Rehabilitation Manual.* New York: Churchill Livingstone, 1999.

Klein L, Rajan JC. The biology of aging human collagen. In Nelson CL, Dwyer AP (eds). *The Aging Musculoskeletal System—Physiologic and Pathological Problems.* Lexington, MA: DC Heath, 1984.

Koeller W, Muehlhaus S, Meier W, Hartmann F. Biomechanical properties of human intervertebral discs subjected to axial dynamic compression—Influence of age and degeneration. *J Biomech* 19:807–816, 1986.

Lanyon LE. Strain related bone modeling and remodeling. *Top Geriatr Rehabil* 413–24, 1989.

Lanyon LE. Using functional loading to influence bone mass and architecture objectives, mechanisms, and relationship with estrogen of the mechanically adaptive process in bone. *Bone* 18(suppl):37S–43S, 1996.

LeVeau BF, Bernhardt DB. Developmental biomechanics. *Phys Ther* 64:1874–1882, 1984.

Lewis CB, Bottomley JM. Musculoskeletal changes with age: Clinical implications. In Lewis CB (ed). *Aging, the health care challenge: An interdisciplinary approach to assessment and rehabilitation management of older adults*, 3rd ed. Philadelphia: FA Davis, 1996.

MacKinnon JL. Osteoporosis—A review. *Phys Ther* 68:1533–1540, 1988.

Malina RM, Bouchard C. *Growth, Maturation and Physical Activity*. Champaign, IL: Human Kinetics, 1991.

Martin AD, Brown E. The effects of physical activity on the human skeleton. *Top Geriatr Rehabil* 4: 25–35, 1989.

Moore KL, Persaud TVN. *The Developing Human: Clinically Oriented Embryology*, 6th ed. Philadelphia: WB Saunders, 1998.

Norkin C, Levangie P. *Joint Structure and Function: A Comprehensive Analysis*, 2nd ed. Philadelphia: FA Davis, 1992.

Ogden JA. Development and growth of the hip. In Katz JF, Siffert RS (eds). *Management of Hip Disorders in Children*. Philadelphia: JB Lippincott, 1983.

Orwoll ES, Ferar J, Oviatt SK, et al. The relationship of swimming exercise to bone mass in men and women. *Arch Intern Med* 149:2197–2200, 1989.

Parfitt AM. Genetic effects on bone mass and turnover: Relevance to black/white differences. *J Am Coll Nutr* 16:325–333, 1997.

Pickles B. Biological aspects of aging. In Jackson O (ed). *Physical Therapy of the Geriatric Patient*, 2nd ed. New York: Churchill Livingston, 1989, pp 27–76.

Prior JC, Barr SI, Chow R, Faulkner RA. Physical activity as therapy for osteoporosis. *Can Med Assoc J* 155:940–944, 1996.

Raab DM, Smith EL. Exercise and aging: Effects on bone. *Top Geriatr Rehabil* 1:31–39, 1985.

Ryan AJ. The role of viscosity in injury prevention. In Ryan AJ and Allman FL (eds). *Sports Medicine*, 2nd ed. San Diego: Academic Press, 1989.

Sinclair D, Dangerfield P. *Human Growth After Birth*, 6th ed. New York: Oxford University Press, 1998.

Smith AD. Children and sports. In Scoles P (ed). *Pediatric Orthopedics in Clinical Practice*, 2nd ed. Chicago: Year Book, 1988.

Smith DW. Recognizable patterns of human deformation: Identification and management of mechanical effects on morphogenesis. *Major Probl Clin Pediatr* 21:1–151, 1981.

Snow CM. Exercise and bone mass in young and premenopausal women. *Bone* 18(suppl):51S–55S, 1996.

Spirduso WW. *Physical Dimensions of Aging*. Champaign, IL: Human Kinetics, 1995.

Staheli LT. Orthopedics in adolescence. *Dev Med Child Neurol* 25:806–818, 1983.

Thibodeau GA, Patton KT. *Anatomy and Physiology*, 4th ed. St. Louis: Mosby, 1999.

VanderWeil CJ. Chemistry and biochemistry of cartilage and synovial fluid. In Wilson FC (ed). *The Musculoskeletal System—Basic Processes and Disorders*, 2nd ed. Philadelphia: JB Lippincott, 1983.

Walker J. Musculoskeletal development: A review. *Phys Ther* 71:878–889, 1991.

Welten DC, Kemper HC, Post GB, et al. Weight-bearing activity during youth is a more important factor for peak bone mass than calcium intake. *J Bone Miner Res* 9:1089–1096, 1994.

Whitbourne SK. *The Aging Body—Physiological Changes and Psychological Consequences*. New York: Springer-Verlag, 1985.

Wojtys EM. Sports injuries in the immature athlete. *Orthop Clin North Am* 18:689–708, 1987.

Suzanne "Tink" Martin
Patricia A. Wilder

Chapter

7 Muscle System Changes

OBJECTIVES

After studying this chapter, the reader will be able to:

1 Define the basic characteristics of skeletal muscle morphology and organization.

2 Describe the basic physiology of skeletal muscle contraction.

3 Discuss the development changes in skeletal muscle across the life span.

4 Identify the functional implications of age-related changes in skeletal muscles.

Muscle is the largest tissue mass in the body. There are three types of muscles: voluntary (skeletal), involuntary (smooth), and cardiac. These three types of muscle are further divided into two subtypes of muscle: striated and nonstriated. Smooth muscle is the single example of the nonstriated type and is found in the walls of the digestive system, urinary bladder, and blood vessels. Smooth muscle contraction in these structures decreases their diameter. The cells are 10 to 600 μm in length and 2 to 12 μm in diameter. They are spindle shaped and have a single, centrally placed nucleus.

Cardiac and skeletal muscles are composed of striated muscle. Cardiac muscle is a special form of striated muscle found only in the heart. Its arrangement of contractile proteins is identical to that of skeletal muscle, but the arrangement of fibers is different. Cardiac cells are joined together by specialized intercellular junctions that are visible in the light microscope as dark heavy lines between the cells. The cells are irregularly shaped and usually contain a single, centrally placed nucleus.

Skeletal muscle, the focus of this chapter, is generally considered the main energy-consuming tissue of the body and provides the propulsive force to move about and to perform physical activities. Skeletal muscle is also known as voluntary, striated, striped, or segmental muscle. Approximately 20% of the energy produced during muscle contraction is used to produce movement; the remainder is lost as heat.

There are more than 500 skeletal muscles in the body. On a microscopic level, muscle cells are considered to be cylindrical. They range from 1 to 40 μm in length and from 10 to 100 μm in diameter. The cells are multinucleated, with the nuclei located at the periphery of the cell or just beneath the *sarcolemma*, or plasma membrane. External to the sarcolemma is a highly glycosy-

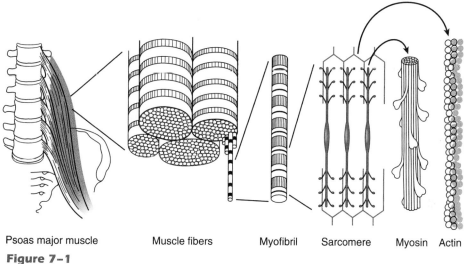

Psoas major muscle   Muscle fibers   Myofibril   Sarcomere   Myosin   Actin

Figure 7–1

Macroscopic to microscopic organization of mature skeletal muscle. (From Porterfield JA, DeRosa C. *Mechanical Low Back Pain: Perspectives in Functional Anatomy*, 2nd ed. Philadelphia: WB Saunders, 1998, p 55.)

lated layer of collagen fibers called the *external lamina;* it is the external lamina that completely ensheathes each cell. This layer also contains proteins that function as enzymes.

Organization of Mature Skeletal Muscle

The organization of skeletal muscle from macroscopic to microscopic levels is illustrated in Figure 7–1. A more detailed view of the micro-organization is provided in Figure 7–2. The entire muscle is encased in a thick connective sheath of collagen fibers and fibroblasts called the *epimysium*. Extensions of this sheath extend into the interior of the muscle, subdividing it into small bundles

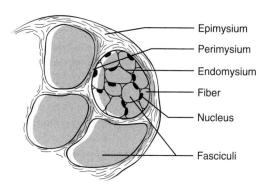

Epimysium

Perimysium

Endomysium

Fiber

Nucleus

Fasciculi

Figure 7–2

Micro-organization of skeletal muscle.

or groups of myofibers called *fasciculi*. Each bundle or fasciculus is surrounded by a layer of connective tissue called the *perimysium*. Within the fasciculus, each individual muscle myofibril is surrounded by a layer of connective tissue called the *endomysium*. The endomysium is rich in capillaries and, to a lesser extent, nerve fibers. All connective tissue coverings ultimately come together at the tendinous junction; the tendon transmits all contractile forces generated by the muscle fibers to the bone.

Each individual myofiber is filled with cylindric bundles of myofibrils that are made up of myofilaments (see Fig. 7–1). Each myofilament is divided into segments by a Z *line;* between these Z lines, filaments of actin and myosin are arranged in parallel groupings. Actin, the thinner filament, originates at the Z line; myosin is the thicker filament. During muscle contraction, as two Z lines move closer together, the actin and myosin filaments do not contract but rather slide over each other. The area from one Z line to the next Z line constitutes a sarcomere, which is the basic contractile unit of the muscle fiber (Fig. 7–3). The alternating light and dark pattern in the sarcomere reflects the amount of overlap of the actin and myosin filaments. The A band is a wide dark band in which thick filaments are located. A light band, the I band, lies between A bands and contains thin filaments that do not overlap the thick filaments. The Z line divides the I band and marks the division between sarcomeres. The H band occupies the space between the thin filaments and therefore contains only thick filaments.

Figure 7–3, a sagittal section of a muscle bundle, shows the arrangement of the *sarcoplasmic reticulum* (SR), a system of membranous anastomosing channels intimately associated with the surface of each myofibril. Calcium ions (Ca^{2+}) necessary for muscle contraction are released from the SR and then resorbed by the SR. Figure 7–3 also illustrates the arrangement of the *trans-*

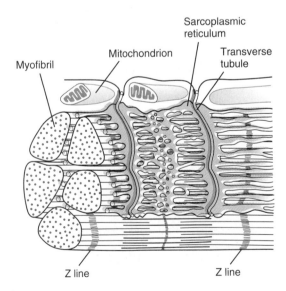

Figure 7–3

Transverse tubule sarcoplasmic reticulum system. (From Porterfield JA, DeRosa C. *Mechanical Low Back Pain: Perspectives in Functional Anatomy*, 2nd ed. Philadelphia: WB Saunders, 1998, p 57.)

verse tubular system (T tubules). T tubules are extensions of the sarcolemma deep into the interior of the muscle fiber. The function of the T tubules is to extend the wave of depolarization that initiates muscle contraction throughout all the myofibrils of the muscle.

EXCITATION-CONTRACTION COUPLING

Excitation-contraction coupling is the mechanism that links plasma membrane stimulation with cross-bridge force production. The muscle receives a neural signal and converts that signal into mechanical force. The *neuromuscular junction*, the point of contact between the axon of the alpha motor nerve and the surface of the muscle fiber, has a number of morphological and biochemical specializations. These specializations directly mediate the transfer of electric impulse of the nerve to the myofiber. Figure 7–4 illustrates the expansion of an axon into a foot plate that comes to rest in a depression of the surface of

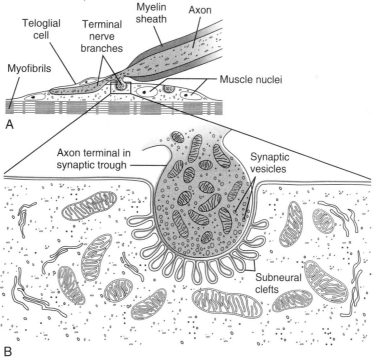

Figure 7–4

Neuromuscular junction: different views of the motor endplate. *A,* Longitudinal section through the endplate. *B,* Electron micrographic appearance of the contact point between one of the axon terminals and the muscle fiber membrane, representing the rectangular area shown in *A.* (Modified from Fawcett DW. *Bloom and Fawcett: Textbook of Histology,* 11th ed. Philadelphia, WB Saunders, 1986, p 290 [after Couteaux].)

the myofiber called a *junctional fold*. The membranes of the nerve and muscle fiber do not come into contact but are separated by a narrow space called the *synaptic cleft*.

The foot plate contains large numbers of small membrane-bound vesicles called *synaptic vessels;* these vessels contain the chemical transmitter *acetylcholine* (ACh). When an action potential passes down the motor axon and reaches the nerve ending, the synaptic vesicles fuse with the presynaptic membrane, thereby emptying their contents, ACh, into the synaptic cleft. Most of the ACh is immediately hydrolyzed by *acetylcholinesterase* (AChE). The remaining ACh molecules diffuse across the synaptic cleft, where they bind to *ACh receptors* in the muscle membrane. This bonding induces the formation of an action potential that sweeps down the surface of the myofiber.

Contraction refers to activation of the cross-bridge cycle. As repolarization occurs for muscle contraction, Ca^{2+} activates the attractive forces between the filaments of actin and myosin. However, the process of contraction will continue only if there is energy; this energy is derived from the high-energy bonds of adenosine triphosphate (ATP), which are degraded to adenosine diphosphate (ADP). In the relaxed state the bulbous heads of the myosin filaments are in close association with the actin filaments but do not touch them (Fig. 7–5A). However, in the presence of Ca^{2+} and ATP, the heads of the myosin molecules form cross-bridges with active sites on the thin filaments of actin. The head of the myosin contains adenosinetriphosphatase (ATPase), which breaks down the ATP. The resulting energy produces a conformational change in the myosin head region that exerts a directional force on the actin filament. As a result, the actin filaments are drawn toward the center of the sarcomere, overlapping the myosin filament. The net result is shortening of the sarcomere, or contraction of the muscle. One ATP is needed for each cross-bridge cycle.

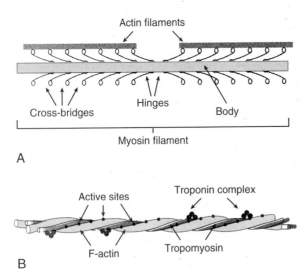

A

B

Figure 7–5

A, The contraction apparatus: many myosin molecules combine to form a myosin filament. In a relaxed state, the bulbous heads of the myosin filaments are in close association with the actin filaments but do not touch them. The cross-bridges and the interaction between the heads of the cross-bridges and adjacent actin filaments are shown. *B*, The actin filament is composed of two strands of F-actin and tropomyosin. Attached to one end of each tropomyosin molecule is a troponin complex that initiates contraction. (From Guyton AC, Hall JE. *Textbook of Medical Physiology*, 9th ed. Philadelphia: WB Saunders, 1996, pp 76–77.)

Every muscle fiber contains the needed ingredients for contraction: ATP, actin, and myosin. What prevents a resting muscle from contracting on its own? Two proteins are present in the actin that prevent cross-bridge formation when the muscle is at rest. These proteins are troponin and tropomyosin and are located on the thin filaments (Fig. 7–5B). The tropomyosin partially covers the myosin binding sites on the actin. Troponin is responsible for maintaining a lock on these binding sites. When calcium binds to a specific site on troponin, this unlocks the myosin-binding site on the actin and allows cross-bridge formation. After cross-bridge formation during the contraction phase of excitation-contraction coupling, relaxation occurs.

In summary, there are 11 major physiological events from excitation to contraction to relaxation:

Excitation

1. A wave of depolarization spreads down the motor axon to the neuromuscular junction.
2. ACh is released from the synaptic terminals and diffuses across the synaptic cleft.
3. ACh combines with receptors in the sarcolemma of the muscle fibril and depolarizes the muscle cell membrane.
4. An action potential spreads inward along the T tubules.
5. Depolarization of the SR occurs.
6. Ca^{2+} is released from the SR.

Contraction

7. Ca^{2+} binds to troponin C.
8. Cross-bridges are formed between the myosin and actin heads, and ATP breaks down.
9. There is a conformational change of the myosin molecule leading to sliding of the actin filaments across the myosin, a shortening of the sarcomere.

Relaxation

10. AChE hydrolyzes ACh to stop the wave of depolarization.
11. SR resorbs all Ca^{2+}, cross-bridge links are broken, and the muscle relaxes.

MUSCLE FIBER TYPES

All human muscles are a mixture of three fiber types: I, IIa, and IIb (Vander et al, 2001). Muscle fibers can be classified according to the maximal velocity of shortening as either slow or fast and by the pathway used to form ATP. ATP is available from creatine phosphate stored in the muscle. Creatine phosphate is a high-energy compound that transfers organic phosphate to ADP to produce ATP (creatine phosphate + ADP = ATP + creatine). Creatine phosphate is responsible for maintaining sufficiently high levels of ATP for muscle contraction to take place. All muscle fiber types use this source of ATP.

Type I muscle fibers are classified as slow oxidative because they use slow glycolysis and oxidative phosphorylation to produce ATP. Slow-twitch, type I fibers have a small diameter, with large amounts of oxidative enzymes and an extensive capillary density. Type I fibers are best suited for activities required in repetitive, lower-force contractions and are considered fatigue resistant. Only slow fibers are found in extraocular and middle ear muscles. Most "postural" muscles, such as those associated with the spinal column or the lower extremities, are composed predominantly of slow-twitch, or type I, fibers. Force is maintained economically by having lower myosin ATPase activity than the fast-twitch fibers. The soleus muscle has a preponderance of slow-twitch muscle fibers and therefore is considered a postural muscle used for prolonged lower extremity activity to support the body against gravity.

Type II muscle fibers are fast-twitch fibers. Type IIa fibers are small in diameter with many mitochondria and are oxidative. Type IIa fibers are also called fast oxidative-glycolytic because they can use both aerobic and anaerobic metabolism. These fiber types are found in some ocular muscles and demonstrate fine, fast movements almost continuously. When glucose is quickly broken down without oxygen present, large amounts of lactate are produced along with ATP. Type IIb fibers have large diameters and are glycolytic. They have a high capacity for anaerobic metabolism. Type IIb fibers have few mitochondria and narrow Z lines. Both of these fast-twitch fibers are suited for short bursts of powerful activity, although the type IIa fibers are more fatigue resistant. The contractile speed and twitch duration of type IIa are between those of type I and type IIb fibers. The gastrocnemius muscle has a preponderance of fast-twitch fibers. This gives the muscle its capacity for very forceful and rapid contractions, which are used for jumping.

ISOMETRIC TWITCH CURVE

A *twitch* is the mechanical response of a single muscle fiber to an action potential (Vander et al, 2001). All muscle fibers respond with the characteristic isometric twitch curve when stimulated. The course of the cycle, however, is not the same for all muscle fiber types. Where calcium ATPase activity is greater, as in fast-twitch fibers, the contraction time is as short as 10 milliseconds. When calcium ATPase activity is less, as in slow-twitch fibers, contraction time can last 100 milliseconds or longer. Figure 7–6 compares an isometric twitch curve in young and old adults.

MOTOR UNIT

The functional unit of a muscle is the *motor unit*, which is defined as a single nerve cell body and its axon plus all muscle fibers innervated by the axon's branches. All the muscle fibers of a motor unit are of the same fiber type. Each muscle fiber receives innervation from one neuron. The intensity of a muscle contraction is graded by the number of motor units recruited and the rate of

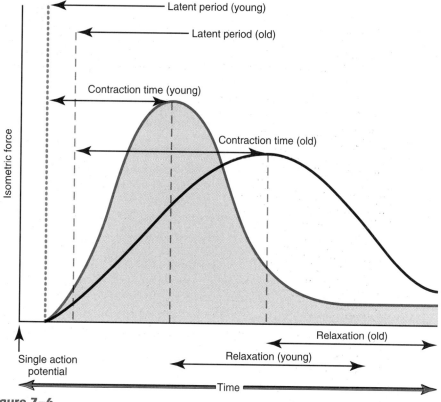

Figure 7–6

Comparison of isometric twitch curves in a young and an old adult. The response of a single muscle fiber to an action potential in a young adult is compared with that of an old adult. All three phases of the curve—latency, contraction, and relaxation—are lengthened in older adults compared with young adults. The amplitude is also reduced in the older adult.

firing. The number of muscle fibers in a motor unit varies according to the muscle. For example, in the large muscles of the lower limb, motor units range in size from approximately 500 to 1000 fibers. In contrast, the small muscles in the hand or the extraocular muscles have motor units that range in size from approximately 10 to 100 fibers. These muscles are capable of producing very fine movements such as typing, tying a bow, or making small adjustments of the eye.

Recruitment is the process of increasing the number of motor units contracting within a muscle at a given time (Vander et al, 2001). The process of recruitment follows the size principle, with the small motor units being recruited before the larger motor units. The small motor neurons innervated by slow oxidative type I fibers are fired first, followed by fast oxidative, type IIa, and finally, the fast glycolytic type IIb fibers.

Skeletal Muscle Development

PRENATAL

To understand some of the age-related changes in skeletal muscle, it is important to study the events of skeletal muscle development. The muscular system develops from mesoderm, except for the muscles of the iris, which develop from neuroectoderm (Uusitalo and Kivela, 1995). The events of mesenchymal tissue differentiation into muscle fiber are depicted in Figure 7–7. The important cell types to be considered are myoblasts, myotubes, myofibers, fibroblasts, and satellite cells (Colling-Saltin, 1980).

The *myoblast* is the major cell type found in areas of muscle formation. Myoblasts appear to be produced from muscle stem cells in the mesoderm (Miller et al, 1999; O'Rahilly and Muller, 1996). Myoblasts are spindle-shaped cells with centrally placed elongated nuclei. These cells do not contain organized contractile proteins. During development, myoblasts align into chain-like configurations parallel to the long axis of the limb. Subsequent to alignment, the basement membranes of the myoblasts fuse to form large, multinucleated cylinders called *myotubes*. Each syncytium (the multinucleate mass of protoplasm produced by cell merging) contains a varying number of nuclei ranging up to several hundred. Cellular fusion via disintegration of the plasma membranes of adjacent myoblasts and myotubes is at present the explanation for how striated muscle cells become multinucleated (Minguetti and Mair, 1986).

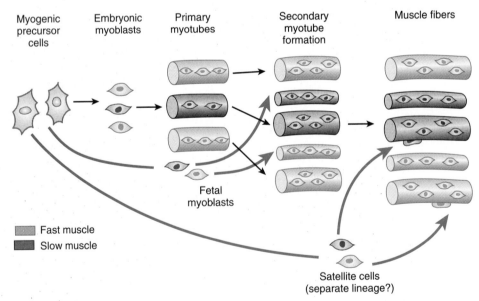

Figure 7–7

Stages in the formation of primary and secondary muscle fibers. A family of embryonic myoblasts contributes to the formation of the primary myotubes, and fetal myoblasts contribute to secondary myotubes. The origin of satellite cells is still unresolved. (From Carlson BM. *Human Embryology & Developmental Biology*, 2nd ed. St. Louis: Mosby, 1999, p 177.)

Myotubes are immature multinucleated muscle cells. Nuclei are centrally located in these elongated cylindrical cells. Contractile proteins are rapidly synthesized and become evident as striated fibrils in the peripheral cytoplasm. There are two types of myotubes: primary and secondary. Primary myotubes are the first to develop prenatally at 5 weeks of gestation. A few weeks later, the secondary myotubes develop. By 20 weeks of gestation, the majority of myotubes have fused to form *myofibers* (Mastaglia, 1974). *Myofibers* are mature multinucleated muscle cells. Myofibers contain the characteristic striations, or sarcomeres, of skeletal muscle. All nuclei are peripherally located and closely apposed to the sarcolemma or plasma membrane of the cell.

The *fibroblasts* are the flattened, irregularly shaped cells found in association with the developing myofibers. During the early stages of development, these cells provide an extracellular matrix on which the connective tissue framework of a muscle is developed. Fibroblasts form the perimysium and epimysium.

The last cell type to be discussed is the *satellite cell*. These mononucleated, spindle-shaped cells are closely associated with the surface of the myofibers. They are found between the plasmalemma and endomysium of the myofibers and can be positively identified only with the electron microscope (see Fig. 7–7). Satellite cells play an integral role in normal muscle growth during the postnatal period and in the repair of muscle following injury. At birth, satellite cell nuclei account for over 30% of the total myofiber nuclei (Schultz and Lipton, 1982).

The role of the satellite cells during normal postnatal growth is to supply nuclei to the enlarging fibers. Although myoblasts constitute a rapidly proliferating cell population during embryonic development, once incorporated into the syncytium of a myofiber, they no longer replicate DNA or divide. The nuclei are permanently postmitotic once they become part of the syncytium. Nevertheless, when myofibers increase in size during growth, the number of nuclei increases, in some cases more than 100 times. This increase in myonuclei depends on the satellite cells associated with the fiber. These cells are continually dividing; after a mitotic division, one or both of the daughter cells fuse with the fiber, thereby injecting an additional nucleus into the syncytium. Likewise, in the event of massive injury to the muscle, myofibers usually die. New muscle fibers can be formed by surviving satellite cells. These cells undergo differentiation much like the primitive myoblasts by repeating the embryonic events leading to muscle formation. In this manner, the damaged muscle is repaired or replaced. Although the ability of the satellite cells is significant, the damaged muscle may not fully regain its strength (Vander et al, 2001). The muscle compensates for residual loss of tissue by increasing the size of the remaining fibers.

As stated previously, muscle tissue develops from primitive cells called myoblasts, which are derived from mesenchymal cells. The muscles (myotomes) and bony segments (sclerotomes) of the vertebral column and overlying skin (dermatomes) are derived from somites, paired masses of mesoderm that lie on either side of the neural tube. Each segmental myotome separates into an epaxial and a hypaxial division. Myoblasts from the epaxial division become the extensor muscles of the neck and vertebral column (Fig. 7–8). Myoblasts from the hypaxial division become the accessory muscles of the neck and the lateral and ventral trunk muscles. The muscles of the extremities develop from myoblasts located within the limb region that surround the developing bones (in situ). Some of the precursor myogenic cells in the limb buds come from somites (Moore and Persaud, 1998).

Changes in Fiber Types

Muscle is developed from two distinct lineages: the primary and secondary myotubes. Primary myotubes develop and differentiate into muscle fibers without neural input; however, secondary myotubes require neural input for development. Generally, primary myotubes become type I fibers and secondary myotubes become type II fibers. Because type I fibers are innervated before type II fibers, they are the first ones to be seen in the fetus. Type II fibers are generally not identified until 30 or 31 weeks of gestation (Grinnell, 1995). Studies have concluded that between 31 and 37 weeks of gestation, type II fibers constitute about 25% of the muscle fibers present in the fetus (Malina and Bouchard, 1991). It was once believed that there was an equal number of type I and II fibers at birth (Colling-Saltin, 1980), but evidence appears not to substantiate the claim (Elder and Kakulas, 1993).

Development and Migration of Fibers

Nearly all skeletal muscles are present and in essence exhibit a mature form at the end of the embryonic period (8 weeks of gestation). Approximately six fundamental processes occur during the first 8 weeks of development. The formation of a muscle is the result of one or more of these processes. The six fundamental processes as described by Crelin (1981) are as follows:

1. The direction of the muscle fibers may change from the original craniocaudal orientation in the myotome. Only a few muscles retain their initial fiber orientation (parallel to the long axis of the body); examples of these are the rectus abdominis and the erector spinae.
2. Portions of successive myotomes commonly fuse to form a single composite muscle. An example of this process is the rectus abdominis. This muscle is formed by the fusion of the ventral portions of the last six or seven thoracic myotomes.
3. A myotome may split longitudinally into two or more parts that become separate muscles; examples of this process are the trapezius and the sternocleidomastoid muscles.
4. The original myotome masses may split into two or more layers. The intercostal muscles are the derivatives of single myotomes which split into two layers, the external and the internal intercostal muscles.
5. A portion of the muscle or all of the muscle may degenerate. The degenerated muscle leaves a sheet of connective tissue known as an *aponeurosis.* The epicranial aponeurosis connecting the frontal and occipital portions of the occipitofrontalis muscle is an example of this particular process.

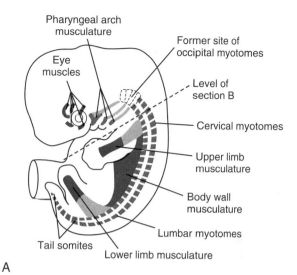

A

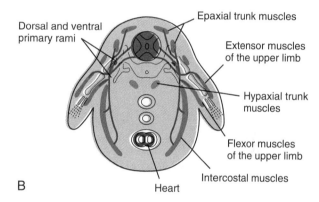

B

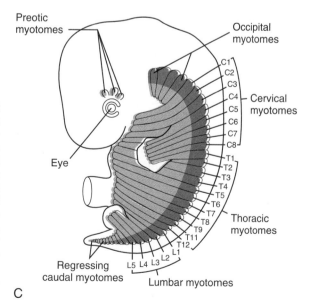

C

Figure 7–8

A, Sketch of an embryo (about 41 days), showing the myotomes and developing muscular system. *B,* Transverse section of the embryo, illustrating the epaxial and hypaxial derivatives of a myotome. *C,* Six-week embryo showing the myotome regions of the somites that give rise to most skeletal muscles. (From Moore KL, Persaud TVN. *Before We Are Born: Essentials of Embryology and Birth Defects,* 5th ed. Philadelphia: WB Saunders, 1998, pp 401–402.)

6. The last process involves muscle migration of a myotome from its site of formation to a more remote region. The formation of the muscles of the upper chest is an example of this process. The serratus anterior muscle migrates to the thoracic region and attaches ultimately to the scapula and the upper eight or nine ribs. This muscle migration takes with it the fifth, sixth, and seventh cervical spinal nerves for innervation. The migration of the latissimus dorsi muscle is even more extensive. This migration carries with it its seventh and eighth cervical spinal nerve innervations to attach ultimately to the humerus, the lower thoracic and lumbar vertebrae, the last three or four ribs, and the crest of the ilium of the pelvis.

In muscle development, a wide range of variation of these six processes can occur without interfering with an individual's normal functional ability.

Control of Muscle Development and Differentiation

Differentiation into fiber types occurs about the same time as fibers are being innervated. The primary myotubes are innervated first. The formation of the myoneural junction is initiated with the development of ACh receptors in the periphery of the myotubes around 8 weeks of gestation. This coincides with the earliest fetal movement observed in the intercostal muscles (Hesselmans et al, 1993). Prenatally, each motor end plate receives multiple axons. This polyneuronal innervation insures that there will be at least one axon for every muscle fiber. Between 16 and 25 weeks of gestation, there is a dying back of extra connections and thus a transition to mononeuronal innervation indicative of the classic motor unit (Hesselmans et al, 1993). During the last half of gestation, there is also a tremendous increase in the number and size of muscle fibers. The increase in number is primarily from secondary myotubes. Fifteen percent of the body mass in the fetus midway through pregnancy is attributable to muscle. Muscle mass accounts for 25% of a person's body weight at birth.

Control of development and differentiation of the muscle cell, during both the fetal period and the neonatal period, are strongly determined by what is inherited and genetically coded in the nucleus of the muscle cell (Colling-Saltin, 1980). Researchers agree that genetic coding is responsible for muscle fiber differentiation (Grinnell, 1995). Primary myotubes develop and differentiate into both slow (type I) and fast fiber types (types IIa and IIb) without nervous input. Secondary myotubes are more dependent on nervous input and differentiate into fast fiber types (types IIa and IIb) (Grinnell, 1995; Grove, 1989).

INFANCY TO ADOLESCENCE

The growth of skeletal muscles in the first year of life is the result of an increase in both the number of muscle fibers and the size of the individual fibers. Although the greatest increase in the number of muscle fibers occurs before birth, an increase in muscle fiber number does occur during the first year of postnatal development. The increase in fiber number is achieved by differentiation of myoblasts into secondary myotubes or by division of already existing cells (Mastaglia, 1974). After birth, the growth of the muscle comes mainly from an increase in size of the individual fibers. The average muscle fiber size at birth is around 12 μm.

Differentiation of muscle fibers continues into postnatal life. At birth, the distribution of type I fibers ranges from 28% to 41% in various skeletal muscles. Intercostal and diaphragm muscles demonstrate adult-like distribution of type I fibers by 2 and 7 months, respectively (Keens et al, 1978). The soleus achieves its type I predominance by 8 to 10 months of age (Elder and Kakulas, 1993). Proportions of different types of fibers also vary considerably among individuals for a given skeletal muscle. For example, a standard deviation of about 15% is observed in the percentage of type I fibers in the vastus lateralis muscle of young men (the mean is about 50%) (Malina and Bouchard, 1991). In a later study of growth and development of the vastus lateralis, Lexell and colleagues (1992) found significantly higher distribution of type I fibers in children (5 to 15 years) than in adults. Furthermore, adult distributions of type I fibers were demonstrated in the vastus lateralis, biceps brachii, and triceps brachii of a 16-year-old (Elder and Kakulas, 1993). The adult distribution was not found in a 15-year-old, which might suggest a change occurs relative to puberty. Changes in fiber type differentiation continue postnatally, even into the period preceding young adulthood.

The changes in contractile properties of skeletal muscle follow the differentiation of fiber types. The contractile properties of certain muscles slow postnatally, somewhere between 6 weeks and 3 years of age (Gatev et al, 1977). Whether the slowing of the contractile properties is caused by this differentiation is not certain (Elder and Kakulas, 1993). The muscles that become postural muscles develop adult slow-twitch characteristics as motor development proceeds. The characteristics of slow-twitch fibers are their slow speed of contraction and longer relaxation times.

Muscle maturation occurs in childhood. Contractile properties of muscle are measured by maximal twitch tension, time to peak tension, and half-relaxation times. Soleus muscle relaxation time was studied as a measure of muscle dynamics in children 3 to 10 years of age (Lin et al, 1994). Researchers found that a child's muscles are initially slow to relax after contraction but that relaxation speed doubles between 3 and 10 years of age. These values reach adult rates at age 10. In further examination of this phenomenon, the investigators found that the speed of contraction improved because of the ability of the muscle to relax more quickly (Lin et al, 1996). A possible mechanism for the change in muscle dynamics with age may be a change in the calcium reuptake mechanism of the SR. Furthermore, the change to an adult muscle phenotype of relaxation appears complete at age 10, the same time at which fiber diameter differences are apparent in males and females (Brooke and Engel, 1969).

Strength gains in children follow a typical growth curve for height and weight. Changes in strength are associated with increases in muscle size and muscle maturation. There are several characteristics of strength that may determine how strong someone will be at a given age, including the cross-sectional area of the muscle, the age of the individual, the gender of the individual, the body size or type, and the fiber type and size of the muscle being assessed. Muscle mass is gained before strength (Malina, 1986). Although muscle makes up only 25% of body mass at birth, the proportion of muscle mass increases 5 times in boys and 3.5 times in girls in the progression from childhood to adulthood. Children are stronger than infants, and adolescents are stronger than children. In absolute terms, muscle strength increases linearly with chronologic age from childhood to age 12 or 13 (Beunen and Thomis, 2000).

Mean levels of isometric strength increase gradually between 3 and 6 years. Small gender differences are present (Beunen and Thomis, 2000). Boys as young as 3 years of age are stronger than girls of the same age. This trend continues and intensifies at puberty (Malina, 1986). Static strength in boys continues to increase linearly from 6 to 13 years, followed by a spurt that continues through the late teens.

ADOLESCENCE AND ADULTHOOD

Puberty marks an increase in growth of the musculoskeletal systems. As the skeleton grows, the muscles have to lengthen to re-establish the appropriate length-tension relationship. The resting length of a muscle affects the amount of tension that can be generated. At rest, the majority of skeletal muscles are near the optimal length for force production. Separation of the attachments of the muscles as the skeleton grows appears to be a strong stimulus for muscle growth (Sinclair and Dangerfield, 1998). Muscles add sarcomeres and fibrils to achieve a new length (Malina, 1986). Greater muscle growth is seen in males than females because of the effects of steadily rising levels of testosterone.

Strength in Relation to Age

Strength is seen to increase linearly between the ages of 6 and 18 years (Fig. 7–9). Boys appear to have a strength spurt during the adolescent years, which is due to hormone production. Although testosterone is the most likely reason why males increase muscle mass more than do females, other hormones play a role. Growth hormone, insulin, and thyroid hormones are important for somatic and muscle growth. With increasing age, the percentage of girls whose performance on strength tests equals or exceeds that of boys declines considerably. After age 16, the strength of an average boy is greater than that of the strongest girl. Although growth studies generally stop at age 18, strength continues to increase into the 20s, especially for men.

Strength appears to peak in the 30s and to not decline until the 50s (Larsson et al, 1979). There is a 30% decline from age 50 to 70 years and a more rapid decline after 70 (Connelly, 2000; Vandervoort and McComas, 1986). There is a decrease in both isometric and dynamic strength, but relatively speaking, eccentric strength is better maintained in older adults than is concentric strength (Evans, 1995; Lexell, 1995).

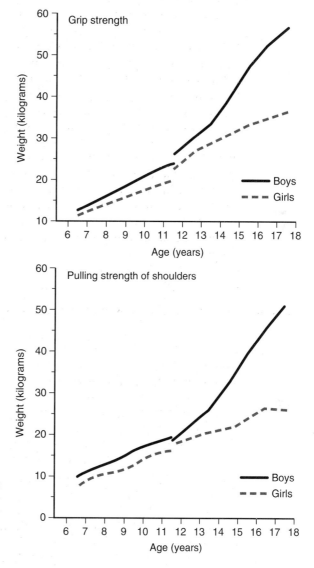

Figure 7–9

Mean grip strength and pulling strength between 6 and 18 years of age. (From Malina RM, Bouchard C. *Growth, Maturation and Physical Activity*. Champaign, IL: Human Kinetics, 1991, p 191.)

Firing Rates and Contractile Properties

Muscles speed up during the first 20 years of life with a documented decline seen in the proportion of type I muscle fibers in the vastus lateralis (Lexell et al, 1992). Elder and Kakulas (1993) postulated that over the course of development from infancy to childhood and into adulthood, muscles undergo a fast-slow-fast phenotype to meet the demands of motor development. The phenotype of a muscle reflects its functional use, not necessarily its developmental characteristics or genotype. In infancy, the slow-twitch characteristics of postural muscle have not yet developed, so muscle response is characterized by fast-twitch responses. Infants make rapid, reflexive movements. By childhood, the muscles that function predominantly as slow-twitch, type I muscles have completed their maturation and are used appropriately for balance and postural holding. The muscles that are predominantly fast-twitch do not exhibit adult proportions of type II fibers until young adulthood. For example, the proportion of type II (fast-twitch) fibers in the vastus lateralis increases from approximately 35% at age 5 to 50% at age 20 (Lexell et al, 1992).

The increase in muscle cross-sectional area of the vastus lateralis from childhood to adulthood is due to an increase in fiber size and a transformation of type I fibers to type II fibers (Lexell et al, 1992). In a study of more than 100 healthy individuals from 20 to 100 years of age, Vandervoort and McComas (1986) found a gradual lengthening of twitch contraction and an increase in half-relaxation times.

Motor neurons control the biochemical and physiological properties of the skeletal muscle they innervate. Once muscle fiber differentiation has occurred, neural input makes a tremendous difference in the way the muscle functions (muscle phenotype). Studies conducted on adults reveal that by switching a nerve (cross-innervation) from a fast-twitch (type II) glycolytic muscle to a slow-twitch (type I) oxidative muscle, the oxidative muscle becomes glycolytic. The reverse is also true (Bishop, 1982). The expression of muscle fiber type in adults is dependent on innervation regardless of whether that muscle fiber was originally derived from a primary or a secondary myotube.

OLDER ADULTHOOD

Development of Sarcopenia

The muscle wasting associated with the aging process is referred to as *sarcopenia* (Evans, 1995). Sarcopenia is present in 6% to 15% of older adults (Melton et al, 2000). No distinct patterns of muscular loss are clearly apparent. Some reports state that muscle loss is greater in the lower extremities, with the thigh muscles exhibiting greatest loss. However, functional patterns of the subjects involved in these reports were not well controlled. Actually, because the various muscles of the body are composed of different proportions of the three basic fiber types and are subjected to different degrees of functional demands, it should not be surprising that different muscles show different rates and magnitudes of muscle loss. The degree of muscle loss associated with aging may be partially related to the activity level of the individual (see Functional Implications).

Mechanism of Muscle Loss

The etiology of the muscle loss associated with advanced aging has been attributed to loss of contractile proteins, decline in circulating hormones, and changes in the nervous system, specifically the motor unit.

Age-associated loss of muscle mass is associated with a decline in the number and size of muscle fibers (Lexell, 1995). The changes in the muscle are a result of neural changes in the motor unit. Motor units lose 1% of their total number yearly beginning in the 20s. The rate of loss increases after age 60

(Thomlinson and Irving, 1977). Loss of motor neurons orphans muscle fibers. Abandoned muscle fibers are partially reinnervated by surviving motor neurons. As a result, there is a decline in functional motor units and an increase in the innervation ratio. The process of denervation and reinnervation is called *motor unit remodeling*. For example, if the motor unit originally consisted of 1 motor nerve and 50 muscle fibers, after motor unit remodeling, the ratio would be 1 motor nerve to 75 or 100 fibers. As a result of motor unit remodeling, the number of fibers innervated by a motor neuron increases so that the remaining motor units exert, on average, greater amounts of force. With aging, a selective denervation of type II fibers occurs with reinnervation by slow motor neurons (Roos et al, 1997). Physiologically, they become slow motor units. The functional significance of the reorganization is that the nervous system may have to alter its strategies for controlling muscle force (Enoka, 1997).

Structural changes also occur in the muscle itself. There are changes in the mitochondria, T tubules, and the SR (Guttman and Hazlikova, 1976). Connective tissue increases in the area of the endomysium, the location of the capillary bed. In addition, the basement membrane increases in thickness around both the capillary and the myofiber. The net result of these changes (all mainly at the level of the endomysium) is an increase in diffusion distances, possibly producing an age-related hypoxia. It is unknown whether chemical changes in the basement membrane, for example, may produce a selective barrier to certain essential molecules required by the muscle fibers. Muscle protein synthesis rates decline in muscle with old age. This decline has been associated with age-related loss in muscle strength and aerobic exercise tolerance (Proctor et al, 1998; Yarasheski et al, 1999). The decline in protein synthesis in muscle has been related to declines in insulin-like growth factor, testosterone, and dehydroepiandrosterone (DHEA) sulfate (Proctor et al, 1998).

Changes in Contractile Properties

The ability of muscle to generate force is reduced with age (Connelly et al, 1999). Although not generally accepted, some report a reduction in force by as much as 20% per unit of cross-sectional area (Jubrias et al, 1997; Rice, 2000). Others report that the absolute amount of force remains the same but that the speed with which that force is generated declines (Gross et al, 1998; Larsson et al, 1979). According to Patten and Craik (2000), contraction time increases by 45%, whereas there is a 32% reduction in twitch force and a 206% increase in half-relaxation time. Spirduso (1995) notes that elders have less difficulty with eccentric contractions than with concentric contractions. If there is selective loss of type I fibers, that could explain why muscles generate force more slowly but also relax more slowly. Not all muscles are equally affected by age. A discussion of muscle function at the motor unit level is given by Rice (2000).

Changes in Force Control and Firing Rate

Force control is lessened in the older adult because of the greater number of low threshold (type I) motor units compared with the number found in younger adults. Older adults may use more co-contraction during low-force isometric contractions (Grabiner and Enoka, 1995). Motor unit firing rates appear to generally be reduced with aging, but the changes seem to be task and muscle specific. The number of studies is limited, and they use different techniques. The subjects vary in age and physical status. The decrease in the firing rate could be due to the larger motor units seen in the older adult and the reduced excitability of the corticospinal tract or a decrease in central drive (Connelly et al, 1999; Rice, 2000).

Motor unit firing rates appear to slow with age and to exhibit greater variability (Roos et al, 1997; Soderberg et al, 1991). Changes in motor unit firing rate are related to the amount of effort required for an activity or task because force output is modulated in part by the motor unit firing. Kamen and associates (1995) reported a considerable decrease in motor unit discharge rate with maximal effort contractions. Soderberg and colleagues (1991) saw only a tendency toward a decrease in submaximal levels of work. Nelson and co-workers (1984), as well as Soderberg and colleagues (1991), documented the variability of motor unit firing rates with age.

Other Changes Associated with Age

Collagen. As we age, the amount of connective tissue increases, mostly at the level of the endomysium. Collagen obtained from old muscle is less soluble and exhibits increased resistance to degradative enzymes such as collagenase. Changes in the collagen are consistent with increased cross-linking or additional bonds between the collagen molecules and would explain the increase in stiffness of old muscle. As muscle fibers are lost and replaced by fat and collagen, the volume or girth of the muscle as measured anthropometrically may not demonstrate an actual reduction in muscle mass.

Motor End Plate. Changes in one part of the motor unit affect other parts of the motor unit. Motor end plates remodel continuously during normal aging, with changes seen in presynaptic and postsynaptic components (Lexell, 1997). The number of synaptic vesicles is increased with age, but they are found in tight clusters, suggesting that they have undergone agglutination. The synaptic cleft becomes enlarged, and the enlarged area is filled with thickened basal lamina. In addition, the junctional folds appear unfolded, and the plasma membrane of the muscle fiber appears thickened.

Age-Related Changes to the Isometric Twitch Curve

In general, in the older adult the three phases of the isotonic twitch curve are prolonged. The amplitude of the curve is also reduced (see Fig. 7–6).

In phase I, *the latency phase*, the latent period of the twitch curve is prolonged. A major factor contributing to the increased latency period is a 10% to 15% reduction in nerve conduction velocity. Once the impulse reaches the nerve terminal, portions of the following scenario may also play a role in further increasing the latency period. The nerve impulse should cause the release of ACh from the synaptic vesicles. However, because many of the vesicles are clumped, the process of release is slowed, and the amount of ACh that is ultimately released is reduced. Because the synaptic cleft is enlarged, it takes longer for the substance to diffuse across the cleft to the postsynaptic membrane. The increased basement membrane material adds a further diffusion barrier. Once the ACh molecules have reached the postsynaptic membrane, there are fewer receptors for binding because of the unfolding of the synaptic folds. Membrane characteristics of the thickened sarcolemma may have changed sufficiently to decrease conduction velocity of muscle depolarization.

Phase II, *the contraction phase,* is also prolonged. Maximum contraction potentials are prolonged up to six times in aged individuals. Several factors may contribute to this increase. A disorganization of the myofilament lattice has been observed with use of the electron microscope and may indicate disruption of the contractile process at the molecular level. Calcium-activated ATPase activity is decreased with age. In addition, the levels of creatine phosphate are reduced with age. Interestingly, although creatine phosphate decreases with age, the levels of creatine remain constant. Thus, the rate at which creatine is rephosphorylated is compromised with age. Finally, there is a reduced uptake of calcium by the SR.

Phase III, *the relaxation phase,* is also prolonged. The amount of AChE at the neuromuscular junction is reduced. The net result is an increase in the time required to hydrolyze the ACh, allowing depolarization of the sarcolemma to continue.

Functional Implications

Changes occurring in the development of skeletal muscle tissue across the life span have functional and clinical implications for our muscle strength, endurance, and power. Clinical Implications—Muscle Strength Acquisition Across the Life Span outlines markers for promoting strength and related training and exercise programs along the developmental continuum.

Muscle strength is an expression of muscular force, or the individual's capacity to develop tension against an external resistance. The literature defines several types of strength: static, power, and dynamic (Beunen and Thomis, 2000). *Static, or isometric, strength* is the maximal voluntary force produced against an external resistance without any change in muscle length. It is generally measured in specific muscle groups, such as those in the hand, by grip strength or isokinetically in the quadriceps or hamstrings. *Power* is explosive strength or the ability of muscles to produce a certain amount of force in the shortest amount of time. It is measured as a function of strength. *Dynamic strength* is the force generated by repetitive contractions of a muscle. Therefore, it is closely linked to muscular endurance. Dynamic strength is also known as functional strength in the physical fitness literature.

Muscle endurance is the ability to repeat or maintain muscular contractions over time. It is believed that the capacity of a muscle to increase in muscular endurance is related to the ability of the muscle to utilize oxygen, or the *oxidative metabolism* of the muscle. This ability is related to the individual's

CLINICAL IMPLICATIONS
Muscle Strength Acquisition Across the Life Span

Strength acquisition follows a general growth curve as seen in other anthropometric measures such as height and weight. Children at or after puberty demonstrate changes in muscle mass and muscle strength.

Children

- Static strength and power in children may be determined more by genetic factors than is muscle endurance.
- Children can increase strength and endurance as a result of regular participation in a program of progressive resistance training.
- An exercise prescription for a child should focus on higher repetitions and moderate resistance during the initial training period (Faigenbaum et al, 1999).

Adolescents

- Muscle mass in adolescence increases before strength. Peak muscle mass occurs during and after peak weight gain, but maximum strength does not occur until after the peak velocity of growth in height and weight.
- Prepubescent and early postpubescent boys and girls increased strength after participating in a 12-week strength training program using progressive resistive exercise (Lillegard et al, 1997).
- Adolescents have an increased risk for musculoskeletal injury such as apophyseal avulsion during periods of rapid growth. This risk can be countered with a good stretching program.
- Physiological mismatching is possible between 13 and 17 years of age and may increase the risk of injury due to differences in body size, age, and maturity status.

Adults

- Maximum strength is achieved in the 30s and maintained until the 50s.
- Strength training results in improved performance in trained and untrained individuals.
- Eight weeks of heavy resistance training resulted in significant increases in strength and speed of muscle contraction (Schmidtbleicher and Haralambie, 1981).
- Strength training needs to be specific to the task, such as speed, power, and endurance.

Older Adults

- Limb muscle strength declines in the elderly (Bohannon, 1997; Kivinen et al, 1998).
- Participation in a regular exercise program is effective in combating the functional declines associated with aging.

- Resistance training of moderate to high intensity is a safe and effective means of increasing strength in women up to 96 years of age (Foster-Burns, 1999).
- Upper and lower body strength and gait speed can be improved over a 12-week period of twice weekly resistance training in adults over 65 years of age. The individuals participated in a 6-month maintenance phase in which they were trained in Tai Chi (Verfaillie et al, 1997).
- Physically frail institutionalized elderly demonstrate significant strength gains in response to high-intensity progressive resistance training over a 10-week period (Fiatarone et al, 1994).
- Frailty and advanced age are not a contraindication to exercise. A sedentary lifestyle is far more dangerous than activity in the older adult.

maximal oxygen uptake, or $\dot{V}O_{2max}$, levels. This is defined as the transport of oxygen from the atmosphere for utilization by the mitochondria of the muscle and is related to individual cardiovascular efficiency (Frontera and Evans, 1986). (Further discussion is found in Chapter 15.) Muscle fatigue is the reduced ability to achieve the same amount of force output (Brown, 2000). Fatigue is related to endurance but is not the same thing. Although endurance is related to the aerobic capacity of the muscle, fatigue may be the result of a failure of motor unit recruitment or altered excitation-contraction coupling. There are many central and peripheral sites that can be responsible for muscle fatigue.

CHILDHOOD AND ADOLESCENCE

Information on strength measures is not very extensive for early childhood; more information is available for the middle childhood and adolescent years. It is clear that muscular strength increases gradually during early infancy and early childhood. Longitudinal studies show that the adolescent growth spurt in isometric strength occurs within 1.5 years before the age at peak height velocity and may coincide with peak weight velocity (Beunen and Malina, 1988). In girls, there is improvement in strength through about 15 years of age but no clear evidence of a spurt (Malina and Bouchard, 1991). Strength and body size and muscle mass are related. Because boys are usually bigger than girls and have more muscle mass, boys are stronger. When strength is measured per unit body size, boys are stronger in the upper body and trunk than girls. There is little difference in lower body strength when controlled for body size (Malina and Bouchard, 1991). Power as measured by the ability to perform a vertical jump or a standing long jump shows increases in boys and girls from 6 to 12 or 13 years. After 13, boys continue to improve and girls' scores level off. Others have noted an adolescent spurt in explosive strength in boys.

Children typically participate in short bursts of highly intense activity. During short intense bouts of exercise, children have a lesser ability to generate mechanical energy from chemical energy sources (Van Praagh, 2000). These exercise needs can more easily be met by anaerobic energy production. Anaer-obic function in children improves faster than can be accounted for by growth alone (Rowland, 1996). Genetics, fiber type differentiation, and hormonal influ-ences all contribute to the development of anaerobic muscle function (Van Praagh, 2000).

"Energy for skeletal muscle contraction in activities lasting more than several minutes is derived from aerobic metabolism" (Rowland, 1996, p 73). Muscular endurance improves linearly with age from 5 to 13 or 14 years in boys, followed by a spurt similar to that for static muscular strength. Muscular endurance also increases with age in girls, but there is no clear evidence of a spurt like that seen in boys (Malina and Bouchard, 1991). Faigenbaum and associates (1999) compared the effect of two exercise prescriptions on a small group of children ranging in age from 5.2 to 11.8 years. The children exercised in a community youth center twice a week for 8 weeks. One group performed low repetitions against a heavy load, and the other performed high repetitions against a moderate load. The control group did no resistance training. Strength and endurance of leg extension increased in both exercise groups. Endurance increased to a significantly greater degree in the group performing high repeti-tions against a moderate load.

Genetic factors contribute to muscle strength development and perform-ance. Static strength and power in children may be determined more by ge-netic factors than is muscle endurance. During growth, the genetic influence on strength development is strong. Body mass and height are most directly re-lated to strength. Genes seem to play a greater role in strength development in males than in females (Beunen and Thomis, 2000). At puberty, the interaction among height, body mass, and biological maturity explains the majority of strength differences seen with age.

Strength can be increased in children before puberty through the use of resistance training. However, the increase in muscle strength occurs without much increase in muscle size (Rowland, 1996). Strength gains after a weight training program are only somewhat genetically determined (Beunen and Thomis, 2000). Lillegard and colleague (1997) studied the efficacy of strength training in children 9.5 to 14.5 years old. Strength gains were seen in males and females in the experimental group; the males demonstrated greater strength gains. Motor performance was also significantly improved in three of the five measures.

Skeletal age can be related to chronological age to determine whether a child is an early, an average, or a late maturer. The relationship between a child's bone age (how old the skeleton is based on a standard set of radio-graphs) and the child's chronological age determines the maturity category. If the child's chronological age and skeletal (bone) age are within 1 year of each other, the child is an average maturer. If the bone age is greater than the chronological age by more than 1 year, the child is an early maturer. If the bone age is less than the chronological age by more than 1 year, the child is a late maturer. The relationship between skeletal age and strength (static and explosive) is significant between 13 and 17 years of age. The difference in maturation explains why children of the same age can be so disparate in body growth. Although those individuals who mature early do appear to have a strength advantage during this time, the advantage disappears by adulthood (Katzmarzyk et al, 1997; Lefevre, et al, 1990).

ADULTHOOD AND AGING

Strength in men is maximal between the ages of 30 and 35 years. Larsson and coworkers (1979) reported an increase in quadriceps strength up to 30 years and a decline after age 50. Generally, strength declines by 30% between age 50 and 70 (Connelly, 2000; Mazzeo et al, 1998). Data from cross-sectional studies indicate a 15% decline in the 50s and 60s with a greater decline after 70 years of age (Mazzeo et al, 1998). A person 80 years of age may have lost so much strength that she may have barely enough strength to get out of a chair (Alexander et al, 1997).

Adults have the ability to improve strength by resistance training. Training needs to be specific to the muscle function to be improved—static strength, power, or endurance. Training also needs to be specific to the type of task being performed. Once a strength base is established, specific power or endurance training can be followed.

Researchers agree that the rate of decline in muscular strength with age appears to be slightly less in the upper extremities (i.e., small muscle groups) than in the legs (i.e., large muscle groups) (Lexell, 1993). Larsson and colleagues (1982) evaluated 114 males, ages 11 to 70 years, for both static and dynamic lower extremity strength. Both strength and speed of contraction were found to decline with age. Studies of women indicate similar findings—muscle strength, both static and dynamic, decreases with age (Lexell, 1995). Women are weaker than men in muscular strength (Lexell, 1995). Women also demonstrate the decrement in strength earlier than do men (Phillips et al, 2000). About 50% of an individual's muscle strength is lost by the age of 70 years. There is a curvilinear relationship between maximum voluntary isometric strength and age in healthy adults (Krishnathasan and Vandervoort, 2000) (Fig. 7–10). Some of the strength loss in individuals may be related to activity or fitness level of the individual. If an individual remains active, the amount of muscle strength loss may be less (Table 7–1).

Loss of strength is associated with a loss of function in older adults. The strength-function relationship is also curvilinear. As noted by Buchner and de Lateur (1991), there appears to be a minimum amount of strength required for a given task; this threshold may vary from task to task. Strong correlations between strength and function may exist only in individuals who have less than the "threshold" amount of strength. The amount of strength and the mode of muscle contraction—isometric, concentric, or eccentric—are specific to the task to be performed. For example, isometric hip abductor strength may be more representative of the force that needs to be generated during single limb stance than a concentric contraction of the same muscle group. By using the best measure of strength for a particular task, Chandler and coworkers

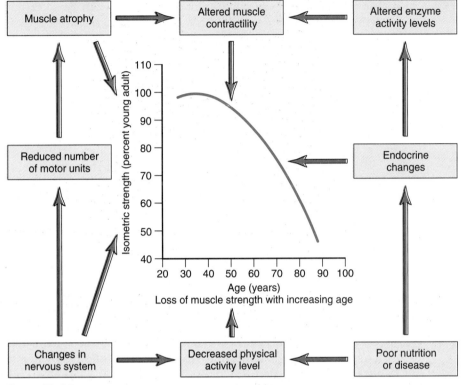

Figure 7–10

Relationship between age and maximal isometric muscle strength in healthy adults. The decline with age does not become apparent until the sixth decade. Note the curvilinear pattern, which is steeper for concentric strength (muscle shortening during contraction) but less affected by age for eccentric strength (active muscle is lengthened by external resistance). Many mechanisms contribute to the loss of muscle strength with aging, including muscle atrophy that is likely genetically controlled and muscle loss due to inactivity in sedentary individuals. (Modified from Vandervoort AA. Biological and physiological changes. In Pickles B, Compton A, Cott CA, et al (eds). *Physiotherapy With Older People*. Philadelphia: WB Saunders, 1995, p 73.)

(1998) were able to predict the relative strength of the correlations between muscle strength and certain functional activities.

Muscle power also relates to the ability to perform functional skills. As stated earlier, power diminishes with age. "Power is a function of the fiber composition and the oxidative capacity of a muscle" (Rice, 2000, p 75). The loss of power with age is associated with a decline in tension produced, a decline in optimal velocity, and energy availability (Faulkner and Brooks, 1995). All of these can be related to a loss of the fast-twitch, type II muscle fibers. Men appear to be affected more by the loss of power with age than do women. The loss of power can be as much as 10% greater than the loss of strength (Metter et al, 1997). Still, the degree of functional loss depends on many factors, including the activity level of the individual. Declines in strength

TABLE 7-1

Strength Changes In Older Adulthood

Better Relative Maintenance	Greater Relative Decline
Muscles used in activities of daily living	Muscles used infrequently in specialized activities
Isometric strength	Dynamic strength
Eccentric contractions	Concentric contractions
Slow-velocity contractions	Rapid-velocity contractions
Repeated low-level contractions	Power production
Strength using small joint angles	Strength using large joint angles
Strength in males	Strength in females

Spirduso WW. *Physical Dimensions of Aging.* Champaign, IL: Human Kinetics, 1995.

and power are the result of a decrease in muscle quantity (reduction in muscle fiber numbers) and altered muscle quality. Velocity-specific resistance training for improvement in power is controversial (see Kraemer and Newton [2000] for a further discussion of the concept).

Endurance is related to the "use it or lose it" concept and can be assessed by looking at muscle fatigue. Aging has little effect on muscle fatigability during voluntary contractions if the exercise is done using a constant amount of force (Faulkner and Brooks, 1995). Lindstrom and colleagues (1997) found no difference in fatigue rate between young and old individuals on an isokinetic test of knee extension. The preponderance of slow-twitch motor units in older adults may maintain the active state of the muscle for a longer time and assist in prolonging force production. "The higher the proportion of type I fibers, the better the endurance capacity of that muscle" (Brown, 2000, p 260).

Factors related to muscle fatigue and endurance are strength, muscle mass, and aerobic conditioning. The age-related loss of muscle mass and subsequent loss of strength contribute to difficulty in sustaining muscular work needed for activities of daily living. Despite the fact that Lindstrom and colleagues (1997) found no difference in rates of fatigue between young and old adults, there is a very real association between the amount of lean body mass and the ability to perform routine tasks of daily living (Ringsberg et al, 1999). Muscular contractions can affect the circulation of a muscle, as previously described, and may result in fatigue. Individuals who are conditioned will not fatigue as quickly as individuals who are deconditioned. Being sedentary is considered a real danger to an older person because of the effect inactivity has on decreasing aerobic fitness.

STRENGTH TRAINING IN OLDER ADULTS

Older adults can improve muscular strength and endurance and substantially increase their functional capacity. Strength training helps offset the loss of muscle and the decline in strength seen with normal aging, according to the

American College of Sports Medicine's position paper (Mazzeo et al, 1998). Older adults should participate in aerobic activities, strength training, and exercises for postural stability and flexibility. Vandervoort (2000) states that the benefits and guidelines for strength training in older individuals can be summed up by, again, the old adage "use it or lose it."

In a compilation of information on strengthening in older adults, Brown (2000) remarks that exercise is efficacious even in the oldest old. She further comments that physical frailty can be delayed by increasing the activity level of the elder. Chandler and colleagues (1998) demonstrated that functional improvements in mobility and performance are associated with increased strength. Older adults were able to improve transfers, stair climbing, and gait speed after a 10-week program of progressive resistive exercise. Strength improvement in older adults appears to be the result of improved neural activation (Brown, 2000).

Eccentric loading of muscles is recommended for older adults by Krishnathasan and Vandervoort (2000). They believe that older adults should take advantage of their relatively higher eccentric strength. The eccentric part of the training program, as they describe, is implemented after a strength base has been established. Eventually, the eccentric training involves using weights that are greater than what the person can lift and lengthening the time it takes to eccentrically "let go" of the muscle.

Older adults can improve their aerobic capacity to the same degree as young adults, about 15% to 25% over baseline. Those adults who are more sedentary may make larger gains because of a more severely depressed baseline (Lexell, 2000). More-conditioned individuals, such as master athletes, may not demonstrate as much change. Aerobic exercise and endurance training can increase $\dot{V}O_{2max}$, which typically declines with age. For example, the maximum amount of oxygen available to a 75-year-old master athlete may be 85 mL/min/kg compared with 15 mL/min/kg for a debilitated 75-year-old person. If 12 mL/min/kg is required to walk at 3 miles per hour, it would "cost" the athlete 14% of $\dot{V}O_{2max}$ compared with 80% for the debilitated older adult. Aerobic exercise improves the ability of the muscle to utilize oxygen. Endurance training increases $\dot{V}O_{2max}$ by increasing cardiac output or by widening the arterial-to-venous oxygen difference (Thompson, 2000). (For additional discussion on cardiovascular changes with aging and fitness issues, see Chapters 8 and 15.)

Summary

Many factors can influence muscle development both before and after birth, including genetics, nutrition, and activity levels. Muscle maturation occurs in childhood, and the rate of that maturation may limit the speed and dexterity with which a child can perform motor tasks. Strength development in childhood and adolescence increases with age (Beunen and Thomis, 2000). Anaerobic function also improves during the same time period (Van Praagh, 2000). Physiological mismatching can occur in adolescence, when skeletal growth temporarily outstrips the ability of limb muscles to lengthen. Strength gains increase with age to maturity and then decline.

After the age of 50, the loss of muscle mass known as sarcopenia can affect strength and functional abilities. As we age, maintaining functional independence has a great deal to do with remaining physically active. During the 1990s, key research has been published on the effects of strength training in older adults. Knowledge of how and why weakness occurs is far more abundant than in previous decades. Age-related changes in muscle cannot be stopped, but they can be slowed. The only known way to slow them is to maintain a healthy nutritional status and to exercise on a regular basis. Human muscle remains responsive to these factors throughout the life span. Even aged muscle is trainable with the appropriate endurance and resistance goals. As part of our role as advocates for healthy aging, we refer you to a publication from the National Institutes of Health (2000) called *Exercise: A Guide from the National Institute on Aging*, which is designed to motivate older adults to exercise.

References

Alexander NB, Schultz AB, Ashton-Miller JA, et al. Muscle strength and rising from a chair in older adults. *Muscle Nerve* 5(suppl):S56–S59, 1997.

Beunen G, Malina RM. Growth and physical performance relative to the timing of the adolescent growth spurt. *Exerc Sport Sci Rev* 16:503–540, 1988.

Beunen G, Thomis M. Muscular strength development in children and adolescents. *Pediatr Exerc Sci* 12:174–197, 2000.

Bishop B. *Basic Neurophysiology*. Garden City, NY: Medical Examination Publishing, 1982.

Bohannon RW. Reference values for extremity muscle strength obtained by hand held dynamometry from adults aged 20–79 years. *Arch Phys Med Rehab* 78:26–32, 1997.

Brooke MH, Engel WK. Histographic analyses of human muscle biopsies with regard to fiber types: 4. Children's biopsies. *Neurology* 19:591–605, 1969.

Brown MB. Strength training and aging. *Top Geriatr Rehabil* 15:1–5, 2000.

Buchner DM, de Lateur BJ. The importance of skeletal muscle strength to physical function in older adults. *Ann Behav Med* 13:91–98, 1991.

Chandler JM, Duncan PW, Kochersberger G, Studenski S. Is lower extremity strength gain associated with improvement in physical performance and disability in frail, community dwelling elders? *Arch Phys Med Rehabil* 79:24–30, 1998.

Colling-Saltin AS. Skeletal muscle development in the human fetus and during childhood. In Berg K, Eriksson BO (eds). *Children and Exercise IX*, Baltimore, MD: University Park Press, 1980, pp 193–207.

Connelly DM. Resisted exercise training of institutionalized older adults for improved strength and functional mobility: A review. *Top Geriatr Rehabil* 15:6–28, 2000.

Connelly, DM, Rice CL, Roos MR, Vandervoort AA. Motor unit firing rates and contractile properties in tibialis anterior of young and old men. *J Appl Physiol* 87:843–852, 1999.

Crelin ES. Development of the musculoskeletal system. *Clin Symp* 33:2–36, 1981.

Elder GC, Kakulas BA. Histochemical and contractile property changes during human muscle development. *Muscle Nerve* 16:1246–1253, 1993.

Enoka RM. Neural strategies in the control of muscle force. *Muscle Nerve* 5(suppl):S66–S69, 1997.

Evans W. What is sarcopenia? *J Gerontol* 50A(special issue):5–8, 1995.

Faigenbaum AD, Westcott WL, Loud RL, Long C. The effects of different resistance training protocols on muscular strength and endurance development in children. *Pediatrics* 104:e5, 1999.

Faulkner JA, Brooks SV. Muscle fatigue in old animals: Unique aspects of fatigue in elderly humans. *Adv Exp Med Biol* 384:471–480, 1995.

Fiatarone MA, O'Neill EF, Ryan ND, et al. Exercise training and nutritional supplementation for physical frailty in very elderly people. *N Engl J Med* 330:1769–1775, 1994.

Foster-Burns SB. Sarcopenia and decreased muscle strength in the elderly woman: Resistance training as a safe and effective intervention. *J Women Aging* 11:75–78, 1999.

Frontera WR, Evans WJ. Exercise performance and endurance training in the elderly. *Top Geriatr Rehabil* 2:17–32, 1986.

Gatev V, Stamatova L, Angelova B. Contraction time in skeletal muscles of normal children. *Electromyogr Clin Neurophysiol* 17:441–452, 1977.

Grabiner MD, Enoka RM. Changes in movement capabilities with aging. *Exerc Sports Sci Rev* 23:65–104, 1995.

Grinnell AD. Dynamics of nerve-muscle interaction in developing and mature neuromuscular junctions. *Physiol Rev* 75:789–834, 1995.

Gross MM, Stevenson PJ, Charette LS, et al. Effect of muscle strength and movement speed on the biomechanics of rising from a chair in healthy elderly and young women. *Gait Posture* 8:175–185, 1998.

Grove BK. Muscle differentiation and the origin of muscle fiber diversity. *Crit Rev Neurobiol* 4:201–234, 1989.

Guttman E, Hazlikova V. Fast and slow motor units and aging. *J Gerontol* 22:280–300, 1976.

Hesselmans LF, Jennekens FG, Van Den Oord CJ, et al. Development of innervation of skeletal muscle fibers in man: Relation to acetylcholine receptors. *Anat Record* 236:553–562, 1993.

Jubrias SA, Odderson IR, Esselman PC, Conley KE. Decline in isokinetic force with age: Muscle cross-sectional area and specific force. *Eur J Physiol* 434:246–253, 1997.

Kamen G, Sison SV, Du DCC, Patten C. Motor unit discharge behavior in older adults during maximal effort contractions. *J Appl Physiol* 79:1908–1913, 1995.

Katzmarzyk PT, Malina RM, Beunen GP. The contribution of biological maturation to the strength and motor fitness of children. *Ann Hum Biol* 24:493–505, 1997.

Keens TG, Bryan AC, Levison H, Ianuzzo CD. Developmental pattern of muscle fiber types in human ventilatory muscles. *J Appl Physiol* 44:909–913, 1978.

Kivinen P, Sulkava R, Halonen P, Nissinen A. Self-reported and performance-based functional status and associated factors among elderly men: The Finnish cohorts of the Seven Countries Study. *J Clin Epidemiol* 51:1243–1252, 1998.

Kraemer WJ, Newton RU. Training for muscular power. *Phys Med Rehabil Clin North Am* 11:341–368, 2000.

Krishnathasan D, Vandervoort AA. Eccentric strength training prescription for older adults. *Top Geriatr Rehabil* 15:29–40, 2000.

Larsson L, Grimby G, Karlsson J. Muscle strength and speed of movement in relation to age and muscle morphology. *J Appl Physiol* 46:451–456, 1979.

Lefevre JG, Beunen G, Steens G, et al. Motor performance during adolescence and age thirty as related to age at peak height velocity. *Ann Hum Biol* 17:423–434, 1990.

Lexell J. Ageing and human muscle: Observations from Sweden. *Can J Appl Physiol* 18:2–18, 1993.

Lexell J. Human aging, muscle mass, and fiber type composition. *J Gerontol* 50A(special issue):11–16, 1995.

Lexell J. Evidence for nervous system degeneration with advancing age. *J Nutr* 127:1011S–1013S, 1997.

Lexell J. Strength training and muscle hypertrophy in older men and women. *Top Geriatr Rehabil* 15:41–46, 2000.

Lexell J, Sjostrom M, Nordlund A, Taylor CC. Growth and development of human muscle: A quantitative morphological study of whole vastus lateralis from childhood to adult age. *Muscle Nerve* 15:4040–4049, 1992.

Lillegard WA, Brown EW, Wilson DJ, et al. Efficacy of strength training in prepubescent to early postpubescent males and females: Effects of gender and maturity. *Pediatr Rehabil* 1:147–157, 1997.

Lin J-P, Brown JK, Walsh EG. Physiological maturation of muscles in childhood. *Lancet* 343:1386–1389, 1994.

Lin J-P, Brown JK, Walsh EG. The maturation of motor dexterity, or why Johnny can't go any faster. *Dev Med Child Neurol* 38:244–254, 1996.

Lindstrom B, Lexell J, Gerdle B, Downham D. Skeletal muscle fatigue and endurance in young and old men and women. *J Gerontol* 52:B59–B66, 1997.

Malina RM. Growth of muscle and muscle mass. In Faulkner R, Tanner JM (eds). *Human Growth: A Comprehensive Treatise, Vol. 2: Postnatal Growth.* New York: Plenum Press, 1986, pp 77–99.

Malina RM, Bouchard C. *Growth, Maturation and Physical Activity.* Champaign, IL: Human Kinetics, 1991.

Mastaglia FL. The growth and development of the skeletal muscles. In Davis JA, Dobbing J (eds). *Scientific Foundations of Paediatrics.* Philadelphia: WB Saunders, 1974, pp 348–375.

Mazzeo RS, Cavanagh P, Evans WJ, et al. American College of Sports Medicine position on exercise and physical activity for older adults. *Med Sci Sports Exerc* 30:992–1008, 1998.

Melton LJ 3rd, Khosla S, Crowson CS, et al. Epidemiology of sarcopenia. *J Am Geriatr Soc* 48:625–630, 2000.

Metter EF, Conwit R, Tobin J, Fozard JL. Age-associated loss of power and strength in the upper extremities in women and men. *J Gerontol Biol Sci Med Sci* 52:B267–B276, 1997.

Miller JB, Schaefer L, Dominov JA. Seeking muscle stem cells. *Curr Top Dev Biol* 43:191–219, 1999.

Minguetti G, Mair WG. Ultrastructure of developing human muscle: The problem of multinucleation of striated muscle cells. *Arq Neuropsiquiatr* 44:1–14, 1986.

Moore KL, Persaud TVN. *Before We Are Born: Essential of Embryology and Birth Defects*, 5th ed. Philadelphia: WB Saunders, 1998.

National Institutes of Health. *Exercise: A Guide from the National Institute on Aging.* Washington, DC: U.S. Government Printing Office, 2000, publication No. NIH 99-4258.

Nelson RM, Soderberg GL, Urbscheit NL. Alteration of motor unit discharge characteristics in aged humans. *Phys Ther* 64:29–34, 1984.

O'Rahilly R, Muller F. *Human Embryology and Teratology*, 2nd ed. New York: Wiley-Liss, 1996.

Patten C and Craik R. Sensorimotor changes and adaptation in the older adult. In Guccione AA (ed). *Geriatric Physical Therapy*, 2nd ed. St. Louis: Mosby, 2000, pp 78–112.

Phillips BA, Lo SK, Mastaglia FL. Muscle force measured using "break" testing with a hand-held myometer in normal subjects aged 20–69 years. *Arch Phys Med Rehab* 81:653–661, 2000.

Proctor DN, Balagopal P, Nair KS. Age-related sarcopenia in humans is associated with reduced synthetic rates of specific muscle proteins. *J Nutr* 128(2 suppl):351S–355S, 1998.

Rice CL. Muscle function at the motor unit level: Consequences of aging. *Top Geriatr Rehabil* 15:70–82, 2000.

Ringsberg K, Gerdhem P, Johansson J, Obrant KJ. Is there a relationship between balance, gait performance and muscular strength in 75-year-old women? *Age Ageing* 28:289–293, 1999.

Roos MR, Rice CL, Vandervoort AA. Age-related change in motor unit function. *Muscle Nerve* 20:679–690, 1997.

Rowland TW. *Developmental Exercise Physiology.* Champaign, Ill: Human Kinetics, 1996.

Schmidtbleicher D, Haralambie G. Changes in contractile properties of muscle after strength training in man. *Eur J Appl Physiol* 46:221–228, 1981.

Schultz E, Lipton BH. Skeletal muscle satellite cells: Changes in proliferation potential as a function of age. *Mech Aging Dev* 20:377–383, 1982.

Sinclair D, Dangerfield P. *Human Growth After Birth*, 6th ed. Oxford, England: Oxford University Press, 1998.

Soderberg GL, Minor SC, Nelson RM. A comparison of motor unit behaviour in young and aged subjects. *Age Ageing* 20:8–15, 1991.

Spirduso WW. *Physical Dimensions of Aging.* Champaign, II: Human Kinetics, 1995.

Thompson LV. Physiological changes associated with aging. In Guccione AA (ed). *Geriatric Physical Therapy*, 2nd ed. St. Louis: Mosby, 2000, pp 28–55.

Thomlinson BE, Irving D. The numbers of limb motor neurons in the human lumbosacral cord throughout life. *J Neurol Sci* 34:213–260, 1977.

Uusitalo M, Kivela T. Development of cytoskeleton in neuroectodermally derived epithelial and muscle cells of human eye. *Invest Ophthalmol Vis Sci* 36:2584, 1995.

Vander A, Sherman J, Luciano D. *Human Physiology*, 8th ed. Boston: McGraw-Hill, 2001.

Vandervoort AA. Introduction. *Top Geriatr Rehabil* 15:vi–viii, 2000.

Vandervoort AA, McComas AJ. Contractile changes in opposing muscles of the human ankle joint with aging. *J Appl Physiol* 61:361–367, 1986.

Van Praagh E. Development of anaerobic function during childhood and adolescence. *Pediatr Exerc Sci* 12:150–173, 2000.

Verfaillie DF, Nichols JF, Turkel E, Hovell MF. Effects of resistance, balance, and gait training on reduction of risk factors leading to falls in elders. *J Aging Phys Activ* 5:213–228, 1997.

Yarasheski KE, Pak-Loduca J, Hasten DL, et al. Resistance exercise training increases mixed muscle protein synthesis rate in frail women and men $\geq$ 76 yr old. *Am J Phyiol* 277(1 Pt 1):E118–E125, 1999.

8 Cardiovascular and Pulmonary Systems Changes

OBJECTIVES

After studying this chapter, the reader will be able to:

1 Describe structural and functional characteristics of the cardiovascular and pulmonary systems as they relate to physical functioning.

2 Discuss age-related structural and functional characteristics of the cardiovascular and pulmonary systems.

3 Relate age-related changes in the cardiovascular and pulmonary systems to physical functioning.

Together, the cardiovascular and pulmonary systems deliver necessary nutrients and oxygen to body tissues, as well as remove waste products. Blood, circulating through the vascular system, provides the transport system for these substances. Oxygen is delivered to the blood via the pulmonary system. An understanding of the structure, function, and development of these two systems as they relate to physical function is important to our ability to assess and promote functional movement development across the life span.

Components of the Cardiovascular and Pulmonary Systems

CARDIOVASCULAR SYSTEM

Components

The cardiovascular system is made up of the heart and the vascular network. Its purpose is to pump blood and to deliver it throughout the body. The blood is pumped from the heart through a high-pressure arterial system to the target organs. There, nutrients and waste products are exchanged between capillaries and tissue. The low-pressure venous system then returns blood to the heart. *Heart rate* refers to the number of times the heart beats per minute; *stroke volume* refers to the amount of blood that is pumped from the ventricle with each heartbeat. By multiplying heart rate by stroke volume, one can determine

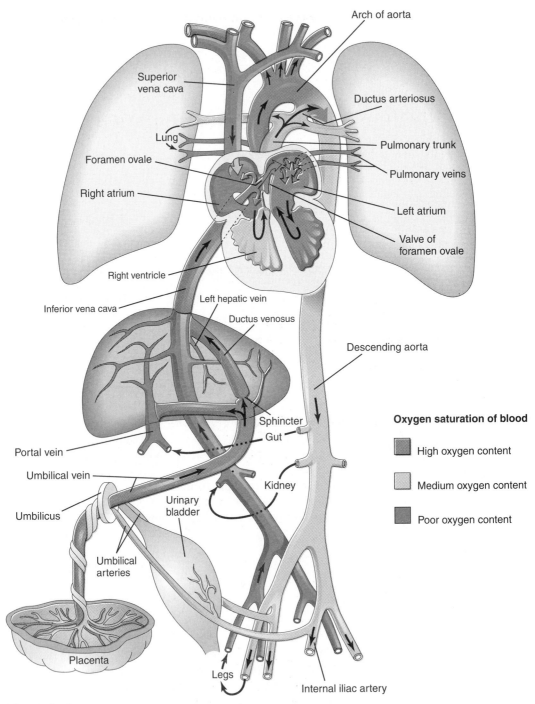

Figure 8–1

Schematic of the fetal circulation. The shades of blue (dark to light) indicate the oxygen saturation of the blood, and the *arrows* show the course of the blood from the placenta to the heart. The organs are not drawn to scale. Three shunts permit most of the blood to bypass the liver and lungs: (1) ductus venosus, (2) foramen ovale, and (3) ductus arteriosus. The poorly oxygenated blood returns to the placenta for oxygen and nutrients through the umbilical arteries. (From Moore KL, Persaud TVN. *Before We Are Born: Essentials of Embryology and Birth Defects*, 5th ed. Philadelphia: WB Saunders, 1998, p 370.)

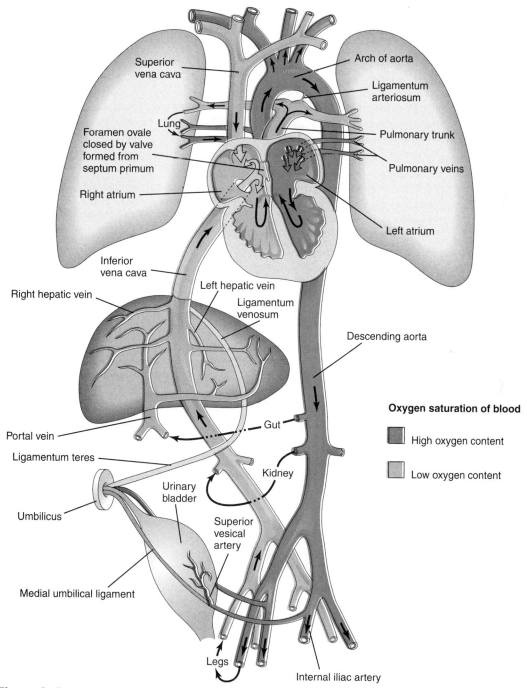

Figure 8–2

Schematic of the neonatal circulation. The adult derivatives of the fetal vessels and structures that become nonfunctional at birth are also shown. The *arrows* indicate the course of the blood in the infant. The organs are not drawn to scale. After birth, the three shunts that short-circuited the blood during fetal life cease to function, and the pulmonary and systemic circulations separate. (From Moore KL, Persaud TVN. *Before We Are Born: Essentials of Embryology and Birth Defects,* 5th ed. Philadelphia: WB Saunders, 1998, p 371.)

the amount of blood pumped from the ventricles in 1 minute, which is referred to as *cardiac output.*

The Heart

The heart is made up of four chambers and acts as the pump of the cardiovascular system. Each of the chambers, the right and left atria and ventricles, are individual pumps, but their actions are coordinated. Figure 8–1 depicts the prenatal circulation that short-circuits the circulation via three shunts that permit most of the blood to bypass the liver and lungs: (1) ductus venosus, (2) foramen ovale, and (3) ductus arteriosus. Poorly oxygenated blood returns to the placenta for oxygen and nutrients through the umbilical arteries (Moore and Persaud, 1998). Dramatic changes occur in the cardiovascular and pulmonary systems at birth when the infant's lungs fill with air. The shunts are no longer needed and immediately start to close. Figure 8–2 illustrates postnatal circulation of blood through the heart, lungs, and periphery. After birth, the atria move blood into the ventricles, which then pump with sufficient force to deliver blood to the lungs and the periphery. The chambers of the right side of the heart receive blood from the periphery and pump it to the lungs to be oxygenated. The chambers on the left side of the heart then receive the oxygenated blood and pump it through the aorta to the systemic circulation. Valves in the heart ensure unidirectional blood flow. The tricuspid and mitral valves, found between the atria and ventricles, prevent blood from flowing back into the atria during ventricular contraction. The aortic and pulmonary valves, also called the *semilunar valves,* prevent blood from flowing back into the ventricles from the aorta and pulmonary artery.

Structurally, the heart is made up of three layers, which are also called *tunics* (Fig. 8–3). The inner layer, the *endocardium,* is made up of a single layer of squamous endothelial cells and a layer of connective tissue. The connective tissue contains blood vessels, nerves, and branches of the conducting system of the heart. The middle layer, the *myocardium,* is the thick muscular layer of the heart and is richly supplied with capillaries. Cardiac muscle cells in the myocardium are able to conduct electricity, but they also have a long refractory period, allowing them to maintain rhythmic heart contraction. The outer layer, the *epicardium,* is made up of loose connective tissue and fat that is covered by simple squamous epithelium. Large blood vessels, such as the coronary arteries, and nerves that supply the heart are found in the epicardium.

Contraction of the heart muscle is controlled by the cardiac conducting system, which consists of the sinoatrial node, atrioventricular node, and atrioventricular bundle of His (Fig. 8–4). The conduction system contains specialized cardiac muscle cells that carry impulses faster than other myocardial cells. The stimulus for cardiac contraction originates in the sinoatrial node, the pacemaker of the heart. The sinoatrial node is supplied by the nodal artery, a branch of the right carotid artery. Autonomic nerve and ganglion cells are also found near and in the node. These cells influence the circulatory and nervous system and help regulate heart rate and contractility. The atrioventricular node receives the impulse from the sinoatrial node and delays it slightly, allowing

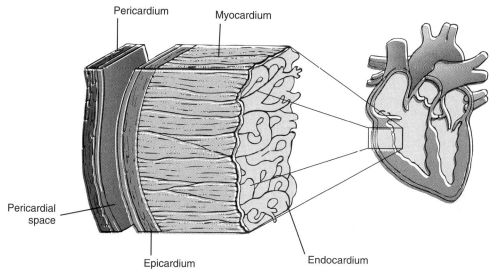

Figure 8–3

Layers of the heart. (From Black JM, Matassarin-Jacobs E. *Medical-Surgical Nursing: Clinical Management for Continuity of Care,* 5th ed. Philadelphia: WB Saunders, 1997, p 1192.)

the atria time to empty before the ventricles contract. The atrioventricular bundle of His and its branches then carry the stimulus to the ventricles. From there, the contractile stimulus is transmitted from one cardiac muscle fiber to another, resulting in a wave of cardiac contraction. The conduction system of the heart is a coordinating system. Each part of it can conduct or initiate an impulse on its own, but because the sinoatrial node fires first, the rhythm is

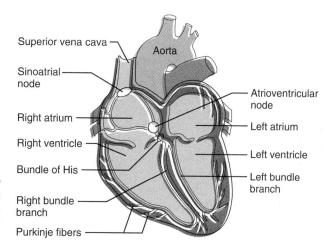

Figure 8–4

The conducting system of the heart. (From Gartner LP, Hiatt JL. *Color Textbook of Histology,* 2nd ed. Philadelphia: WB Saunders, 2001, p 267.)

controlled. When the sinoatrial node is not functioning properly, cardiac arrhythmias occur.

The Vascular System

Three main types of vessels make up the vascular system: *arteries, capillaries,* and *veins.* Arteries and veins are structurally similar to the heart in that they are made up of three concentric layers (Fig. 8–5). The inner layer, *tunica intima,* is made up of a layer of endothelial cells and a subendothelial layer of elastic connective tissue. Some smooth muscle cells are also found in the subendothelial layer. The middle layer, *tunica media,* consists of concentric layers of smooth muscle cells, elastic fibers, collagen fibers, and proteoglycans. The outer layer, *tunica adventitia,* is made up of fibroelastic connective tissue. The fibers are arranged parallel to the vessel and become continuous with the connective tissue of the organ through which the vessel is running. Small blood vessels, *vasa vasorum,* are found in the media and adventitia layers of large vessels. They nourish the thicker layers of the vessel, where sufficient nutrition cannot be supplied by diffusion from the circulating blood.

Arteries carry blood from the heart to the rest of the body and minimize fluctuations in pressure caused by the heartbeat. For instance, when the ventricles contract, the arteries are stretched, decreasing pressure. When the ventricles relax, the arteries return to their original size and maintain the level of pressure.

Arteries can be divided into three groups. The large elastic arteries, called *conducting arteries,* include the aorta and its main branches. The tunica media of these vessels is made up of layers of elastic membrane, which makes them efficient at absorbing the pressure changes that accompany each heartbeat. The number of layers increases from 40 layers in the newborn to 70 layers in the adult. The second category, the *muscular,* or *distributing arteries,* are branches of the large elastic arteries that supply blood to the organs and extremities. The tunica media of the distributing arteries is made of up to 40 layers of smooth muscle cells that regulate blood flow in response to nervous system or hormonal input. Connective tissue, including elastic and collagen fibers, can be found between the muscular layers. The third category of arteries, the *arterioles,* are small vessels that deliver blood to the capillaries. The tunica intima of the arteriole consists of a layer of endothelium and an internal elastic membrane. The tunica media is made of one to five layers of smooth muscle cells and a few elastic fibers. Vasoconstriction and vasodilation of the arterioles control the systemic blood pressure so that only a slow steady stream of blood enters the capillaries. The arterioles are innervated by the autonomic nervous system and can quickly react to functional needs of the tissue.

Capillaries provide a site for the exchange of nutrients and waste products between the blood and the tissue, connect the arterial and venous systems, and contain a large volume of the blood in the body. The capillary itself is a small vessel, made up of a single layer of endothelial cells surrounded by a thin layer of collagen fibers. A very large network of capillaries branches off the arteriole system; the surface area of the capillary network is 60,000 miles

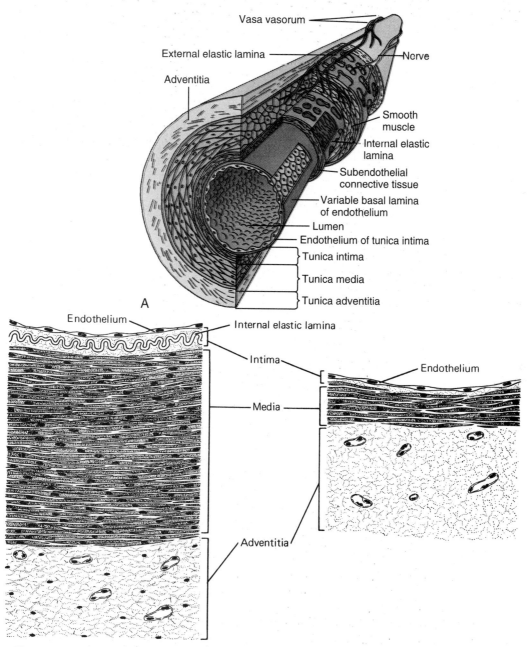

Figure 8–5

A, Diagram of a typical artery showing the three layers: tunica intima, tunica media, and tunica adventitia. *B*, Comparison of muscular artery (*left*) and accompanying vein (*right*). (*A*, From Gartner LP, Hiatt JL. *Color Textbook of Histology*. Philadelphia: WB Saunders, 1997, p 213; *B*, from Junqueira LC, Carneiro J, Kelley RO. *Basic Histology*, 7th edition. Norwalk, CT: Appleton & Lange, 1992.)

(Junqueira et al, 1998). Areas of the body with high metabolic needs, such as the lungs, liver, kidneys, and skeletal muscle, have large capillary networks.

Veins are responsible for carrying blood back to the heart and for the transport of waste products from the tissue. Seventy percent of the total blood volume can be found in the venous system of the body (Junqueira et al, 1989). Veins have larger diameters and thinner walls than do arteries. Because of their size and the large number of veins that make up the venous system, blood flows back to the heart slowly and at low pressure.

Veins can be divided into three major categories by size. *Venules,* the smallest veins, receive blood from the capillaries. The diameter of the venule is greater than that of the capillary and serves to slow the rate of blood flow. As the venule size increases, layers of connective tissue and then smooth muscle cells are added. When the size of the venule is approximately 50 μm, elastic fibers and smooth muscle fibers can be found between the tunica intima and the tunica adventitia. At greater than 200 μm, muscle fibers make up the tunica media of the venule (Leeson et al, 1988). The next category of *small to medium-sized* veins includes most named veins in the body and their branches. These veins contain valves that maintain unidirectional flow of blood. The tunica intima and tunica media are thin, whereas the tunica adventitia is thick. The *large veins* make up the third category of veins and include the superior vena cava, inferior vena cava, portal vein, pulmonary veins, abdominal veins, and main tributaries. The tunica adventitia is the thickest and most developed component of these veins, containing longitudinal bundles of smooth muscle fibers. These muscle cells strengthen the venous wall and help to prevent distension.

Control

Regulation of heart rate and dilation/constriction of the vessels of the vascular system are influenced by the autonomic nervous system and by the presence of chemicals in the circulation. Nervous system control originates in the medulla and is carried via the sympathetic and parasympathetic branches of the autonomic nervous system.

Autonomic fibers are found within the cardiac conducting system. Sympathetic input to the heart increases the rate and strength of cardiac contraction via the release of catecholamines (epinephrine and norepinephrine). Sympathetic innervation of smooth muscle cells in the tunica media of the arteries and the tunica media and tunica adventitia of the veins stimulates vasoconstriction. Parasympathetic input to the heart is received via the vagus nerve and slows the heart rate by releasing acetylcholine. Skeletal muscle arteries also dilate in response to parasympathetic input.

The vascular system relates sensory information to the nervous system through the stretch-sensitive *baroreceptors,* found in the aorta and carotid sinus, and the *chemoreceptors,* found in the carotid and aortic bodies. These receptors react to changes in blood pressure, levels of oxygen and carbon dioxide in the circulating blood, and acidity (pH) of the blood.

Mechanics of Circulation

Blood flow is regulated by pressures exerted by the various structures in the system. Within the heart, *preload* is the amount of pressure necessary to stretch the ventricles during cardiac filling. *Afterload* is the amount of pressure that must be exerted by the ventricles to overcome aortic pressure, open the aortic valve, and push the blood out toward the periphery. The vessels then continue to control blood flow, not only because of the neural and chemical influences described here but also because of their physical properties. Length and diameter of the vessels help to determine peripheral vascular resistance and to influence the speed of blood flow. Blood pressure is actually the pressure exerted by the blood on the vessels as it flows through them.

For efficient mechanical control of blood flow, the blood pressure must be sufficient for blood to flow through the system and must stretch the ventricles during preload. It must likewise not be so high that afterload is increased, making the ventricles work harder to overcome aortic pressure and to empty. In individuals with *hypertension* (high blood pressure), the chronic increased aortic pressure eventually leads to left ventricular hypertrophy because the ventricle has been working so hard to maintain adequate stroke volume. This can eventually contribute to congestive heart failure.

PULMONARY SYSTEM

Components

The pulmonary system consists of the lungs and the structures that connect the lungs to the external environment. It is a closed system, open to the external environment only at the nose and mouth.

The system can be divided into two major structural parts: the conducting portion and the respiratory portion (Fig. 8–6). Functionally, the pulmonary system can be divided into the ventilatory pump and the respiratory component.

Conducting Portion

When considering the structural components of the pulmonary system, the conducting portion of the pulmonary system provides a pathway for air to travel between the environment and the lungs. In this portion, no gas exchange takes place, but the air is cleaned, moistened, and warmed. The conducting portion of the pulmonary system includes the nose, pharynx, larynx, and trachea and portions of the bronchial tree in the lungs. The conducting portion of the bronchial tree includes the two main bronchi, bronchi to the main lobes and to the segments of the lungs, and bronchioles. The diameter of these conducting tubes decreases with each successive branching, helping to regulate the flow of air during inspiration and expiration. The *bronchi* are made up of hyaline cartilage and smooth muscle cells. The muscle cells are arranged in spirals and increase in number closer to the respiratory portion of

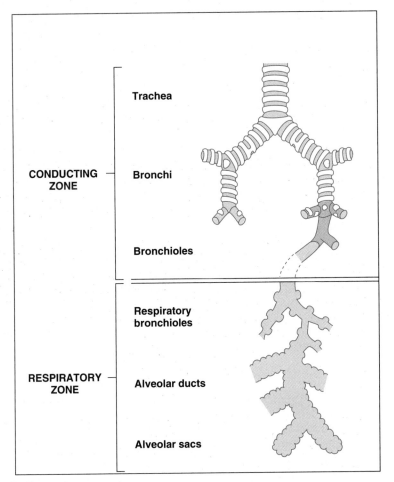

Figure 8–6

The main divisions of the pulmonary system: the conducting portion and the respiratory portion. (From Costanzo LS. *Physiology*. Philadelphia: WB Saunders, 1998, p 164.)

the pulmonary system. The *bronchioles* are made up of smooth muscle cells and elastic fibers. Sympathetic nervous system input via the vagus nerve influences contraction of the smooth muscle cells and changes in length and diameter of the conducting vessels in the bronchial tree.

Respiratory Portion

The respiratory portion of the pulmonary system includes the remaining branches of the bronchial tree, alveolar ducts, alveolar sacs, and alveoli. As air is moved through these structures, gas exchange takes place. Respiratory bronchioles differ from conducting bronchioles because they have alveoli along their walls. Alveoli are small air sacs where gas exchange can take place. At the alveolar level, only a very thin barrier is found between the air and the circulating blood. Alveoli are not only found in the respiratory bronchioles; large numbers of alveoli branch off of the alveolar ducts and alveolar sacs. If the total alveolar surface could be flattened out, 150 m^2 of surface area would be available for gas exchange (Leeson et al, 1988). *Alveolar sucs* (clusters of alveoli) and alveoli branch off of alveolar ducts, which contain smooth muscle cells, elastic fibers, and collagen fibers. Elastic and reticular fibers are found where the alveoli arise from the respiratory bronchioles, alveolar ducts, or alveolar sacs. The elastic fibers help to open the alveoli during inspiration and allow recoil during exhalation. Reticular fibers help maintain the shape of the alveoli.

Alveolar epithelium is made up of two types of cells. *Type I* alveolar cells are flat and thin respiratory epithelial cells, providing a large surface area for gas exchange. *Type II* cells are responsible for the production of surfactant, the detergent-like substance that mixes with water to decrease the alveolar surface tension. The decreased surface tension allows the alveoli to open more easily during respiration. Without surfactant, alveolar collapse can occur. This is especially important for the newborn—lack of surfactant in the premature infant results in respiratory distress. Surfactant is constantly produced and turned over throughout life.

Air can also move from one part of the respiratory system to another via collateral ventilation mechanisms. Two mechanisms of collateral ventilation are pores of Kohn and Lambert's canals. *Pores of Kohn* are gaps in the alveolar walls that provide an opening from one alveolus and its neighbor. *Lambert's canals,* or *channels,* are small pathways from the respiratory bronchi to nearby alveoli. Little is known about these structures, so the functional significance of their absence can only be hypothesized.

Ventilatory Pump

In considering the functional components of the pulmonary system, the ventilatory pump component controls the flow of gases. It is made up of the respiratory muscles, thorax, diaphragm, and abdominal compartments.

Respiratory Component

The respiratory component is the site of gas exchange and consists of the lungs, intrapulmonary airways, and intrapulmonary vessels.

Control and Regulation

Ventilation is controlled by input from the respiratory center of the central nervous system, located in the brain stem. Chemoreceptors detect changes in blood levels of oxygen and carbon dioxide, as well as the pH of the blood, stimulating appropriate respiratory changes. Proprioceptive input from stretch receptors in the lungs also stimulates respiration.

The pulmonary system is innervated by the parasympathetic and sympathetic branches of the autonomic nervous system. Parasympathetic input results in bronchial constriction, whereas sympathetic input results in bronchodilation. Sensory and motor nerve fibers are found in the lung to the level of the terminal bronchioles. Some studies have reported sensory endings to the level of the alveoli and suggest that these receptors are responsible for increased levels of surfactant secretion with nervous stimulation (Leeson et al, 1988).

Mechanics of Ventilation

The lungs, thorax, intercostal muscles, and diaphragm provide a pumping action that transports gas between the environment and the alveoli. During inspiration, the intercostal muscles contract to elevate the rib cage. The diaphragm also contracts, increasing the diameter of the thoracic cavity. This muscle activity expands the pleural cavity and results in increased negative pressure in the thoracic cavity. Atmospheric air rushes in and the lungs expand. Bronchi and bronchioles increase in diameter. The expansion of the lungs activates stretch receptors, inhibiting inspiration. Exhalation occurs passively, with muscle relaxation and elastic recoil of the chest wall. Inhibitory input to inspiration is decreased, once again activating inspiration.

The ability of the musculoskeletal pump to transport inspiratory and expiratory gases is influenced by the compliance and resistance of the chest wall and lungs. Flexibility of the joints of the thoracic cavity contributes to achieving optimal expansion of the space. Resistance and elasticity of the pulmonary tissues must be overcome by contraction of the respiratory muscles, diaphragm, intercostal muscles, and accessory muscles of respiration. Resistance of the conducting airways also affects the amount of work necessary to deliver air to the respiratory system.

The amount of air contained in the lungs is defined by various functional volumes (Fig. 8–7). The maximal amount of air that can be contained in the lungs is referred to as the *total lung capacity*. The amount of air moved during resting inspiration and exhalation is referred to as the *tidal volume* (V_T). The additional inspired air that can be taken into the lungs with a deep breath is called the *inspiratory reserve volume* (IRV); the additional air that can be pushed out of the lungs with forced exhalation is called the *expiratory reserve volume* (ERV). The sum of these three volumes is called the *vital capacity* (VC). The *residual volume* (RV) is the amount of air that is left in the lungs after exhalation. *Minute ventilation* (MV) is the total amount of air exchanged by the pulmonary system in 1 minute.

Resistance and compliance factors, the breathing rate, and the amount of air being moved with each breath determine the energy cost of breathing. The pulmonary system itself requires oxygen to fuel the work of breathing. The source of that oxygen is the bronchial arteries, which deliver blood from the aorta to the lung tissue. Blood is then returned to the heart via the pulmonary and bronchial veins.

A second source of pulmonary circulation originates in the pulmonary artery, which carries deoxygenated blood from the right ventricle to the lungs. This artery branches in conjunction with the bronchial tree to the level of the respiratory bronchioles. From here, a capillary network is formed, accompanying the alveoli. Other branches from the pulmonary artery are sent to the

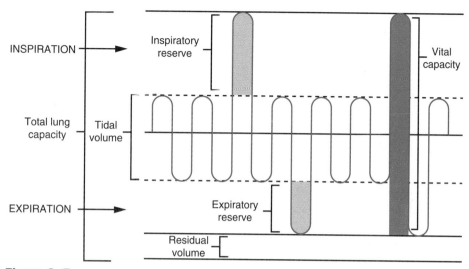

Figure 8–7

Functional lung volumes.

periphery of the lungs. Pulmonary venules arise from the capillary network and branch into successively larger veins through the bronchial tree. The pulmonary veins carry the blood back to the heart.

Development of the Cardiovascular and Pulmonary Systems Across the Life Span

PRENATAL PERIOD

Cardiovascular System

The cardiovascular system is the earliest system of the body to function in the developing embryo, with blood circulation starting in the third week of gestation. Functionally, this circulation is necessary because the embryo has grown, and simple diffusion of nutrients and waste products across cell membranes can no longer meet nutritional demands.

The heart is developed as a recognizable structure between 20 and 50 gestational days. By the end of the third week of gestation, a primitive heart tube has been formed from clusters of mesoderm cells. As this tube elongates, a series of dilatations and constrictions differentiate the vessel into an atrium, a ventricle, the truncus arteriosus, and the sinus venosus (Fig. 8–8). The sinus venosus functions early as the pacemaker of the conducting system of the heart and is the precursor to the sinoatrial node, atrioventricular node, and bundle of His. At approximately four weeks of gestation, areas of swelling form on the walls of the atrioventricular canal. These swellings, called *endocardial cushions*, grow together during the fifth week of gestation and begin to

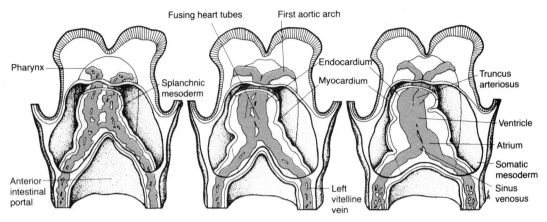

Figure 8-8

Early fetal development of the heart. (Adapted from Moore KL, Persaud TVN. *The Developing Humans,* 6th ed. Philadelphia: WB Saunders, 1998, p 356.)

divide the heart into left and right chambers. The primitive atrium is also divided into two chambers by the formation of the septum primum and the septum secundum. An oval opening left between the interatrial septae, called the *foramen ovale,* is important for fetal circulation. Near the end of the fourth week of gestation, contractions of the heart coordinate unidirectional flow of blood. By the seventh week, the heart tube has become a four-chambered vessel (Fig. 8–9).

The embryo's primitive heart tube establishes links with its blood vessels and with the placenta as early as 13 to 15 days of gestation. Circulation is then established between the mother and the embryo, ensuring the exchange of nutrients and waste products. Maternal nutrients and oxygen are transported to the fetus via the umbilical vein; waste products and carbon dioxide are removed via the umbilical artery. By the fifth week of development, embryonic vessel formation is underway.

Vascular development begins with the differentiation of mesodermal cells into vessels. This process is called *vasculogenesis* and occurs only during the embryonic period. Larger vascular networks in organs such as the liver and endocardium of the heart are formed by vasculogenesis. Further development of the vessels occurs as branches are formed from existing vessels. This process is called *angiogenesis* and can occur in embryonic development as well as throughout the life span. Embryonically, angiogenesis occurs in organs such as the brain and kidney. Throughout the life span, angiogenesis plays a role in healing (Baldwin, 1996).

The fetus receives all necessary oxygen from the mother; little blood flow is necessary through the lungs (see Fig. 8–1). The foramen ovale and ductus arteriosus in the fetal heart allow blood to circumvent the pulmonary system. The *foramen ovale* shunts blood from the right to the left atrium. The *ductus*

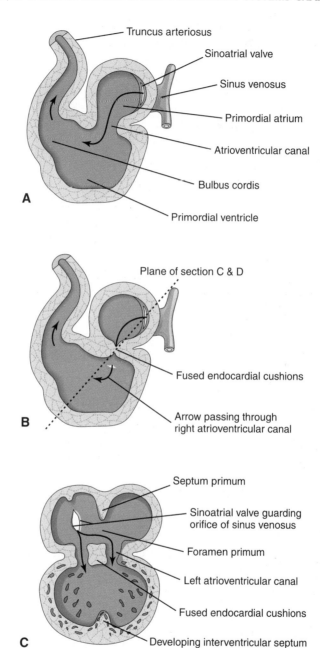

Figure 8-9

Schematic sketches of fetal heart development. *A* and *B,* Sagittal sections of the heart during the fourth and fifth weeks, illustrating blood flow through the heart and division of the atrioventricular canal. *C,* Coronal section of the heart at the plane shown in *B.* Note that the interatrial and interventricular septa have also started to develop.

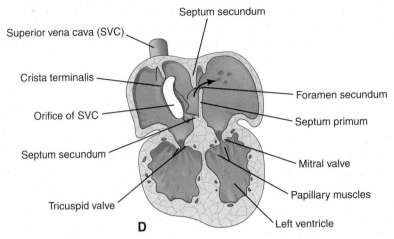

Figure 8–9 *Continued.*

D, At about 8 weeks, after the heart is partitioned into four chambers. (From Moore KL, Persaud TVN. *Before We Are Born: Essentials of Embryology and Birth Defects,* 5th ed. Philadelphia: WB Saunders, 1998, pp 342–343.)

arteriosus shunts blood from the right ventricle to the pulmonary artery and the aorta. These two shunts will close at birth, allowing blood to enter the pulmonary circulation. Fetal hemoglobin levels are higher than postnatal hemoglobin levels. This is necessary because the oxygen saturation of blood coming to the fetus from the umbilical vein is only 70% compared with an arterial blood oxygen saturation of 97% after birth. By having an increased hemoglobin level, the fetus has a greater capacity to carry oxygen to the tissues.

Pulmonary System

The pulmonary system of the embryo arises from both endodermal and mesodermal germ cells and first appears in the fourth week of gestation. Endodermal cells from the primitive pharynx form the epithelial lining of trachea, larynx, bronchi, and lungs. Mesoderm surrounding the developing lung buds contributes to the development of smooth muscle, connective tissue, and cartilage within these structures.

Early development of the fetal pulmonary system is shown in Figure 8–10. At 28 days of gestation, *bronchial buds* have developed at the end of the laryngotracheal tube and have divided into the right and left lung buds. At 35 days, secondary bronchi have appeared. By 42 days, all of the branches of the conducting airways are formed. Between 42 and 56 days of gestation, branching had continued to the level of at least two respiratory bronchioles. Formation of the pulmonary arterial tree accompanies the branching of the respiratory tree.

The bronchial epithelium thins and flattens, increasing the diameter of the

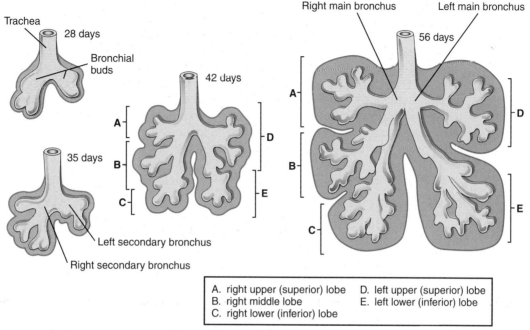

A. right upper (superior) lobe   D. left upper (superior) lobe
B. right middle lobe   E. left lower (inferior) lobe
C. right lower (inferior) lobe

Figure 8-10

Successive stages in the development of bronchi and lungs. (From Moore KL, Persaud TVN. *Before We Are Born: Essentials of Embryology and Birth Defects*, 5th ed. Philadelphia: WB Saunders, 1998, p 247.)

bronchi and terminal bronchioles. Capillaries also appear in the epithelium. From 24 weeks of gestation until birth, development of the *terminal respiratory units* continues. These may also be referred to as *terminal sacs* or *primitive alveoli*. Type II epithelial cells appear in the lining of the primitive alveoli. Primitive alveoli continue to multiply in the last few weeks of the normal gestational period. The structure of the primitive alveoli becomes more complex, and the number of alveoli continues to increase after birth until approximately 8 years of age (Moore and Persaud, 1998).

Type II epithelial cells appear in the lining of the primitive alveoli, and surfactant production begins at approximately 24 weeks of gestation. Surfactant is necessary for maximum lung expansion after birth. Once surfactant is produced, the amniotic fluid begins to contain lecithin, a phospholipid. The ratio of two types of phospholipids, lecithin and sphingomyelin (L/S ratio), is used as an index of lung maturity. A ratio of 2:1 or greater indicates that the lungs are mature and that the risk of development of hyaline membrane disease in the fetus is less than 5% (Burgess and Chernick, 1986). In this disease, the lungs collapse easily because of a lack of surfactant. By 26 to 28 weeks of gestation, the fetus has sufficient vascularized terminal sacs and surfactant to survive if born prematurely. Premature neonates cannot survive without an adequate pulmonary vasculature and sufficient surfactant, because the lungs will not have the ability to provide adequate gas exchange (Moore and Persaud, 1998).

The intrauterine lung is not responsible for gas exchange. Weak attempts at fetal breathing appear to be in preparation for respiration after birth. Instead, the lung tissue secretes liquid that is swallowed or added to amniotic fluid. This fluid production slows shortly before birth so that the lungs are only 50% filled with fluid at birth (Moore and Persaud, 1998). This fluid has to be removed as the lungs inflate after birth. Like the cardiovascular system, the pulmonary system undergoes dramatic change in the moments after birth.

INFANCY AND YOUNG CHILDHOOD

Cardiovascular and Pulmonary Adjustments at Birth

Immediately after birth, blood must be circulated to the lung tissue, and the lungs must inflate. Much of the fluid that fills the lungs is pushed out through the nose and mouth as a result of pressure on the thorax during the birth process; remaining fluid can be drained by the pulmonary vasculature and lymphatic system (Moore and Persaud, 1998). With each of the first breaths, more and more air is retained in the lungs, building up the newborn's functional residual capacity (residual volume plus expiratory reserve volume). With inspiration, alveolar expansion occurs, delivering oxygenated air to the alveoli (Murray, 1986).

After birth, blood must be shunted into the pulmonary circulation to receive oxygen from the alveoli. As the lungs expand, pulmonary vascular resistance decreases, and blood flow to the lungs increases. With the occlusion of the umbilical cord, the ductus venosus, which had delivered blood from the umbilical vein to the inferior vena cava, closes. This results in decreased pressure in the inferior vena cava and right atrium. As left atrial pressure becomes greater than right atrial pressure, the foramen ovale closes. Another circulatory change occurs as increased systemic and aortic pressures pump the blood toward the pulmonary artery, reversing the direction of blood flow through the ductus arteriosus. The ductus arteriosus constricts and eventually closes (see Figs. 8-1 and 8-2).

Cardiovascular System

The newborn heart lies horizontally in the chest cavity, but as the lungs expand and the chest cavity grows, a more vertical position is assumed. Irregularity in the electrocardiogram of the newborn is not unusual, because stabilization of the autonomic nervous system, conductivity of cardiac muscle fibers, heart position, and hemodynamics are not yet completed (Malina and Bouchard, 1991).

Heart size increases at a rate similar to that of the increase in fat-free body weight. Heart volumes are approximately 40 mL at birth, 80 mL at 6 months, and 160 mL by 2 years of age. The ratio of heart volume to body weight remains constant at approximately 10 mL/kg body weight. Although there is no increase in the number of cardiac muscle fibers (myocytes) as the heart grows, the cross-sectional area of the fibers increases.

Several changes in the myocyte are noted during development, allowing the mature myocyte to contract with more force than the immature myocyte. Immature myocytes are spherical, whereas mature myocytes are more rectangular. As myocytes mature, the number of myofibrils per cross-sectional area increases, and with increased myofibrils, the contractile properties of the myocyte increase. Myofibrils in immature myocytes are also randomly arranged, but as myocytes mature, the myofibrils assume a parallel orientation and increase force-generating potential (Anderson, 1996).

The vascularization of the heart muscle increases from one vessel for six muscle fibers in the newborn to one vessel for each muscle fiber, as seen in the adult. At birth, the thicknesses of the right and left ventricle walls are equal, but as the left ventricle starts pumping against increased pressure, the left ventricular wall increases in size and becomes approximately twice as thick as the right ventricular wall by adulthood (Sinclair and Dangerfield, 1998).

Arteries and veins also increase in size as body weight and height increase. As increased functional demands are placed on the vessels, the thickness of the vessel wall increases. Development of smooth muscle within the walls of the vessels occurs more slowly. No muscle cells are present at birth in the alveolar blood vessels. Muscle cells can be seen in pulmonary vasculature at the level of the respiratory bronchiole by 4 months of age and at the alveolar ducts by 3 years of age. Some alveolar arteries have muscle cells in their walls at 10 years, but others do not complete this process until 19 years of age (Murray, 1986).

The heart rate and stroke volume of infants and young children are very different from those of adults. Because stroke volume is related to heart size, the smaller the heart, the less blood that can be pumped with each heart beat. At birth, stroke volume is only 3 to 4 mL, whereas it may be 40 mL in the preadolescent and 60 mL in the young adult. To compensate for smaller stroke volumes, children demonstrate higher heart rates than adults. Table 8–1 provides both mean resting heart rates and normal ranges of heart rate. Boys and girls younger than 10 years have similar heart rates, but after puberty, girls' heart rates are slightly higher than those of boys (Malina and Bouchard, 1991).

Blood pressure also changes from infancy through childhood. These changes are related to ongoing development of (1) the autonomic nervous system, (2) peripheral vascular resistance, and (3) body mass. Blood pressure increases in children are strongly related to increases in height and weight. Diastolic blood pressure values appear to vary in relation to height, whereas systolic blood pressure values are related to both height and weight (Gerber and Stern, 1999). Mean systolic blood pressure values increase with age in children (see Table 8–1). Diastolic blood pressure is reported to be relatively constant through childhood (Malina and Bouchard, 1991).

Blood volume also increases with body size; the total blood volume of the newborn is 300 to 400 mL, whereas the adolescent or young adult has approximately 5 L of blood. Hemoglobin levels in the blood also vary with age,

TABLE 8–1

Measures of Cardiovascular and Pulmonary Function Across the Life Span

Age	Resting Heart Rate (mean beats/min)	Resting Heart Rate (range, beats/min)	Systolic Blood Pressure (mean mm Hg)	Systolic Blood Pressure (range, mm Hg)	Diastolic Blood Pressure (mean mm Hg)	Diastolic Blood Pressure (range, mm Hg)	Respiratory Rate (range, breaths/min)
Newborn	120–125	70–90	73	54–92	55	38–72	30–40
1 Year	120	80–160	90	71–109	56	39–73	20–40
2 Years	110	80–130	91	72–110	56	39–72	25–32
6 Years	100	75–115	96	77–115	57	41–74	21–26
10 years	90	70–110	102	84–121	62	45–79	20–26
16 Years	80 (girls) 75 (boys)	60–100 (girls) 55–95 (boys)	117	98–136	67	49–85	16–20
Adult	74–76	60–100	120–125 (20–45 years) 135–140 (45–65 years)	*	80 (20–45 years) 85 (45–65 years)	*	10–20
Older adults (>65 years)	74–76	60–100	150	*	85	*	*

*Data unavailable.

Data from Jarvis C. *Physical Examination and Health Assessment*, 3rd ed. Philadelphia: WB Saunders, 1996, pp 186–187; Paz JC, Panik M. *Acute Care Handbook for Physical Therapists*. Woburn, MA: Butterworth-Heinemann, 1997, p 370 (source: Bullock B. *Pathophysiology: Adaptations and Alterations in Function*, 4th ed. Philadelphia: Lippincott, 1996); Wong DL, Perry SE. *Maternal Child Nursing Care*, St. Louis, Mosby, 1998, pp 1790–1791 (sources: Gillette PC. Dysrhythmias. In Adams FH, et al (eds). *Moss' Heart Disease in Infants, Children, and Adolescents*, 4th ed. Baltimore: Williams and Wilkins, 1989; Rosner B. *Data from Second Task Force on Blood Pressure Control in Children*. Bethesda, MD: National Heart, Lung and Blood Institute, 1987).

affecting the oxygen-carrying capacity of the blood. In the newborn, hemoglobin levels are high (20 g/100 mL), but they fall to 10 g/100 mL by 3 to 6 months of age. Hemoglobin values then slowly increase with age to adult levels of 16 g/100 mL for men and 14 g/100 mL for women (Malina and Bouchard, 1991). As discussed, the newborn's hemoglobin level is high due to the lower oxygen saturation of the blood in the umbilical vein.

Pulmonary System

Ventilatory Pump Development

From a mechanical point of view, the shape of the chest wall and limitations in posture and movement affect the infant's breathing efficiency. At birth, the infant maintains a posture of shoulder elevation, limiting the cervical dimensions of the thorax. The ribs are made up primarily of cartilage and are in a horizontal position, giving the lower thorax a circular dimension (Fig. 8–11). This results in a relatively flexible thorax and affects the alignment of the diaphragm. The diaphragm and other ventilatory muscles of the newborn are made up of more type IIa muscle fibers than type I muscle fibers, affecting muscle strength and endurance (Bourgeois and Zadai, 2000). The structural immaturity of the thorax, combined with a lack of development and control of the ventilatory muscles, prevents the infant from stabilizing the rib cage and effectively using the diaphragm to breathe.

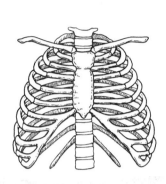
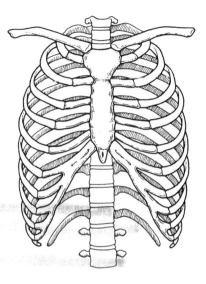

Figure 8–11

Comparison of the infant thorax (*left*) with the mature thorax (*right*). A major difference between the infant and mature adult thorax, other than the size, is the orientation of the ribs. The ribs are oriented horizontally in the infant thorax but are angled downward in the adult.

As the infant learns to move the head and upper body against gravity and to reach in the first 3 to 6 months, muscular development allows increased expansion and use of the upper chest in breathing. In the second half of the first year, the infant learns to sit, stand, and walk, systematically overcoming the force of gravity. As the upright sitting position is assumed, the force of gravity and forces from developing abdominal musculature will pull the ribs downward into a more angular position. This not only expands the thoracic cavity but also increases spacing between the ribs, allowing the intercostal muscles to work more efficiently. Throughout childhood, the rib cage becomes more rigid as osteophytes are laid down to replace cartilage. With growth, the diaphragm is pulled into a dome shape that improves the length-tension relationship of the muscle and improves function. Active use of the abdominal muscles stabilizes the rib cage within the more rigid thorax, providing a stable base for diaphragmatic action (Massery, 1991).

Respiratory System Development

Only a small percentage of the total number of alveoli to be developed are present at birth. From birth to 3 years of age, some of the nonrespiratory bronchioles in the conducting airway system that were formed prenatally are converted to respiratory bronchioles. This increases the gas exchange capacity of the lungs (Bourgeois and Zadai, 2000). New alveoli continue to develop until approximately 8 years of age, when the adult number of 300 million alveoli is attained (DeCesare and Graybill, 1990). The size and complexity of the alveoli increase throughout infancy and childhood, increasing the available surface area for air exchange. The growth of the alveolar surface appears to be related to the increased oxygen demand of working tissue. The pulmonary arterial and venous vasculature develops concurrently with the development of alveoli.

The conducting and respiratory airways increase in length and diameter until growth of the thoracic cavity is complete. Children under age 5 years have a larger number of small airways that are less than 2 mm in diameter. For example, 50% of airways in the neonate and 20% of airways in the adult have diameters of less than 2 mm (DeCesare and Graybill, 1990). Small airways can be problematic in two ways. First, they offer increased resistance to airflow, thereby increasing the work of breathing. Second, they are very easily obstructed by foreign objects.

The bronchioles and alveoli of infants and young children are weaker and less efficient than those of adults. Smooth muscle in the walls of the bronchioles does not develop until the child is 3 to 4 years old. As a result, the airway is more susceptible to collapse, thus trapping air. The development of elastic tissue in the alveoli may be incomplete until after adolescence; this means decreased lung compliance and distensibility for infants and young children. This makes it harder for the infant and small child to fully inflate their lungs and maintain lung volume. In children younger than 7 years, decreased elastic recoil causes the airways to close at greater lung volume than in older children and adults. When combined with small airway size, this relative lack of recoil places young children more at risk for complications from small airway diseases such as bronchiolitis (DeCesare and Graybill, 1990).

One other structural difference between the pulmonary systems of children and adults is the absence of collateral ventilation mechanisms in children. This decreased collateral circulation may increase the risk of respiratory infection and atelectasis in children. Pores of Kohn have not been seen in children younger than 6 years. Lambert's canals are not thought to develop until at least 6 to 8 years of age (Boyden, 1977; Meyrick and Reid, 1977).

In summary, the development of the lungs into their adult form continues well into childhood. Lung volume increases proportionally with increases in body size and increases as the number of alveoli increases (Malina and Bouchard, 1991). Vital capacity values are related to height. Size of the conducting airways is related to stature, and the total number of alveoli an individual develops is proportional to height, which reinforces the relationship between lung volume and body size (Murray, 1986). In the first year of life, the infant has little pulmonary reserve and must increase breathing frequency to meet demands for increased oxygen. Inspiratory and expiratory reserve volumes sufficient to meet increased needs are evident at about 1 year of age.

Differences between the child's and the adult's pulmonary function are seen in breathing pattern and in breathing frequency. The newborn infant undergoes dramatic changes in intrathoracic pressure, lung inflation, and pulmonary circulation. It is not unusual to observe irregular breathing patterns, including periods of apnea, during this time. Small airway size, together with the limited number of developed alveoli, leave the young infant with a small lung volume. As a result, the newborn's respiratory rate is higher than at any other time in the life span (see Table 8–1).

ADOLESCENCE

Growth and functional changes of the cardiovascular and pulmonary systems continue through childhood and into adolescence. During the adolescent growth spurt, gender differences in cardiovascular and pulmonary function become apparent.

The amount of muscle in the heart increases, resulting in increased blood pressure and decreased heart rate (Sinclair and Dangerfield, 1998). Increased blood pressure is primarily related to increased body weight. In girls, blood pressure increases during their prepubertal growth spurt and then levels off. In boys, blood pressure gradually increases with lean body mass through 18 years of age. By the end of adolescence, systolic and diastolic blood pressures of boys become slightly greater than those of girls (Malina and Bouchard, 1991). Gender differences in heart rate are also reported: the basal heart rate of girls is 3 to 5 beats per minute faster than that of boys. Stroke volume also increases but does not appear to be related only to heart size. In the year preceding the peak height velocity, stroke volume changes appear to be related to an increased arterial-venous oxygen difference. This implies that more oxygen is being extracted by the tissues, which may be due to age-related changes in muscle mass, muscle enzyme profusion, and the ratio of capillaries to muscle fiber. In the year after peak height velocity, increased stroke volume may be related to an increased cardiac preload condition with increased venous return (Cunningham et al, 1984).

The adolescent growth spurt is also reflected in lung size and lung volume. Proximal airways and vasculature increase in size. Alveoli become larger, and greater amounts of elastic fiber can be found in the alveolar wall. The capillaries in the alveolar region also become larger, supporting increased gas exchange. By age 19, muscle is developed in the walls of the arteries found at the alveoli, increasing the efficient control of blood flow by vasodilation and vasoconstriction (Davis and Dobbings, 1981).

ADULTHOOD AND AGING

Normal function of the cardiovascular and pulmonary systems in early and middle adulthood is described in the beginning of this chapter. Heart size and weight may continue to increase in adulthood, primarily because of fat deposition (Sinclair and Dangerfield, 1998). Some gender differences in function of the cardiovascular and pulmonary systems do exist. Stroke volume, residual lung volume, mean heart weight, and body surface area are greater in men than in women (Payne and Isaacs, 1987). Age-related changes in mean heart weight are not demonstrated in men, but in women, the mean heart weight increases between the fourth and seventh decades of life (Kitzman and Edwards, 1990). During submaximal exercise, the cardiac output of women is 5%

to 10% greater than that of men. This may be related to stroke volume differences and the fact that women have slightly less hemoglobin (14 g/100 mL blood) than men (15 to 16 g/100 mL blood).

With increasing age, anatomic and physiologic changes in the cardiovascular and pulmonary systems are seen. At least initially, these age-related changes do not seem to significantly interfere with function. Functional losses are more evident beginning in the seventh decade of life (Cunningham and Paterson, 1990). It is also difficult to differentiate cardiovascular and pulmonary changes related purely to aging from those due to asymptomatic disease or deconditioning. As discussed in Chapter 15, it is thought that physically active adults can minimize the impact of aging on cardiovascular and pulmonary function.

Cardiovascular System

The Heart

Structural changes are seen in the heart and cardiac cells with aging. In general, the number of myocytes decreases, whereas their size increases. In the myocardium, increasing amounts of elastic tissue, fat, and collagen contribute to increased stiffness and decreased compliance of the ventricles. Cross-linkage of collagen in the myocardium also contributes to increased stiffness. Accumulation of lipofuscin, a pigment deposit thought to be related to wear and tear, is also seen near the nuclei of the cardiac muscle cells, resulting in a darkening of the myocardium. It is not known whether increased lipofuscin has any functional significance. Other subcellular changes in the cell nucleus and mitochondria affect the ability of the myocyte to function (Thompson, 2000).

Thickening of the left ventricular wall by approximately 25% is reported, between the second and seventh decade (Peel, 1990; Wei, 1986), but whether the thickening is really of the ventricular wall as opposed to the ventricular septum is controversial (Kitzman and Edwards, 1990). Some of this thickening may be related to hypertrophy of the myocytes secondary to the increased demand on the heart necessary to pump blood through a less-compliant vascular system. The volume of the left ventricle is slightly decreased, and the left atrium is slightly dilated. In the endocardium, thickened areas of elastic and collagen fibers can be noted, especially in the atria. Fragmentation and disorganization of elastic, collagen, and muscle fibers also occur (Peel, 1990; Wei, 1986). Increased fat is found within the epicardium, especially over the right ventricle and in the atrioventricular groove (Kitzman and Edwards, 1990).

With aging, changes are also seen in the heart valves and in the conduction system. The valves become thickened and calcified. Collagen and lipid accumulation, as well as calcification, within the aortic and mitral valves impairs the ability of the valves to completely close. Valvular changes contribute to the increased incidence of heart murmur in the older adult population. Collagen and fat are also laid down in the left bundle branches of the conduction system. By age 60, the number of pacemaker cells in the sinoatrial node begins to decrease; by age 75, less than 10% of the number of sinoatrial node cells found in the adult heart are seen (Peel, 1990; Wei, 1986). Cellular loss is also noted in the atrioventricular node and bundle of His. These changes in the conduction system may contribute to the increased incidence of premature ventricular complexes and differences seen on the older adult's electrocardiogram. The QRS wave shifts to the left, and ST-segment depression is seen.

The Vasculature

The vasculature undergoes change throughout life, with vessels becoming thicker, more rigid, and more dilated. In general, the vascular course becomes more tortuous. Changes attributed to aging are initially seen in the coronary arteries at approximately 20 years of age and in the remainder of the arterial system after 40 years of age. Dilation occurs in proximal arteries such as the aorta, whereas thickening of the arterial wall predominates in the peripheral arteries. Elastic arteries change more than muscular arteries, with irregular thickening of elastic tissue, fragmenting of elastic fibers, lipid infiltration, and calcification. These changes are seen earliest in the proximal portions of the large arteries (Wei, 1986). The older vessel is thickened and less elastic, which results in less compliance. *Arteriosclerosis* refers to decreased compliance of the arteries, which is a normal consequence of age-related changes in the arterial walls (Zadia, 1986). This is contrasted to atherosclerosis, a pathologic deposition of fatty plaques on the inner layer of the vessel, which also results in increased resistance to blood flow through the vessel. Research has shown that regular aerobic, endurance exercise can minimize the age-related changes in central arterial compliance. This possibly reflects the mechanism by which exercise decreases the risk of cardiovascular disease in older adults (Tanaka et al, 2000).

Functional Changes

The changes in the cardiovascular system associated with aging functionally affect the heart rate, blood pressure, stroke volume, and adaptability of the system to stress. The structural changes of the left ventricular wall reduce the ability of the ventricle to fill and contract. These changes do not have much effect on an individual at rest or during light exercise, but maximal exercise capacity decreases.

The sensitivity of regulatory mechanisms, such as the baroreceptors, is diminished in the older individual, affecting adaptability of the cardiovascular system to stressful situations such as cough, the Valsalva maneuver, and orthostasis. Increased plasma catecholamine levels and decreased end-organ responsiveness to adrenergic stimulation also affect the ability of the system to increase heart rate, contractility of the heart, and vasodilation of the vessels in response to stress. Because of decreased adaptability, the heart takes longer to reach a steady state or to recover from exercise.

The resting heart rate changes minimally with aging, but maximal heart rate decreases. Because heart rate varies with several factors, including level of fitness, a wide range of resting heart rates are within normal limits for the older adult (see Table 8–1). The decrease in the maximal heart rate may be related to (1) decreased activity of the cardiac pacemaker, (2) decreased sensitivity to catecholamines, and (3) increased ventricular filling time. Increased ventricular filling time results from decreased ventricular compliance. Contraction time and diastole may also be increased because of slowed calcium uptake in the sarcoplasmic reticulum of the cardiac cells. Because of poor calcium transport and storage, the heart muscle will take longer to reach peak tension and to relax.

During aging, maximal stroke volume decreases, with older adults experiencing a 10% to 20% decrease in stroke volume at high workload (Shephard, 1987). Factors that influence a decline in stroke volume are listed in Table 8–2 (Irwin and Zadai, 1990; Shephard, 1985). Decreased venous tone, slowed relaxation of the ventricles, thickening of the mitral valve, and left ventricular stiffness may result in a decreased preload condition. The filling rate of the 65- to 80-year-old heart has been shown to be 50% of that of 25- to 40-year-old subjects (Gerstenblith et al, 1977). Stiffening of the aorta and major arteries, increased systemic blood pressure, and poor perfusion of the skeletal muscle contribute to an increase in afterload (Shephard, 1987; Wei, 1986).

At rest and during exercise, blood pressure increases through adulthood and older adulthood. Blood pressure remains significantly related to adiposity through adulthood (Gerber and Stern, 1999). Systolic blood pressure rises more than diastolic blood pressure (see Table 8–1). A blood pressure of 120/80 mm Hg is considered normal in the younger adult, and a systolic blood pressure of 150 mm Hg would be considered indicative of hypertension. In an older adult, a systolic blood pressure of 150 mm Hg would be considered normal. This normal increase in blood pressure is related to reduced compliance within the vascular system and the decreasing size of the vascular bed. Shephard (1987) and Peel (1990) report that blood pressure changes with aging are not seen in all populations, leaving a question about whether they are really a consequence of aging. Low-intensity aerobic training in older adult hypertensive

TABLE 8–2

Factors Leading to Decreased Stroke Volume During High Workload in Older Adults

Decreased cardiac compliance
Decreased cardiac contractility
  Loss of cardiac muscle fibers
  Increased connective tissue in myocardium
Poor myocardial perfusion
Increased peripheral resistance
  Varicose veins
  Decreased venous tone
  Stiffening of the aorta and major arteries
Slowed ventricular relaxation
Increased systemic blood pressure
Poor perfusion of skeletal muscle
Decreased sensitivity to sympathetic input

patients has also been shown to lower blood pressure, with these patients returning to a pretraining level of blood pressure when exercise was discontinued (Motoyama et al, 1998). This finding seems to reflect that lifestyle factors may also play a role in determining the blood pressure of the older adult.

Delivery of oxygen to the peripheral tissues is altered with aging. The efficiency of oxygen extraction from the blood at the tissue level decreases with age, narrowing the arterial-venous oxygen difference. Loss of muscle strength, decreased muscle enzyme levels, and diminished size of the capillary network that perfuses muscle limit oxygen extraction from the circulating blood. Other vascular changes with aging, obstruction of major vessels, and decreased levels of hemoglobin are also factors (Shephard, 1985, 1987). With increasing age, increased obesity, and decreased efficiency of sweating, blood is shunted away from the muscles and to the skin, assisting in body cooling. This also reduces blood flow to the tissues and contributes to the decreased efficiency of oxygen extraction.

Pulmonary System

Both the ventilatory pump and respiratory system are affected by aging. Because of this, older adults are at increased risk for respiratory failure because of changes in the lung. Risk of ventilatory failure also increases because of changes in the ventilatory pump (Rossi et al, 1996).

Ventilatory Pump Changes

Structural changes occur with aging and create a stiffer bony thorax, which increases the work of breathing. The thorax becomes shortened vertically and larger in the anterior-posterior dimension. Thoracic kyphosis and decreased mobility of the joints allow rib rotation. Rib decalcification, increased calcification of rib cartilage, and changes in the articulation between the ribs and vertebrae may also contribute to increased stiffness. Elasticity of cartilage and collagen in the annulus fibrosus decreases, and loss of fluid from the nucleus pulposus results in a flattened, less-resilient disk. Because of the resting position of the thorax, the intrathoracic pressure at end-expiration is higher, again increasing airway resistance and effort during breathing. Functionally, these changes result in decreased chest wall expansion during breathing. In a young adult, a 40% change in lung volume is noted with thoracic expansion, but only a 30% change is seen in older adults (Rossi et al, 1996).

Elasticity and compliance are also decreased within the lung because of changes in collagen and elastin. Cross-linkage of collagen is seen, and there is a loss of elastin in the airways and blood vessels. This results in decreased recoil of the lung, especially at higher lung volumes (Rossi et al, 1996). In the conducting airways, elasticity of bronchial cartilage is diminished. This results in a slightly increased diameter of the large airways. Hyaline cartilage structures in the trachea may become ossified. Bronchial mucous glands increase in number, thickening the mucus layer in the airway and offering more resistance to airflow. The number and thickness of elastic fibers in the walls of smaller airways decrease, again increasing the resistance to airflow and diminishing elastic recoil of the lungs. As elastic recoil of the lungs is diminished, residual volume increases and vital capacity is reduced. Lungs, alveoli, and alveolar ducts enlarge with age. As a result, more time is needed for inspired air to reach the alveolar area. Decreased elasticity of the alveoli makes them susceptible to collapse on expiration.

Respiratory muscles become less efficient with age. Inspiratory muscle strength and endurance appear to decrease (Rossi et al, 1996). Structural changes in the thoracic cavity alter the length-tension relationship of the respiratory muscles, increasing the work of breathing. For example, the resting position of the diaphragm changes as the thoracic height decreases and diameter increases. Increased residual volume of the aging lung will also affect the resting position of the diaphragm. The abdominal muscles become less effective at stabilizing the diaphragm. Because of these changes, the older adult has to increase breathing rate rather than tidal volume to increase minute ventilation. This also increases the work of breathing (Frontera and Evans, 1986).

Respiratory System Changes

Many changes are noted in the aging lung. The loss of elastic recoil of the lung, as mentioned earlier, decreases effectiveness of the ventilatory pump. The alveolar surface area also changes. A loss of surface area results from a decrease in the actual number of alveoli per unit of lung volume, loss of alveolar wall tissue, and increased size of the respiratory bronchioles, alveolar sacs, and alveolar ducts.

The pulmonary vasculature undergoes the same changes within its vascular wall that were discussed earlier. The capillary bed at the alveolar interface becomes smaller, which, when combined with increased alveolar size, limits the diffusing capacity of the system. Pulmonary blood flow and blood volume within the capillary bed decrease. As a result, pulmonary gas exchange is affected. The alveolar-to-arteriole oxygen gradient increases as the arterial Po_2 decreases. The decrease in Po_2 with age has been well documented (Murray, 1986), but recent references note a decrease in Po_2 until the age of 70 to 75 years, after which Po_2 plateaus (Rossi et al, 1996). Arterial Pco_2 remains constant throughout adulthood.

Functionally, the impact of these changes is reflected in lung volumes and arterial blood gas values at rest and during exercise. Although total lung capacity does not change, vital capacity decreases while functional residual capacity and residual volume increase. By 70 years of age, vital capacity is reported to decrease to 75% of earlier values, and residual volume increases by 50% (Murray, 1986). Inspiratory and expiratory reserve volumes also decrease because of the decreased elasticity of the lung. The loss of elasticity causes the airways to close at a higher volume during expiration, which affects the amount of oxygenated air that is distributed to the tissue. The pulmonary system works harder to deliver less oxygen to the tissues in older adults.

Functional Implications of Changes in the Cardiovascular and Pulmonary Systems

Because of anatomic and physiologic differences in the cardiovascular and pulmonary systems of the infant, child, adolescent, and adult, function and efficiency differ in each age group. Through childhood, most changes are related to changes in body size. Gender differences become apparent in adolescence. In adulthood and older adulthood, effects of environment and normal aging alter the efficiency and capacity of the cardiovascular and pulmonary systems. Lifestyle habits that affect respiratory system function in older adults include nutrition, smoking habits, and exercise. In the presence of protein malnutrition, muscle atrophy may be seen in the respiratory muscles. Smoking has a negative affect on both the cardiovascular and pulmonary systems.

Efficiency of the cardiovascular and pulmonary system is reflected in measures such as cardiac output, minute ventilation, and maximal aerobic capacity. *Cardiac output* is a measure of the efficiency of the cardiovascular system. *Minute ventilation,* the volume of air moved into the lungs in 1 minute, is a measure of the efficiency of the pulmonary system. These two measures, when considered with the ability of working tissue to utilize oxygen for energy production, indicate an individual's *maximal aerobic capacity,* or level of cardiovascular and pulmonary fitness.

Cardiac output varies with an individual's age. The cardiac output of children is less than that of adults both at rest and during exercise. Small heart size limits stroke volume to such a degree that even the increased heart rate of children cannot compensate. Functionally, the lower cardiac output does not affect a child's level of activity, because even with less hemoglobin than an adult, the child efficiently extracts oxygen from the blood. In addition, the small body size of children and their ability to easily dissipate heat over their relatively large body surface area enable them to function with the smaller cardiac output. Cardiac output increases as the body grows. In young adults, cardiac output during maximal exercise limits endurance (Shepard, 1985). With aging, both maximal heart rate and maximal stroke volume are decreased. Because cardiac output during maximal exercise is the product of these two values, it also decreases with age.

Oxygen transportation to working tissues is another important factor in determining an individual's maximal aerobic capacity. Efficient ventilation carries inspired air to a well-developed and expanded alveolar network. Efficient circulation provides sufficient oxygenated blood to the pulmonary capillary network and to the capillaries of working tissues. Factors such as airway resistance, compliance of the thorax, functioning of the respiratory muscles, and compliance/elasticity of the lung and airways affect efficiency. The functional volumes of air in the lungs, such as the tidal volume, vary with the demands placed on the pulmonary system. As more oxygen is required during light to moderate exercise, tidal volume increases (Murray, 1986).

Changes in the functional lung volumes and decreased efficiency of the respiratory muscles reduce an older individual's ability to increase tidal volume and minute ventilation in response to exercise. During exercise, maximal oxygen uptake is decreased 25% by age 65 and 50% by age 75 (Shephard, 1987). Both the decrease in cardiac output and the diminished ability of the peripheral tissues (muscle) to extract oxygen contribute to the decrease in maximal oxygen uptake. The pulmonary system is less able to adapt to stress because of (1) the loss of elastic recoil and chest wall compliance, (2) changes in central nervous system control, (3) innervation of respiratory muscles, and (4) impaired perception of carbon dioxide levels. Breathing frequency is increased in an attempt to provide necessary oxygen transport. The inability of the pulmonary system to meet needs is also thought to limit exercise in the older individual (Peel, 1990; Shephard, 1985). These changes are minimized in the healthy, active, nonsmoking older adult, and endurance training is thought to improve inspiratory muscle strength and lung function (McArdle et al, 1996; Shephard, 1987).

Cardiovascular and pulmonary efficiency contributes to an individual's level of physical fitness. Fitness is a measure of a person's functional ability and health. Clinically, cardiovascular disease is a significant problem for adults. Risk factors for cardiovascular disease can sometimes be identified in young children. It is important to consider cardiovascular and pulmonary development and function across the life span as clinicians work with their clients to prevent cardiovascular disease and to minimize the effects of aging on these systems. A more extensive discussion of fitness issues across the life span, including the effects of exercise and training on the body systems, can be found in Chapter 15.

Summary

The cardiovascular and pulmonary systems work closely together to provide the food and fuel necessary for physical function. Changes in these systems over the life span can alter the functional ability of the systems as well as those of the individual. Some of these changes appear to be the result of normal development, whereas others may be determined by lifestyle choices. Research shows that regular physical activity can have a positive impact on function and health and that exercise at any age is important to maintain these two important systems at maximal efficiency.

References

Anderson PAW. The heart and development. *Semin Perinatol* 20:482–509, 1996.

Baldwin HS. Early embryonic vascular development. *Cardiovasc Res* 31:E34–E45, 1996.

Bourgeois MS, Zadai CC. Impaired ventilation and respiration in the older adult. In Guccione AA (ed). *Geriatric Physical Therapy*, 2nd ed. St. Louis: Mosby, 2000, pp 226–244.

Boyden EA. Development and growth of the airways. In Hodson WA (ed). *Development of the Lung*. New York: Marcel Dekker, 1977, pp 3–35.

Burgess WE, Chernick V. *Respiratory Therapy in Newborn Infants and Children*, 2nd ed. New York: Thieme, 1986.

Cunningham DA, Paterson DH. Discussion: Exercise, fitness and aging. In Bouchard C, Shephard RJ, Stephens T, et al (eds). *Exercise, Fitness and Health: A Consensus of Current Knowledge.* Champaign, IL: Human Kinetics, 1990, pp 699–704.

Cunningham DA, Paterson DH, Blimke CJR. The development of the cardiorespiratory system with growth and physical activity. In Boileau RA (ed). *Advances in Pediatric Sport Science, vol 1: Biological Issues.* Champaign, IL: Human Kinetics, 1984, pp 85–116.

Davis JA, Dobbings J. *Scientific Foundations of Pediatrics.* Baltimore: University Park Press, 1981.

DeCesare JA, Graybill CA. Physical therapy for the child with respiratory dysfunction. In Irwin S, Tecklin JS (eds). *Cardiopulmonary Physical Therapy*, 2nd ed. St. Louis: Mosby, 1990, pp 417–460.

Frontera WR, Evans WJ. Exercise performance and endurance training in the elderly. *Top Geriatr Rehabil* 2:17–32, 1986.

Gerber LM, Stern PM. Relationship of body size and body mass to blood pressure: Sex-specific and developmental influences. *Hum Biol* 71:505–528, 1999.

Gerstenblith G, Frederiksen J, Yin FCP, et al. Echocardiographic assessment of a normal adult aging population. *Circulation* 56:273–278, 1977.

Irwin SC, Zadai CC. Cardiopulmonary rehabilitation of the geriatric patient. In Lewis CB (ed). *Aging: The Health Care Challenge*, 2nd ed. Philadelphia: FA Davis, 1990, pp 181–211.

Jarvis C. *Physical Examination and Health Assessment*, 3rd ed. Philadelphia: WB Saunders, 1996, pp 186–187.

Junqueira LC, Carneiro J, Kelley RO. *Basic Histology*, 9th ed. Norwalk, CT: Appleton and Lange, 1998.

Kitzman DW, Edwards WD. Minireview: Age-related changes in the anatomy of the normal human heart. *J Geriatr Med Sci* 45:33–39, 1990.

Leeson TS, Leeson CR, Paparo AA. *Text/Atlas of Histology.* Philadelphia: WB Saunders, 1988.

Malina RM, Bouchard C. *Growth, Maturation and Physical Activity.* Champaign, IL: Human Kinetics, 1991, pp 151–167.

Massery M. Chest development as a component of normal motor development: Implications for pediatric physical therapists. *Pediatr Phys Ther* 3:3–8, 1991.

McArdle WD, Katch FL, Katch VL. *Exercise Physiology: Energy, Nutrition and Human Performance*, 4th ed. Philadelphia: Lea & Febiger, 1996.

Meyrick B, Reid LM. Ultrastructure of alveolar lining and its development. In Hodson WA (ed). *Development of the Lung.* New York: Marcel Dekker, 1977, pp 135–214.

Moore KL, Persaud TVN. *Before We Are Born: Essentials of Embryology and Birth Defects*, 5th ed. Philadelphia: WB Saunders, 1998.

Motoyama M, Sunami Y, Kinoshita F, et al. Blood pressure lowering effect of low intensity aerobic training in elderly hypertensive patients. *Med Sci Sports Exerc* 30:818–823, 1998.

Murray JF. *The Normal Lung*, 2nd ed. Philadelphia: WB Saunders, 1986.

Payne VG, Isaacs LD. *Human Motor Development: A Life Span Approach.* Mountain View, CA: Mayfield Publishers, 1987.

Peel C. Cardiopulmonary changes with aging. In Irwin S, Tecklin JS (eds). *Cardiopulmonary Physical Therapy*, 2nd ed. St. Louis: Mosby, 1990, pp 477–489.

Rosner B. *Data from Second Tack Force on Blood Pressure Control in Children.* Bethesda, MD: National Heart, Lung and Blood Institute, 1987.

Rossi A, Ganassini A, Tantacci C, Grassi V. Aging and the respiratory system. *Aging Clin Exp Res* 8:143–161, 1996.

Shephard RJ. The cardiovascular benefits of exercise in the elderly. *Top Geriatr Rehabil* 1:1–10, 1985.

Shephard RJ. *Exercise Physiology.* Toronto: BC Decker, 1987.

Sinclair D, Dangerfield P. *Human Growth After Birth*, 6th ed. New York: Oxford University Press, 1998.

Tanaka H, Dinenno FA, Monahan KD, et al. Aging, habitual exercise and dynamic arterial compliance. *Circulation* 102:1270–1275, 2000.

Thompson LV. Physiological changes associated with aging. In Guccione AA (ed). *Geriatric Physical Therapy*, 2nd ed. St. Louis: Mosby, 2000, pp 28–55.

Wei JY. Cardiovascular anatomic and physiologic changes with age. *Top Geriatr Rehabil* 2:10–16, 1986.

Wong DL, Perry SE. *Maternal Child Nursing Care*. St. Louis: Mosby, 1998, pp 1790–1791.

Zadai CC. Cardiopulmonary issues in the geriatric population: Implications for rehabilitation. *Top Geriatr Rehabil* 2:1–9, 1986.

Chapter

9 Nervous System Changes

OBJECTIVES

After studying this chapter, the reader will be able to:

1 Describe the roles of the nervous system.

2 Delineate components of the nervous system.

3 Describe the general organization of the nervous system.

4 Discuss unique structural and functional changes of the nervous system in the developing fetus, infant, child, adolescent, adult, and older adult.

5 Relate nervous system changes over time to functional differences in movement, cognition, and motivation.

6 Incorporate issues of life-span development of the nervous system into patient examination and intervention.

The nervous system is frequently referred to as the *command center for human function.* It not only receives information but also integrates all incoming messages to orchestrate fluid, appropriate responses. The nervous system truly oversees other body systems as they cooperate to perform day-to-day activities and controls the major functions of moving, thinking, and feeling.

Movement is controlled when the nervous system functions as an initiator, a modulator, and a comparator, activating the muscular and skeletal systems. Movement is not the product of any one system, nor does one system act in isolation from the others to produce movement. Attention is necessary for motor function. Absence of movement might result from a problem in the skeletal, muscular, cardiopulmonary, or nervous system. For example, in either muscle disease (e.g., muscular dystrophy) or peripheral nerve injury, the end result is movement dysfunction.

A unique role of the nervous system is thought processing—that is, cognition or intelligence. Psychological theorists such as Erikson have little to say about how the brain "thinks." Physiologists believe that the ability of the brain to form memories is a mechanism for intelligence. Memory formation is contingent on an individual's level of alertness and ability to focus attention. Memory formation occurs in an area of the brain called the *hippocampus* (Zaidel, 1995). The frontal area of the brain has been linked to abstract thought and personality. After head trauma, a patient's sensory, motor, and cognitive deficits can be attributed to the damaged area of the brain. In other areas of the brain, called *association areas*, sensory input is connected to meaning. For example, in the visual association areas, visual input is connected with the memory and names of shapes.

Another important aspect of nervous system control is its role in motivation and emotions. One of the oldest parts of the brain, called the *limbic system*, is responsible for attending to sensory and motor cues; monitoring basic drives for food, water, and sexual gratification; and attaching emotional meaning to actions. The ability of the nervous system to react to these cues is not well understood. Emotions can be powerful motivation for movement. The affective component of movement dysfunction is often the most difficult to deal with, as when trying to motivate a person to perform better physically.

Components of the Nervous System

At the cellular level, the nervous system is made up of two different types of cells: nerve cells (neurons) and glial cells (neuroglia). Both cell types are derived from embryonic ectoderm. *Neurons* allow the nervous system to communicate and to direct movement activities. *Neuroglia* provide support and protection for neurons. On a larger scale, structures such as the brain, spinal cord, and peripheral nerves make up the functional infrastructure of the nervous system.

NEURONS

Neurons are complex structures that form the major communication system of the body. As shown in Figure 9–1, a typical motor neuron is made up of a cell body, which can be thought of as a processing center; multiple *dendrites* that extend from the cell body and receive incoming stimuli, and an *axon*, a long process sheathed in myelin that singularly conducts nerve impulses to other neurons, muscles, or glands. Neurons vary in size and shape according to their function, such as pyramidal neurons found in the cerebral cortex. The structure often reflects the role the neuron plays in the communications network of the nervous system.

There are four types of neurons: bipolar, multipolar, pseudounipolar, and unipolar (Fig. 9–2). The *bipolar* neuron has two processes—an axon and a dendrite. These sensory neurons are found in the vestibular, cochlear, and olfactory areas. Most *multipolar* neurons are motor neurons with multiple dendrites that emerge from one side of the cell body and one axon on the opposite side. The *pseudounipolar* neuron develops from a bipolar neuron. It falsely appears to have one process when, in reality, it has two that extend together from the cell body and then branch; both processes are covered by a myelin sheath and can send nerve impulses, but the peripheral branch displays small dendrites. A true *unipolar* neuron is marked by a single process and is present in humans only during the embryonic stage.

Dendrites are branched to receive multiple inputs from other neurons. The pattern of branching indicates the purpose of the neuron. The neuron communicates by initiating a signal, called an *action potential*. An action potential is

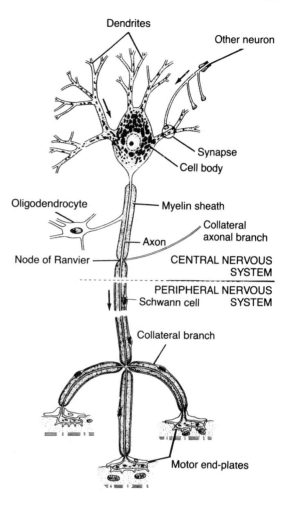

Figure 9–1

Schematic drawing of a motor neuron. The myelin sheath is produced by oligodendrocytes in the central nervous system and by Schwann cells in the peripheral nervous system. The *arrows* show the direction of the nerve impulse. (From Junqueira LC, Carneiro J, Kelley RO. *Basic Histology*, 6th ed. Norwalk, CT: Appleton & Lange, 1992, Fig. 9–1, p. 164. Copyright © by McGraw-Hill, Inc. Used by permission of McGraw-Hill Book Company.)

generated by changing the resting electric potential of the cell membrane. Normal resting membrane potential is about −70 mV and is controlled by charged ions such as K⁺, Na⁺, Cl⁻, and HCO₃⁻. An action potential is generated at a certain membrane potential called *threshold*. The flow of positively charged sodium ions into the cell decreases the membrane potential (depolarization). Depolarization can be triggered by many different events such as synaptic input, a receptor potential generated by a specialized sensory receptor, or innate pacemaker activity. Once the membrane is sufficiently depolarized, the action potential is generated. After depolarization, there is a period during which the cell membrane is unable to react, called a *refractory period*. The axon or nerve fiber terminates in an end bulb that synapses with a target cell. Axons can also branch to transmit signals to more than one target cell or more than one location on a target cell. An axon can generate up to 1000 action potentials per second.

Myelin is a lipid and protein substance that covers axons and increases the

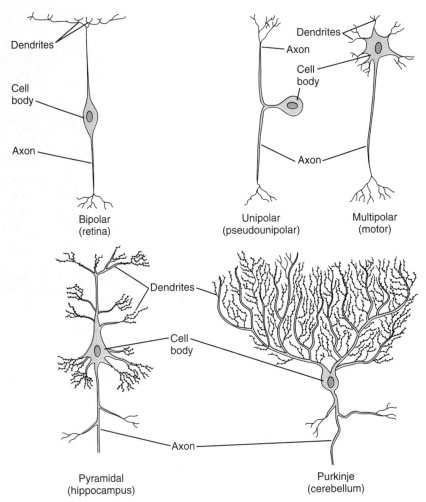

Figure 9–2

Diagram of various types of neurons. (From Gartner LP, Hiatt JL. *Color Textbook of Histology,* 2nd ed. Philadelphia: WB Saunders, 2001, p 187.)

speed of nerve impulse conduction. In the central nervous system (CNS), myelin is produced by glial cells called *oligodendrocytes;* in the peripheral nervous system (PNS), myelin is produced by Schwann cells (see Fig. 9–1). The myelin laid down by the Schwann cells is interrupted at set intervals along the nerve called *nodes of Ranvier* (Fig. 9–3). At these nodes, the action potential can be boosted to keep it from fading out as it journeys along the nerve fiber. Conduction in myelinated peripheral nerves is called *leaping* (or *saltation*) because the current flow can be detected only at the nodes (Fig. 9–3). How fast impulses can be conducted depends on whether the nerve is myelinated or unmyelinated and on the diameter of the nerve fiber.

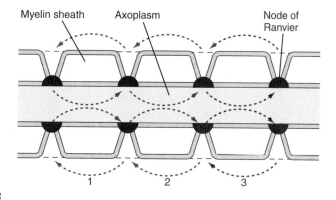

Figure 9–3

Saltatory conduction along a myelinated axon. (Redrawn from Guyton AC, Hall JE. *Textbook of Medical Physiology*, 9th ed. Philadelphia: WB Saunders, 1996, p 70.)

Nerve fibers can be classified on the basis of their size and ability to conduct impulses, as outlined in Table 9–1. For example, type A fibers are myelinated with large diameters and conduct at high speed (12 to 120 m/sec). Type B fibers have smaller diameters and a medium rate of conduction (3 to 15 m/sec). Type C fibers are smaller still and unmyelinated, with a conduction rate of only 0.5 to 2 m/sec.

NEUROGLIA

Neuroglia provide support, nutrition, and protection to the neurons and can be thought of as the connective tissue of the nervous system. Neurons do not survive in tissue cultures unless neuroglia are present. Metabolically, neuroglia assist in regulating the concentration of sodium and potassium ions in the intracellular space; these ions affect the performance of the nerve cell. Unlike neurons, they cannot transmit electric impulses, but they do retain the ability to divide throughout the life of the organism. Injury to the CNS typically triggers glial cell proliferation as a means of repair. Normally, there are approximately 10 glial cells to every neuron, but because glia are smaller than

TABLE 9–1

Nerve Fiber Types

Types	Diameter (mm)	Conduction Velocity (m/sec)
A	12–20	70–120
B	<3	3–15
C	0.4–1.2	0.5–2

Modified from Ganong WF. *Review of Medical Phsyiology*, 16th ed. Norwalk, CT: Appleton & Lange, 1993.

neurons, they account for only half the volume of nervous tissue. Three types of neuroglia are (1) macroglia, which include astrocytes and oligodendrocytes, (2) microglia, and (3) ependymal cells.

The largest neuroglia, the *astrocytes*, provide a vascular link via foot-like projections between blood vessels, the brain, and the spinal cord. In the brain, protoplasmic astrocytes are part of the blood-brain barrier, which regulates the influx of vital nutrients and keeps out harmful substances. The "foot processes" surround the outside of capillary endothelial cells (Fig. 9–4) and may assist in the formation and maintenance of the blood-brain barrier. In preterm infants, this barrier has not been formed. Therefore, foreign matter such as meconium, the first stool, may be deposited in brain structures and cause movement dysfunction (Volpe, 1995).

Astrocytes are also present in the spinal cord. They lend structural support to the nervous system and may eliminate interference or cross-talk in

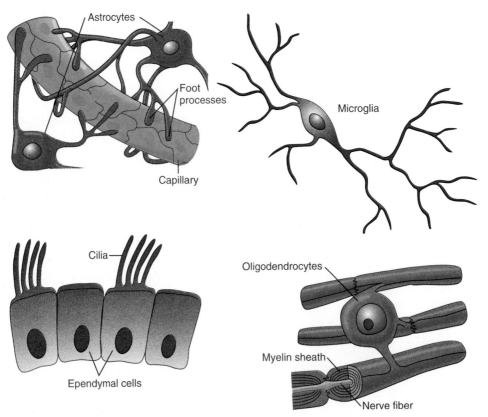

Figure 9–4

The four types of neuroglial cells: astrocytes, microglia, oligodendrocytes, and ependymal cells. (From Copstead LEC, Banasik JL. *Pathophysiology: Biological and Behavioral Perspectives,* 2nd ed. Philadelphia: WB Saunders, 2000, p 987.)

nerve cell transmission. In injury, astrocytes and microglia clean up debris. Fibrous astrocytes fill in the space left by an injury and produce a glial scar, which can actually interfere with healing by blocking reestablishment of synaptic connections.

Oligodendrocytes produce the myelin that covers the neural processes of the CNS (see Fig. 9–4). The large number of this type of glial cell is a hallmark of the increasing evolutionary complexity of the nervous system.

Microglia are derived from mesenchyme and can be found scattered throughout the CNS (see Fig. 9–4). As the major scavenger cells (macrophages), they migrate to any area of injury to remove cellular debris, regardless of whether the spinal cord or brain is damaged. These small cells develop late in the fetal period after the CNS has been supplied by blood vessels.

Ependymal cells line the cavities of the brain and spinal cord and are in constant contact with cerebrospinal fluid (CSF) (see Fig. 9–4). Because some ependymal cells have cilia, movement of the CSF is possible. A special ependymal cell, called a *tanycyte*, relays chemical information from the CSF to the capillary system surrounding the pituitary gland, which is important for regulation of circulating hormones.

CENTRAL NERVOUS SYSTEM

The brain, brain stem, and spinal cord are collectively referred to as the CNS. The brain consists of two cerebral hemispheres, or cortices, the *brain stem* and the *cerebellum*. The surface of each hemisphere of the cortex is convoluted and has elevated areas called *gyri* and grooves called *sulci*. Each hemisphere of the cortex is divided into five lobes: frontal, parietal, temporal, occipital, and limbic (Fig. 9–5). In addition, the five lobes are responsible for different body functions (Table 9–2). The areas that are directly related to processing sensory and motor information or coordinating movement are known as primary and association sensory (or motor) areas (Fig. 9–6 and Table 9–3).

The cerebral hemispheres are also organized into horizontal layers characterized by a different distribution of neurons and glial cells, depending on the part of the cortex studied. A mark of brain maturity is the establishment of these layers. Cell bodies of neurons with similar functions form groups within the CNS called *nuclei*, many of which are in the cerebral hemispheres.

The concept that each side of the brain is specialized to perform certain functions has been widely accepted. Although the two cerebral hemispheres appear to be mirror images of each other, gross anatomical differences have been demonstrated by Geschwind and Levitsky (1968). Research has established that the processing and production of language are localized in the left hemisphere and spatial abilities are localized in the right (Table 9–4). The differences are likely to be related to handedness, because 95% of the population is left hemisphere, or right side, dominant (Purves et al, 1997). The asymmetry of the two hemispheres is present even in infants.

The nervous system is somatotopically organized to relay signals through-

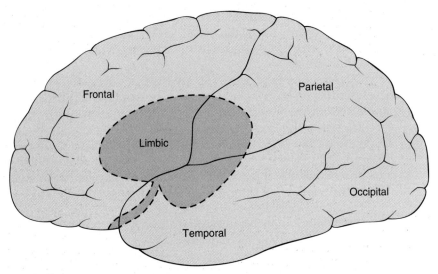

Figure 9–5

The lobes of the brain. The limbic lobe is depicted by a *dashed line* because it is internal to the other four lobes.

TABLE 9–2

Functions of the Lobes of the Cortex of the Brain

Lobe	Structure	Function
Frontal	Primary motor cortex	Voluntary controlled movements
	Premotor area	Control of trunk and girdle muscles, anticipatory postural adjustments
	Supplementary area	Initiation of movement; orientation of eyes and head; and bilateral, sequential movement
	Broca's area in left hemisphere	Motor programming of speech
	Same are in right hemisphere	Nonverbal communication
Temporal	Primary auditory cortex	Discriminates loudness and pitch of sounds
	Wernicke's area	Hears and comprehends spoken language; intelligence
Parietal	Primary somatosensory cortex	Discriminates texture, shape, and size of objects
	Primary vestibular cortex	Distinguishes head movements and head positions
Occipital	Primary visual cortex	Differentiates intensity of light, shape, size, and location of objects
Limbic	Anterior temporal lobe and inferior frontal lobe	Emotion, motivation, processing of memory; motivational drive to learn

Data from Guyton AC, Hall JE. *Textbook of Medical Physiology*, 9th ed. Philadelphia: WB Saunders, 1966; Lundy-Ekman L. *Neuroscience: Fundamentals for Rehabilitation*. Philadelphia: WB Saunders, 1998; Purves D, Augustine GJ, Fitzpatrick LC, et al. *Neuroscience*. Sunderland, MA: Sinauer Associates, 1997.

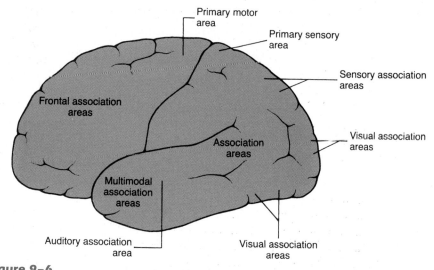

Figure 9–6

Primary and association sensory and motor areas of the brain.

out the body. Somatotopic arrangement of neurons in pathways allows for the localization of somatosensory stimulation. These topographic maps allow specialized axons from one part of the body to be in proximity to axons carrying related signals from adjacent parts of the body. This is true in both the motor and sensory cortices, where the parts of the body are represented. The size of the part is directly related to the functional importance of the part. For exam-

TABLE 9–3

Association Areas of the Brain

Association Area	Location	Function
Frontal	Prefrontal area	Goal-oriented behavior, self-awareness; elaboration of thought
Temporal	Temporal lobe	Recognition of faces or objects
Parietal	Posterior parietal lobe in right hemisphere	Attention to both sides of the body
	Posterior parietal lobe in left hemisphere	Attention to right side of the body
Parietoccipitotemporal	Junction of parietal, temporal, and occipital lobes	Interpretive meaning from sensory signals; sensory integration, problem solving, understanding spatial relationships
Limbic	Anterior temporal and inferior frontal lobes	Emotion, motivation, processing of memory

Data from Purves D, Augustine GJ, Fitzpatrick LC, et al. *Neuroscience.* Sunderland, MA: Sinauer Associates, 1997.

TABLE 9–4

Behaviors Attributed to the Left and Right Hemispheres of the Brain

Behavior	Left Hemisphere	Right Hemisphere
Cognitive style	Processing information in a sequential, linear manner	Processing information in a simultaneous, holistic, or gestalt manner
	Observing and analyzing details	Grasping overall organization or pattern
Perception/cognition	Processing and producing language	Processing nonverbal stimuli (environmental sounds, speech intonations, complex shapes, designs)
		Visual-spatial perception
		Drawing inferences, synthesizing information
Academic skills	Reading: sound-symbol relationships, word recognition, reading comprehension	Mathematical reasoning and judgment
		Alignment of numerals in calculations
	Performing mathematical calculations	
Motor	Sequencing movements	Sustaining a movement or posture
	Performing movements and gestures to command	
Emotions	Expression of positive emotions	Expression of negative emotions
		Perception of emotion

From O'Sullivan SB, Schmitz TJ. *Physical Rehabilitation: Assessment and Treatment*, 3rd ed. Philadelphia: FA Davis, 1994, p 337.

ple, the sensory homunculus seen in Figure 9–7 depicts a caricature of a human being with oversized lips and thumb. The same type of organizational relationship is present in the visual cortex as a visuotopic map and in the auditory cortex as a tonotopic map. This type of mapping occurs at every level of the nervous system.

The internal capsule, diencephalon, and the basal ganglia lie deep within the brain. These subcortical structures are important for functional movement. The *internal capsule* consists of descending axons from the motor areas of the cerebral cortex and ascending fibers from the thalamus and sensory and motor areas of the spinal cord. The capsule is uniquely shaped like a crescent with an anterior and a posterior limb. Because so many fibers are concentrated within a small space, injury to this structure can be devastating. The capsule lies just lateral to the diencephalon.

The *diencephalon* consists of the thalamus and the hypothalamus (Fig. 9–8). The thalamus is a large collection of nuclei that can be divided into three groups based on their main functions: (1) relay nuclei, (2) association nuclei, and (3) nonspecific nuclei. All sensory systems except for the olfactory relay information through the thalamus to the cortex. Information from the basal ganglia and the cerebellum is also processed in the thalamus. Association nuclei integrate touch and visual information, in addition to processing emo-

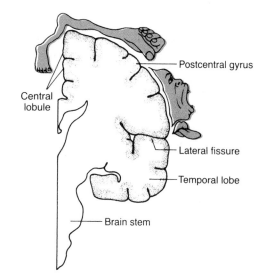

Central lobule

Postcentral gyrus

Lateral fissure

Temporal lobe

Brain stem

Figure 9–7

Sensory homunculus.

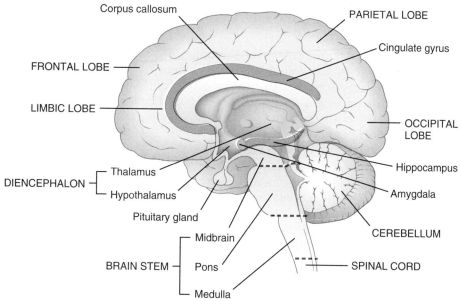

Corpus callosum

PARIETAL LOBE

Cingulate gyrus

FRONTAL LOBE

LIMBIC LOBE

OCCIPITAL LOBE

Hippocampus

DIENCEPHALON — Thalamus

Hypothalamus

Amygdala

Pituitary gland

CEREBELLUM

Midbrain

BRAIN STEM — Pons

SPINAL CORD

Medulla

Figure 9–8

Schematic midsagittal view of the brain shows the relationship between the cerebral cortex, cerebellum, spinal cord, and brain stem and the subcortical structures important to functional movement.

tional and memory information. Nonspecific nuclei are important for regulating consciousness, arousal, and attention (Lundy-Ekman, 1998). The hypothalamus, named because of its anatomic relationship just inferior to the thalamus, is responsible for maintaining homeostasis. The hypothalamus integrates behavior and visceral functions by controlling eating, reproduction, and diurnal rhythms (see Chapter 11).

The *basal ganglia* are another group of nuclei found at the base of the cerebrum. This subcortical structure is in reality a group of structures composed of the caudate, putamen, globus pallidus, substantia nigra, and subthalamic nuclei. The basal ganglia regulate posture, muscle tone, and force production and are involved in cognitive functions related to movement. These related functions include motivation, memory for location of objects, changing behavior based on task demands, and awareness of body position in space (Alexander et al, 1990).

The *limbic system* is very complex. It consists of many interconnected structures, including the amygdala, hippocampus, and cingulate gyrus (see Fig. 9–8). Other areas of the cortex and the thalamus are involved in addition to the hypothalamus. The system is situated above the brain stem and below the cortex. The limbic system regulates visceral and hormonal functions such as eating, drinking, and reproduction. The role of the limbic system in memory is discussed at the end of this chapter.

The *cerebellum* is also made up of two hemispheres connected by a vermis. The cerebellar hemispheres are located inferior to the occipital lobes of the cerebral hemispheres and posterior to the brain stem (see Fig. 9–8). Despite its small size, the cerebellum contains over half of all the neurons in the brain (Ghez and Thack, 2000). The cerebellum is involved in the initiation and timing of movements and in monitoring postural tone. By receiving sensory input from the vestibular, auditory, and visual systems, as well as from the spinal cord, it compares actual with anticipated motor performance, thereby functioning as a comparator. The cerebellum receives input from the cerebral cortex via nuclei in the pons, part of the brain stem. The cerebellum influences nuclei in the thalamus and brain stem to control movement, and its circuits are modified during motor learning.

Functionally, the cerebellum can be divided into three parts based on where it receives inputs. These three parts of the cerebellum are called the cerebrocerebellum, spinocerebellum, and vestibulocerebellum and are associated with different types of movements. Equilibrium is regulated by the *vestibulocerebellum* due to its direct connections with the vestibular receptors and nuclei. The vestibulocerebellum provides anticipatory control for balance during voluntary movement. The *spinocerebellum* has connections to the spinal cord and regulates ongoing gross limb movements. The *cerebrocerebellum* is connected indirectly to the cerebral cortex and regulates fine, distal voluntary movements of the limbs.

The brain stem is located between the base of the cerebrum and the spinal cord. As such it represents a transition between the brain and the spinal cord (see Fig. 9–8). Its structures include the midbrain, pons, and medulla moving from the brain above to the spinal cord below. The *midbrain* connects the diencephalon to the pons and acts as a conduit for tracts between the cerebrum and the spinal cord or cerebellum. Reflex centers for visual, auditory, and tactile responses are found in the midbrain. The red nucleus receives information from the cerebellum and the cerebral cortex and connects to the spinal cord via the rubrospinal tract. Activity in this tract contributes to upper limb flexion.

The *pons* contains bundles of axons traveling between the cerebellum and the remainder of the nervous system to assist the medulla in regulating the rate of breathing. Reflex centers in the pons assist with orientation of the head in response to auditory and vestibular stimulation. Cranial nerves V through VIII, which provide sensory and motor information to and from the face, are located in the pons. The cochlear and vestibular nuclei are located at the junction of the pons and the medulla. Postural muscle activity is controlled partially by tracts arising from these vestibular nuclei and connecting to the spinal cord.

The *medulla* houses nuclei that control and coordinate cardiovascular responses, breathing, and swallowing. This is accomplished by the action of cranial nerves VII through X and XII (see Chapter 10 for a complete list of cranial nerves and functions). The medulla contributes to the control of eye and head movements, which may be observed when head turning in an infant results in extension of the face arm (the arm toward which the face is turned) and flexion of the skull arm. This asymmetrical tonic neck reflex (ATNR) requires circuits in the medulla (Lundy-Ekman, 1998). The eyes also turn toward the extended arm.

Loosely arranged groups of neurons within the core of the brain stem are responsible for keeping us alert to novel stimuli or for picking up information pertinent to movement safety. This group of neurons is called the *reticular activating system*. This system regulates the level of consciousness as well as the daily cycle of arousal, which includes periods of sleep and waking. Consciousness is governed by the reticular activating system, its ascending system that projects to the cortex, thalamus, and the basal forebrain (anterior to the hypothalamus). These latter structures constitute the cerebral part of the consciousness system (Lundy-Ekman, 1998). Cortical arousal levels are influenced by the activity in specific brain stem nuclei, including the raphe nuclei, the pons-midbrain junction nuclei, and the locus ceruleus.

The brain stem, specifically the reticular activating system, produces generalized arousal and integrates all sensory information and cortical input. Another part of the reticular formation contains autonomic nuclei, which are needed to sustain life. And still another part regulates the flow of information regarding pain, level of awareness, and somatic motor activity. The brain stem acts to filter sensory input, such as pain, to the cortex.

The spinal cord is made up of groups of axons, called *tracts*, that ascend or descend within the spinal cord and relay input to and from CNS structures. Figure 9–9 depicts cross sections through the spinal cord with representative ascending and descending tracts. Ascending tracts carry sensory information,

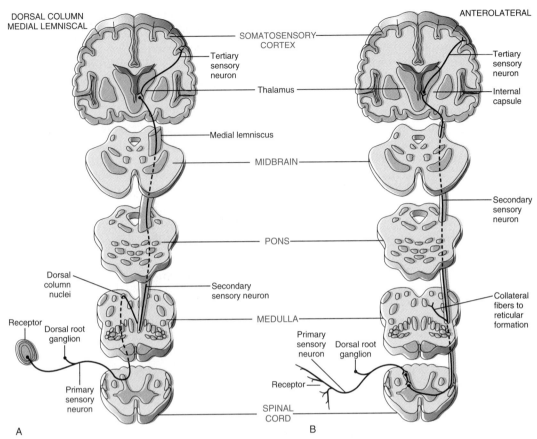

Figure 9–9

Comparison of two major ascending somatosensory tracts: *A*, dorsal column, receiving impulses related to movement, position, touch, and vibration; *B*, anterolateral tract, receiving impulses for pain and temperature.

and descending tracts direct movement. The two primary ascending tracts are the dorsal column and the anterolateral tract (Fig. 9–9*A*, *B*). The dorsal or posterior columns carry information about position sense (proprioception), two-point discrimination, deep touch, and vibration. The fibers of this tract cross in the brain stem (medulla). The anterolateral or spinothalamic tract carries pain and temperature sensations to the thalamus for awareness. The fibers enter the spinal cord, synapse, and cross to the other side within three segments. Light touch and pressure are carried in the dorsal and ventral columns. The descending corticospinal tract carries impulses from the cortex, cerebellum, and basal ganglia down the spinal tract that synapse on cell bodies of motor neurons to control distal muscle movement in the arms, fingers, legs, and feet (Fig. 9–9*C*).

The tracts surround a central butterfly-shaped area that consists of inter-

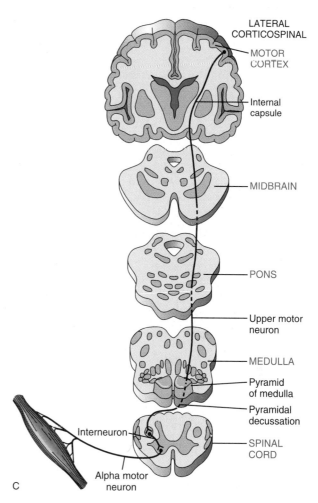

Figure 9–9 *Continued*

C, descending corticospinal tract directing impulses from the brain downward to control distal muscle movement. (From Copstead LEC, Banasik JL. *Pathophysiology: Biological and Behavioral Perspectives*, 2nd ed. Philadelphia: WB Saunders, 2000, pp 996 and 998.)

neurons, neuronal cell bodies, dendrites, and glial cells (Fig. 9–10). This H-shaped area is composed of gray matter and is divided into anterior and posterior "horns." The lower portion is the anterior horn, and the upper portion is the posterior horn. Cell bodies of motor neurons send out axons via the ventral roots to striated muscle. The position of a motor neuron within the anterior horn correlates with the location of the muscle groups it innervates (see Fig. 9–9C). Neurons in the posterior horn receive sensory information via the posterior roots of the spinal nerves (see Fig. 9–10).

One of the major descending tracts originates in the frontal lobe from the primary motor cortex, the premotor cortex, and the supplementary motor cortex. This efferent or motor tract is the corticospinal tract. The tract travels from the cortex to the brain stem, where it crosses to the other side. It is located in the dorsal lateral portion of the gray matter of the spinal cord. It synapses on interneurons, which then synapse on anterior horn cells within

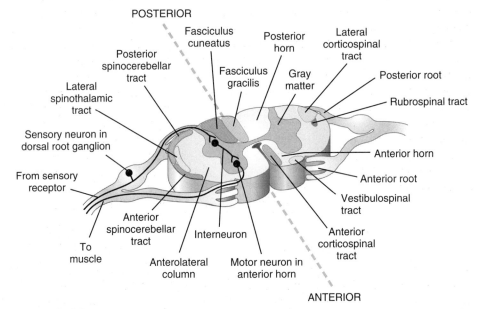

POSTERIOR

Figure 9–10

Diagram showing a cross section of the spinal cord with the major ascending (sensory) and descending (motor) tracts.

the anterior horn of the spinal cord. Axons of anterior horn cells innervate skeletal or striated muscle. Alpha motor neurons are lower motor neurons and have classically been referred to as the *final common path for motor behavior* (Sherrington, 1947). The corticospinal tract is essential for planning, initiating, and coordinating voluntary movement (Purves et al, 1997).

The second major set of descending motor tracts is from the reticular formation and the vestibular nucleus. The vestibular nucleus sends fibers to the spinal cord with information about movements generated in response to sensory signals of a postural disturbance. This provides a feedback mechanism for postural control. The reticular formation is involved in providing feedforward control of posture. It anticipates a change in body posture and acts to ready posture for movement. Gross motor movements can be controlled by these brain stem pathways, but the motor cortex connections to the alpha motor neuron are necessary for fine, fractionated extremity movements.

PERIPHERAL NERVOUS SYSTEM

The cranial and peripheral nerves along with their accompanying nerve ganglia are referred to as the peripheral nervous system (PNS). *Ganglia* are groups of neuron cell bodies outside the CNS. Cranial nerves from the brain stem innervate head and neck muscles involved in vital functions. Some cranial nerves also connect special sensory receptors with the brain. All 31 pairs of

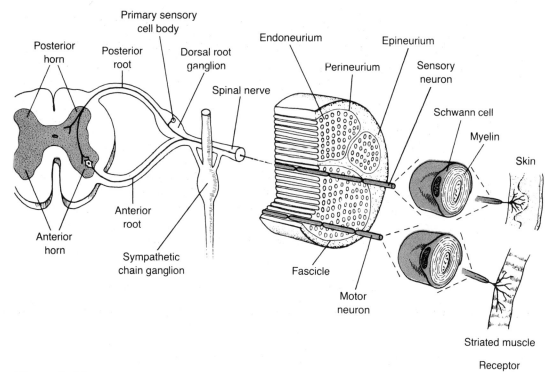

Figure 9–11

Schematic representation of the peripheral nervous system and the transition to the central nervous system. (Redrawn from Farber S. *Neurorehabilitation: A Multisensory Approach.* Philadelphia: WB Saunders, 1982, p 17; Ham AW. *Histology,* 6th ed. Philadelphia: JB Lippincott, 1969; and Junqueira LC, Carneiro J, Kelley RO. *Basic Histology,* 6th ed. Norwalk, CT: Appleton & Lange, 1989, p 177. Copyright © by McGraw-Hill, Inc. Used by permission of McGraw-Hill Book Company.

spinal nerves are part of the PNS and have sensory and motor components. The cell bodies of the sensory neurons are located outside the spinal cord, in the dorsal root ganglion. The peripheral process extends from the receptor to the cell body in the ganglion, and the central process (axon) goes from the ganglion into the CNS (Fig. 9–11).

Continuing proximally in Figure 9–11, the peripheral nerve and groups of nerve fibers are surrounded by specialized interstitial connective tissue. The *epineurium* covers the entire peripheral nerve; the *perineurium* surrounds bundles of nerve fibers called *fascicles;* and the *endoneurium* surrounds each individual nerve fiber. As seen in Figure 9–12, the bundles combine to form common nerves such as the sciatic nerve in the lower extremity or the radial nerve in the upper extremity.

A motor unit consists of an alpha neuron and the muscle fibers it innervates. Alpha motor neurons are multipolar neurons located in the anterior horn of the spinal cord with axons that innervate skeletal muscle fibers. Alpha motor neurons are also called *lower motor neurons* or the *final common path for*

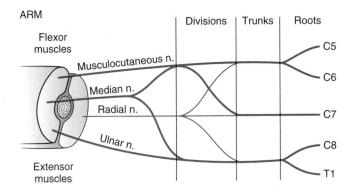

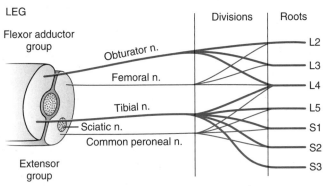

Figure 9–12

Relationship of common nerves to bundles of nerve roots from which they are derived. (Redrawn from Williams PL, Wendell-Smith CP, Treadgold S. *Basic Human Embryology,* 3rd ed. London: Pitman, 1984.)

motor behavior. All fibers connected to one alpha motor neuron contract together. Therefore, the sensitivity of a motor unit depends on the number of muscle fibers that the branches of its axon contacts. Which motor unit is more sensitive—one that innervates 6 muscle fibers or one that innervates 200 muscle fibers? The lower the innervation ratio of axon to fiber, the more easily a discrete movement can be produced. Eye muscles have a lower innervation ratio than do large lower extremity muscles. Three types of motor units that are related to the characteristics displayed by the motor fibers are recognized: fast fatigable (FF), fatigue-resistant (FR), and slow (S). The differences between these types are based on speed of contraction, force generated, and fatigability. Table 9–5 describes the motor unit characteristics and relationship to muscle fiber types.

The *efferent (motor) peripheral system* can be divided into the somatic nervous system and the autonomic nervous system (ANS); the major differences

TABLE 9–5

Motor Unit Characteristics and Relationship to Muscle Fiber Types

Motor Unit Type	Speed of Contraction	Force of Contraction	Fatigue	Muscle Fiber Type
Slow	Slow	Smallest	Highly resistant (>1 hr)	I
Fatigue resistant	Fast	Intermediate	Intermediate	IIa
Fast fatigable	Fastest	Largest	Several minutes	IIb

Data from Purves D, Augustine GJ, Fitzpatrick LC, et al (eds). *Neuroscience.* Sunderland, MA: Sinauer Associates, 1997; Spirduso WW. *Physical Dimensions of Aging.* Champaign, IL: Human Kinetics, 1995.

of each system are outlined in Table 9–6. The *somatic efferent system* conducts impulses to skeletal muscle; the *autonomic efferent system* conducts the impulses to smooth muscle, cardiac muscle, and glands. Both the somatic and the autonomic systems produce muscular contractions and change the rate of those contractions, but only the autonomic system causes the secretion of hormones.

The ANS is primarily responsible for maintaining an internal balance of visceral functions related to the heart, smooth muscle, and glands. It consists of three divisions: sympathetic, parasympathetic, and enteric. The sympathetic and parasympathetic divisions use acetylcholine as a neurotransmitter at the preganglionic synapse, as diagrammed in Figure 9–13. The parasympathetic division also uses acetylcholine at postganglionic synapses, whereas the sympathetic division uses norepinephrine to transmit nerve impulses to effector organs. The cell bodies of the sympathetic division are found in the thoracolumbar segments of the spinal cord. The sympathetic ganglia are adjacent to the thoracolumbar spinal cord in paired "sympathetic trunks," which then connect to an effector organ. The cell bodies of the parasympathetic division are in the cranial and sacral regions of the spinal cord. The parasympathetic ganglia usually lie within the effector organ. Some effects of ANS activity are outlined in Table 9–7.

The third division of the ANS is contained within the walls of the gastro-

TABLE 9–6

Differences Between Somatic Efferent and Autonomic Nervous Systems

Somatic Nervous System	Autonomic Nervous System
Consists of a single neuron between the central nervous system and the effector organ	Has a two-neuron chain (connected by a synapse) between the central nervous system and the effector organ
Innervates skeletal muscle	Innervates smooth or cardiac muscle or gland cells
Always leads to excitation of the muscle	Can lead to excitation or to inhibition of the effector cells

Modified from Vander A, Herman JH, Luciano DS. *Human Physiology: The Mechanism of Body Function,* 4th ed. New York: McGraw-Hill, 1985, p 184, Table 8–3. Copyright © by McGraw-Hill, Inc. Used by permission of McGraw-Hill Book Company.

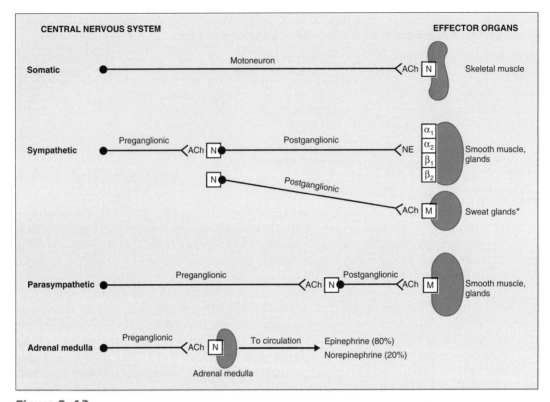

Figure 9–13

Organization of the autonomic nervous system. (From Costanzo LS. *Physiology*. Philadelphia: WB Saunders, 1998, p 40.)

intestinal (GI) tract and controls digestive function. In fact, this self-contained nervous system contains close to 100 million neurons, about the same or more than the number in the spinal cord (Guyton and Hall, 1996; Purves et al, 1997). Although the GI tract receives both sympathetic and parasympathetic input, because of the built-in neural network, it acts independently to some degree. The release of over a dozen neurotransmitters by different types of enteric neurons has been documented (Guyton and Hall, 1996) (see Chapter 11).

Communication Within the Nervous System

The nervous system is connected via synapses. As the system matures, more and more connections are made. A labyrinth of relay stations with an infinite number of ways to take in, disseminate, and combine information is formed (Fig. 9–14). Dendritic branching increases the synaptic potential of the nervous system (Fig. 9–15). It occurs after initial pathways are formed and provides a mechanism for intercommunication between brain structures. The increasing density and complexity of these structures is a mark of advanced communica-

TABLE 9–7

Selected Effects of Autonomic Nervous System Activity

Organ	Effect of Sympathetic Stimulation	Effect of Parasympathetic Stimulation
Eye		
Pupil	Decrease dilation	Decrease constriction
Heart		
SA node	Increase heart rate	Decrease heart rate
Muscle	Increase rate and force	Decrease rate and force
Arterioles	Constriction	Dilation
Veins	Constriction	None
Lungs		
Bronchi	Dilation	Constriction
Gut		
Lumen	Decrease peristalsis	Increase peristalsis
Sphincter	Increase tone (usually)	Relax tone (usually)
Liver	Release glucose	Slight glucose synthesis
Kidney	Decrease output and renin secretion	None
Bladder	Relax detrusor muscle	Contract detrusor muscle
	Contract trigone muscle	Relax trigone muscle
Glands		
Lacrimal	None/slight secretion	Copious secretion
Sweat	Copious sweat	Sweaty palms of hands
Basal metabolism	Increase	None

tion seen in phylogenetically higher animals. Synaptic remodeling occurs throughout the life span in response to experience.

SYNAPSES

Neuron-to-neuron transmission of nerve impulses occurs at an interneuronal junction called a *synapse*. The direction of synaptic transmission determines where the impulses will go within the nervous system. There are two basic types of synapses: chemical and electrical. Electrical synapses are referred to as *gap junctions*. Only a very few are present in the human nervous system, which uses predominantly chemical synapses that are activated by substances called *neurotransmitters*.

More than 40 different chemical substances have been classified as neurotransmitters. A few of the best known are acetylcholine, norepinephrine, serotonin, glutamate, gamma-aminobutyric acid (GABA), and dopamine. These are small-molecule, rapid-acting neurotransmitters that are manufactured by the neurons that release them. When an action potential reaches the end of an axon, it triggers the release of neurotransmitter from synaptic vesicles. Sodium

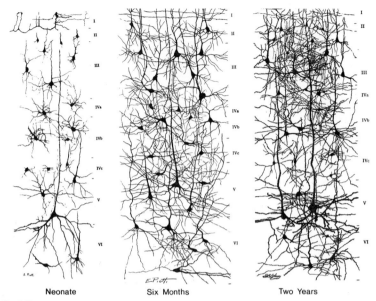

Neonate	Six Months	Two Years

Figure 9–14

Dendritic growth in the visual cortex of an infant. (Reprinted by permission of the publisher from THE POSTNATAL DEVELOPMENT OF THE HUMAN CEREBRAL CORTEX, VOL I-VIII by Jesse LeRoy Conel, Cambridge, MA: Harvard University Press, Copyright © 1939, 1975 by the President and Fellows of Harvard College.)

ions facilitate the depolarization of the presynaptic membrane, and calcium ions facilitate the release of the neurotransmitter. The transmitter diffuses across the space between the two neurons and binds to receptors on the postsynaptic neuron membrane. At many types of synapses, surplus neurotransmitter is broken down in the cleft by enzymes and recycled by the presynaptic neuron or by glial cell uptake.

Neurons can synapse on other neurons called *interneurons*, or they can synapse on muscle or glands. Interneurons are a major source of synaptic input to motor neurons. "Spinal cord interneurons receive sensory inputs as well as descending projections from higher centers and provide much of the reflexive coordination between muscle groups that is essential for movement" (Purves et al, 1997, p 291). In addition, signals received from interneurons can facilitate or inhibit the firing of motor neurons.

Each group of axons or tract of the CNS has its own characteristic way of sending and receiving nerve signals and coding information. The intensity of a nerve signal depends on the number of nerve fibers activated. The more fibers used, the stronger is the signal. This is called *spatial summation.*

Information from nerve fibers can also be varied by the pattern of neuron firing. The frequency of the firing and the time between firings is called *temporal summation,* the sum of the signals over time. Temporal summation might work like this: "dot, dot, space" means pressure, and "dot, space, dot" means light touch. The more different ways of coding information, the better

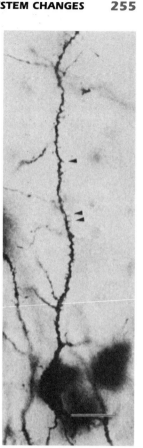

Figure 9–15

Portion of the apical dendritic of a pyramidal neuron illustrating dendritic spines. Golgi-Cox stain, human cerebral cortex; bar represents 20 μm. (From Burt AM. *Textbook of Neuroanatomy.* Philadelphia: WB Saunders, 1993, p 40.)

the organism is able to discriminate one sensation from another, in this case, pressure from light touch.

CORTICAL CONNECTIONS

Communication within the nervous system takes place via one of three ways: by association fibers, by commissural fibers, and by projection fibers. *Association areas* are cortical areas responsible for horizontally linking different parts of the cortex. The parietal, temporal, and occipital association areas are involved in perception. The sensory association cortex is responsible for interfacing sensory information from the three lobes to perceive and to attach meaning to sensory input, such as identifying shapes by touch. The thalamus and other nuclei in the brain stem relay sensory information to association areas for perceptual judgments. The prefrontal and the limbic association areas are concerned with movement and motivation, respectively (see Table 9–3).

Information is communicated not only within the hemispheres but also between the right and left hemispheres. A large group of nerve fibers, called the *corpus callosum*, transmits information between similar areas of the two sides of the brain (see Fig. 9–8). For example, the anterior part of the corpus callosum transmits from the anterior cortex of one side to the anterior cortex of the opposite side.

Information is also shared vertically, up and down the neural axis, by tracts and nuclei that connect the cortex and the spinal cord. Afferent fibers bring sensory input into the spinal cord via the posterior root and connect with or continue as ascending tracts that carry information to various parts of the brain. Efferent fibers carry out commands from the motor cortex and prefrontal cortex, which travel in descending tracts to the anterior horn of the spinal cord.

Adaptation of the Nervous System

NEURAL PLASTICITY

Neural plasticity is the ability of the nervous system to change. Hypothetically, the nervous system can adapt throughout the life span, but plasticity appears to be greatest when the nervous system is developing. The concept of plasticity includes the ability of the nervous system to make structural changes in response to internal or external demands. Bishop and Craik (1982) defined the period during which each type of nerve cell is able to change as the *critical period*. Activity-dependent changes in neural circuitry usually occur during a restricted time in development, or critical period, when the organism is particularly sensitive to the effects of experience (Purves et al, 1997).

After birth, the nervous system continues to mature. Although most of the 100 billion neurons are already formed at birth, neurons continue to make connections with other structures through dendritic branching and by remodeling other connections. Neuronal projections compete for synaptic sites during critical periods (Lundy-Ekman, 1998). Postnatal experience plays a major role in further inducing developmental changes in the pattern of synaptic connections of the system. Development and experience interact to produce change.

Experience is critical to development. Two types of neural plasticity have been described in the literature (Black, 1998). Unfortunately, the names given to them are confusing. One is *experience-expectant*, and the other is *experience-dependent*. In the course of typical prenatal and postnatal development, the infant is expected to be exposed to sufficient environmental stimuli at appropriate times. In fact, if the infant is not exposed to the proper quality and quantity of input, development will not proceed normally. This type of *experience-expectant* neural plasticity is exemplified in the sensory systems that are ready to function at birth but require experience with light and sound to complete maturation. Deprivation during critical time periods can result in the lack of expected development of vision and hearing.

Experience-dependent neural plasticity allows the nervous system to incorporate other types of information from environmental experiences that are relatively unpredictable and idiosyncratic. These experiences are unique to the individual and depend on the context in which development occurs, such as the physical, social, and cultural environment. Lebeer (1998) referred to this as *ecological plasticity*. Climate, social expectation, and child-rearing practices can alter movement experiences. What each child learns depends on the unique physical challenges encountered. Similarly, not every child experiences the same exact words, but every child does learn language. Motor learning is an example of experience-dependent neural plasticity.

NEURON CELL DEATH

Neuron cell death is an important occurrence in the development of the nervous system because the nervous system initially overproduces neurons. This overproduction ensures a sufficient number of neurons to complete the "wiring" of the organism and to support optimal function. Regressive phenomena take place at the end of neuron development and can result in cell loss as high as 70% (Rabinowicz et al, 1996). Two regressive processes mold the developing nervous system. One is *apoptosis,* or programmed cell death, and the other is *axon retraction.* Apoptosis is a naturally occurring phenomenon within the nerve cell that is different from cell death that occurs secondary to injury or disease. The metabolic state of the extracellular environment appears to strongly influence this process. Those neurons deprived of trophic support, that is, those not nourished, degenerate and die. The trimming of extraneous axon connections, or *axon retraction*, occurs without harm to the cell of origin and allows for sculpting of the nervous system.

RESPONSE TO INJURY

Plasticity includes the ability of damaged neurons or nerve tracts to adapt. Adaptability within the CNS is functionally limited to reorganization, because regeneration could not occur. Typically, when a neuron dies, it is not replaced except by glial cells. Researchers have shown, however, that new neurons can be produced in the hippocampus of adults (Kempermann and Gage, 1999). The functional ability of these neurons has yet to be proved. Additional neuron damage or death can occur due to excitotoxicity, during which time synaptic activity can contribute to ischemic injury. Excess secretion of the excitatory neurotransmitter glutamate can cause destruction and death of previously injured neurons. Therefore, blockage of glutamate receptors after the onset of an insult could rescue neurons from destruction (Purves et al, 1997). Adjacent neurons that are not directly injured may become inhibited from functioning. The development of collateral sprouting as a recovery phenomenon is seen in the brain, spinal cord, and PNS. Damaged axons can sprout new processes, which can lead to new synapse formation. Theoretically, therapy attempts to use this reorganization for the recovery of function. Therapy is also postulated to disinhibit intact neurons in adjacent areas (Held and Pay, 1999). *Disinhibition* is the removal of inhibition.

    The PNS retains the ability to regenerate, as evidenced by a return of muscle function after some types of peripheral nerve lesion. When peripheral nerve damage is severe enough to disrupt the myelin sheath and the axon, the axon will degenerate back to the node of Ranvier that is most proximal to the injury. This is called wallerian degeneration. After a time, the axon will regrow and try to reestablish contact. The path of nerve growth can be followed by the Tinel sign (a tingling when the nerve is tapped) as the severed nerve grows and reestablishes contact with its receptor. In the most severe peripheral nerve injury, surgical intervention is required to reestablish the connection.

Summary of Structure and Function

Neurons are the means by which the nervous system communicates. All information is received by specialized receptors and transmitted along several distinct pathways to various regions of the brain, where it is interpreted, acted on, stored, or ignored. Structurally, neurons are produced to match their functions within the nervous system. Neurons increase their ability to communicate by the branching of dendrites and making of new synaptic connections. This branching can be very sophisticated and is related to the amount of information that can be processed. Complexity in dendrite formation is a mark of advanced evolution. Fewer dendritic spines are seen in individuals with mental retardation (Purpura, 1974). Neurons exhibit plasticity but until recently were not thought to be able to divide, with the exception of olfactory neurons (Kempermann and Gage, 1999). Research continues to analyze the structural and functional responses of the nervous system when it is damaged and to delineate the factors that influence a person's potential for recovery.

Life-Span Changes

PRENATAL PERIOD

The CNS develops from specialized ectoderm at 3 weeks of gestation when the neural tube is formed. The brain is created from the cranial two thirds, and the spinal cord from the caudal one third, of the neural tube by the end of the fourth week of gestation, 1 month before the mother feels the fetus move (Moore and Persaud, 1998). When this process is disturbed, severe brain and spinal cord anomalies such as anencephaly and myelomeningocele may result. During the fourth week of gestation, the embryo develops head and tail folds due to rapid growth of the cranial region and spinal cord. The head continues to enlarge during the succeeding weeks, with the brain being folded back onto itself. By 8 weeks, the head of the embryo is half the size of the body. At the end of the eighth week, the fetus looks definitely human and has completed the most critical period of CNS development.

Development of the nervous system is a complicated process. Via cytogenesis or cell production, the maximum number of neurons and glia are produced. Neurons of the spinal cord and brain stem are generated by the 10th week. The neurons of the forebrain, including the cerebral hemispheres, are produced by 20 weeks (Evrard and Minkowski, 1989). During histogenesis, or tissue formation, the structures of the brain and spinal cord are formed. Neurons move or migrate to their correct location within the nervous system, where they differentiate into different nerve cell types, form synaptic connections, and enlarge. Neuronal targets produce trophic substances that guide neuronal connections. Neuronal connections need to have the correct number of axons so that axons innervate the correct number of target cells (Purves et al, 1997). Initially, there is polyneuronal innervation of prenatal muscle fibers compared with the 1:1 relationship seen in postnatal life (Lundy-Ekman, 1998).

Nerve cell types are genetically determined. Therefore, the size and shape of the nerve cell, the pattern of axon or dendrite branching, and even the type of neurotransmitter a neuron will use are innately determined. The cerebral cortex begins as one layer only a few cells thick, known as the *germinal zone* (Green, 1998). Nerve cell classes in the newest part of the cerebral cortex are produced in a set sequence. Cell generation order and cell position in the cortex have an inside-out relationship because of the mechanism of cell migration. The cells formed earliest occupy the deepest layer of the cortex; the cells formed later occupy progressively more superficial layers (Evrard and Minkowski, 1989). These cells migrate using a system of guides, the radial glial fibers, which extend from the surface of the ventricles to the surface of the cortex. Structurally, the six layers of the cortex are completed during the last months of gestation and the first postnatal months of life (Green, 1998).

The first endocrine gland, the thyroid, develops at 24 days (Moore and Persaud, 1998). By the 11th week, it begins to secrete thyroxin, a hormone necessary for proper brain growth. This hormone triggers the cessation of nerve cell proliferation and initiates nerve cell migration (Ford and Cramer, 1977). Without thyroid hormone, axons are poorly myelinated and neurons do not completely branch. Too little hormone produces cretinism, which arrests mental and physical development.

Neuroglia form from the neuroepithelium as early as 3 weeks, although proliferation does not start until 18 weeks of gestation (Herschkowitz, 1989). Microglia appear to be derived from mesenchymal cells late in the fetal period after blood vessels have established their connections. Glial tissue provides a kind of road map for migrating neurons within the brain (Brittis and Silver, 1994). The migration appears to be facilitated by some type of chemical affinity between neuronal and glial surfaces, at least in the cerebellum (Evrard and Minkowski, 1989).

Internal brain structures such as the thalamus and hypothalamus are present at 7 weeks of gestation. The internal structure of the spinal cord is achieved by 10 weeks. During the next 5 to 15 weeks, general structural features—sulci and gyri, cervical and lumbar enlargements of the spinal cord—are attained (Moore and Persaud, 1998). The 12 pairs of cranial nerves emerge during the fifth and sixth weeks of gestation.

In addition to giving rise to the neural tube, the neural plate gives rise to neural crest cells, which are the precursors of the PNS. The PNS begins as paired masses of neural crest cells, one on each side of the neural tube, that differentiate into the sensory ganglia of the spinal nerves. The neural crest cells in the brain region migrate to form sensory ganglia for cranial nerves V, VII, VIII, IX, and X (Moore and Persaud, 1998). Other structures also are produced from the neural crest cells: Schwann cells, meninges (the connective tissue covering of the brain), and many musculoskeletal components of the head.

Motor nerve fibers begin to appear in the spinal cord at the end of the fourth week of gestation, forming the spinal nerves. Next, the dorsal nerve root (consisting of sensory fibers) appears. It is made up of the axons of neural crest cells that have migrated to the dorsolateral part of the spinal cord, forming a spinal ganglion. The spinal nerves exit between the vertebrae, elongate, and grow into the limb buds, where they supply muscles that are differentiated from *mesenchyme* (Fig. 9–16). The muscles innervated by segments of the spinal nerve are referred to as *myotomes*. Skin innervation occurs in the same segmental fashion, resulting in *dermatomes*.

The relationship between the spinal roots and the vertebral column is shown in Figures 9–17 and 9–18. Any root above C8 exits above the vertebra of the corresponding number; any root below C8 exits below the vertebra of the corresponding number. This change in relationship is due to differential growth of the spinal cord and vertebral column (see Fig. 9–18).

Synapse formation occurs relatively late in the development of the nervous system, just before 6 to 7 weeks. Synapse formation is highly variable in pattern and distribution. The development of connections between the sensory

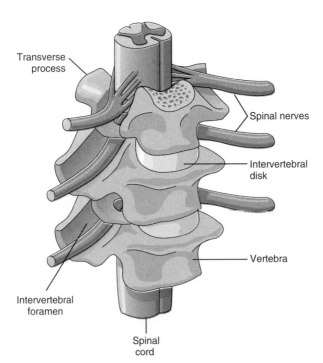

Transverse process

Spinal nerves

Intervertebral disk

Vertebra

Intervertebral foramen

Spinal cord

Figure 9–16

As the spinal cord travels down the vertebral column, spinal nerves exit at the intersections of each two vertebrae. (From Copstead LEC, Banasik JL. *Pathophysiology: Biological and Behavioral Perspectives*, 2nd ed. Philadelphia: WB Saunders, 2000, p 978.)

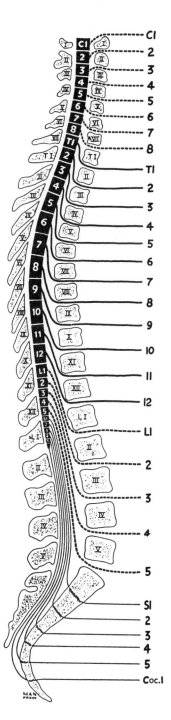

Figure 9–17

Intervertebral relationship of spinal nerves. The bodies and spinous processes of the vertebrae are indicated by roman numerals. Spinal segments and spinal nerves are indicated by arabic numerals and letters. (Redrawn from Haymaker W, Woodhall B. *Peripheral Nerve Injuries: Principles of Diagnoses,* 2nd ed. Philadelphia: WB Saunders, 1953, p 32.)

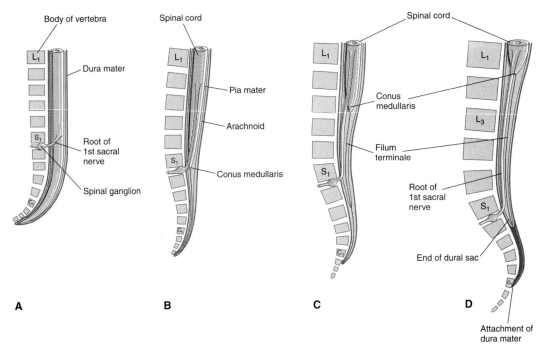

Figure 9–18

Diagrams showing the position of the caudal end of the spinal cord in relation to the vertebral column and meninges at various stages of development. The increasing inclination of the root of the first sacral nerve is also illustrated. *A,* Eight weeks. *B,* Twenty-four weeks. *C,* Newborn. *D,* Adult. (From Moore KL, Persaud TVN. *Before We Are Born,* 5th ed. Philadelphia: WB Saunders, 1998, p 432.)

neurons and the motor neurons is critical to laying the framework for spinal reflexes and for the pairing of sensory and motor information. A spinal reflex is the pairing of a sensory neuron and a motor neuron so that incoming stimuli produce a motor response. Once established, spinal reflexes are permanent (Sperry, 1959) and considered "hard-wired." Reflexes can be monosynaptic or polysynaptic—that is, they can involve one or more than one synapse. The establishment of reflex connections provides the fetus and eventually the infant with survival reflexes such as suck-swallow, rooting, and gag. Fetal movement begins in utero at about 6 to 7 weeks of gestation. Reflex movements in response to touch have been chronicled as early as 7 to 8 weeks of gestation. Reflex connections are established in utero in a cephalocaudal direction; arm withdrawal occurs earlier than leg withdrawal.

As another late-stage phenomenon of neural development, myelination starts after neuron formation (8 to 16 weeks of gestation) and overlaps with neuron migration (12 to 20 weeks of gestation). Myelination occurs first in those areas of the nervous system that will be used first. Myelin is initially laid down in the cervical part of the spinal medulla and in the cranial nerves related to sucking and swallowing, abilities needed for survival. The first axons to be myelinated are the anterior (motor) roots of the spinal cord at about 4 months of gestation. One month later, the posterior, or sensory, roots begin the process. Myelin is deposited as a sheath or covering in the spinal cord at the same time that functional connections (i.e., synapses) are being formed (Martinez, 1989). The vestibulocochlear system (cranial nerve VIII) is myelinated at the end of the fifth month of gestation (Almli and Mohr, 1995) and is related to awareness of head and body position in space.

Rapid periods of growth such as those seen in the fetal period are critical periods when the nervous system is most vulnerable to damage. Malnutrition or trauma can have dramatic effects on the developing system. The nervous system requires adequate nutrition for cell formation and myelination to occur (Wiggins et al, 1984). For example, lipids in the form of fatty acids must be transported through the blood-brain barrier because there are no endogenous fats in the brain (Bourre, 1989). A lack of nutrition results in a decrease in the number of synapses formed and in the amount of dendritic branching and myelination (Herschkowitz, 1989).

INFANCY AND YOUNG CHILDHOOD

At birth, the brain is one fourth the weight of the adult brain, whereas the head is already 70% of its adult size. Critical periods for brain growth occur between 3 and 10 months and between 15 and 24 months of age (Rabinowicz, 1996). Brain weight doubles by 6 months of age and is half the weight of the adult brain. Malnutrition during the first 2 years of life reduces the number of glial cells formed (Dobbing, 1984), which may result in poorer vascular support for nervous system function. The relationship of brain weight and brain growth is depicted in Figure 9–19. Children who are malnourished before 3 years of age reportedly have impaired motor ability (Kretchmer, 1989).

Brain metabolism changes with CNS maturation during infancy. Tracking glucose metabolism in the brain postnatally provides another means to document functional maturation. The pattern of activity, that is, where glucose is being utilized, corresponds to the areas of the brain that are maturing. In the newborn, the highest activity is found in the primary motor and sensory cortex, thalamus, brain stem, and midline of the cerebellum. By 2 to 3 months, increases in glucose utilization are evident in the parietal, temporal, and primary visual cortex; basal ganglia; and cerebellar hemispheres. The frontal cortex is the last area to demonstrate increased glucose use. The increase begins between 6 and 8 months, and by 8 to 12 months, utilization is widespread in the frontal lobes (Chugani, 1998). The increase in glucose use in the frontal lobes also corresponds to the expansion of dendritic branching and capillary networks in the frontal lobe (Diemer, 1968; Schade and van Groenigen, 1961).

The cerebral metabolic rate of glucose utilization in infancy is 30% lower than that in adulthood (Chugani, 1998). Figure 9–20 depicts the changes that occur in the metabolic rate of glucose utilization of the brain over time and compares the relative rate of use between children and adults. These changes

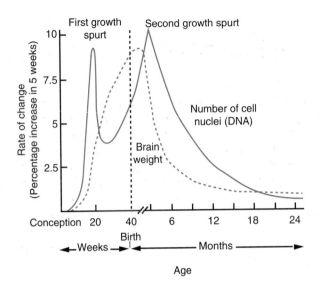

Figure 9–19

Relationship of brain weight *(dotted line)* and growth *(solid line)*. The DNA curve has two peaks: one reflecting neuron multiplication, and the other reflecting glial multiplication. (Modified from Dobbing J. Undernutrition and the developing brain. *Am J Dis Child* 120:411–415, 1970, copyright 1970, American Medical Association; Trevarthen CB. Neuroembryology and the development of perceptual mechanisms. In Falkner FT, Tanner JM [eds]. *Human Growth.* New York: Plenum Press, 1986.)

over time partially mirror the time course for synaptogenesis. Synaptic proliferation occurs in the period between birth and 4 years of age. A period of leveling off follows during middle childhood. The decline at adolescence is due to synaptic elimination that occurs in the cortex with a further diminishment of energy requirements to adulthood (Chugani, 1994).

Myelination of the PNS is largely complete at birth (Bishop and Craik, 1982), allowing the newborn immediate access to information about the environment through touch, motion, smell, and taste. The infant uses these sensory cues to carry out vital functions of eating, breathing, sleeping, and excreting. All cranial nerves (with the exception of the optic nerve) are completely myeli-

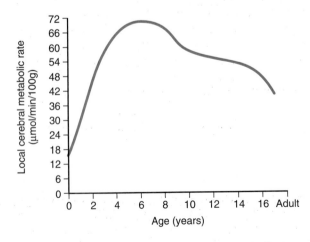

Figure 9–20

Brain metabolism rate of glucose utilization. (Adapted from Chugani HT. A critical period of brain development: Studies of cerebral glucose utilization with PET. *Prev Med* 27:184–188, 1998.)

nated at birth. The richness of the experiences that a child is exposed to during the first 3 years of life can be critical to cognitive development (Kotulak, 1998).

Within the brain, myelination continues into young adulthood. Although the PNS is ready to function at birth, myelination has been occurring for only 2 months in the brain (assuming that the infant is born at term, 40 weeks of gestation). The primary motor cortex develops ahead of the primary sensory cortex. The rates of myelination are related to when these areas reach adult levels of function (Bronson, 1982). Figure 9–21 shows when some major struc-

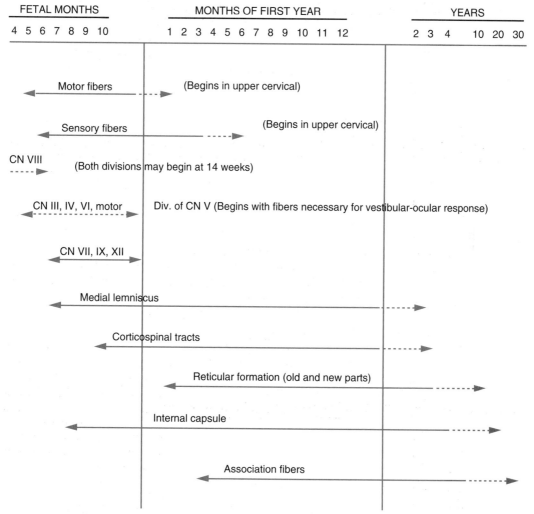

Figure 9–21

Timetable of myelination of selected nervous system structures. (Modified from Yakovlev PI, Lecours AR. The myelogenetic cycles of regional maturation of the brain. In Minkowski A [ed]. *Regional Development of the Brain in Early Life.* Oxford: Blackwell, 1967.)

tures undergo myelination. The midbrain and spinal cord are the most advanced portions at birth in terms of myelination, which may account for early descriptions of infants as functioning only on a brain stem level. Early myelination of the brain stem supports the many vital functions controlled there and accounts for the fact that the newborn sleeps most of the time and is totally dependent on caregivers.

The first 2 months after birth are considered a period of CNS organization. During this time, the infant establishes physiologic control of sleep and wakefulness as evidenced by the relationship between sleep states and electroencephalographic patterns, and by increasing the number and duration of periods of alertness. Social behavior begins around 2 months of age with the advent of the social smile. Circadian rhythm, or the 24-hour biologic cycle, is established between 2 and 4 months of age without regard for night and day (Stratton, 1982). In other words, this is a time when infants can get their days and nights mixed up.

ANS changes occur during the first year of life as the newborn responds more via the sympathetic nervous system to ever-changing stressors such as light, gravity, and air. As internal body processes (e.g., GI motility) stabilize, behavioral responses gradually become more characteristic of the parasympathetic nervous system, which maintains the status quo or steady state.

Nerve conduction velocity increases over time in both skin and muscle fibers because of the change to saltatory conduction and the increase in nerve fiber diameter with age. Values for nerve conduction speed change remarkably quickly after birth. For example, ulnar nerve conduction in infants and young children increases from 30 to 50 m/sec from birth to 9 months of age and reaches adult values (60 m/sec) by 3 years of age (Thomas and Lambert, 1960).

Brain structures are ready to support the development of function during the first year of life. The major efferent (motor) tract, the corticospinal tract, begins myelination 1 month before birth and completes the process by 1 year. The corticospinal tract in the newborn has not yet innervated the anterior horn, so during the first 6 months of life the infant demonstrates a Babinski sign (Lundy-Ekman, 1998). Stroking the foot from the heel results in extension of the great toe. Although presence of this sign in individuals older than 6 months is indicative of corticospinal tract damage, in a young infant it is a sign of immaturity (Purves et al, 1997). The sensory area of the brain catches up to the motor area by the age of 2. During the second year of life, the increasing speed and complexity of movement may be related to myelination. The process slows after 2 years and is mostly complete by 10 years of age.

Brain growth during childhood is thought to coincide with the stages of cognitive development as described by Piaget (1952) and the development of language (Hallett and Proctor, 1996). The infant's brain weight at 1 year is 60% of its adult weight, a gain of 10% in 6 months. During the next year, growth continues until 75% of adult brain weight is reached by age 2. The relationship of brain weight, age, and language acquisition is shown in Table 9–8. Myelination of structures that support speech development, such as the tectum, an integration center for auditory information, and the striatum, an integration

TABLE 9–8

Relationship of Age, Brain Weight, and Language Acquisition

Age	Brain Weight (% of adult weight)	Language Level
Birth	25	Crying; no words
1 yr	60	Average age of first spoken word
18 mo to 2 yr	75	Two-word combinations
3 yr	80	Phrases and short sentences
6 yr	90	Five- to six-word sentences
Puberty	100	Abstract language concepts

center for language, occurs within the first year of life. Myelination of the striatum by 1 year of age coincides with the child's first spoken word. The pattern and density of dendritic branching have also been linked to language development, especially the specialization of the left hemisphere as the language center in the majority of individuals (Hallett and Proctor, 1996). A 2-year-old child can put together two-word combinations and by age 3 can speak in phrases and short sentences.

CHILDHOOD AND ADOLESCENCE

Children develop fundamental skills such as jumping, throwing, catching, and balancing in early childhood (3 to 6 years). From 6 to 10 years of age, these skills become refined as the nervous system continues to increase the speed of conduction of nerve impulses through ongoing myelination, and motor control becomes more automatic. The adolescent may continue to improve motor skills with practice. The amount of change after adolescence is highly variable and depends more on practice, instruction, motivation, and innate ability.

To achieve its adult weight, the brain undergoes additional critical periods during growth spurts at 6 to 8 years, 10 to 12 years, and around 18 years of age. Despite the fact that children exhibit a partially mature corticospinal tract between 6 and 9 years of age, the ability to conduct nervous impulses at adult-like speeds is not sufficient for proficient motor performance. A group of young school-age children could not perform a motor task as well as adults (Heinen et al, 1998). Myelination continues in the sensorimotor systems, including secondary cortical areas. The last areas to be myelinated are the association cortices in the frontal, parietal, and temporal lobes, along with other association fibers. This process continues through adulthood (Green, 1998).

Language development continues to be related to brain growth. At 6 years of age, 90% of the adult brain weight is achieved and the child speaks in five- to six-word sentences. At puberty, adult brain weight is attained and abstract language concepts such as the use of complex clauses are demonstrated. The corticospinal tract is morphologically mature by 10 years of age but not electrophysiologically mature until age 13 (Heinen et al, 1998; Nezu et al, 1997).

Low-frequency electroencephalographic rhythms change to adult high-frequency rhythms by 10 to 13 years of age (Valadian and Porter, 1977). Dendritic branching reaches adult levels of complexity from 12 to 16 years of age (Hallet and Proctor, 1996).

The brain directs other body systems to change at puberty via hormonal influences. These changes include, but are not limited to, development of the secondary sex characteristics, changes in body composition, and the onset of menses (see Chapter 11).

ADULTHOOD

The majority of individuals between the ages of 20 and 29 years are at the peak of their ability to perform physically. Those involved in sports, such as recent Olympic competitors, are even younger. The nervous system begins to decline in adulthood. Brain weight and volume decline linearly with age in the average population (Duara et al, 1985). Beginning at age 20, brain weight declines (Duara et al, 1985), the cortex thins (Magnotta et al, 1999), and the number of glial cells changes depending on type. Astrocytes and microglia increase and oligodendrocytes decrease (Willott, 1999). Much of the loss of brain mass occurs in the white matter with an age-related decline in brain weight and size related to the loss of myelin (Patten and Craik, 2000). How much decline is necessary before functional abilities are affected is not known. We do know that age-related changes in the nervous system have far-reaching effects on all systems of the body.

CNS changes related to aging are not the same for every part of the brain. Aging affects the frontal and temporal lobes more than the parietal lobes (Jack et al, 1997). Positron emission tomography scans show decreased brain glucose metabolism in both of these areas in older individuals compared with young adults (DeSanti et al, 1995; Eberling et al, 1995). Previous reports of neuron loss from other areas of the cortex, such as the primary motor and sensory areas of the cortex, have not been substantiated by further research. Subcortical areas such as the thalamus, striatum, and locus ceruleus are more likely to lose neurons with aging (Kemper, 1994). Computed tomography scans confirm that atrophy of the brain occurs with aging (Stafford et al, 1988). In addition, there is ventricular enlargement. Cerebral volume declines by 11% in relation to cranial volume between the ages of 20 and 30 (Yamamura et al, 1980). A greater decline in brain volume has been reported in women than in men beginning in their 40s. Birge (1998) reported on research findings in women that the loss primarily affects the hippocampus (in the temporal lobe) and parietal lobe. A total of about 15% of brain weight and volume is lost throughout the life span, beginning in middle adulthood (Double, 1996). The amount of these decreases is moderated by overall good health and varies according to the area of the brain studied. There is considerable interindividual variability in the patterns of brain changes (Whitbourne, 1999).

The hippocampus, a part of the limbic system associated with memory, has been reported to show a 30% decrease in neurons beginning after the age of 30 (Mouritzen Dam, 1979). This is due to the loss of pyramidal cells, which play an important role in memory and learning (Fox and Adler, 1999). As stated, research has shown that new neurons are produced in the hippocampus in adulthood (Kempermann and Gage, 1999).

In contrast to a litany of decreases in large populations of cells, the absence of significant age-related neuron cell loss has been documented in some discrete brain structures. The basal ganglia, which implement movement programs, maintain stability during adulthood (Whitbourne, 1996). Some brain stem nuclei show little or no neuron loss as a result of aging (Konigsmark and Murphy, 1970).

In the adult, nerve conduction velocity of peripheral nerves decreases (Schaumburg et al, 1983). The speed with which sensory nerves conduct impulses begins to decline after 30 years of age (Buchtal et al, 1984). Motor nerve conduction velocity, according to Schaumburg et al (1983), decreases by 1 m/sec per decade after 15 to 24 years of age. Therefore, sensory information continues to come into the nervous system, albeit more slowly.

The nervous system changes that result from aging begin at age 20. Brain weight and thickness of the cortex decline, whereas the number of glial cells increases. Whether the number of neurons increases, decreases, or stays the same with reduced neuron size is still being debated. Despite all of these occurrences, few overall changes in the structure of the brain and nervous system exceed 25% of the total area, except in disease states, and only during the last few months of life (Cotman and Holets, 1985). The built-in redundancy of the nervous system by way of synaptic plasticity is such that even if neurons are lost in one place, other connections may be gained. Most areas of the brain stem that deal with vital functions are stable throughout adulthood and show minimal change with aging.

OLDER ADULTHOOD

A major problem with identifying primary aging changes in the nervous system is that it is impossible to know with any degree of certainty if these are signs of preclinical pathology. The potential that both intrinsic and extrinsic environmental factors can produce changes with aging further compound the problem of identifying what are primary aging changes. Some degree of brain volume and neuron loss is probably inevitable, but it is not possible to state unequivocally what is "normal" or "typical" because universal or primary aging changes are difficult to separate from those that are harbingers of pathology. A cross-sectional comparison of a normal brain and an aging brain is shown in Figure 9–22.

Age-related decline in brain weight and volume is accompanied by neuronal atrophy, cell death, and ventricular enlargement. Gyral atrophy includes loss of gray and white matter, whereas white matter loss includes the loss of myelin. Significant differences in brain volume are seen between young-old, middle-old, and old-old subjects (Mueller et al, 1998). Mueller and associates (1998) have also shown volume loss to be minimal after age 65 with decline

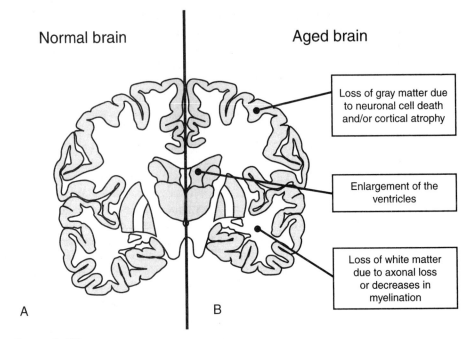

Normal brain

Aged brain

Loss of gray matter due
to neuronal cell death
and/or cortical atrophy

Enlargement of the
ventricles

Loss of white matter
due to axonal loss
or decreases in
myelination

A

B

Figure 9–22

Comparison of a normal and an aged brain. *A,* A normal hemisection of the human cortex. *B,* Aged human cortex. Researchers have observed several age-related gross anatomic changes, including a loss or atrophy of cortical neurons, a decrease in white matter (due to axonal or myelin loss), and an enlargement of the ventricles. (From Fox CM, Alder RN. Neural mechanisms of aging. In Cohen H [ed]. *Neuroscience for Rehabilitation,* 2nd ed. Philadelphia: Lippincott Williams & Wilkins, 1999, p 404.)

progressing at small constant rates from young-old to middle-old to old-old. The rate of loss is small and constant in the healthy older adults.

Myriad changes happen within the nervous system during the early and middle part of adulthood, and even more significant changes are seen in older adulthood. Terry and colleagues (1987) studied 51 brains from normal individuals aged 24 to 100 years and found that the overall total number of neurons, neuron density, and percentage of cell area occupied remained unchanged. A striking reduction in neuron size, however, was noted, along with a minor degree of neuronal loss when the entire cortex was considered. Large neurons in the frontal and temporal lobes shrank, whereas the number of smaller neurons increased (Terry et al, 1987). Haug and colleagues (1984) and Haug (1985) concluded that the total number of neurons in the cortex does not change during the aging process and that the dominant age-related change is neuronal shrinkage.

Morgan (1989) considered the loss of neuron size and aging a possible explanation for forgetfulness in older adulthood. Minor to moderate neuron loss and the loss of the ability of dendrites to produce new spines (sprouting) have been reported in many parts of the brain, but the link to a decline in function is far from apparent. Structural losses may be a result of an age-dependent decline in use, because dendrites continue to grow into old age. Synaptic remodeling and growth also occur late in adulthood (Herschkowitz, 1989). Synaptic plasticity can be assessed using positron emission tomography as a measure of cognitive reserve capacity. Dendritic complexity in older individuals who are cognitively intact supports the idea that the nervous system is still able to adapt well into the 70s (Mrak et al, 1997).

Myelination continues into adulthood in those areas responsible for integrating information for purposeful action, the association areas of the brain. The commissures that provide interhemispheric communication are essential to human memory (Zaidel, 1995). Minor changes in electroencephalographic patterns, such as a slowing of the alpha waves, have been reported (Friedlander, 1958). Additional evidence, however, suggests that no significant changes in pattern occur with age (Shigeta et al, 1995). In fact, the temporal wave slowing so often attributed to normal aging has been linked to pathological brain changes (Keefover, 1999). The cerebellum also shows age-related changes that could be associated with declines in posture, balance, and gait seen in the older adult. Although not proved to be cause and effect, the decrease in Purkinje cells and the fact that the cerebellum is highly myelinated seem to indicate a potential correlation may be found. Any significant loss of neurons would be expected to cause an increase in glial cells (Mrak et al, 1997). A decrease in glial cells, however, has been reported in connection with the destruction of the myelin sheaths of some nerves. More importantly, it is thought that structural changes in several types of glial cells may have a greater effect on neuron function if, over time, such changes interfere with the transport of vital nutrients from the surrounding blood supply to the neuron (Whitbourne, 1996).

Brain function as measured by glucose metabolism shows a 6% decline from ages 20 to 67 years (Petit-Taboue et al, 1998). Mielke and coworkers (1998) have attributed "normal aging of the brain [to be] predominantly characterized by metabolic changes in the prefrontal cortex." The frontal lobes appear to be an area of the brain affected early and extensively by aging according to some researchers (Luszcz and Bryan, 1999; Woodruff-Pak, 1997). Indeed, studies of age-related memory loss show a decline with age that is related to the frontal lobe executive function abilities. Others have shown that higher-order association areas lose more neurons than the primary motor or visual cortex area during aging (Brody and Vijayashanker, 1977; Kemper, 1994).

Cerebral blood flow has been shown to decrease with age in some studies and not in others. This paradox appears to be related to a decrease in sensory function or the presence of arteriosclerosis. According to Duara and colleagues (1985), measures of brain metabolism made without sensory input control are skewed and therefore will show a decrease with age. If the amount of sensory input is controlled for, as in their study, no change in brain metabolism is seen. This may illustrate the adage "use it or lose it."

The hippocampus exhibits a number of neurofibrillary tangles (NFTs) within the neuron cell body as a result of aging (Bell and Ball, 1990). Although the incidence of NFTs increases with age in the healthy brain, an even greater incidence is seen in patients with dementia (Mrak et al, 1997). Neuritic or senile plaques and lipofuscin accumulation are additional cellular hallmarks of aging. A *senile plaque* is a thickened mass of degenerating *neurites* (small axons, some dendrites, astrocytes) with an *amyloid* (starchy glycoprotein) deposit in the center. Neuritic plaques occur as a result of pathologic aging and are some of the earliest neuropathologic hallmarks of Alzheimer's disease (AD) (Haroutunian et al, 1998).

The role of lipofuscin in normal aging is not clear at this time. Lipofuscin is a pigment associated with aging. It accumulates in some neurons and tissues and not in others. The amount of lipofuscin had previously been thought to roughly correlate to the degree of dementia in AD (Brody and Vijayashanker, 1977), but that has been linked to oxidative damage in neurons and may serve as a marker of age-related stress on cells. Oxidative stress has been implicated as a possible mechanism of aging (Yin, 1996).

On a biochemical level, the loss of enzymes involved in neurotransmitter synthesis has been documented along with a moderate loss of receptor sites for certain neurotransmitters in both the CNS and the PNS (Rogers and Bloom, 1985; Strong, 1998). A decline in motor system performance has been linked to a steady decrease in dopamine uptake sites due to age-related loss of axons in basal ganglia pathways (Volkow et al, 1998). Loss of serotonin receptors in the cortex has been postulated to predispose older individuals to depression and cognitive impairment (Strong, 1998). Cholinergic function declines in patients with AD; therefore, deficits in cholinergic function are also related to cognitive impairment. Specifically, the muscarinic type of cholinergic receptors decreases by 50% to 60% in the caudate, putamen, hippocampus, and frontal cortex between the ages of 4 and 93 years (DeKosky and Palmer, 1994). The declines in the serotonergic and cholinergic systems may play a role in cognitive decline associated with pathologic aging.

Modest declines in dopamine content of the basal ganglia have been measured after midlife (DeKosky and Palmer, 1994). This 25% loss is in sharp contrast to the losses exhibited with severe lesions involving the basal ganglia or in Parkinson's disease. The age-related alterations in the basal ganglia resemble those that occur in Parkinson's disease, but the cell dropout is not as severe. Despite the similarity of brain cell degeneration, the causes for the changes are likely to be different (Hubble, 1998).

Aging changes in the ANS can be linked to changes in the sensitivity of sympathetic receptors to circulating neurotransmitters. *Aging* has been described as a hyperadrenergic state because of the more intense cardiac and vascular sympathetic responses seen in older adults (Katzman and Terry, 1983). Although increased levels of norepinephrine have been documented in older subjects, Whitbourne (1996) postulated that the increase in circulating neurotransmitters could be an adaptive response to a decrease in receptor sensitivity, as seen in aging cardiac muscle. No consistent age-related changes in norepinephrine have been documented (Strong, 1998).

Peripherally, over age 60, the loss of motor neurons and myelinated anterior root fibers contributes significantly to the gradual loss of muscle mass and strength seen with aging (Lexell, 1997). Decreased awareness of touch and vibration are two documented peripheral changes that occur by the age of 70 (Potvin et al, 1980). The concept of "use it or lose it" cannot be overlooked when assessing the competence of any body system to adapt over time. It is especially true for the nervous system. As we age, lifestyles and habits formed early in life will be what motivate, inspire, and provide an impetus to move. If exercise, fitness, and health are valued and the individual stays physically fit and actively participates in life, how will the outcome differ?

Functional Implications

Two aspects of nervous system function—reaction time and cognition—are used to illustrate the relationship between nervous system development and acquisition of function. Reaction time is a measure of nervous system efficiency during movement. *Cognition* is that function of our brain that enables interaction with the environment. It is a complex brain function, whereas *reaction time* is a simple function. Both aspects of nervous system function—cognition and reaction time—change over time.

REACTION TIME

The batter sees the ball, swings, and hits the ball. *Reaction time* is defined as the amount of time between presentation of a stimulus and the motor response. As would be expected, the reaction time of children is slower than that of adults (Eaton and Ritchot, 1995). Reaction time improves as the child develops more complex skills such as catching and hitting. Physical maturation affects information processing speed in 9- and 10-year-olds, with early maturers being faster than late maturers (Eaton and Ritchot, 1995). Reaction time peaks in young adulthood and then declines; it is slowed 15% to 30% in older persons (Willott, 1999).

A simple response time (SRT) test measures reaction speed when only one response is required from a stimulus, such as hitting a key when a light flashes. Fast test responses are reported for subjects in their 20s, with the greatest consistency of response seen in subjects in their 30s. Responses on SRT tests slow with age (Birren and Fisher, 1995). A 20% increase in reaction time is seen in 60-year-old subjects compared with 20-year-old subjects (Birren et al, 1979). Slowing reaction time or psychomotor speed has been recognized as a universal behavioral change in aging (Kail and Salthouse, 1994).

Reaction time consists of three parts: (1) sensory transmission of input, (2) motor execution time, and (3) central processing (Schaie and Willis, 1996). The latter component makes up 80% of the total reaction time. Reaction time requires attention because attention is a prerequisite for sensory information to get into working memory, a concept that is discussed under cognition. Investigators using electromyography separate premotor time from motor time. *Premotor time* is the time between the stimulus and electromyographic activity and reflects the neural component of reaction time. Premotor time represents components 1 and 3. *Motor time* is defined as the time between the electromyographic activity and the movement and therefore reflects the muscular component of reaction time.

Both premotor and motor times are related to chronologic age. Premotor time (the neural component) is slower in all older individuals regardless of task. Motor time (the motor component) depends more on the type of task, especially the amount of muscular force required. Simple tasks such as hand movement show more age-related effects on the premotor time (Welford, 1984); jumping (Onishi, 1966) and movement against resistance (Singleton, 1954) show more age-related effects on the motor time. The more complicated the task, the more likely it is to be influenced by age-related change. In general, the more complicated the decision or task, the bigger is the difference seen in the reaction time of young and old persons (Spirduso, 1995).

Complex or choice reaction time studies involve a choice between two responses. Light and Spirduso (1990) confirmed that as the task becomes more complex, reaction time increases with the increasing age of the individual. In a complex task such as trying to recover balance, an individual's risk of falling increases with age. After the age of 60, reaction time variability increases relative to that of younger individuals. When Fozard and colleagues (1994) compared simple and choice reaction times in a group of men and women ranging in age from 20 to 90 years, however, they found only slight slowing of simple reaction time but more dramatic slowing in choice reaction time.

Health and exercise may modify age-related changes in reaction time (Emery et al, 1995). When the level of physical activity of the individual is considered, active older subjects have been found to have faster reaction times than sedentary older subjects (Spirduso, 1980). Also, variability within older subjects increases such that on a day-to-day basis, responses are not as consistent as they are in younger individuals. The rate of slowing depends a great deal on the task (Stine-Morrow and Soederberg Miller, 1999). Thus, results involving reaction time in the elderly must be regarded cautiously.

Central and peripheral factors contribute to the slowing of reaction time. Laufer and Schweitz (1968) reported that only 4% of the change in reaction time in aging individuals can be accounted for by the decrease in motor nerve conduction velocity, and 10% can be accounted for by the decrease in sensory nerve conduction velocity. The greater contribution to slowing comes from the central factors or premotor components. These premotor components include stimulus identification and processing, response selection, and response programming. Older subjects process sensory information for an aiming task, similar to younger subjects but at a lower speed (Chaput and Proteau, 1996). Slowness is related to changes in neural pathways in the brain and brain stem that integrate sensory and motor information (Woodruff-Pak, 1997).

ATTENTION, LEARNING, AND MEMORY

Cognition is the process of knowing and the application of that knowledge is intelligence. Cognitive processes include selective attention, learning, and memory. Executive functions performed by the brain involve goal-directed, conscious decision-making and strategy selection. These functions require attention to select features on which to make decisions, to resolve conflicts, and to plan new actions. The ability to change the structure of the nervous system in response to experience is the basis for learning and memory (Bertoni-Freddari et al, 1996).

Self-Control

Executive or focal attention is related to a human's ability to assess the many conflicting details of the environment and self and then make choices that influence cognitive and emotional function. Posner and Rothbart (1998) posited that the ability to attend develops during the first year of life and is initially demonstrated by the infant's self-regulation of her own distress. Infants can consistently self-calm at 3 to 4 months when their attention is distracted. Posner and Rothbart (1998) further hypothesized that the mechanism used by infants to cope with feelings of distress, or self-regulate, is transferred and applied to the control of cognition during later infancy and childhood. The development of self-control begins in infancy with the regulation of distress and may involve interaction between areas in the frontal lobe, specifically the cingulate and the amygdala. For example, an 18-month-old shows context sensitive learning when visually attending to the surroundings. Spatial locations are learned when the frontal areas of the brain develop a functional visual field. The development of self-control progresses slowly in early life, continues throughout adolescence, and becomes mutable during adulthood (Posner and Rothbart, 1998).

Self-control is needed for attention, and attention is needed for learning. Executive attention undergoes a dramatic change around 30 months of age. Patterns of response change, with older children becoming more accurate. Casey and coworkers (1997) showed a significant correlation between the ability to perform tasks that relied on attentional control and the size of the right anterior cingulate in children aged 5.3 to 16 years. Further refinement of the attentional system occurs in adulthood.

Memory

The developmental psychologist Piaget (1952) attributed the origin of intelligence to the pairing of sensory and motor experiences. He viewed cognitive development as necessary for memory development. The nervous system controls cognition by processing thought and memory. According to Guyton and Hall (1996), "A thought reflects a pattern" of stimulation of the cortex, thalamus, limbic system, and reticular formation of the brain stem. Physiologically, memories are produced by changes in the ability of one neuron to transmit to another neuron across a synapse, producing a "memory trace." Movement of energy leaves a residue by which use of the pathway can be assessed; think of a thermogram, in which greater intensity of the color denotes warmth and increased blood flow. Memories can be considered immediate, short term, or long term depending on their duration. Immediate memories last for only a few seconds or a few minutes. Short-term memories can last for days or weeks but will eventually be lost if they are not converted to long-term memory. Long-term memory can be recalled years later and is thought to result from structural changes at the level of the synapses that influence signal conduction (Lynch, 1998).

Types of Memory

There are two types of memory and learning: implicit and explicit. *Implicit,* or procedural, memory relies on performance of procedural skills, which include forms of perceptual and motor learning that do not require verbal expression but are exhibited by alterations in task performance. An example is matching shapes to a template. Researchers have shown that infants as young as 3 months remember a particular motor event. Rovee-Collier (1987) experimented with connecting an infant's arm or leg to a mobile with a ribbon. The infant learned to move the mobile and even remembered which arm or leg to move after a short time had passed. Implicit memory is unconscious memory and is related to the cerebellum and striatum (caudate and putamen) (Nelson, 1995, 1998).

Explicit, or declarative, memory is the learning of facts and experiences that can be reported verbally, such as naming body parts, state capitals, or muscle origins and insertions. Explicit memory is conscious memory. It depends on structures in the medial part of the temporal lobe, including the hippocampus (Nelson, 1995, 1998). Because relative value is placed on this type of learning, the limbic system becomes involved. Declarative learning and memory allow for categoric aspects of higher cognitive and affective (emotional) processing such as abstract thought.

The development of memory occurs throughout life (Table 9–9). Before 6 months of age, there is no conscious memory, only a learned adaptive response. After 6 months of age, an infant learns object permanence, so that he knows that an object does not disappear when it is out of sight. Conscious, explicit memory is demonstrated as early as 7 months, but recall of events is minimal until a child is about 3 years of age. Conscious memory may be related to the linguistic ability of the child.

Between 5 and 7 years of age, the child begins to relate past and present memories and to reason more efficiently (Mussen et al, 1974). Children no longer just monitor perceptual information, such as size, shape, and color, but correlate perceptual information (e.g., "all round objects made of rubber bounce, whereas round stones do not"). They continue to pick up and reflect on relevant perceptual cues to solve increasingly complex problems or to perform tasks after the age of 6 or 7 years (Paris and Lindauer, 1982). Around the age of 9 or 10 years, children begin to direct their thinking. They can evaluate, plan, and refine their own thinking about how best to solve a problem. Being able to think about thinking is called *metacognition,* a term that subsumes elaborate executive functions. The ability to think about remembering is called *metamemory.* We practice metacognition when encountering a patient with an undefined movement dysfunction and thinking of ways to

TABLE 9-9

Types of Memory

Type	Age	Neural Structures	Examples
Implicit (procedural)	First few months	Striatum (caudate and putamen); olivary-cerebellar complex	Procedural learning Conditioning
Preexplicit	Before 8 mo	Hippocampus and temporal lobe	Attention Recognition memory Novelty detection
Explicit (declarative)	Begins at 8–12 mo	Limbic and temporal lobe	Event sequence Novelty preference
Working	Begins at 8–12 mo; increases at 6–24 yr	Prefrontal lobes	Relate past events to present
Long-term	Over life span	Hippocampus; basal ganglia, cerebellum, premotor cortex	Word meaning Motor behavior

Data from Nelson CA. The ontogeny of human memory: A cognitive neuroscience perspective. *Dev Psych* 31:723–738, 1995; Purves D, Nelson CA. The nature of early memory. *Prev Med* 27:172–179, 1998; Augustine GJ, Fitzpatrick LC, et al. *Neuroscience.* Sunderland, MA: Sinauer Associates, 1997; Swanson HL. What develops in working memory? A life span perspective. *Dev Psych* 35(4):986–1000, 1999.

approach the patient's problem. We practice metamemory when planning for a test by reviewing what one does and does not know.

With aging, there is a decrease in complex cognitive skills involving memory. As you may recall, there are three phases of memory—immediate, short term, and long term. The frontal lobes are affected early by aging, and therefore the cognitive processes collectively referred to as *executive functions* are also affected (Woodruff-Pak, 1997). Certain aspects of short-term memory are impaired with age. There are many components of short-term memory related to the types of tasks the person is asked to perform. Memory loss appears to involve only recent events, leaving immediate and long-term memory intact (Keefover, 1998). Free recall, episodic, explicit, and working memory all show a decline with age; Table 9–10 provides a description of these components of short-term memory. New information can be registered and retrieved, but new information is forgotten more quickly. The speed with which information is processed slows with age and is a fundamental cause of age-related decline in memory (Luszcz and Byran, 1999).

Working memory is most affected by aging because information must not only be retained but also be manipulated or changed to be retrieved. This activity requires that information storage occur at the same time as acquisition of new data, something that is difficult for the older learner. Older adults appear to have to redistribute resources from storage to allocation to keep up. Changes in memory abilities need to be considered when giving verbal direction to older patients with movement dysfunction. Written instructions that

TABLE 9–10

Memory Functions and Their Sensitivity to the Aging Process

Type of Memory Function	Description	Declines with Age
Registration or immediate	Retention for seconds	No
Delayed recall, short-term, secondary, or intermediate	Retention for minutes to hours	Yes
Free recall	Items recalled without benefit of cues or associated stimuli	Yes
Episodic	Recollection of context-specific information (e.g., word lists recall after a 5-minute delay)	Yes
Semantic	Retrieval of vocabulary or general knowledge	Min.
Explicit	Conscious recall of specified information	Yes
Implicit	Unconscious recollection of facts/skills acquired during earlier exposures	No
Working	Retention of information for manipulation or transformation	Yes
Primary	Simple recall of nontransformed data	Min.
Long-term or permanent	Retention for months to years	Min.

Min., minimal.
Modified from Keefover RW. Aging and cognition. *Neurol Clin* 16:635–648, 1998.

parallel the verbal instructions are often critical to provide adequate carryover in a home program.

INTELLIGENCE

Cognition is functionally reflected in intelligence. Horn and Donaldson (1980) described two types of intellectual ability: fluid intelligence and crystallized intelligence. *Fluid intelligence* is the ability to form novel associations, to reason logically, and to solve problems. It can be measured by looking at reaction time and memory. Fluid intelligence peaks in the early 20s and declines throughout adulthood (see Fig. 2–7). *Crystallized intelligence* is experiential learning, education, and stored information. It is the ability to use judgment to decide on a course of action. This type of intelligence incorporates a lifetime of decision making and is postulated to improve with age (Horn and Donaldson, 1980).

According to measures of intelligence, intellectual ability peaks between ages 20 and 30 and is maintained until at least 75 years of age (Katzman and Terry, 1983). Despite all we do know about the aging changes related to cognition or intelligence, we do not understand why some older individuals remain alert, sharp, and active participants in the world around them and others lose touch, disengage, or show signs of dementia. To date, there is insufficient research to relate loss of neurons from the nervous system to functional decline in cognitive function in healthy aging individuals. Intellectual changes seen in later life that are considered "normal" include (1) slowing of reaction time or cognitive processing, (2) decline in fluid intelligence, and (3) impairment in some aspects of short-term memory (Keefover, 1999).

ALZHEIMER'S DISEASE

AD is a progressive degenerative dementia that is the fourth leading cause of death in adults (Fuller, 1998). A major reason that memory loss is so feared by the elderly is because of the association between memory loss and AD. AD is characterized by a slow decline in memory, cognition, and functional abilities. The presence of NFTs inside the neurons and of neuritic plaques outside the neurons is a hallmark of the neuropathology of AD. This involvement is most often seen in the temporal and parietal lobes with extension into the frontal region (Davis, 1999) (Fig. 9–23).

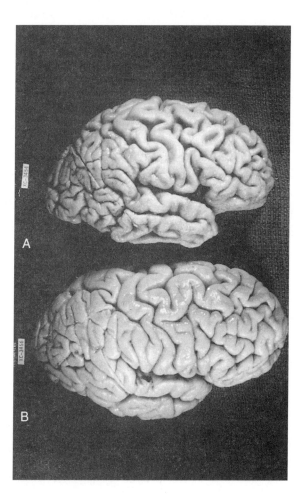

Figure 9–23

Pathologic changes seen in Alzheimer's disease. *A,* Alzheimer's diseased brain shows reduced size, narrow gyri, and wide sulci in frontal and temporal lobes. *B,* Age- and sex-matched control. (From Damjanov I, Linder J [eds.] *Anderson's Pathology,* 10th ed. St. Louis: Mosby, 1996.)

Age and genetics are two risk factors for the development of AD. With increased age comes an increased risk of AD; the prevalence goes up with each decade. Aging contributes to an increased potential for neuronal injury. If neuronal repair is inadequate, as is supposed in AD, this defective response could lead to aberrations in the processing of beta-amyloid precursor proteins. Amyloid, an insoluble fibrous substance, makes up the core of the plaques. Tangles tend to form in cortical areas that have the least myelin and a greater degree of dendritic plasticity (Arendt et al, 1998). The genes associated with the amyloid precursor protein on chromosome 21 and presenilin-1 and -2 are involved in only a small percentage of cases of AD. These patients present with an earlier onset, before the age of 60.

Not all memory loss is pathological. In a study using a series of memory tasks, Carlesimo and colleagues (1998) demonstrated quantitative and qualitative differences in memory loss between normal and pathological aging. They noted a progressive decline in episodic memory with age in all groups of normal aging individuals. The group with AD showed an even greater decline in the learning of a word list than did the normal groups. This is "consistent with the view that a sort of continuum exists between memory changes resulting from normal aging and the memory impairment due to AD" (Carlesimo et al, 1998, p 26). Two other aspects of memory showed specific deterioration in the AD group, whereas the performance of normally aging individuals remained stable—these aspects are episodic memory or word recall and semantic memory. It was hypothesized that these tasks required more attention and allocation of processing resources than individuals with AD possess. Last, procedural learning tasks were found to be unaffected by either aging or dementia. In Clinical Implications: Alzheimer's Disease—A Variation of Normal Aging? the neurologic changes associated with normal aging are compared with those seen in AD.

Other researchers who study memory in aging and dementia dispute the idea of the existence of a continuum of decline. Most notable, Salthouse (1996) documented the role of speed in mediating the memory abilities of adults. When speed of processing is taken into account, the age-related variance in memory is eliminated or considerably reduced. Sliwinski and Buschke (1997) examined the role of processing speed as a modifying variable, which might explain differences seen on memory tasks with increasing age and in the presence of dementia. They found that processing speed did not affect the memory impairment seen in dementia and therefore concluded that the memory impairments seen in aging and dementia are qualitatively different.

Summary

When looking at the function of the nervous system, we must understand that it is constantly changing in response to environmental demands, both from within and from without. The degree of adaptation and accommodation varies from one person to another. Movement, language, and cognitive changes that occur across the life span are based on the interaction between the structure

CLINICAL IMPLICATIONS
Alzheimer's Disease—A Variation of Normal Aging?

Alzheimer's disease (AD) is the most common form of progressive degenerative dementia. There are presently 4 million people with AD in the United States, and it is the fourth leading cause of death in adults (Fuller, 1998). Diagnosis is based on a history of progressive deterioration in at least two aspects of cognition, one of which is typically memory. If we live long enough, is dementia of the Alzheimer's type inevitable? There are reports of increased risk in individuals over age 90 (Ritchie and Kildea, 1995). However, there are differences between normal aging and AD; differences are seen in the areas of the brain that are involved and the structural and functional changes that occur (Birge, 1998; Carlesimo et al, 1998; Davis, 1999; Fuller, 1998; Haroutunian et al, 1998, 1999; McDougall, 1996; Strong, 1998).

Normal Aging

- Changes in frontal cortex and subcortical areas
- Diffuse amyloid B protein deposition; some neurofibrillary tangles (NFTs) in limbic structures, almost none in neocortical structures
- No language impairment
- No change in implicit memory or learning
- Word recall declines
- Semantic memory stable
- Older adults use list making as a memory strategy
- No consistent change in neurotransmitters
- Estrogen deficiency speeds aging effects on memory in women

Alzheimer's Disease

- Changes in association areas in temporal, parietal, and frontal lobes
- Dense NFTs and neuritic plaques in all limbic structures; density related to severity of dementia
- Loss of word finding; inability to remember names, anomia; receptive aphasia
- Loss of ability to learn new information
- Word recall declines greater than normal
- Semantic memory declines
- Older adults use rehearsal as a memory strategy; external cues do not help
- Decreased activity in cholinergic neurons; norepinephrine and serotonin decreased in early onset
- Women have a two to three times greater prevalence

and function of the nervous system. How and why we move, talk, and think depend on the integrity of our nervous system. Our ability to learn and to adapt to the environment reflects the development of our unique nervous system characteristics across the life span. Our ability to perform the functions of the nervous system—thinking, talking, and reacting—continue as long as our system's reserves are maintained and not compromised by disease.

REFERENCES

Alexander GE, Crutcher MD, DeLong MR. Basal ganglia-thalamocortical circuits: Parallel substrates for motor, oculomotor, "prefrontal" and "limbic" functions. *Prog Brain Res* 85:119–146, 1990.

Almli CR, Moore NM. Normal sequential behavior and physiological changes throughout the developmental arc. In Umphred DA (ed). *Neurological Rehabilitation*, 3rd ed. St. Louis: CV Mosby, 1995, pp 33–65.

Arendt T, Bruckner MK, Gert HJ, Marcova L. Cortical distribution of neurofibrillary tangles in Alzheimer's disease matches the pattern of neurons that retain their capacity of plastic remodeling in the adult brain. *Neuroscience* 83:991–1002, 1998.

Bell MA, Ball MJ. Neuritic plaques and vessels of visual cortex in aging and Alzheimer's dementia. *Neurobiol Aging* 11:359–370, 1990.

Bertoni-Freddari C, Fattoretti P, Paoloni R, et al. Synaptic structural dynamics and aging. *Gerontology* 42:170–180, 1996.

Birge SJ. Hormones and the aging brain. *Geriatrics* 53(suppl 1):S28–S30, 1998.

Birren JE, Fisher LM. Aging and speed of behavior: Possible consequences for psychological functioning. *Annu Rev Psych* 110:1571–1576, 1995.

Birren JE, Woods AM, Williams MV. Speed of behavior as an indicator of age changes and the integrity of the nervous system. In Hoffmeister F, Muller C (eds). *Brain Function in Old Age.* New York: Springer-Verlag, 1979, pp 10–44.

Bishop B, Craik RL. *Neural Plasticity.* Washington, DC: American Physical Therapy Association, 1982.

Black JE. How a child builds its brain: Some lessons from animal studies of neural plasticity. *Prev Med* 27:168–171, 1998.

Bourre JM. Developmental synthesis of myelin lipids: Origin of fatty acids-specific role of nutrition. In Evrard P, Minkowski A (eds). *Developmental Neurobiology*, Vol 12, Nestle Nutrition Workshop Series. New York: Raven Press, 1989, pp 111–154.

Brittis PA, Sliver J. Exogenous glycosaminoglycans induce complete inversion of retinal ganglion cell bodies and their axons within the retinal neuroepithelium. *Proc Natl Acad Sci USA* 91: 7539–7542, 1994.

Brody H, Vijayashanker N: Anatomical changes in the nervous system. In Finch CE, Hay-Flick L (eds). *Handbook of Biology and Aging.* New York: Van Nostrand Reinhold, 1977, pp 241–256.

Bronson GW. Structure, status and characteristics of the nervous system at birth. In Stratton P (ed). *Psychobiology of the Human Newborn.* New York: Wiley, 1982, pp 99–118.

Buchtal F, Rosenfalck A, Behse F. Sensory potentials of normal and diseased nerves. In Dyck PJ, Thomas PK, Griffin JW, et al (eds). *Peripheral Neuropathy*, 2rd ed. Philadelphia: WB Saunders, 1984, pp 442–464.

Carlesimo GA, Mauri M, Graceffa A, et al. Memory performances in young, elderly, and very old healthy individuals versus patients with Alzheimer's disease: Evidence for discontinuity between normal and pathological aging. *J Clin Exp Neuropsychol* 20:14–29, 1998.

Casey BJ, Trainor R, Giedd J, et al. The role of the anterior cingulate in automatic and controlled processes: A developmental neuroanatomical study. *Dev Psychobiol* 3:61–69, 1997.

Chaput S, Proteau L. Aging and motor control. *J Gerontol B Psychol Sci Soc Sci* 51:P346–P355, 1996.

Chugani HT. Development of regional brain glucose metabolism in relation to behavior and plasticity. In Dawson G, Fischer KW (eds). *Human Behavior and the Developing Brain*. New York: Guilford, 1994, pp 153–175.

Chugani HT. A critical period of brain development: Studies of cerebral glucose utilization with PET. *Prev Med* 27:184–188, 1998.

Cotman CW, Holets VR. Structural changes at synapses with age: Plasticity and regeneration. In Finch CE, Schneider EL (eds). *Handbook of the Biology of Aging*. New York: Van Nostrand Reinhold, 1985, pp 617–644.

Davis KL. Alzheimer's disease: Seeking new ways to preserve brain function. *Geriatrics* 54:42–47, 1999.

DeKosky ST, Palmer AM. Neurochemistry of aging. In Albert ML, Knoefel JE (eds). *Clinical Neurology of Aging*, 2nd ed. New York: Oxford University Press, 1994, pp 79–101.

DeSanti S, de Leon MJ, Convit A, et al. Age-related changes in brain: II. Positron emission tomography of frontal and temporal lobe glucose metabolism in normal subjects. *Psychiatr Q* 66:357–370, 1995.

Diemer K. Capillarisation and oxygen supply of the brain. In Lubbers DW, Luft EC, Thews G, Witzleb E (eds). *Oxygen Transport in Blood and Tissue*. Stuttgart: Thieme, 1968, pp 118–123.

Dobbing J. Infant nutrition and later achievement. *Nutr Rev* 42:1–7, 1984.

Double KL, et al. Topography of brain atrophy during normal aging and Alzheimer's disease. *Neurobiol Aging* 17:513–521, 1996.

Duara R, London ED, Rapoport SI. Changes in structure and energy metabolism of the aging brain. In Finch CE, Schneider EL (eds). *Handbook of the Biology of Aging*. New York: Van Nostrand Reinhold, 1985, pp 595–616.

Eaton WO, Ritchot KFM. Physical maturation and information-processing speed in middle childhood. *Dev Psychol* 31:967–972, 1995.

Eberling JL, Nordahl TE, Kusubov N, et al. Reduced temporal lobe glucose metabolism in aging. *J Neuroimaging* 5:178–182, 1995.

Emery CF, Huppert FA, Schein RL. Relationships among age, exercise, health, and cognitive function in a British sample. *Gerontologist* 35:378–385, 1995.

Evrard P, Minkowski A (eds). *Developmental Neurobiology*, Vol 12, Nestle Nutrition Workshop Series. New York: Raven Press, 1989.

Farber S. *Neurorehabilitation: A Multisensory Approach*. Philadelphia: WB Saunders, 1982, p 17.

Ford DH, Cramer EB. Developing nervous system in relationship to thyroid hormone. In Grave GD (ed). *Thyroid Hormones and Brain Development*. New York: Raven Press, 1977, pp 1–18.

Fox CM, Adler RN. Neural mechanism of aging. In Cohen H (ed). *Neuroscience for Rehabilitation*, 2nd ed. Philadelphia: Lippincott Williams & Wilkins, 1999, pp 401–418.

Fozard JL, Vercruyssen M, Reynolds SL, et al. Age differences and changes in reaction time: The Baltimore Longitudinal Study of Aging. *J Gerontol B Psychol Sci Soc Sci* 49:P179–P189, 1994.

Friedlander WJ. Electroencephalographic alpha rate in adults as a function of age. *Geriatrics* 13:29–31, 1958.

Fuller KS. Degenerative diseases of the central nervous system. In Goodman CG, Boissonnault WG (eds). *Pathology: Implications for the Physical Therapist*. Philadelphia: WB Saunders, 1998, pp 723–747.

Geschwind N, Levitsky W. Human brain: Left-right asymmetries in temporal speech regions. *Science* 161:186–187, 1968.

Ghez C, Thack WT. The cerebellum. In Kandel ER, Schwarz JH, Jessell TM (eds). *Principles of Neural Science*, 4th ed. New York: McGraw-Hill, 2000, pp 832–852.

Green E. Developmental neurology. In Stokes M. *Neurological Physiotherapy*. St. Louis: Mosby, 1998, pp 215–228.

Guyton AC, Hall JE. *Textbook of Medical Physiology*, 9th ed. Philadelphia: WB Saunders, 1996.

Hallett T, Proctor A. Maturation of the central nervous system as related to communication and cognitive development. *Inf Young Child* 8:1–15, 1996.

Haroutunian V, Perl DP, Purohit DP, et al. Regional distribution of neuritic plaques in the nondemented elderly and subjects with very mild Alzheimer disease. *Arch Neurol* 55:1185–1191, 1998.

Haroutunian V, Purohit DP, Perl DP, et al. Neurofibrillary tangles in nondemented elderly subjects and very mild Alzheimer disease. *Arch Neurol* 56:713–718, 1999.

Haug J. Are neurons of the human cerebral cortex really lost during aging? A morphometric examination. In Traber J, Gispen WH (eds). *Senile Dementia of the Alzheimer Type*. New York: Springer-Verlag, 1985, pp 150–163.

Haug J, Kuhl S, Mecke E, et al. The significance of morphometric procedures in the investigation of age changes in cytoarchitectonic structures of human brain. *J Hirnforsch* 25:353–374, 1984.

Heinen F, Fietek UM, Berweck S, et al. Fast corticospinal system and motor performance in children: Conduction proceeds skill. *Pediatr Neurol* 19:217–221, 1998.

Held JM, Pay T. Recovery of function after brain damage. In Cohen H (ed). *Neuroscience for Rehabilitation*, 2nd ed. Philadelphia: Lippincott Williams & Wilkins, 1999, pp 419–439.

Herschkowitz N. Brain development and nutrition. In Evrard P, Minkowski A (eds). *Developmental Neurobiology*, Vol 12, Nestle Nutrition Workshop Series. New York: Raven Press, 1989, pp 297–304.

Horn JL, Donaldson G. Cognitive development in adulthood. In Brim OG, Kagan J (eds). *Constancy and Change in Human Development*. Cambridge, MA: Harvard University Press, 1980, pp 445–529.

Hubble JP. Aging and the basal ganglia. *Neurol Clin* 16:649–657, 1998.

Jack CR Jr, Petersen RC, Xu YC, et al. Medial temporal atrophy on MRI in normal aging and very mild Alzheimer's disease. *Neurology* 49:786–794, 1997.

Kail RV, Salthouse TA. Processing speed as a mental capacity. *Acta Psychol* 86:199–225, 1994.

Katzman R, Terry RD. Normal aging of the nervous system. In Katzman R, Terry RD (eds). *The Neurology of Aging*. Philadelphia: FA Davis, 1983, pp 15–50.

Keefover RW. Aging and cognition. *Neurol Clin* 16:625–648, 1998.

Kemper TL: Neuroanatomical and neuropathological changes during aging and dementia. In Albert ML, Knoefel JE (eds). *Clinical Neurology of Aging*. New York: Oxford University Press, 1994, pp 3–67.

Kempermann G, Gage FH. New nerve cells for the adult brain. *Sci Am* May:48–53, 1999.

Konigsmark BW, Murphy EA. Neuronal population in the human brain. *Nature* 228:1335–1336, 1970.

Kotulak R. Inside the brain: Revolutionary discoveries of how the mind works. *Prev Med* 27:246–247, 1998.

Kretchmer N. Nutritional influences on neurological development: A contemplative essay. In Evrard P, Minkowski A (eds). *Developmental Neurobiology*, Vol 12, Nestle Nutrition Workshop Series. New York: Raven Press, 1989, pp 261–264.

Laufer AC, Schweitz B. Neuromuscular response tests as predictors of sensory-motor performance in aging individuals. *Am J Phys Med* 47:250–263, 1968.

Lebeer J. How much brain does a mind need? Scientific, clinical and educational implication of ecological plasticity. *Dev Med Child Neur* 40:352–357, 1998.

Lexell J. Evidence for nervous system degeneration with advancing age. *J Nutr* 127:1011S–1013S, 1997.

Light KE, Spirduso WW. Effects of adult aging on the movement complexity factor of response programming. *J Gerontol* 45:P107–P109, 1990.

Lundy-Ekman L. *Neuroscience: Fundamentals for Rehabilitation*. Philadelphia: WB Saunders, 1998.

Luszcz MA, Bryan J. Toward understanding age-related memory loss in late adulthood. *Gerontology* 45:2–9, 1999.

Lynch G. Memory and the brain: Unexpected chemistries and a new pharmacology. *Neurobiol Learn Mem* 70:82–100, 1998.

Magnotta VA, Andreasen NC, Schultz SK, et al. Quantitative in vivo measurement of gyrification in the human brain: Changes associated with aging. *Cereb Cortex* 9:151–160, 1999.

Martinez M. Biochemical changes during early myelination of the human brain. In Evrard P, Minkowski A (eds). *Developmental Neurobiology*, Vol 12, Nestle Nutrition Workshop Series. New York: Raven Press, 1989, pp 185–200.

McDougall GJ. Predictors of the use of memory improvement strategies by older adults. *Rehab Nurs* 21:202–209, 1996.

Mielke R, Kessler J, Szelies B, et al. Normal and pathological aging: Findings of positron-emission-tomography. *J Neural Transm* 105:821–837, 1998.

Moore KL, Persaud TVN. *The Developing Human: Clinically Oriented Embryology*, 6th ed. Philadelphia: WB Saunders, 1998.

Morgan DG. Consideration in the treatment of neurological disorders with trophic factors. *Neurobiol Aging* 10:547–549, 1989.

Mouritzen Dam A. The density of neurons in the human hippocampus. *Neuropathol Appl Neurobiol* 5:249–264, 1979.

Mrak RE, Griffin ST, Graham DI. Aging-associated changes in human brain. *J Neuropathol Exp Neurol* 56:1269–1275, 1997.

Mueller EA, Moore MM, Kerr DC, et al. Brain volume preserved in healthy elderly through the eleventh decade. *Neurol* 51:1555–1562, 1998.

Mussen PH, Conger JJ, Kagan J (eds). *Child Development and Personality*, 4th ed. New York: Harper & Row, 1974.

Nelson CA. The ontogeny of human memory: A cognitive neuroscience perspective. *Dev Psychol* 31:723–738, 1995.

Nelson CA. The nature of early memory. *Prev Med* 27:172–179, 1998.

Nezu A, Kimura S, Uehara S, et al. Magnetic stimulation of motor cortex in children: Maturity of corticospinal pathway and problem of clinical application. *Brain Dev* 19:176–180, 1997.

Onishi N. Changes of the jumping reaction time in relation to age. *J Sci Labour* 42:5–16, 1966.

Paris SC, Lindauer BK. The development of cognitive skills during childhood. In Wolman BB (ed). *Handbook of Developmental Psychology*. Englewood Cliffs, NJ: Prentice-Hall, 1982, pp 333–349.

Patten C, Craik RL. Sensorimotor changes and adaptation in the older adult. In Guccione AA (ed). *Geriatric Physical Therapy*, 2nd ed. St. Louis: Mosby, 2000, pp 78–109.

Petit-Taboue MC, Landeau B, Desson JF, et al. Effects of healthy aging on regional cerebral metabolic rate of glucose assessed with statistical parametric mapping. *Neuroimage* 7:176–184, 1998.

Piaget J. *Origins of Intelligence*. New York: WW Norton, 1952.

Posner MI, Rothbart MK. Attention, self-regulation and consciousness. *Phil Trans R Soc Lond B* 353:1915–1927, 1998.

Potvin AR, Syndulko K, Tourtellote WW, et al. Human neurologic function and the aging process. *J Am Geriatr Soc* 28:1–9, 1980.

Purpura D. Dendritic spine "dysgenesis" and mental retardation. *Science* 186:1126–1128, 1974.

Purves D, Augustine GJ, Fitzpatrick LC, et al (eds). *Neuroscience*. Sunderland, MA: Sinauer Associates, 1997.

Rabinowicz T, De Courten-Myers G, McDonald-Comber Petetot J, et al. Human cortex development: Estimates of neuronal numbers indicate major loss late in gestation. *J Neuropathol Exp Neurol* 55:320–328, 1996.

Ritchie K, Kildea D. Is senile dementia "age-related" or "ageing-related"? Evidence from meta-analysis of dementia prevalence in the oldest old. *Lancet* 346:931–934, 1995.

Rogers J, Bloom FE. Neurotransmitter metabolism and function in the aging nervous system. In Finch CE, Schneider EL (eds). *Handbook of the Biology of Aging*. New York: Van Nostrand Reinhold, 1985, pp 645–691.

Rovee-Collier C. Learning and memory in children. In Osofsky JD (ed). *Handbook of Infant Development*, 2nd ed. New York: J Wiley and Sons, 1987, pp 98–148.

Salthouse TA. The processing-speed theory of adult age differences in cognition. *Psychol Rev* 103:403–428, 1996.

Schade JP, van Groenigen WB. Structural organization of the human cerebral cortex. *Acta Anat* 47:74–111, 1961.

Schaie KW, Willis SL (eds). *Adult Development and Aging*, 4th ed. New York: Harper Collins, 1996.

Schaumburg HH, Spencer PS, Ochoa J. The aging human peripheral nervous system. In Katzman R, Terry RD (eds). *The Neurology of Aging*. Philadelphia, FA Davis, 1983, pp 111–122.

Sherrington CS. *The Integrative Action of the Nervous System*. London: Cambridge University, 1947.

Shigeta M, Julin P, Almkvist O, et al. EEG in successful aging: A 5 year follow-up study from the eighth to the ninth decade of life. *Electroencephalogr Clin Neurophysiol* 95:77–83, 1995.

Singleton WT. The change of movement timing with age. *Br J Psychol* 45:166–172, 1954.

Sliwinski M, Buschke H. Processing speed and memory in aging and dementia. *J Gerontol B Psychol Sci Soc Sci* 52B:P308–P318, 1997.

Sperry R. Growth of nerve circuits. *Sci Am* 201:5–68, 1959.

Spirduso WW. Physical fitness, aging and psychomotor speed: A review. *J Gerontol* 35:850–865, 1980.

Spirduso WW. *Physical Dimensions of Aging.* Champaign, IL: Human Kinetics, 1995.

Stafford JL, Albert MS, Naeser MA, et al. Age-related differences in computed tomographic scan measurements. *Arch Neurol* 45:409–415, 1988.

Stine-Morrow EAL, Soederberg Miller LM. Basic cognitive processes. In Cavanaugh JC, Whitbourne SK (eds). *Gerontology: An Interdisciplinary Perspective.* New York: Oxford University Press, 1999, pp 186–212.

Stratton P. Rhythmic functions in the newborn. In Stratton P (ed). *Psychobiology of the Human Newborn.* New York: J Wiley and Sons, 1982, pp 119–145.

Strong R. Neurochemical changes in the aging human brain: Implications for behavioral impairment and neurodegenerative disease. *Geriatrics* 53(suppl 1):S9–S12, 1998.

Terry RD, De Teresa R, Hansen LA. Neocortical cell counts in normal human adult aging. *Ann Neurol* 21:530–539, 1987.

Thomas JE, Lambert EH. Ulnar nerve conduction velocity and H-reflex in infants and children. *J Appl Phys* 15:1–9, 1960.

Valadian I, Porter D. *Physical Growth and Development from Conception to Maturity.* Boston: Little, Brown, 1977.

Volkow ND, Gur RC, Wang G-J, et al. Association between decline in brain dopamine activity with age and cognitive and motor impairment in healthy individuals. *Am J Psychiatry* 155:344–349, 1998.

Volpe JJ. *Neurology of the Newborn,* 3rd ed. Philadelphia: WB Saunders, 1995.

Welford AT. Between bodily changes and performance some possible reasons for slowing with age. *Exp Aging Res* 10:73–88, 1984.

Whitbourne SK. *The Aging Individual: Physical and Psychological Perspectives.* New York: Springer, 1996.

Whitbourne SK. Physical changes. In Cavanaugh JC, Whitbourne SK (eds). *Gerontology: An Interdisciplinary Perspective.* New York: Oxford University Press, 1999, pp 91–122.

Wiggins RC, Fuller G, Enna SJ. Undernutrition and the development of brain neurotransmitter systems. *Life Sci* 35:2085–2094, 1984.

Willott JF. *Neurogerontology.* New York: Springer, 1999.

Woodruff-Pak DS. *The Neuropsychology of Aging.* Malden, MA: Blackwell, 1997.

Yamamura H, Ito M, Kubota K, Matsuzawa T. Brain atrophy during aging: A quantitative study with computed tomography. *J Gerontol* 35:492–498, 1980.

Yin D. Biochemical basis of lipofuscin, ceroid, and age pigment-like fluorophores. *Free Radic Biol Med* 21:871–888, 1996.

Zaidel DW. The case for a relationship between human memory, hippocampus and corpus callosum. *Biol Res* 28:51–57, 1995.

10 Sensory System Changes

OBJECTIVES

After studying this chapter, the reader will be able to:

1 Discuss the role of sensation in perception and movement.

2 Describe common characteristics of sensory systems.

3 Describe age-related sensory changes across the life span.

4 Relate sensory function to state and novelty of stimulus.

5 Correlate sensory changes with function across the life span.

Our senses provide the only means of communicating with and about the world around us. The psychologist J. J. Gibson (1966) introduced the concept of *affordance* to describe the complementary effect of the environment on the developing organism. Sensation affords interaction between the infant and the environment, as well as interaction between the environment and the infant in such a manner that both are changed The environment includes the biophysical and sociocultural surroundings that affect movement outcome (Fig. 10–1). These surroundings can also encompass people and objects. No wonder Piaget (1952) described the origins of intelligence as the sensorimotor period. An infant's initial foray into the world is guided by sensations that are paired with movement to initiate communication, motor control, and intelligence.

Because the sensory system is part of the nervous system, sensory and motor systems have a common goal—movement production. The role of sensory input in the development and control of posture and movement is well documented (Nougier et al, 1998; Shumway-Cook and Woollacott, 1995). Initially, sensory input is paired with motor output, resulting in reflexes such as rooting and flexor withdrawal. Infants learn to maintain their posture and balance in response to sensory input with the development of *postural reactions* that automatically occur to maintain the alignment of the head and trunk in response to a weight shift; these include protective extension of the extremities, righting, and equilibrium reactions of the head and trunk. Automatic postural reactions in response to anteroposterior body sway (postural sway) are governed by somatosensory, vestibular, and visual input (see Chapter 12).

Sensory input aids the process of learning movement by providing feedback for movement accuracy, such as in reaching for or rolling toward a

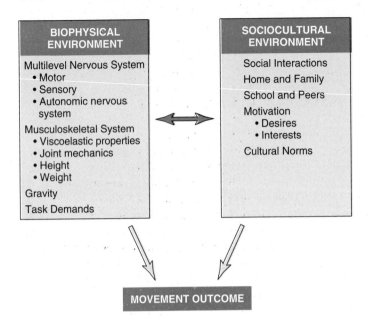

Figure 10–1

Environmental factors that affect movement outcome.

desired object. Once movement is learned, sensation may not be as necessary for the movement to occur. When movement becomes more automatic, however, sensation becomes an anticipatory signal to move, for example, gathering your things when you hear the bell ring at the end of class or changing your walk to a run when you think you may miss your bus. The way a movement feels can be recalled when playing a once-forgotten piano piece or riding a bicycle. Once you learn, you do not forget how, although execution may be impaired through nervous or muscular system deficits.

Sensory systems are important to functional movement. The majority of what we know about the senses comes from research with animals and infants. We also need to understand the age-related changes in sensory function across the life span, including the importance of state and stimulus novelty. The normally expected changes with age in sensory awareness are just beginning to be distinguished from pathological changes, and our knowledge of the functional implication of age-related sensory deficits for movement is still preliminary.

Characteristics of Sensory Systems

Sensation entails the reception of afferent stimuli from both the internal milieu of the body and the external world. To receive input, the body must be sufficiently aroused The state of arousal that an infant experiences will determine the level of responsivity to sensory stimuli. A patient in a coma may respond only to painful stimuli. With recovery, sensory awareness grows. Reception of sensory stimuli does not always imply that the sensation reaches conscious awareness. Each sensory system has its own unique set of receptors and pathways it travels to reach conscious awareness.

The senses monitor internal processes related to vital functions such as breathing, eating, sleeping, and excreting, as well as produce arousal in the form of general alerting, sexual responses, and fight-or-flight reactions. The arousal functions are choreographed by various subsystems of the nervous system (central, peripheral, and autonomic) in concert with the brain stem reticular activating, hypothalamic, and limbic systems. The interpretation of sensory stimuli is often determined by the state of the autonomic nervous system. Think of how slowly you respond to the alarm clock in the morning when you have an 8 o'clock class. Your parasympathetic system predominates during vegetative functions such as sleep, but you animatedly respond to cold water when showering, a sympathetic response to a brief cold stimulus.

Sensory input comes in via special receptors, is conveyed by nerve fibers, and is disseminated to appropriate regions of the central nervous system (CNS). For example, your eye picks up a moving image and relays the information to the brain, which identifies a hummingbird. In the meantime, your eye muscles track the bird's movements while you safely continue your forward progression on the nature path. Different sensory receptors have sent a variety of messages to the brain that have been interpreted and have resulted in an adaptive response to allow you to enjoy a pleasurable activity while continuing a motor task.

A sensory system is basically a three-neuron system (Fig. 10–2). The primary sensory neuron transmits the signal along a primary afferent axon toward the CNS. In the peripheral nervous system, cell bodies are located in the sensory ganglia. The axon of the sensory neuron enters the spinal cord and synapses with a secondary, or second-order, sensory neuron, usually in the thalamus, and then travels on to a third-order neuron along specific neural pathways, or *tracts*. Sensory neural pathways are made up of synaptically interconnected interneurons. Some pathways relay information from only one type of sensory receptor such as mechanoreceptors; others carry information about pain and temperature. All sensory systems have the ability to transform one type of energy (the stimulus) into an electrical signal, code for specific qualities of the stimulus, be represented topographically on many levels of the

Figure 10–2

Three neuron nervous system. (Redrawn from Romero-Sierra C. *Neuroanatomy: A Conceptual Approach.* New York: Churchill Livingstone, 1986.)

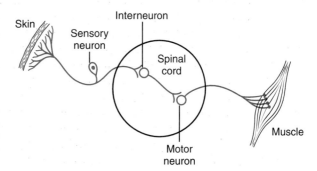

nervous system, integrate information between one or more sensory systems, and participate in motor responses.

TYPES OF RECEPTORS

A *sensory receptor* is a peripheral ending of an afferent nerve fiber or the receptor cell associated with it. Each sensory modality is served by one or more receptors that are sensitive to a particular form of physical energy, such as mechanical, thermal, or chemical energy (Table 10–1). In general, there are two main categories of receptors: generalized and specialized. *Generalized receptors* are somatic receptors and motion receptors. *Specialized receptors* are those involved in the special senses of vision, hearing, taste, and smell.

THE SENSES

Somatic Senses

Touch, temperature, pain, and awareness of body position (proprioception) are conveyed by mechanoreceptors, thermoreceptors, and nociceptors. Touch and proprioception contribute to the development of body scheme and awareness of our relationship to the outside world. Touch defines the limits of the body and provides information about people and objects in the environment. Temperature detection ensures survival and efficient physiological function of the body. Pain protects the body from too much pressure, as from sitting too long in one position, and from overexposure to sun, snow, or chemicals. Somatic

TABLE 10–1

Sensory Systems

Modality	Stimulus	Receptor Type	Receptors
Somatic	Mechanical, thermal	Mechanoreceptors, thermoreceptors, nociceptors	Dorsal root ganglion neurons
Proprioceptive	Limb positions, muscle tension, joint angulation	Mechanoreceptors	Muscle spindles, Golgi tendon organs, joint receptors
Motion	Head movement	Mechanoreceptors	Hair cells, semicircular canals
Vision	Light	Photoreceptors	Rods, cones
Hearing	Sounds	Mechanoreceptors	Hair cells (cochlea)
Taste	Chemical	Chemoreceptors	Taste buds
Smell	Chemical	Chemoreceptors	Olfactory sensory neurons

Modified from Martin JH. Coding and processing of sensory information. In Kandel ER, Schwartz JH, Jessell TM (eds). *Principles of Neural Science*, 3rd ed. Norwalk, CT: Appleton & Lange, 1991, Table 23–1, p 334. Copyright © by McGraw Hill, Inc. Used by permission of McGraw-Hill Book Company.

receptors convey pressure, vibration, temperature, pain, and some proprioceptive information about the body.

Free nerve endings are found in the skin, muscle, joints, and viscera. These nociceptors convey noxious stimuli. As such, they can respond to mechanical, thermal, and chemical stimuli, either on the skin or internally at the periosteum, arterial walls, and joint surfaces. Thermoreception also occurs by activating free, unencapsulated nerve endings. Thermoreceptors detect hot and cold by responding to changes in their own metabolic rate relative to actual temperature changes in the ambient air. Extremes of hot or cold can be detected as pain through the stimulation of pain receptors in addition to the temperature receptors.

The majority of *mechanoreceptors* are encapsulated and include *pacinian corpuscles, Meissner's corpuscles, Merkel's disks,* and *Ruffini endings.* Pacinian corpuscles respond to tissue vibration and rapid changes in the mechanical state of the tissues (Guyton and Hall, 1996). Meissner's corpuscles are sensitive to light touch and vibration, whereas Merkel's disks respond to pressure. The latter receptor is found in hairy skin, and the former two receptors are found primarily in hairless skin. Ruffini endings convey stretch of the skin.

Muscle spindles and Golgi tendon organs are examples of mechanoreceptors but are also classified as proprioceptors. Proprioceptive receptors detect the position of body parts in space and are found in the vestibular part of the ear as well as in muscles, tendons, and joints. Muscle spindles provide information about limb position (Matthews, 1988), whereas joint receptors relay knowledge of joint angulation, especially at end ranges. It is likely that the muscle spindle also detects rate of movement. More than half of the innervation to a muscle conveys information to and from the muscle spindles, the body's primary source of proprioceptive information (Boyd, 1985). The Golgi tendon organ, located in the muscle tendon, detects tension generated by the contraction or stretch of that muscle and safeguards the muscle from overwork by inhibiting or stopping the muscle from contracting. Various sensory receptors are shown in Figures 10–3 and 10–4.

Motion Sense

The ear is a special part of our anatomy that is crucial to motion sense as well as the sense of hearing. It is, therefore, important to understand its various parts and how they work (Fig. 10–5). The vestibular system relays input about the body's relationship to gravity, head position, and head movement. Although it is considered part of proprioception in some regards, it is discussed separately because of its intimate relationship to movement. Vestibular receptors in the inner ear provide information about head position and head movement in space. Vestibular information is used to update postural tone and equilibrium and to ensure gaze stability during head movements (Fisher et al, 1991). Gaze stability allows the eyes to fix on an image even though the head is moving. The vestibular system resolves intersensory conflicts about balance. If the proprioceptors think the body is not moving and the eyes think the

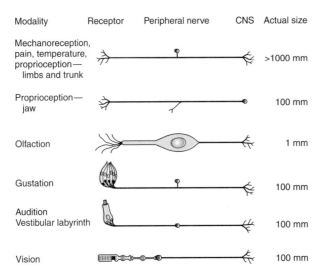

Modality	Receptor	Peripheral nerve	CNS	Actual size
Mechanoreception, pain, temperature, proprioception— limbs and trunk				>1000 mm
Proprioception— jaw				100 mm
Olfaction				1 mm
Gustation				100 mm
Audition Vestibular labyrinth				100 mm
Vision				100 mm

Figure 10–3

Various sensory receptors that have different structures and organization. (Redrawn from Martin JH. Coding and processing of sensory information. In Kandel ER, Schwartz JH, Jessell TM [eds]. *Principles of Neural Science*, 3rd ed. Norwalk, CT: Appleton & Lange, 1991, Fig. 23–5, p 333. Copyright © by McGraw-Hill, Inc. Used by permission of McGraw-Hill Book Company.)

body is moving, the input of the vestibular system decides what the real situation is and relays information to appropriate motor centers.

The vestibular receptors are located within the membranous labyrinth of the inner ear. The labyrinth is made up of three fluid-filled semicircular ducts and the utricle and saccule (Fig. 10–6). The vestibular receptors are specialized hair cells located in the ampullae of the semicircular ducts and the maculae of the saccule and utricle (Fig. 10–7). The semicircular ducts respond to angular head movement. The saccule and utricle detect gravity; the utricle also monitors the position of the head when you are upright, and the saccule monitors it

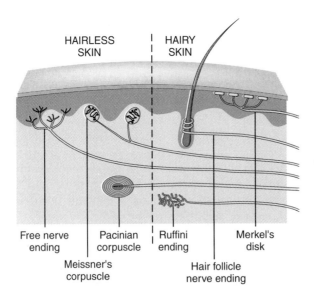

Figure 10–4

Cutaneous receptors include the free nerve ending, Meissner's corpuscle, and Pacinian corpuscle found in hairless skin and the Ruffini ending and Merkel's disk in hairy skin. (From Lundy-Ekman L. *Neuroscience Fundamentals for Rehabilitation*. Philadelphia: WB Saunders, 1998, p 88.)

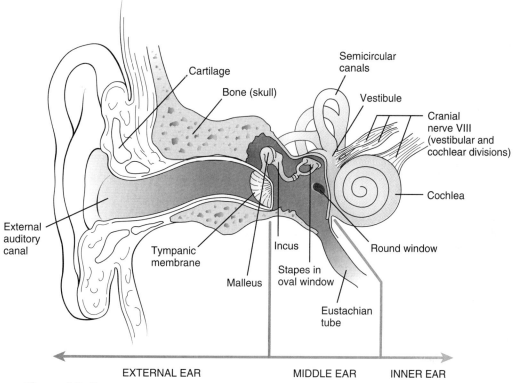

Figure 10-5

Anatomy of the ear. (Redrawn from Applegate E. *The Anatomy and Physiology Learning System,* 2nd ed. Philadelphia: WB Saunders, 2000, p 194.)

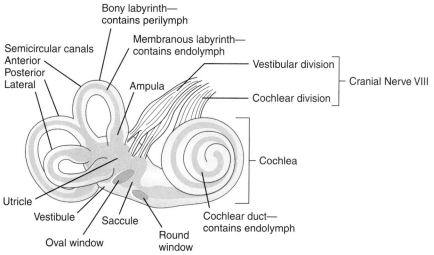

Figure 10-6

Labyrinths of the inner ear. (Redrawn from Applegate E. *The Anatomy and Physiology Learning System,* 2nd ed. Philadelphia: WB Saunders, 2000, p 195.)

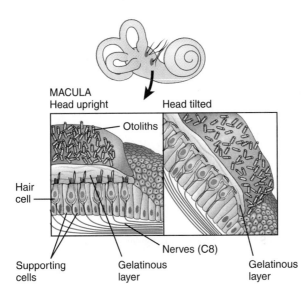

Figure 10–7

Structure of the macula. (Redrawn from Applegate E. *The Anatomy and Physiology Learning System,* 2nd ed. Philadelphia: WB Saunders, 2000, p 198.)

when you are lying down. Both respond to linear acceleration from the deflection of the hair cells. The three semicircular ducts are oriented at right angles to each other and respond to angular acceleration. When these paired structures are stimulated, the hair cells (receptors) are deformed (bent). They transmit electrical signals via the vestibular part of cranial nerve VIII to the vestibular ganglion and on to the vestibular nuclei in the medulla and vestibulocerebellum. These relay nuclei also communicate with the cervical spinal cord, oculomotor system, cerebellum, vestibular nuclei of the other side of the body, brain stem reticular formation, thalamus, and hypothalamus. Although the vestibular system exerts an influence on all other sensory systems (Ayres, 1972; Fisher et al, 1991), it exerts more influence on the motor systems by contributing to postural tone. Postural tone is sufficient muscle tone to sustain a posture.

Special Senses

Vision, hearing, taste, and smell are considered the traditional special senses and are linked to specific cranial nerves (Table 10–2). Specialized receptors found in the eye, ear, tongue, and nose are specifically and uniquely designed to sense light, sound, taste, and odors. The distance receptors—vision and hearing—have been the most thoroughly studied.

Vision is the most complex special sense. The sharpness of vision (acuity) and the ability to focus on near and far objects (accommodation) are functions of the structure of the eye. The eye is the organ of sight, but the photoreceptors are the rods and cones within the retina of the eye. After light passes through the lens of the eye, it passes over layers of cells to the back of the eye, where it is detected by the rods and cones. A very small area of the retina called the *macula* is capable of detailed and acute vision. The center of this small area, the fovea, consists of only cones. Pigment made by the receptors is

TABLE 10–2

Cranial Nerves

Cranial Nerve	Component	Function
I: Olfactory	S	Smell
II: Optic	S	Vision
III: Oculomotor	M	Eye muscles
IV: Trochlear	M	Eye muscles
V: Trigeminal	S	Face, tongue, and meninges
	M	Chewing and tympanic reflex
VI: Abducens	M	Eye muscles
VII: Facial	S	Taste
	M	Facial muscles
	A	Nasal and salivary glands
VIII: Vestibulocochlear	S	Linear and angular acceleration, head position in space, hearing
IX: Glossopharyngeal	S	Taste, pharyngeal sensation, chemoreception, and baro-reception
	M	Swallowing muscles
	A	Parotid gland
X: Vagus	S	Visceral sensation, except pain
	M	Pharyngeal and laryngeal muscles
	A	Smooth muscles in respiratory, cardiovascular, and gastrointestinal tract
XI: Spinal accessory	M	Neck muscles
XII: Hypoglossal	M	Tongue muscles

A, autonomic parasympathetic; M, motor; S, sensory.
Modified from Farber S. *Neurorehabilitation*. Philadelphia: WB Saunders, 1982, pp 53–54.

broken down by light energy and subsequently produces a nerve impulse. The eye is innervated by cranial nerve II, the optic nerve; the eye muscles are innervated by cranial nerves III, IV, and VI. Visual recognition of objects and the interpretation of their meaning involve the occipital cortex and the limbic system.

Hearing is possible because sound waves are transformed into vibration in the ear. Sound is captured by the external ear and funneled to the eardrum, or tympanic membrane. Three small bones form the ossicular chain (the malleus, incus, and stapes) and are linked to transmit the sound vibration from the tympanic membrane to the cochlea in the inner ear (Fig. 10–8). Remember that the cochlea is embedded in the temporal bone or bony labyrinth and is a set of fluid-filled coiled tubes. The sound wave travels along the basilar (bottom) membrane of the cochlear duct like a ripple of water on a pond. The hair cells of the organ of Corti lying on the basilar membrane receive the vibration and generate nerve impulses in the auditory division of cranial nerve VIII. The signals are conveyed via complex connections in the brain stem to the cerebral cortex, where sound is perceived and the meaning can be interpreted.

Taste and smell are involved in the vital functions of eating and smelling

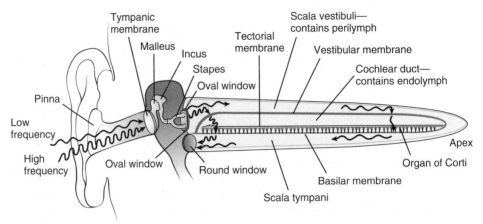

Figure 10–8

Schematic model of the auditory system peripheral apparatus showing an uncoiled cochlea with the pathway of the pressure waves vibrating against the basilar membrane of the organ of Corti and its enclosed hair cells. (Redrawn from Applegate E. *The Anatomy and Physiology Learning System,* 2nd ed. Philadelphia: WB Saunders, 2000, p 197.)

and are considered near and far receptors, respectively. These receptors are the only ones that are continually being replaced. Substances in the mouth enter taste pores and interact with the membranes of the taste receptors (buds). The chemical stimulus is transduced into taste sensation. There are four primary taste sensations: sweet, sour, bitter, and salty. There also is a continuum of tastes, with multiple receptor sites coding for sweetness. Taste buds are found in special skin structures called *papillae,* which are innervated by branches of cranial nerves VII, IX, and X. Three distinct types of papillae are present in humans and located on different parts of the tongue, soft palate, and epiglottis.

Smell is the most primitive special sense. It has a direct connection to the limbic, or emotional, system as well as to the cortex. The olfactory receptor is a remarkably simple structure found in the olfactory mucosa. Olfactory hairs, or cilia, project into the mucus, react to odors, and stimulate the olfactory cells. As a bipolar neuron, the olfactory receptor is the actual cell body of the sensory neuron. The receptor can be replaced if damaged. Its axon forms cranial nerve I.

Transduction and Coding

Sensory receptors transform mechanical, heat, sound, or light energy into electrical signals. The process used to convert one type of energy, such as sound, into an electrical signal is called *transduction.* Changing physical energy into usable neural impulses is necessary for each sensory modality (e.g., touch, pain, temperature) to be coded for intensity, duration, and location. Each sensory modality has unique features in transduction and coding and to some extent exhibits differences in anatomical and physiological development that affect our perception of any given sensory stimulus. Everyone feels pain, but there are individual differences in the way each of us perceives and tolerates pain.

Receptors also have the ability to adapt to stimulation. In other words, the receptor has some way to code for the frequency of stimulation. Rapid-adapting receptors can detect rapid stimulation and respond with many action potentials. Slow-adapting receptors respond to sustained stimuli such as gravity with fewer action potentials.

Representation

Areas of the body are represented in the brain according to their relative importance to function. For example, the sensory cortex is topically arranged so that somatic information from one part of the body is transmitted to a specific part of the cortex. This is referred to as a *somatotopic (neural) map*. The same type of mapping is found in other sensory systems. For example, in the auditory system, high-frequency sound is detected at the base of the cochlea, and low-frequency sound is detected at the apex of the cochlea. Each frequency is transmitted to a different part of the thalamus and then on to a specific part of the auditory cortex to be heard (tonotopic mapping).

The area of the body served by a sensory receptor is called a *receptor field*. The size of the area is determined by the branching of the dendrites at the end of the afferent neuron. Think of a receptor field as the shade produced by a tree's branches—the more branches, the greater the area that is shaded; the denser the branches, the darker is the shaded area. Just as two trees close together may have overlapping areas of shade, receptor fields can also overlap. Receptor fields are the means by which the nervous system keeps track of the location (on the body) of the stimulus.

Organization of these receptor fields provides the nervous system with a representation of the body. The map must be represented at each level of the nervous system. For example, to detect being touched, receptors pick up the information and relay it to the thalamus and on to the appropriate part of the sensory cortex. The stimulus is identified and localized If we are touched at two points at the same time and the distance between the two points is sufficient to be in two different receptive fields, the phenomenon of *two-point discrimination* occurs.

Specific pathways subserve specific sensory modalities. For example, the dorsal column medial lemniscal system transmits tactile, proprioceptive, and vibratory information; the lateral spinothalamic tract carries crude touch, pain, and temperature information. These pathways usually travel to the brain stem and thalamus and on to the primary sensory cortex. The dorsal columns are more discriminating in function.

Perception and Integration

Sensory input plays a major role in perceptual development. When meaning is attached to sensory information, sensation becomes *perception*. *Self-perception* is the ability to distinguish the self from other objects within the environment. Sensory information is shared between senses to provide for the identification and manipulation of objects and people within the environment. Detection, awareness, and localization come before discrimination. *Sensory integration* is the ability to use sensory information to move efficiently. *Integration* means a putting together of many sensory inputs for the purpose of adapting to the task at hand. Integration enhances the adaptiveness or effectiveness of an individual's response. An individual who has difficulty processing any of the many sensory inputs might exhibit difficulty in planning or executing certain tasks.

There are three types of sensory integration. *Intrasensory* integration occurs when information is shared within the same sensory system. Input from both eyes provides for the perception of depth. *Intersensory* integration occurs when two different sensory systems combine to impart a richer understanding than could be provided by only one sensory dimension. For example, touch and proprioception combine to provide a sense of body scheme. The last type, *sensorimotor* integration, involves the interaction of sensory and motor systems, as with the combining of vision and movement to draw or write. The combination of head turning, looking, and hearing to localize an auditory cue is another example. The linking of movement awareness and language results in the establishment of directionality, or the ability of the child to use spatial cues. Others have called this *spatial cognition*.

The role of *sensation* in perceptual organization was defined by Ayres (1972) as being able to make use of sensory information. A later definition explains that the sensory information from within the body and from the environment is processed to allow the individual to move effectively within the environment (Ayres, 1989). Sensory integration is an adaptive phenomenon that takes place within the context of a specific task and environment. It is one thing to maneuver a wheelchair through an obstacle course and quite another to walk on the deck of a rolling ship in a storm.

Cortical and subcortical structures participate in sensory integration. Association cortices, the thalamus, and the brain stem reticular system can process, amplify or dampen, and direct sensory information to other areas of the brain. The thalamus relays the sensory stimulus to the cortex as well as to appropriate association areas to plan a response. Recognition and interpretation of the stimulus occur in the primary sensory cortex, such as the realization that you have been touched and the quality of that touch (gentle or rough). The touch is further interpreted in the higher association areas as emotionally pleasing or dangerous. In an open system, interconnected structures regulate and organize sensory input into a conceptual whole to allow us to identify shapes by touch. This ability is called *stereognosis*. Perceptual abilities and sensory integration develop over time and reflect the increasing adaptation of the individual to the environment.

Life-Span Changes

PRENATAL PERIOD

The senses of touch, motion (vestibular), smell, and taste are ready to function at birth, as evidenced by the complete myelination of their respective neural pathways. Vision and audition are capable of some level of function at birth but require additional time and environmental experience to complete myelination and maturation of central pathways. The sensory systems develop in utero in the following order: touch, motion, smell, hearing, vision, taste, and proprioception.

Somatic Senses

The fetus develops the ability to respond to touch around the mouth as early as 7½ weeks of gestation (Hooker, 1952). The earliest response to touch is avoidance, or turning away. By 17 weeks, cutaneous sensation spreads to the entire body with the exception of the top and back of the head; these areas are subjected to the most sensory input during delivery.

Proprioceptive receptors are well developed by mid-fetal life (Lowrey, 1986). Tapping, stretching, or even a change in amniotic fluid pressure can cause a response in the fetus (Windle, 1940). Muscle spindles are known to differentiate between 11 and 12 weeks (Bergstrom and Bergstrom, 1963, cited in Wyke, 1975). The Golgi tendon organ does not differentiate until 16 weeks of gestation. Pacinian corpuscles are found in the distal parts of limbs at 20 weeks of gestation but are immature.

Motion Sense

The vestibular apparatus begins as a thickening of ectoderm, or placode, in the primitive ear early in the fourth week of gestation. A *placode* is a common precursor of most sensory organs. The semicircular canals, utricle, and saccule are completely formed at 9½ weeks of gestation (Humphrey, 1965). The fetus moves constantly in utero, and the vestibular apparatus provides information about that movement. This is the first sensory system to be myelinated and the first to function. The fetus shows a generalized body response to changes in body position, including the ability to right the head. Movement in utero has been linked to later movement competence (Milani-Comparetti, 1981).

Special Senses

Vision

The eyes also develop during the fourth week of gestation from a placode that forms a vesicle. The optic vesicle folds in onto itself to produce a two-layered optic cup, from which the retina is derived The neural cells of the retina differentiate into 10 layers containing photoreceptors (the rods and cones), cell bodies of bipolar neurons, and ganglion cells. Because of the infolding, the photoreceptors are adjacent to the pigment layer. Therefore, light must pass through the retina to reach the receptors.

Neurons in the occipital cortex are organized into their adult layers during the second half of gestation (Meisami and Timiras, 1988), so they are ready to receive input after birth. Myelination begins at the optic chiasm around 13 weeks of gestation, and the rods and cones differentiate at 16 weeks. Light perception is possible in utero (Almli and Mohr, 1995); the fetus exhibits reflexive eye-blinking at 6 months of gestation. Thalamic connections begin to myelinate before term and continue until the fifth postnatal month of life. The thalamic connections, those to the lateral geniculate nucleus, are crucial to the development of more sophisticated visual perceptual abilities. Central visual pathways develop postnatally even though the neurons that constitute these pathways are formed prenatally.

Hearing

The ectoderm of the otic placode forms both the membranous labyrinth of the vestibular system and the structures of the inner ear—the cochlear duct and the organ of Corti—during the fourth week of gestation. The hair cells differentiate by 16 weeks of gestation (Almli and Mohr, 1995). The remaining structures of the ear, including ligaments and muscles, come from the branchial arches. Hearing in utero is possible as early as 24 weeks of gestation and is consistently present after 28 weeks of gestation (Birnholz and Benacerraf, 1983).

Taste

The tongue is developed from the mandibular arch at 26 to 31 days of gestation. Formation is completed by the 37th day; the various types of taste buds reach maturity by 13 weeks of gestation (Meisami and Timiras, 1988). Ingestion of amniotic fluid in utero is thought to contribute to the development of the primitive gut as well as to the regulation of amniotic fluid volume. Taste is functional in utero in the last third of the pregnancy. The amniotic fluid is rich in chemicals such as sugars, salts, acids, and lactate that can be "tasted" by the fetus (Beauchamp et al, 1991). Steiner (1979) reports that infants born at 6 to 7 months of gestation can detect citric acid.

Smell

The olfactory placode also forms during the fourth week of gestation. It is the earliest distance receptor to develop. The fifth cranial nerve innervates the walls of the nose at 5 weeks; the olfactory organ (bulb) is well developed by the fifth and sixth months of gestation. The unmyelinated nerve fibers of cranial nerve I are the olfactory nerve. It is these fibers that end in the olfactory bulb. Olfactory discrimination is possible in preterm infants beyond 29 weeks of gestation (Lowrey, 1986).

INFANCY AND EARLY CHILDHOOD

Complete maturation of sensory pathways after birth is the rule in vision, hearing, and proprioception. Physiological changes occur after birth in all sensory systems, as evidenced by an increase in nerve conduction velocity (time to conduct) with myelination, redistribution of axon branching, and increased synaptic efficacy. Functional changes are apparent as the infant interacts more meaningfully with the world.

State and Novelty

Behavioral state and novelty of stimulus play a role in the infant's level of interest in sensory information. A sleeping or overstimulated infant is not able to react to a new stimulus. On the other hand, a quietly alert infant looking at a mobile will generally become attentive to a new toy. Sensory awareness requires that the infant be sufficiently aroused. The concept of state was first described by Prechtl (1974) as levels of alertness ranging from sleep to crying. The quiet alert state has been deemed the most appropriate for testing an infant's responses to sensory stimulation. Studies show that an infant's state will affect the level of reflex and motor responsiveness (Smith et al, 1982). The ability of the infant to change states smoothly is also an indication of the organization of the CNS.

Many studies of visual preference in infants have pinpointed the role of novelty in gaining attention and producing motor behavior. The behavior may be looking, reaching, vocalizing, or even quieting, but the common denominator is that the infant responds to a certain level of stimulus novelty. For example, when an infant is shown two pictures, the infant typically attends to the new picture. From the earliest moment that the infant is quietly alert, there is the ability to perceive sensory stimuli and to demonstrate preferences. Novelty and complexity guide infants' exploratory behavior (Sahoo, 1998). Learning and adaptation occur much earlier than was once believed. Perceptual abilities once reserved as the province of the older child are consistently being documented in infants. Sensory perception, that is, the ability to attach meaning to sensory information, occurs from the beginning of extrauterine life.

Self-Perception

Infants develop a sense of self as young as 2 to 3 months. Hand-to-mouth and -face behavior is typical in an infant. This cutaneous self-stimulation does not trigger any of the typically observed rooting responses when an external object contacts the same facial location. Rochat and Hespos (1997) suggest that the infant can distinguish between self-touch and environmental touch. The self-stimulation would involve proprioceptive stimulation from self-movement as well as touch. When touching their own face, infants experience a unique sensorimotor event that potentially identifies their body as a differentiated body. Rochat (1998) categorizes infants' self-exploration of their own bodies as visual-proprioceptive calibration: "infants appear fascinated by the simultaneous experience of seeing and feeling the limbs of their own body moving through space" (p 103). Three-month-old infants begin to show systematic visual and proprioceptive self-exploration (Rochat and Morgan, 1995).

Somatic Senses

Touch

The perception of touch and pain is crucial to the newborn's survival. Although the defensive movements to light touch seen in utero fade by birth, the newborn reflexively moves to clear the nose and mouth of any object that obstructs the airway. The first responses to touch are generalized diffuse responses, such as random arm and leg movements. Information from touch is initially used by the infant to locate food. Within a few days after birth, head turning in response to touching the mouth is precisely related to the part of the mouth touched. Although touch and pain are not completely differentiated in the full-term newborn, pain sensitivity has been shown to increase over the first 4 days of life (Kaye and Lipsitt, 1964). Pain receptors are equally prevalent in infants and adults (Anand and Hickey, 1987), with pain sensitivity appearing to increase in the first month of life (Salapatek and Cohen, 1987). Studies of infant circumcision (Gunnar et al, 1981) show that physiological changes in response to the procedure occur and that preterm infants display behavioral and physiological changes in response to painful stimuli (Craig et al, 1993).

Early tactile input plays a role in parent-infant attachment, stress-coping mechanisms, sociability, and cognitive development. The use of tactile input to recognize differences develops gradually; a 1-month-old infant is able to distinguish among pacifier shapes (Meltzoff and Borton, 1979). Prechtl (1958) reports a refinement in the receptive field for touch-mediated reflex responses such as flexor withdrawal. Touch to any part of the leg of a newborn results in a reflexive withdrawal. Gradually, the receptive field becomes limited to the sole of the foot.

Touch sensation can be localized generally at 7 to 9 months; specific localization is demonstrated by 12 to 16 months of age (Lowrey, 1986). General localization is exhibited by the infant's moving the extremity; specific localization involves the infant's touching or looking at the area touched A toddler can touch the place where he was touched and will either rub the area or push away the stimulus. The spot also will be noticed visually, which supports the possibility that intersensory association occurs between touch and vision.

The ability to use touch to identify objects is called *haptic perception* (Gibson, 1966). *Haptic* means "able to lay hold of" and is appropriate because the majority of information about objects comes from manipulation. Nine-month-old infants have been found to possess this ability, as determined by manual exploration (Gottfried and Rose, 1980). When visual information is combined with touch, infants as young as 6 months can pick out toys that were touched previously without being seen (Rose, 1994).

Temperature

The newborn must regulate its own body temperature at birth and is sensitive to the temperature of the ambient air. Responses to changes in air temperature are often seen in common body postures assumed by the infant. Infants who are too warm may appear to be "sunbathing," decrease their calorie intake, sleep, and show peripheral vasodilation. Sweating and panting responses mature later. Conversely, the infant will wake and move about if too cool. Discrimination of hot and cold is possible early on and is characterized by more reactivity to cold. Respiratory changes, limb movement, and state changes have been documented for temperatures varying as little as 5° to 6°.

Proprioception

Proprioception is the foundation for purposeful movements such as imitation, reaching, and locomotion. It is used for action very early after birth, when the tactile and vestibular systems are functioning. The fact that newborn infants imitate mouth opening and tongue protrusion is interpreted as a pairing of visual and proprioceptive input (Meltzoff and Moore, 1977). In the same way a child handles objects to gain haptic perception, infants move to gain proprioceptive information. Self-perception in the infant appears to depend on touch and proprioception (Morgan and Rochat, 1997). Research has shown that reaching behavior in 5-month-olds depends more on the infant's motor ability and proprioception than on visual control; no difference is seen between reaching in the dark and reaching in the light (Sugden, 1986). Vision becomes more important as the system matures, as evidenced by more successful reaching with vision in the 7-month-old (Lasky, 1977; Von Hofsten, 1979).

Achieving and maintaining an upright posture depend on the infant's ability to interpret and respond to information about body sway, which comes from vestibular, visual, and proprioceptive input. Multiple studies have shown that infants use vision proprioceptively in sitting and standing to maintain stable postures (Butterworth and Ciccheti, 1978; Butterworth and Hicks, 1977; Lee and Aaronson, 1974; Sundermier and Woollacott, 1998). When proprioceptive and vestibular input indicated that the body was stable and visual input indicated movement, the majority of subjects made compensatory movements.

Motion Sense

The vestibular system defines the body's relationship to gravity and is completely myelinated at birth. Many of the infant's earliest activities are related to achieving and maintaining stable postures against gravity. Preterm infants were initially found to have delayed vestibular responses to movement (Eviatar et al, 1974), especially preterm infants, who are also small for gestational age. This delay in responding is due to immaturity, not pathology (Ornitz, 1983), and is related to the difficulty preterm infants have in maintaining alert wakefulness. When alert and awake, even preterm infants can demonstrate vestibular responses (Eliot, 1999).

Righting reactions of the head mediated by the labyrinths are possible from birth. The ability to move against gravity continues with the development of trunk righting and progresses to the development of equilibrium reactions. The body appears to seek the most efficient posture to support reaching, manipulation, and locomotion. Infants and children with vestibular problems demonstrate delays in motor function (Kaga, 1999).

Nystagmus is an alternating sequence of fast and slow horizontal eye movements normally seen in response to rotatory movement such as being spun in a swing. This vestibular ocular reflex is not present until a few weeks after birth. The earliest postnatal vestibular ocular reflex is called the *doll's eye phenomenon*. When a normal newborn is held in dorsal suspension and moved horizontally, the eyes appear to move in the opposite direction of the body motion. The eye movement corresponds to the slow component of nystagmus. Persistence of this phenomenon after the first 2 weeks of life indicates serious brain damage. The form and amount of nystagmus normally present in infants change between birth and the first year of life (Eviatar and Eviatar, 1979).

Vestibular sensitivity increases from birth to a peak between 6 and 12 months of age. After this peak, there is a decline to 2½ years and a more gradual decline to puberty. Infants are more sensitive to vestibular input, and that oversensitivity may explain their relative unsteadiness. The slow maturation of vestibular sensitivity is a result of changes in synaptic strength and connectivity in the brain stem and higher centers (Eliot, 1999).

Special Senses

Vision

Newborns were always thought to have relatively poor, if any, visual abilities at birth. However, as technology for testing has become more sophisticated, so has our understanding of the infant's visual system. Newborns have pattern preference and can maintain attention if a stimulus is novel enough or resembles a face. To obtain visual alerting behavior, newborns need to be approached from the side, because they are unable to maintain their heads in the mid-line until 4 months of age. Visual acuity at birth appears to be about 20/800 (Coren et al, 1999), and steadily increases with age. Some authors report that adult levels of vision (20/20) are achieved as early as 1 year (Salapatek and Cohen, 1987), but others use 3 years as the age at which adult resolution is possible (Coren et al, 1999).

The infant sees initially in black and white. As the cones (the color receptors) mature over the first several months, color vision develops. Two-month-olds see two colors, and full-color vision is present by 4 months.

Smooth tracking abilities begin by 2 months of age (Aslin, 1981) and progress over an ever-widening arc as the infant matures and head control is achieved. Accommodation is possible at 2 months but improves to adult levels by 6 months. Depth and size perception begin to develop with the ability to use the two eyes together to converge or diverge on near and far objects. This may be aided by the development of head control in the prone position as the infant practices looking down at his or her hands or up at toys.

Vision provides vital information for balance and head control: "perceptual sensitivity to visual information improves rapidly during the first few months after birth" (Bertenthal et al, 1997, p 1631). Head control contributes to the ability of the infant to visually fix on objects. Conversely, visual fixation contributes to postural stability of the head and neck. Visual information is used to control posture even before infants can sit. Optical flow is detected peripherally by infants and used as a cue to make a compensatory response. "Optical flow refers to the perceived motion of the visual field that results from an individual's own movement through the environment" (Kandel et al, 2000, p 553).

Binocular vision depends on adequate alignment of the eyes. Most infants demonstrate good visual alignment between 3 and 6 months of age. Shimojo and colleagues (1986) postulate that the change in binocular function seen at 3 months is related to the separation of the afferent input from the two eyes into columns within the visual cortex. These bands of cells are known as *ocular dominance columns*. If the input from each eye is the same, the columns will be the same size. Two-year-olds exhibit adult-like binocular vision. Table 10–3 provides a list of changes in visual development along with changes in visual motor behavior.

TABLE 10–3

Visual Development

Age	Visual Development	Visual-Motor Behavior
Newborn	Focal distance 7–10 in 20/800 Acuity	Hands fisted Doll's eye Tracks toy to midline Prefers black and white
1 mo	Focal distance ≥1–3 ft Frontal visual fields mature	Tracks 180 degrees Prefers face to object Tracks horizontally
2 mo	Accommodation develops Depth and size perception developing Dichromatic (red and yellow)	Unilateral hand regard Asymmetrical tonic neck reflex Hands open, manipulates red ring, swipes
3 mo	Head turning with eyes Binocular vision begins Improved visual attention	Strong visual inspection of hands at midline Mouths objects
4 mo	Sees in full color Well-developed binocular vision Accommodates over wide range of distances	Bilateral reach at midline Hits and shakes objects Instinctive grasp Holds one cube
5 mo	Vision directs grasp and manipulation	Turns head to follow vanishing object Raking; holds two cubes
6 mo	Adult accommodation 20/40 Acuity	Tracks objects in all directions Transfers at midline Palmar grasp
7 mo		Transfers hand to hand Radial palmar grasp
8 mo	Macula more mature	Anticipates future position of objects in motion Reaches for hidden objects
9 mo		Radial digital grasp
10 mo		Recognizes object by seeing only part of it Inferior pincer grasp (9–12 mo)
12 mo	20/20 Acuity	Follows rapidly moving objects Visually monitors hand play Neat pincer grasp
2 yr	Adult binocular vision	

Hearing

At birth, the infant physiologically responds to sound by changing respiratory patterns or heart rate. Sensory thresholds are slightly higher than those of adults (Werner and Marean, 1996). Behaviorally, the infant may demonstrate facial grimacing, eye blinking, and crying at loud noises. The auditory system is completely myelinated 1 month after birth. By 3 months of age, head turning to localize sound is well established. In the appropriate state of wakefulness, a newborn may exhibit eye or head turning to sound. New sounds will produce searching behavior in infants older than 4 months and will encourage the infant to babble in vocal play. Vocal imitation follows, with words being produced by the first year. Locke (1997) suggests that the infant's orientation to the voices and location of people speaking may be an important precursor to the development of spoken language.

The 2-year-old develops listening skills, which refine the production of speech and facilitate the rapid acquisition of language. Speech is learned by successive approximations of the correct sound. Basic auditory listening skills are mastered by 3 years of age (Lowrey, 1986). Data from auditory-evoked potentials document adult latency values by the age of 4 years, indicating the early postnatal maturation of the auditory system (Allison et al, 1984).

Ear infections that result in increased fluid in the ear are a common problem in infants and preschoolers. Because fluid in the middle ear can produce a conductive hearing loss, these infections are now treated aggressively. Previously, many children with a chronic ear infection showed delayed development of language. Dynamic balance problems and delays in gross motor development have been reported in children with chronic ear infections (Cohen et al, 1997).

Taste and Smell

These two chemical senses are significant to the newborn. Although obviously linked to feeding, these senses are also involved in parent-infant communication, control of respiration, and cognition (Salapatek and Cohen, 1987). Taste may assist in modulating oral intake, as well as in coordinating breathing and eating. Smell may be related to infant attention, although this has not been adequately studied. Infants may use smell to identify familiar features of the environment, including people, before the visual system is effective in performing this function. A 5-day-old newborn can selectively orient to his or her mother's breast pad based on odor (MacFarlane, 1975). Both taste and smell are functional at birth and quickly become connected to feeding reflexes. Infants discriminate among all four primary taste sensations but prefer to ingest sweet things.

CHILDHOOD AND ADOLESCENCE

Sensory changes continue during childhood and adolescence. It is during childhood that the integration of sensation and movement occurs. The perceptual process, although evident in early development, is further refined by the child's increased ability to attend to more than one characteristic of a stimulus, to attach meaning to sensory stimuli, and to plan a motor response. Cognitive and language development is of paramount importance in developing and verbalizing spatial and directional concepts.

Somatic Senses

The somatic senses of touch and proprioception continue to be refined in childhood. Two-point discrimination is possible by 4 years of age (Hermann et al, 1996). Children can usually identify familiar objects by touch at 5 years of age. Knowledge of where the body is in space and the sequence of movements that must be planned to perform a motor task are based on appropriate interpretation of tactile and proprioceptive input. The ability to motor plan, or *praxis*, emerges during childhood. Tactile and proprioceptive sensation also refine the changing adolescent's body scheme and the affective view of the body.

The coupling of movement and perception is a central process in perceptual development. Bigelow (1981) identified how children use proprioceptive information in visual self-recognition. Children recognized moving images of themselves sooner than they did static pictures, which supports the belief that children move their bodies purposefully to gain proprioceptive information. Thelen (1995) believes that individuals perceive in order to move and move in order to perceive.

Kinesthetic acuity improves with age. *Kinesthetic acuity* is the ability to proprioceptively discriminate differences in location, distance, weight, force, speed, and acceleration of movement. For example, an individual can distinguish objects by weight when held in the hand while blindfolded. Based on research using the Kinesthetic Acuity Test (Elliot et al, 1988), performance in children improves from age 5 through 12 and sometimes beyond. Kinesthetic acuity improves more quickly than kinesthetic memory. Memory for movement is kinesthetic memory. Examples of movement tasks performed from memory are a dance routine and the sequence of step-hopping that occurs in skipping. Adult levels of kinesthetic acuity are achieved by 8 years of age, whereas kinesthetic memory maturity is not usually achieved until age 12 (Gabbard, 1996).

Motion Sense

Vestibular responses change greatly between preadolescence and adulthood (Ornitz, 1983). The most striking maturational changes occur in preschool children (Ornitz et al, 1979). Vestibular sensitivity declines from 2½ years to puberty. Before this period, infants and children engage in repetitive self-stimulation such as rocking in a rocker or spinning themselves. This period of vestibular stimulation begins around 6 to 8 months of age and coincides with a peaking of vestibular sensitivity. With increasing maturation, these behaviors decline. Children have a stronger response to vestibular stimulation than adults, who respond less intensely as the system matures. Maturation is completed between 10 and 14 years of age (Ornitz, 1983).

Special Senses

Vision

Many aspects of visual perception develop in childhood. The child shows refinement of size constancy: the ability to recognize that objects remain the same size even if the distance of the viewer from the object changes. The ability to separate the figure from the background, or *figure-ground perception*, improves with age. By 8 years of age, most children are as good as adults in performing this perceptual task (Williams, 1983).

Visual perception related to object identification, movement, and task performance seems to follow the same trend. By 5 years of age, children demonstrate *visual closure*, or the ability to discern a shape when seeing only part of it. Between 5 and 10 years of age, children accurately track moving objects, such as a softball (Haywood, 1977). Perceptual judgments regarding the size of various objects at different distances become mature at the age of 11 years (Collins, 1976). Adult levels of depth perception are achieved at 12 years of age.

Spatial Awareness

Spatial awareness is the internalization of our own location in space as well as object localization. The teacher stands in front of the students with the blackboard behind her. *Space perception* is the ability to perceive direction or distance. Combining visual information with proprioception allows the child to recognize the location and orientation of objects within the environment. By age 3 to 4 years, most children have conceptualized the spatial dichotomies of over/under, top/bottom, front/back, and in/out. The sequence of acquisition of these spatial directions is vertical to horizontal, then diagonal or oblique (Williams, 1983). Knowledge of the spatial environment is necessary to construct effective motor programs. Objects are first related to the child and later related to other objects. Space perception and spatial awareness are needed for successful execution of a motor program when accommodating to changing environmental demands.

Most 5-year-old children know the right side of the body from the left side. This concept of *laterality* is a conscious internal awareness of the two sides of the body. However, it is not until children are 8 years of age that they consistently and accurately answer questions about right-left discrimination (Gabbard, 1996). It is also at this age that children can begin to relay information in directional terms such as "the playground is on the right."

Directionality, the motor expression of laterality and spatial awareness, develops between 6 and 12 years of age (Long and Looft, 1972). Directionality is initially demonstrated at 6 years when the child mirrors and imitates movement. At 7 years of age, the child uses the body as a directional reference: "The ball is in front of me." Next, the child can reference objects objectively, such as, "The water fountain is on the left." By 10 years of age, the child can identify the right and left of the person opposite him. He will no longer mirror movements but will move the right arm when the other person moves the right arm. At 12 years of age, the child can use a natural frame of reference so that he can describe that the sun sets in the west.

ADULTHOOD AND AGING

Sensory abilities present in adolescence continue to guide motor activities. Despite the continued development of intersensory associations, a decline in sensory function begins in adulthood and progresses with advanced age. Peripheral and central changes are documented in many of the sensory systems. Again, however, these changes are not always directly related to a decline in function, nor are they universal.

Somatic Senses

Some older adults show a diminished ability to detect touch, temperature, pain, and vibration (Kenshalo, 1977). Structural changes in skin such as loss of dermal thickness, decline in nutrient transfer, and loss of collagen and elastin fibers contribute to a decline in the functions of the skin. A nearly 20% loss of dermal thickness in older adults may explain that paper-thin, sometimes translucent quality of their skin. Physiologically, the growth rate, healing response, sensory perception, and thermoregulation of the skin decline (Duthie and Katz, 1998).

The skin receptors responsible for the perception of pressure and light touch, *pacinian* and *Meissner's corpuscles*, decline in number with age. By the ninth decade, they are only one third of their original density. Both of these receptors also undergo morphological or structural changes. Meissner's corpuscles change relative to whether we have performed physical labor. With manual labor, the corpuscles become winding and large; without manual labor, they develop neurofibrillary networks. Regardless of the structural changes, older adults can lose up to 90% of these receptors. *Merkel's disks,* another type of pressure receptor, appear to be unchanged (Meisami, 1994; Weisenberger, 1996).

Compromised thermoregulation can predispose older adults to hypothermia or heat stroke. Control of body temperature regulation by the hypothalamus is altered significantly with age. The ability of the sympathetic nervous system to cause vasoconstriction and impede heat loss is impaired As a result, mild hypothermia occurs in a large number of older adults in cooler rooms, which is why older people accommodate by more often wearing sweaters, coats, and hats. Thermoregulatory deficiency is also a result of a decline in temperature perception (Timiras, 1994).

Effects of aging on pain perception are not clearly understood. Although deep pain perception is known to diminish with age (Katzman and Terry, 1983), conflicting reports in the literature support both a decrease and an increase in superficial sensitivity. In a study by Harkins and associates (1986), age had no main effect on sensitivity, although middle-aged and older adult participants tended to rate the stimulus lower in intensity than did younger adults. Superficial pain probably diminishes with age, but the amount varies individually.

One of the most common sensory losses documented in older adults is the loss of vibratory sensation. Awareness of vibration begins to decline at 50 years of age (Steiness, 1957), with the lower extremities more affected than the upper extremities (Merchut and Toleikis, 1990). Although pacinian corpuscles in the skin are lost with age, Kenshalo (1977) attributes the loss of vibratory sensation to decreased nerve conduction in the lower extremities.

Joint position sense definitely declines with age (Skinner et al, 1984), especially in the lower extremities. Women exhibit an age-related decline in proprioception and static joint position sensation of the knee (Kaplan et al, 1985). Subjects using a visual analogue scale also reported an age-related decline in position sense of the knee (Barrett et al, 1991). Proximal joints may be more sensitive to movement than distal joints (Weisenberger, 1996). Functionally, the decline in proprioception in the lower extremities could impair balance in older adults. Additional age-related changes in somatosensation are listed in Table 10–4.

Motion Sense

Dizziness and vertigo are common disturbances in persons older than 50 years. Structures of the vestibular system such as the hair cells undergo degeneration (Ochs et al, 1985). A 20% to 40% reduction in hair cells has been reported in

TABLE 10–4

Age-Related Changes in Somatosensation

Function	Nature of Change
Touch/pressure	Significant increase in thresholds after age 40 years; lower thresholds in fingers than toes
	Light touch thresholds significantly increase in hands and feet
	Men are generally less sensitive to touch than are women
Vibration	Decreased sensitivity
	Greatest decline after 80 years
Proprioception (passive limb position)	Decreased sensitivity from 20 to 80 years
	Thresholds for lower extremity joints two times greater after 50 years than before 40 years
	More variability in responses
Kinesthesia (active joint motion)	No major changes across 5-year periods
	Few age-related changes generally if minimal memory involved
	Age-related changes increase with greater memory demands

Modified from Williams HG. Aging and eye-hand coordination. In Bard C, Fleury J, Hay L (eds). *Development of Eye-Hand Coordination*. Columbia, SC: University of South Carolina Press, 1990, p 352.

the saccule and utricle and in the semicircular canals, respectively. Neuronal loss has been documented in parts of the vestibular nuclear complex that receive input from the semicircular canals (Lopez et al, 1997). Neural changes in the vestibular nerve are evident in older adults and may begin as early as 40 years of age. By 75 years, the number of myelinated vestibular nerve fibers declines almost 40% (Bergstrom, 1973). The older individual may exhibit dysequilibrium from age-related changes in the peripheral or central vestibular system.

Presbyastasis is the age-related decline in equilibrium or dynamic balance seen when no other pathology is noted (Kennedy and Clemis, 1990). Reliance on vestibular input alone may result in loss of balance and even falls in the older adult (Wolfson et al, 1992). Healthy older adults without general sensory deficits do not exhibit as much of an increase in postural sway as do older adults who show sensory deficits. The latter group is more likely to experience falls (Duncan et al, 1992; Lord et al, 1994; Ring et al, 1989). Postural sway is described in Chapter 12.

Special Senses

Vision

Visual acuity increases in the 20s and 30s, remains stable in the 40s and 50s, and then declines (Pitts, 1982). The most rapid decrease in acuity occurs between 60 to 80 years of age. By 85, there is an 80% loss from the acuity level present at 40 years of age (Weale, 1975). Structural changes in the optical part of the eye contribute to these age-related changes in function. The cornea and lens thicken, the lens curvature decreases, and a yellowish pigment accumulates. Aging changes in the lens protein may be a result of oxidative damage (Timiras, 1994). Table 10–5 lists some age-related changes in vision.

Central vision can be impaired by cataracts, a decrease in the transparency of the lens. The increase in lens density is due to accumulation of pigments. Cataracts begin to form in everyone older than 30 years (Duthie and Katz, 1998). The rate of progression, however, is different for every individual. Most cataracts develop bilaterally in those older than 50 years and are present to some degree in all 70-year-olds (Cleary, 1997). Fully developed cataracts are documented in one third of persons 80 years old (Duthie and Katz, 1998). Visual acuity of 20/50 or worse is an indication for surgical removal. Those with diabetes have a higher incidence of cataracts than do the rest of the population.

Color discrimination in the green-blue end of the spectrum becomes more difficult as the lens of the eye yellows with aging. Pupil size declines with age, allowing less light into the eye. By 60 years of age, retinal illumination is reduced by one third, and the older adult is less able to detect low levels of light. Because of the lens changes, light may be scattered over more of the retinal surface, resulting in glare. Glare introduces extraneous light into the eye and may be particularly troublesome to older adults. Because of retinal sensitivity loss, the elder's eyes are overstimulated by oncoming headlights or sudden flashes of light.

TABLE 10–5

Age-Related Changes in Vision

Function	Nature of Change
General	Decreased transparency of lens Decreased amount of light reaching the eye Decrease in number of macular neurons by almost half from 20 to 80 years
Visual acuity	Usually retained throughout life; slight decrease from 20 to 50 years More rapid decrease from 60 to 80 years; need more light to detect objects
Light adaptation	Sharp decline in ability to quickly adapt from dark to light environments after 40 years; dramatic decrease after 60 years
Contrast sensitivity	Three times as much contrast needed by older individuals as younger ones to perceive a coarsely structured target
Dark adaptation	Little or no change from 20 to 40 years Significant increase in time to adapt after 70; an 80-year-old requires 40+ minutes
Depth perception	Little or no changes to 60+ years Accelerated decrease from 60 to 75 years
Visual information processing	Older individuals are one third slower than younger ones Significant decrease in peripheral and central information between 50 and 60 years

Modified from Williams HG. Aging and eye-hand coordination. In Bard C, Fleury M, Hay L (eds). *Development of Eye-Hand Coordination*. Columbia, SC: University of South Carolina Press, 1990, p 350.

Contrast sensitivity and dark adaptation decline with age. Contrast sensitivity loss causes a loss of depth perception, which can be especially dangerous when going up or down stairs. Adaptation to dim light decreases with age, which can be hazardous when entering a darkened house or a less well illuminated room. A teenager needs only 6 to 7 minutes to adapt to darkness, but an 80-year-old may need more than 40 minutes (Williams, 1990). These changes are related to a decline in the number of receptors and a decreased regeneration capacity of photoreceptor pigment (Meisami, 1994).

Presbyopia is the diminished ability to focus clearly at normal reading distances. One contributing cause is the thickening of the lens due to continued growth of lens fibers (Duthie and Katz, 1998). The ciliary muscle normally acts to change the curvature of the lens to focus the image. With aging, the ciliary muscles become less able to adequately accommodate to distance changes; those over 40 often complain, "My arms are not long enough to read the print of the newspaper." Accommodation difficulties may also impair the older person's ability to read the speedometer in the car because of a decreased ability to change the lens size when switching from far to near vision. Corrective lenses such as bifocals or trifocals become necessary. By the age of 60, when the lens can no longer accommodate, presbyopia exists.

Hearing

Presbycusis, an age-related decline in hearing acuity, is due to a loss of sensory cells in the inner ear or, more specifically, the organ of Corti. Structural changes that contribute to age-related hearing loss include degeneration of the hair cells at the base of the cochlea, degeneration of nerve cells in the spiral ganglia, atrophy of associated vascular and connective tissue, and loss of neurons in the cortical auditory centers (Meisami, 1994). Because the loss typically occurs at the base of the structure, hearing is initially impaired for high-frequency tones such as the whistle of a tea kettle or a doorbell. Speech perception is preserved because speech is heard at lower sound frequencies. This type of hearing loss is associated with aging and can begin as early as 30 years of age and progress until 80.

Presbycusis is more than a simple hearing loss of pure tones. It also involves speech processing and discrimination. Although speech perception is preserved, the ability to discriminate or recognize what is being said decreases. The loss of discrimination is greater than would be expected from the hearing loss alone. Seventy-five percent of adults older than 70 years will exhibit hearing loss of this type.

Researchers (Corso, 1981; Meisami, 1994) have postulated that the losses seen in presbycusis are due not only to a decline in function of the end organ but also to central factors. These factors include lengthier auditory processing of information in the cortex and decreased neuron cell counts in the temporal lobes. Wingfield and coworkers (1985) indicated that processing difficulties common in older adults might be related to a slowing of auditory decoding processes.

Taste and Smell

Taste and smell are intimately linked to the perception of the flavor of food. Age-related deficits may explain reports of flavor changes and food intake by older adults (Rolls, 1999). The loss of taste bud function is documented (Miller, 1988), but recognition of taste, temperature, and viscosity (thickness) of stimuli has been shown to remain stable with age. The functional changes may be more related to changes in taste cell membranes than to an actual loss of taste buds (Patten and Craik, 2000). Pressure detection on the tongue is the only parameter that declines with age (Weiffenbach and Bartoshuk, 1992).

The loss of smell is greater than that of taste (Finkelstein and Schiffman, 1999). In a review, Schiffman (1997) noted that there is a modest loss of taste in normal healthy aging. Smell identification declines progressively with age (Ship, 1999). Memory distortion, changes, or both in the social and emotional context in which eating occurs may also contribute to a decreased perception of the flavor and appeal of food for older adults.

FUNCTIONAL IMPLICATIONS

Impairment of any one sensory system during early development can lead to difficulty in function. Hearing loss affects the development of motor skills and balance (Effgen, 1981; Horak et al, 1988). Because the eighth cranial nerve subserves both hearing and motion sense, it stands to reason that if one part is damaged, the other portion may also be damaged Many children with hearing impairments have poor vestibular function, resulting in balance deficits (Rine et al, 2000). Some children with primarily vestibular deficits are unsafe without protective headgear.

The effects of deficits in tactile, vestibular, and proprioceptive systems on sensory integration are also well documented (Fisher et al, 1991). Deficits are linked to poor body scheme, self-image, difficulty in motor planning, or sequencing movement and balance. Sensory information is used to learn movement. The ability to process sensory information and thus integrate it with movement in a planned and organized manner is important for motor coordination.

The effects of visual deficits on the developmental course were documented by Jan and colleagues (1990). Visually impaired children must substitute auditory cues to direct movement; because so many movements are visually guided, their acquisition of motor milestones is delayed. Children with crossed eyes, or strabismus, may have difficulty in developing head control or mid-line reaching. The earlier that the visual alignment deficits are detected and corrected, the better off children are in terms of upper extremity control.

A decline in function of any one sensory system due to aging can have serious functional implications. For example, presbyopia makes it more difficult for the older adults to read dials on the stove or to do needle work. A decline in depth perception can contribute to an increased potential for falling while going up or down stairs. Presbycusis may isolate an elder from a lively conversation or decrease awareness of a warning siren while driving the automobile with the radio turned on. Food preparation and meal time may be less enjoyable because of age-related changes in smell and taste abilities. Changes in somatosensation in the lower extremities and motion sense may contribute to an increased likelihood of falling or an increased fear of falling, which can lead to hypoactivity. Any or all of the potential sensory changes with aging can curtail an individual's range of movement by increasing dependence on compensatory devices or strategies.

Because vision is so important to development across the life span, two conditions that affect vision, amblyopia and macular degeneration, are discussed in detail. One occurs early in development and is potentially reversible, whereas the other occurs at the end of the life span. Both are examples of sensory changes that can have significant functional implications. An important life skill that can be impeded by either of these conditions is driving. It is our most relied on means of mobility and is prized as a reward by the adolescent, deemed almost as a right of passage. Adults depend on driving to get to and from jobs, appointments, shopping, and leisure activities. Driving becomes a significant quality of life issue as individuals reach older age and strive to maintain independence.

Amblyopia

Amblyopia, or "lazy eye," is a deficit of visual acuity that cannot be corrected with glasses. *Amblyopia* is derived from the Greek word for "blunt or dull sight." The loss can occur in childhood. The brain depends on receiving simultaneous clear focused images from both eyes for the visual pathways to de-

CLINICAL IMPLICATIONS
Amblyopia—A Preventable Loss of Vision

Deprivation of visual input during a critical period can lead to a permanent visual deficit. There are three critical periods for visual acuity: during development from early gestation through 3 to 5 years of age; during a period of deprivation, possible from the first few months to 7 to 8 years of age; and during the recovery period from the time of deprivation into adulthood (Daw, 1998). Many motor and sensory conditions can lead to amblyopia, including strabismus, myopia, astigmatism, cataract, and refractive differences between the two eyes.

Prevention Focuses

- Screening of all children 3 to 4 years of age for amblyopia and strabismus (American Academy of Pediatrics, 1996; US Preventive Services Task Force, 1996); despite a prevalence of 2% to 5% (US Preventive Services Task Force, 1996), many children are not screened
- Development of a gold standard ophthalmologic examination including measurement of visual acuity (Kemper et al, 1999)
- Continued review of screening tests for reliability and validity within primary care settings (Kemper et al, 1999)

velop properly (American Academy of Pediatrics, 1996). Because of difficulty in producing a single image when looking with both eyes, the person with amblyopia elects to see with only one eye to see one image. The lazy eye, if deprived of visual input for sufficient time, will lose sight, and the child will become functionally blind because of a lack of visual cortex development. This problem may be associated with an eye that is deviated in any direction—in, out, up, or down—a condition known as *strabismus*. However, strabismus is not necessarily a cause of amblyopia. In addition, the use of only one eye may not be apparent unless screening is conducted

Amblyopia is the leading cause of loss of vision in one eye in adults between the ages of 20 and 70 (Simmons, 1996). The potential for loss of vision occurs during critical periods in the postnatal development of the visual system. Maturation of the visual system is activity dependent; that is, the eye must be exposed to sensory stimulation to complete its development (see Clinical Implications: Amblyopia—A Preventable Loss of Vision).

Macular Degeneration

The macula is the part of the eye where the most acute vision occurs because it contains the fovea, the central focusing point of the optic system. Age-related maculopathy is more likely to be seen after age 50 (Kliffen et al, 1997). With aging, vascular and nutritional changes can affect the function of the macula. Age-related macular degeneration (AMD) is the late stage of age-related maculopathy and has a prevalence of 15% in adults over the age of 85 (Patten and Craik, 2000). Macular degeneration is the most common cause of irreversible loss of eyesight late in life (Duthie and Katz, 1998).

Clinically, the early stage of AMD is marked by the presence of *drusen,* which are extracellular deposits and pigment abnormalities in the retinal pigment epithelium. There are two types of AMD: a "wet" type and a "dry" type. The latter is much less common, accounting for about 20% of legal blindness (Berger et al, 1999). The dry type is also referred to as *geographic atrophy.* It is responsible for a large number of cases of moderate visual loss in older adults. The wet type includes choroidal neovascularization, pigment epithelial detachment, and disciform scarring. The wet and dry types are seen in late-stage AMD, which is associated with moderate to severe loss of vision (Berger et al, 1999). AMD has no known definitive pathogenesis, although oxidative damage to the retinal pigment epithelium has been hypothesized as a cause. The link between oxidation-induced events and the onset and progression of AMD remains unclear (Winkler et al, 1999).

Macular degeneration begins differently in every person. Some common symptoms include a gradual loss of the ability to see objects clearly, distorted vision, a gradual loss of clear color vision, and a dark or empty area in the center of vision. These symptoms are not unique to AMD but do indicate the need to seek professional assessment. The Amsler grid is an early detection chart that may be used independently, alerting the clinician to changes in vision that should be assessed by an optometrist (Fig. 10–9). The wet type of AMD is caused by the leakage of newly formed blood vessels into the eye. If it is detected early, it can be treated with laser therapy. There is no way to restore central vision once it is lost, but peripheral vision is not damaged and low vision aids can be helpful. It is important to be aware of risk factors and potential prevention strategies (see Clinical Implications: Macular Degeneration—Who Is at Risk?).

Driving

Retention of the ability to drive in older adulthood is a significant quality of life issue. In one study, a group of older adults who chose to stop driving reported experiencing loneliness and isolation as consequences (Johnson, 1998). Healthy older adult drivers drive more slowly, which could reflect their insight into their own limitations (Fitten et al, 1995). Although some report driving skills are preserved in healthy older persons (Carr et al, 1992), others have documented that older healthy drivers make fewer steering corrections and eye-movement excursions than do younger drivers (Perryman and Fitten, 1996).

Three categories of age-related changes can affect driving: sensory, cognitive, and motor function (Table 10–6). Driving is a very visual task. Decline in visual acuity, contrast sensitivity, visual attention, and useful field of view are frequently mentioned as reasons for impaired performance of motor vehicle operational skills (Duthie and Katz, 1998; Owsley and McGwin, 1999; Perryman and Fitten, 1996). *Useful field of view* is defined as "the area of the visual field that is functional for an observer at a given time and for a given task"

CLINICAL IMPLICATIONS
Macular Degeneration—Who Is at Risk?

Age-related macular degeneration (AMD) is the leading cause of legal blindness among older adults in the United States and Europe (Evans and Wormald, 1996; Klein et al, 1995). Unfortunately, few of the many potential risk factors are modifiable. Increased public awareness of AMD as a common cause of irreversible loss of eyesight in older adults may promote further research into the prevention of blindness.

Risk Factors

- *Age:* Women 75 years old or older are twice as likely to develop early AMD and have a seven times greater incidence of later AMD (Klein et al, 1997).
- *Race:* Blacks have a lower prevalence rate than whites (Berger et al, 1999).
- *Heredity:* A positive family history (parent or sibling with AMD) is a strong predictor; Myers (1994) found 100% concordance among identical twins with AMD.
- *Environment:* Cigarette smoking increases the risk (Klein et al, 1998); Hammond and colleagues (1996) found an inverse relationship between cigarette smoking and macular pigment density; light exposure data are inconclusive, but it has been difficult to study lifetime effects of light exposure.

Potential Prevention Strategies

- Wear sunglasses, coated to filter out ultraviolet light, at all times when in the sun.
- Increase intake of carotenoids (sources of vitamin A), which have been found to have a protective effect against AMD (Berger et al, 1999). The consumption of foods rich in carotenoids, such as corn and spinach, promoted the elevation of macular pigment density (Hammond et al, 1997).
- Have regular vision assessments.
- Use an Amsler grid as a means to detect early AMD in those at risk and to recognize progression if already diagnosed (see Fig. 10–9).
- Take a good multivitamin.

(Coren et al, 1999, p 493). The useful field of view becomes smaller in older adults when distractions are present, making visual search less efficient. The presence of cataracts or glaucoma can also restrict an elder's driving and decrease driver safety (McGwin et al, 1998; Owsley et al, 1999).

Cognitive impairments, especially those related to Alzheimer's disease, are associated with an increased risk in driving (Duthie and Katz, 1998). Someone with Alzheimer's disease can be easily distracted, not remember where he or she is going, and may even have a greater decrease in visual-spatial processing and orientation. Drivers with Alzheimer's disease tend to drive faster than do older adults without Alzheimer's disease (Fitten et al, 1995).

Perceptual-motor performance declines as evidenced by a decrease in reaction time. This may be related to difficulty sustaining attention or managing

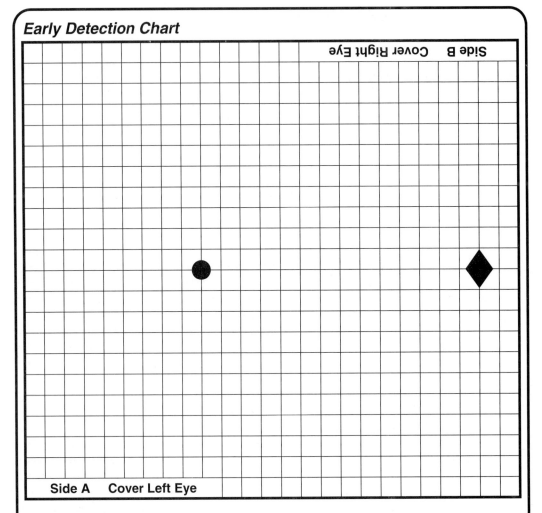

Early Detection Chart

Side B   Cover Right Eye

Side A   Cover Left Eye

Directions for using the chart:

1. Wear your reading glasses or bifocals and have good lighting on card. Hold card facing you so you can read side A. Cover your left eye.

2. Hold card at arm's length and stare only at small dot while bringing chart toward your eye.

3. Pull the card toward you until the large "◆" disappears from view. The lines should look straight and black.

4. If lines appear wavy, grey or fuzzy, draw on top of them and show chart to your optometrist.

5. Turn card upside down to read side B. Close your right eye and follow steps 2, 3 and 4.

Be sure to call your optometrist immediately if you notice a change, or if you don't understand how to use the chart. This screening test does not replace a thorough eye examination by your optometrist.

 American Optometric Association
243 North Lindbergh Blvd., St. Louis, MO 63141

Figure 10–9

Amsler Grid: Early Detection Chart. (From the American Optometric Association.)

TABLE 10–6

Age-Related Physiological Changes That May Affect Driving

Sensory Changes	Cognitive Changes	Psychomotor Changes
Presbycusis (hearing loss)	Distraction by irrelevant stimuli	Slowed speed of behavior
Visual decrements in	Memory retrieval impairment	Decreased reaction time
Static visual acuity	Decline in spatial orientation	Declines* in
Acuity under low illumination	Decreased visual searching	Strength
Resistance to glare	Decreased visuomotor integra-	Range of motion
Contrast sensitivity (static and	tion	Trunk and neck mobility
dynamic)		Proprioception
Visual fields		
Depth perception		

*The contribution of age-related changes versus deconditioning and diseases remains unclear. From Reuben DR. Driving. In Duthie EH Jr, Katz PR. *Practice of Geriatrics,* 3rd ed. Philadelphia: WB Saunders, 1998, p 58.

divided attention for the many visually related driving tasks. A decline in the function of any sensory system, whether peripheral (as in the eye with changes in lens accommodation) or central (as with the processing of sensory information), results in the modification of motor behavior. A decline of visual acuity to 20/50 or less means restriction from driving. The implications of visual difficulties for the ability of the individual to drive (especially at night), to be mobile on uneven terrain, or to be in unfamiliar environments are vast. The impact of the loss of mobility, both real and perceived, can substantially affect an individual's self-image.

Safety is always a concern for older adults. As individuals live longer, there will be greater numbers of geriatric drivers. Remaining independent requires the ability to get to and from the physician's office, grocery store, and friends' and relatives' homes. Maintaining independence by being able to come and go whenever the need arises is important to the average elder. Older drivers are less likely to drive under compromising visual conditions such as at night or in inclement weather. Are older drivers safe? Older drivers have a high crash rate per vehicle mile of travel (McGwin et al, 1998). They are more likely to be fatally injured when involved in a vehicular crash (Cobb and Coughlin, 1997). Difficulty with seeing instrument panels, dealing with glare and haze, and judging vehicle speed have also been reported by older drivers (Scialfa and Thomas, 1994). Because so many problems are related to visually related driving tasks, some states have initiated the use of state-mandated tests of visual acuity in 70-year-old drivers. The testing has been associated with lower fatal crash rates (Levy et al, 1995).

Summary

Sensory input plays an important role in the learning and refinement of movement. The integration of multiple sensory input and the association-coordination of sensory and motor information form the basis for cognition and perception. Sensory input from the external environment initiates the activity that shapes synaptic connections. The autonomic nervous system and the reticular system act as gatekeepers, determining which sensory information reaches consciousness and which is dampened. The thalamus is a central relay station that directs the flow of sensory information to association cortices. All sensory systems have similar characteristics: transduction and coding, representation, and integration at all levels of the nervous system. Sensory systems develop early in utero to be ready to function at birth. Some, such as vision and hearing, must have additional input to completely develop the neural pathway. Sensory abilities change with age; deficits in any sensory system, whether from congenital absence, trauma, or decline with age, can result in functional impairment of movement. Presbyastasis, presbyopia, and presbycusis are all seen in older adults but not to the same degree in all individuals. Age-related changes in the sensory systems, therefore, are neither uniform nor universal.

References

Allison T, Hume AL, Wood CC, Golf WR. Developmental and aging changes in somatosensory, auditory and visual evoked potentials. *Electroencephalogr Clin Neurophysiol* 58:14–24, 1984.

Almli CR, Mohr NM. Normal sequential behavioral and physiological change throughout the developmental arc. In Umphred DA (ed). *Neurological Rehabilitation,* 3rd ed. St. Louis: Mosby, 1995, pp 33–65.

American Academy of Pediatrics, Committee on Practice and Ambulatory Medicine, Section on Ophthalmology. Eye examination and vision screening in infants, children, and young adults. *Pediatrics* 98:153–157, 1996.

Anand KJ, Hickey PR. Pain and its effect in the human neonate and fetus. *N Engl J Med* 31:1321–1329, 1987.

Aslin RN. Development of smooth pursuit in human infants. In Fisher DF, Monty RA, Senders JW (eds). *Eye Movements: Cognition and Visual Perception.* Hillsdale, NJ: Erlbaum, 1981, pp 31–51.

Ayres AJ. *Sensory Integration and Learning Disorders.* Los Angeles: Western Psychological Services, 1972.

Ayres AJ. *Sensory Integration and Praxis Tests.* Los Angeles: Western Psychological Services, 1989.

Barrett DS, Cobb AG, Bently G. Joint proprioception in normal, osteoarthritic and replaced knees. *J Bone Joint Surg* 73B:53–56, 1991.

Beauchamp GK, Cowart BJ, Schmidt HJ. Development of chemosensory sensitivity and preference. In Getchell TV, Doty RL, Bartoshuk LM, Snow JB Jr (eds). *Smell and Taste in Health and Disease.* New York: Raven Press, 1991, pp 405–416.

Berger JW, Fine SL, Maguire MG. *Age-Related Macular Degeneration.* St. Louis: Mosby, 1999.

Bergstrom B. Morphology of the vestibular nerve: III. Analysis of the myelinated vestibular nerve fibers in man at various ages. *Acta Otolaryngol* 76:331–338, 1973.

Bertenthal BI, Rose JL, Bai DL. Perception-action coupling in the development of visual control of posture. *J Exp Psych* 23:1631–1643, 1997.

Bigelow A. The correspondence between self and image movement as a cue to self-recognition for young children. *J Genet Psychol* 139:11–26, 1981.

Birnholz JC, Benacerraf BR. The development of human fetal hearing. *Science* 222:516–518, 1983.

Boyd IA. The isolated mammalian muscle spindle. In Evarts EV, Wise SP, Bousfield D (eds). *The Motor System in Neurobiology.* New York: Elsevier, 1985, pp 154–167.

Butterworth GE, Ciccheti D. Visual calibration of posture in normal and motor retarded Down's syndrome infants. *Perception* 7:513–525, 1978.

Butterworth GE, Hicks L. Visual proprioception and postural stability in infants: A developmental study. *Perception* 6:255–262, 1977.

Carr D, Jackson WJ, Madden DJ, Cohen HJ. The effect of age on driving skills. *J Am Geriatr Soc* 40: 567–573, 1992.

Cleary BL. Age-related changes in the special senses. In Matteson MA, McConnell ES, Linton AD (eds). *Gerontological Nursing*, 2nd ed. Philadelphia: WB Saunders, 1997, pp 385–405.

Cobb RW, Coughlin JF. Regulating older drivers: How are the states coping? *J Aging Soc Policy* 9: 71–87, 1997.

Cohen H, Friedman EM, Lai D, et al. Balance in children with otitis media with effusion. *Int J Pediatr Otorhinolaryngol* 42:107–115, 1997.

Collins JK. Distance perception as a function of age. *Aust J Psychol* 28:109–113, 1976.

Coren S, Ward LM, Enns JT. *Sensation and Perception*, 5th ed. Fort Worth: Harcourt, 1999.

Corso JF. *Aging, Sensory Systems, and Perception*. New York: Praeger, 1981.

Craig KD, Whitfield MF, Grunau RVE, et al. Pain in the preterm neonate: Behavioral and physiological indices. *Pain* 52:238–299, 1993.

Daw NW. Critical periods and amblyopia. *Arch Ophthalmol* 116:502–505, 1998.

Duncan G, Wilson JA, MacLennen WJ, Lewis S. Clinical correlates of sway in elderly people living at home. *Gerontology* 38:160–166, 1992

Duthie EH, Katz PR. *Practice of Geriatrics*, 3rd ed. Philadelphia: WB Saunders, 1998.

Effgen SK. Effect of an exercise program on the static balance of deaf children. *Phys Ther* 61:873–877, 1981.

Eliot L. *What's Going On in There? How the Brain and Mind Work the First Five Years of Life*. New York: Bantam, 1999.

Elliot JM, Connolly KJ, Doyle AJR. Development of kinaesthetic sensitivity and motor performance in children. *Dev Med Child Neurol* 30:80–92, 1988.

Evans J, Wormald R. Is the incidence of registrable age-related macular degeneration increasing? *Br J Ophthalmol* 99:933–943, 1996.

Eviatar L, Eviatar A. The normal nystagmic response of infants to caloric and perrotatory stimulation. *Laryngoscope* 89:1036–1044, 1979.

Eviatar L, Eviatar A, Naaray I. Maturation of neurovestibular responses in infants. *Dev Med Child Neurol* 16:435–446, 1974.

Finkelstein JA, Schiffman SS. Workshop on taste and smell in the elderly: An overview. *Physiol Behav* 66:173–176, 1999.

Fisher AG, Murray EA, Bundy AC (eds). *Sensory Integration: Theory and Practice*. Philadelphia: FA Davis, 1991.

Fitten LF, Perryman KM, Wilkinson CJ, et al. Alzheimer and vascular dementias and driving: A prospective road and laboratory study. *JAMA* 273:1360–1365, 1995.

Gabbard CP. *Lifelong Motor Development*, 2nd ed. Dubuque, IA: Brown and Benchmark, 1996.

Gibson JJ. *The Senses as Perceptual Systems*. Boston: Houghton-Mifflin, 1966.

Gottfried AW, Rose SA. Tactile recognition in infants. *Child Dev* 51:69–74, 1980.

Gunnar M, Fisch,R, Korsvik S, Donhowe JM. The effects of circumcision on serum cortisol and behavior. *Psychoneuroendocrinology* 6:269–275, 1981.

Guyton AC, Hall JE. *Textbook of Medical Physiology*, 8th ed. Philadelphia: WB Saunders, 1996.

Hammond BR Jr, Johnson EF, Russell RM, et al. Dietary modification of human macular pigment density. *Invest Ophthalmol Vis Sci* 38:1795–1801, 1997.

Hammond BR Jr, Wooten BR, Snodderly DM. Cigarette smoking and retinal carotenoids: Implications for age-related macular degeneration. *Vision Res* 36:3003–3009, 1996.

Harkins SW, Price DD, Martelli M. Effects of age on pain perception: Hermonociception. *J Gerontol* 41:58–63, 1986.

Haywood KM. Eye movements during coincidence-anticipation performance. *J Motor Behav* 9:313–318, 1977.

Hermann RP, Novak CB, Mackinnon SE. Establishing normal values of moving two-point discrimination in children and adolescents. *Dev Med Child Neurol* 38:255–261, 1996.

Hooker D. *The Prenatal Origin of Behavior*. Lawrence, KS: University of Kansas Press, 1952.

Horak FB, Shumway-Cook A, Crowe TK, Black FO. Vestibular function and motor proficiency of children with impaired hearing or with learning disability and motor impairments. *Dev Med Child Neurol* 30:64–79, 1988.

Humphrey T. The embryologic differentiation of the vestibular nuclei in man correlated with functional development. In *International Symposium on Vestibular and Oculomotor Problems*. Tokyo, 1965, p 51.

Jan JE, Sykanda A, Groenveld M. Habilitation and rehabilitation of visually impaired and blind children. *Pediatrician* 17:202–207, 1990.

Johnson JE. Urban older adults and the forfeiture of a driver's license. *J Gerontol Nurs* 25:12–18, 1998.

Kaga K. Vestibular compensation in infants and children with congenital and acquired vestibular loss in both ears. *Otorhinolaryngology* 49:215–224, 1999.

Kandel ER, Schwartz JH, Jessell TM. *Principles of Neural Science*, 4th ed. New York: McGraw-Hill, 2000.

Kaplan FS, Nixon JE, Reitz M, et al. Age-related changes in proprioception and sensation of joint position. *Acta Orthop Scand* 56:72–74, 1985.

Katzman R, Terry RD. *The Neurology of Aging*. Philadelphia: FA Davis, 1983.

Kaye H, Lipsitt L. Relationship of electro to actual threshold to basal skin conductance. *Child Dev* 35:1307–1312, 1964.

Kemper AR, Margolis PA, Downs SM, Bordley WC. A systematic review of vision screening tests for the detection of amblyopia. *Pediatrics* 104:1220–1222, 1999.

Kennedy R, Clemis JD. The geriatric auditory and vestibular system. *Otolaryngol Clin North Am* 23: 1075–1082, 1990.

Kenshalo DR. Age changes in touch, vibration, temperature, kinesthesis, and pain sensitivity. In Birren JE, Schaie KW (eds). *Handbook of Psychology of Aging*. New York: Van Nostrand Reinhold, 1977, pp 562–579.

Klein R, Klein BE, Jensen SC, Meuer SM. The five-year incidence and progression of age-related maculopathy: The Beaver Dam Eye Study. *Ophthalmology* 104:7–21, 1997.

Klein R, Klein BEK, Moss SE. Relation of smoking to the incidence of age-related maculopathy: The Beaver Dam Eye Study. *Am J Epidemiol* 147:103–110, 1998.

Klein R, Wang O, Klein BE, et al. The relationship of age-related maculopathy, cataract, and glaucoma to visual acuity. *Invest Ophthalmol Vis Sci* 36:182–191, 1995.

Kliffen M, van der Schaft TL, Mooy CM, de Jong PT. Morphologic changes in age-related maculopathy. *Microsc Res Tech* 36:106–112, 1997.

Lasky RE. The effect of visual feedback of the hand on the reaching and retrieval behaviour of young infants. *Child Dev* 48:112–117, 1977.

Lee DN, Aaronson E. Visual proprioceptive control of standing in infants. *Percept Psychophys* 15: 529–532, 1974.

Levy DT, Vernick JS, Howard KA. Relationship between driver's license renewal policies and fatal crashes involving drivers 70 years or older. *JAMA* 274:1026–1030, 1995.

Locke J. A theory of neurolinguistic development. *Brain Language* 58:265–326, 1997.

Long AB, Looft WR. Development of directionality in children: Ages six through twelve. *Dev Psychol* 6:375–380, 1972.

Lopez I, Honrubia V, Baloh RW. Aging and the vestibular nucleus. *J Vest Res* 7:77–85, 1997.

Lord SR, Ward JA, Williams P, Anstey KJ. Physiological factors associated with falls in older community-dwelling women. *J Am Geriatr Soc* 42:1110–1117, 1994.

Lowrey GH. *Growth and Development of Children*, 8th ed. Chicago: Year Book, 1986.

MacFarlane A. Olfaction in the development of social preferences in the human neonate. *Ciba Found Symp* 33:103–113, 1975.

Matthews PBC. Proprioceptors and their contribution to somatosensory mapping: Complex messages require complex processing. *Can J Physiol Pharmacol* 66:430–438, 1988.

McGwin G Jr, Owsley C, Ball K. Identifying crash involvement among older drivers: Agreement between self-report and state records. *Accid Anal Prev* 30:781–791, 1998.

Meisami E. Aging of the sensory systems. In Timiras PS. *Physiological Basis of Aging and Geriatrics*, 2nd ed. Boca Raton, FL: CRC Press, 1994, pp 115–132.

Meisami E, Timiras PS. *Handbook of Human Growth and Developmental Biology*, Vol I, part B. Boca Raton, FL: CRC Press, 1988.

Meltzoff AN, Borton R. Intermodal matching by human neonates. *Nature* 282:403–404, 1979.

Meltzoff AN, Moore MK. Imitation of facial and manual gestures by human neonates. *Science* 198: 75–78, 1977.

Merchut MT, Toleikis SC. Aging and quantitative sensory thresholds. *Electromyogr Clin Neurophysiol* 30:293–297, 1990.

Milani-Comparetti A. The neurophysiological and clinical implications of studies on fetal motor behavior. *Semin Perinatol* 5:183–189, 1981.

Miller IJ. Human taste bud density across adult age groups. *J Gerontol Biol Sci* 43:26–30, 1988.

Morgan R, Rochat P. Intermodal calibration of the body in early infancy. *Ecol Psychol* 9:1–24, 1997.

Myers SM. A twin study on age-related macular degeneration. *Trans Am Ophthalmol Soc* 92:775–844, 1994.

Nougier V, Bard C, Fleury M, Teasdale N. Contribution of central and peripheral vision to the regulation of stance: Developmental aspects. *J Exp Child Psychol* 68:202–215, 1998.

Ochs A, Newberry J, Lenhardt M, et al. Neural and vestibular aging associated with falls. In Birren JE, Schaie KW (eds). *Handbook of the Psychology of Aging*, 2nd ed. New York: Van Nostrand Reinhold, 1985, pp 378–399.

Ornitz EM. Normal and pathological maturation of vestibular function in the human child. In Romand R (ed). *Development of Auditory and Vestibular Systems*. New York: Academic Press, 1983, pp 479–536.

Ornitz EM, Atwell CW, Walter DO, et al. The maturation of vestibular nystagmus in infancy and childhood. *Acta Otolaryngol* 88:244–256, 1979.

Owsley C, McGwin G Jr. Vision impairment and driving. *Surv Ophthalmol* 43:535–550, 1999.

Owsley C, Stalvey B, Wells J, Sloane ME. Older drivers and cataract: Driving habits and crash risk. *J Gerontol A Biol Sci Med Sci* 54:M203–M211, 1999.

Patten C, Craik RL. Sensorimotor changes and adaptation in the older adult. In Guccione AA (ed). *Geriatric Physical Therapy*, 2nd ed. Philadelphia: WB Saunders, 2000, pp 78–109.

Perryman KM, Fitten LJ. Effects of normal aging on the performance of motor-vehicle operational skills. *J Geriatr Psychiatry Neurol* 9:136–141, 1996.

Piaget J. *Origins of Intelligence*. New York: International University Press, 1952.

Pitts DG. Visual function as a function of age. *J Am Optom Assoc* 53:117–124, 1982.

Prechtl HFR. The directed head turning response and allied movements of the human baby. *Behavior* 13:212–242, 1958.

Prechtl HFR. Behavioral states of the newborn infant (a review). *Brain Res* 76:185–212, 1974.

Rine RM, Cornwall G, Gan K, et al. Evidence of progressive delay of motor development in children with sensorineural hearing loss and concurrent vestibular dysfunction. *Percept Mot Skills* 90:1101–1112, 2000.

Ring C, Nayak USL, Isaacs B. The effect of visual deprivation and proprioceptive change on postural sway in healthy adults. *J Am Geriatr Soc* 37:745–749, 1989.

Rochat P. Self-perception and action in infancy. *Exp Brain Res* 123:102–109, 1998.

Rochat P, Hespos SJ. Differential rooting response by neonates: Evidence for an early sense of self. *Early Dev Parent* 6:105–112, 1997.

Rochat P, Morgan R. Spatial determinants in the perception of self-produced leg movements by 3–5 month-old infants. *Dev Psychol* 31:626–636, 1995.

Rolls BJ. Do chemosensory changes influence food intake in the elderly? *Physiol Behav* 66:193–197, 1999.

Rose SA. From hand to eye: Findings and issues in infant cross-modal transfer. In Lewkowicz DJ, Lickliter R (eds). *The Development of Intersensory Perception*. Hillsdale, NJ: Erlbaum, 1994, pp 265–284.

Sahoo SK. Novelty and complexity in human infants' exploratory behavior. *Percept Mot Skills* 86: 698, 1998.

Salapatek P, Cohen L. *Handbook of Infant Perception: From Sensation to Perception*. New York: Academic Press, 1987.

Scialfa CT, Thomas DM. Age differences in same-different judgments as a function of multidimensional similarity. *J Gerontol* 49:P173–P178, 1994.

Schiffman SS. Taste and smell losses in normal aging and disease. *JAMA* 278:1357–1362, 1997.

Shimojo SJ, Bauer J, O'Connell KM, Held R. Pre-stereoptic binocular vision in infants. *Vision Res* 26:501–510, 1986.

Ship J. The influence of aging on oral health and consequences for taste and smell. *Physiol Behav* 66:209–215, 1999.

Shumway-Cook A, Woollacott MH. *Motor Control: Theory and Practical Applications.* Baltimore: Williams & Wilkins, 1995.

Simmons K. Preschool vision screening: Rationale, methodology and outcome. *Surg Ophthalmol* 41: 3–30, 1996.

Skinner HB, Barrack RL, Cook SD. Age-related decline in proprioception. *Clin Orthop Rel Res* 184: 208–211, 1984.

Smith SL, Gossman M, Canan BC. Selected primitive reflexes in children with cerebral palsy: Consistency of response. *Phys Ther* 62:1115–1120, 1982.

Steiner JE. Human facial expression in response to taste and smell stimulation. *Adv Child Dev* 13: 257–295, 1979.

Steiness I. Vibratory perception in normal subjects. *Acta Med Scand* 158:315–325, 1957.

Sugden DA. The development of proprioceptive control. In Whiting HTA, Wade MG (eds). *Themes in Motor Development.* Boston: Nijhoff, 1986, pp 21–39.

Sundermier L, Woollacott MH. The influence of vision on the automatic postural muscle responses of newly standing and newly walking infants. *Exp Brain Res* 120:537–540, 1998.

Thelen E. Motor development: A new synthesis. *Am Psychol* 50:79–95, 1995.

Timiras PS. *Physiological Basis of Aging and Geriatrics.* Boca Raton, FL: CRC Press, 1994.

Umphred DA. *Neurological Rehabilitation*, 3rd ed. St. Louis: Mosby, 1995.

US Preventive Services Task Force. *Guide to Clinical Preventive Services,* 2nd ed. Alexandria, VA: International Medical Publishing, 1996.

Von Hofsten C. Development of visually directed reaching: The approach phase. *J Hum Mov Stud* 5:160–178, 1979.

Weale RA. Senile changes in visual acuity. *Trans Ophthalmol Soc UK* 95:36–38, 1975.

Weiffenbach JM, Bartoshuk LM. Taste and smell. *Clin Geriatr Med* 8:543–555, 1992.

Weisenberger JM. Touch and proprioception. In Birren JE (ed). *Encyclopedia of Gerontology*, Vol 2. San Diego: Academic Press, 1996, pp 591–603.

Werner LA, Marean GC. *Human Auditory Development.* Boulder, CO: Westview Press, 1996.

Williams HG. *Perceptual and Motor Development.* Englewood Cliffs, NJ: Prentice Hall, 1983.

Williams HG. Aging and eye-hand coordination. In Bard C, Fleury M, Hay L (eds). *Development of Eye-Hand Coordination.* Columbia, SC: University of South Carolina Press, 1990, pp 327–357.

Windle WF. *Physiology of the Fetus.* Philadelphia: WB Saunders, 1940.

Wingfield A, Poon LW, Lombardi L, Lowe D. Speed of processing in normal aging: Effects of speech rate, linguistic structure and processing time. *J Gerontol* 40:579–585, 1985.

Winkler BS, Boulton ME, Gottsch JD, Sternberg P. Oxidative damage and age-related macular degeneration. Available at http://www.molvis/v5/p32/. Accessed 1999.

Wolfson L, Whipple R, Derby CA, et al. A dynamic posturography study of balance in healthy elderly. *Neurology* 42:2069–2075, 1992.

Wyke B. The neurological basis of movement: A developmental review. In Holt KS (ed). *Movement and Child Development.* Philadelphia: JB Lippincott, 1975, pp 19–33.

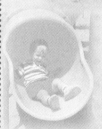

Functional
Movement
Outcomes

Vital Functions

OBJECTIVES

After studying this chapter, the reader will be able to:

1 Describe vital human functions.

2 Define homeostasis.

3 Identify the systems involved in vital functions.

4 Describe the role of the endocrine system in vital functions.

5 Discuss changes in vital functions across the life span.

6 Understand the interactions between vital functions.

We define vital functions as those functions necessary for survival. In humans, vital functions are breathing, sleeping, eating, and eliminating. All of these functions involve multiple systems of the body. And these systems interact to produce functions that support our ability to explore the environment and to experience life. Homeostasis also is important to vital functions because it is the process that keeps the internal environment constant or in balance.

The four vital functions—breathing, sleeping, eating, and eliminating— can be broken down into six processes: ventilation-respiration, sleep-wakefulness, ingestion, digestion, absorption, and excretion. All processes must occur for life to be sustained.

These processes and functions are cyclical. Each process has a rhythm or occurs in a cycle. Breathing brings air in and lets carbon dioxide out; wakefulness and sleep occur in patterns that generally correspond to day and night; food and water are ingested and wastes are eliminated. Circadian rhythms (from *circa*, which means "about," and *dies*, which means "day") are innately directed rhythms that occur every 24 hours. These rhythms affect all aspects of human physiology. Easily recognizable rhythms include the sleep-wake cycle and the cyclical release of hormones. Biologically, the cycles of change seen in these vital functions make it easier to adapt to different environments.

The cyclical nature of the vital functions provides a clue to their control and a way to explain behavior. Hormonal control of cyclical vital functions is mediated by the autonomic nervous system and the endocrine system, which together maintain the body's internal homeostasis. The circadian timing system is a neural system composed of a biological clock with input and output pathways. The central nervous system site of the biological clock in humans is found in the anterior hypothalamus (Moore, 1999; Rivkees, 1997).

The hypothalamus and its related structures oversee the vegetative functions of the brain such as body temperature, thirst and satiation centers, and osmolality of body fluids. These functions are vital to the maintenance of homeostasis and represent basic physiological needs. The human species has a need to drink and to take in salt, to maintain body temperature, to eat, to reproduce, and to respond to stress (Iverson et al, 2000). These basic physiological drives ensure the survival of the species.

The control of vegetative functions is therefore closely related to behavior. In addition to its major role in controlling vegetative and endocrine functions of the body, the hypothalamus controls many aspects of emotional behavior. Because the hypothalamus is a major part of the limbic system, it is not surprising that our emotional state can and does affect basic bodily functions. Homeostasis is disrupted by our thoughts, emotion, and stress, which are manifested in physiological changes in vegetative functions, as anyone nervously waiting for an important interview can attest. The hypothalamus directs its actions through the endocrine and autonomic nervous systems. The latter is discussed in Chapter 9, and the endocrine system is discussed here.

Endocrine System

The endocrine system consists of a collection of glands that manufacture and secrete hormones into the bloodstream. These chemical messengers affect various cells of the body and regulate many aspects of physiological function. The endocrine system plays a role in the rate of growth, basal metabolic rate, stress responses, and reproduction. The endocrine system is second only to the nervous system in terms of its ability to act as a major communication system. It is composed of the pituitary gland, thyroid, parathyroid, adrenal cortex, adrenal medulla, islet cells of the pancreas, secretory cells in the intestines, and the gonads. The hypothalamus is also considered part of the endocrine system because it releases hormones that control the activity of the pituitary gland.

The hypothalamus monitors physiological set points for almost every internal body function. For example, there are set point values for body temperature, blood glucose levels, blood pressure, and salt concentration in the blood. If these values are under or over the normal range, sensing mechanisms relay information to the hypothalamus or subsystems under its control and steps are taken to correct the error. Negative feedback is the most common way in which values are corrected. Set points for regulated variables can be changed or reset. Set points can be changed by external or internal stimuli. Some set points, such as body temperature, display a circadian rhythm; body temperature is higher during the day than during the night.

HOMEOSTATIC CONTROL MECHANISMS

Reflexes control some endocrine functions. A stimulus is received that is interpreted as an error by an integrating center. The integrating center stimulates an effector, which is typically a muscle or a gland, which in turn produces a response that corrects the error, reestablishing homeostasis. The muscle may act to change blood flow to an area to prevent heat loss. The hypothalamus relays commands to the autonomic nervous system to activate heat-gain or heat-loss mechanisms. When an increase in blood sugar is detected, insulin is secreted by the pancreas. The level of glucose in the blood declines and insulin secretion ceases. Negative feedback systems are corrective by nature. An error must be detected for the system to be engaged.

Another way in which homeostasis is controlled by the endocrine system is by local responses. Local homeostatic responses occur within the tissues. For example, skin is damaged by a puncture. The damaged cells in the area release chemicals that assist in preventing further injury. Chemical messengers are used in reflex and local homeostatic responses. There are many categories of chemical messengers. An example of a chemical messenger is human growth factor; there are at least 50 growth factors, so they represent a family of chemical messengers (see Guyton and Hall, 1996, for additional information).

Circadian rhythms provide an anticipatory facet to homeostasis. These rhythms are internally driven by hormones and entrained by external factors. One of the strongest of these cues is the duration of light and dark. Even in the absence of cues, however, the rhythms run free, that is, they maintain the cycle. A biological rhythm is an example of a feedforward system that operates without detectors.

ENDOCRINE CHANGES ACROSS THE LIFE SPAN

Hormones and their roles in growth and development, response to stress, and effects of aging are associated with our body's responses and change as we mature (Tables 11–1 and 11–2).

Prenatal

The endocrine system does play a role in growth in utero after the end of the second month of gestation. The first endocrine gland to form in utero is the thyroid, at 24 days (Moore and Persaud, 1998). The pituitary forms at 4 weeks and is composed of ectoderm from two different sources, which explains why there are two different tissue types (glandular and neural) composing the gland. The function of these tissues contributes to the maximum rate of growth in height of the fetus seen around the fourth month of gestation (Sinclair and Dangerfield, 1998).

Growth hormone has little to no effect on the growth of the fetus in utero. Fetal growth is primarily nutrition dependent and therefore reliant on the mother's nutritional intake and the integrity of the placenta. The sex hormones also play no role in fetal growth.

Infancy Through Adolescence

Growth hormone is the main impetus for postnatal growth (Vander et al, 2001). Whereas it has no effect on fetal growth, growth hormone exerts a profound effect on cell proliferation in target tissues. Too much growth hor-

TABLE 11–1

Hormones Important to Human Growth and Development

Hormone	Function and Impact
Aldosterone	Aldosterone is secreted by the adrenal cortex. It affects how the kidneys handle sodium, potassium, and hydrogen ions. Aldosterone maintains a balance among sodium, water, and potassium. The renin-angiotensin system controls aldosterone secretion. Aldosterone is released during periods of physiological stress to retain water and sodium within the body.
Corticotropin (ACTH)	ACTH is secreted by the anterior pituitary. It improves the mobilization of fat as an energy source, increases the rate of glucose formation, and stimulates the breakdown of proteins. ACTH controls the secretion of cortisol by the adrenal cortex.
Cortisol	Cortisol is secreted by the adrenal cortex in response to stimulation by ACTH secreted from the anterior pituitary. Small amounts of cortisol are needed by the liver to form glucose and to break down stored fat. In this respect, its action is the opposite of insulin. In higher concentrations, cortisol mobilizes fuel sources. It is a stress hormone. Prolonged secretion can cause breakdown of bone and inhibit secretion of growth hormone (GH).
Estrogen	Estrogen is secreted by the ovaries during the follicular phase of the menstrual cycle. Estrogen has far-reaching effects that range from growth and development of the reproductive organs and secondary sex characteristics to protective effects on brain neurons and blood vessels. During puberty, it stimulates an increase in the secretion of GH and the closure of epiphyses.
Glucagon	Glucagon is secreted by the alpha islet cells of the pancreas. All of its effects are on the liver and are directly opposite those of insulin. It stimulates the formation of glucose from liver glycogen stores and amino acids. It also stimulates the breakdown of stored fats. Glucagon secretion increases during exercise to provide glucose to working muscles.
Growth hormone	GH is secreted by the anterior pituitary. It does not affect fetal growth, but it is the primary stimulus for growth from the postnatal period through adolescence. It promotes the maturation and cell division of chondrocytes in the epiphyseal plate, resulting in increased bone length. It stimulates protein synthesis, particularly in muscle. GH decreases the use of carbohydrates and increases the use of fat metabolism for energy production. Intensity and duration of exercise affect its secretion. GH secretion also increases with stress.
Insulin	Insulin is secreted by the beta islet cell of the pancreas. It promotes growth in the fetus by assisting cell differentiation and cell division. Insulin stimulates postnatal growth by causing secretion of insulin growth factor I and promoting protein synthesis. Insulin is the major hormone of metabolism. It is secreted in response to eating even before blood glucose levels rise. Insulin facilitates glucose uptake by muscle. It inhibits the effects of epinephrine and glucagon on fat metabolism. Last, insulin is secreted when blood glucose levels are too high.
Norepinephrine and epinephrine	These hormones are part of a group called catecholamines. Norepinephrine and epinephrine are secreted by the adrenal medulla. They have the same effect as sympathetic nervous system stimulation, but their effects last longer. They increase cardiac contractility, heart rate, and distribution of blood within the vascular system. Epinephrine has a great effect on tissue metabolism and can significantly increase the activity of the body. It increases the breakdown of stored fat into fatty acids and the production of glucose from glycogen in the liver and muscle. The effects of epinephrine on carbohydrate and fat metabolism are opposite those of insulin.

Continued

TABLE 11–1   Continued

Hormones Important to Human Growth and Development

Hormone	Function and Impact
Testosterone	Testosterone is secreted by the Leydig cells of the testes. Differentiation and later growth and function of accessory sex organs depend on testosterone. During puberty, it causes increased secretion of GH. It is needed for the initiation and maintenance of sperm formation and the inducement of secondary sex characteristics. Testosterone promotes protein anabolism, bone growth, and eventual epiphyseal closure.
Thyroid hormones	Thyroid hormones are secreted by the thyroid gland. These hormones are essential for the normal maturation of the nervous system in the fetus and infant. Postnatally, they facilitate secretion of and response to GH and support mental alertness. They are the primary determinant of the basal metabolic rate regardless of age, sex, or body size. Thyroid hormones have a calorigenic effect on the basal metabolic rate, that is, they can determine the rate at which the body produces heat. Last, thyroid hormones actively support the sympathetic nervous system by aiding the synthesis of beta receptors for norepinephrine and epinephrine.
Vasopressin	Antidiuretic hormone (ADH) is secreted by the posterior pituitary. Its secretion is controlled by osmoreceptors in the hypothalamus and the baroreceptors in the cardiovascular system. ADH determines the degree of permeability of the kidneys' collecting ducts, thereby determining the amount of water retained and the fluid volume. During stress or exercise, water retention is increased and fluid volume is maintained. ADH also stimulates secretion of ACTH.

mone can produce gigantism; too little, dwarfism. Secretion of human growth hormone controls the rate of growth and development. It sustains the normal rate of protein synthesis in the body and is needed for cartilage cell proliferation at the epiphyseal plates of bone.

Growth hormone works indirectly on cell division by influencing the liver to secrete insulin-like growth factor I. This growth factor in turn stimulates protein synthesis and impedes protein degradation. Insulin-like growth factor II is also a growth hormone, which plays a role in postnatal growth, but its exact function is unclear. A peak level of insulin-like growth factor is seen in adolescence. Growth hormone and insulin-like growth factor I levels are low during the day, but 1 to 2 hours after falling asleep, large amounts are secreted. The amount of growth hormone produced at night can represent 20% to 40% of the day's total output.

Thyroid and parathyroid hormones are important to the growth of bones, teeth, and the brain. Insufficient thyroid hormone results in retardation of bone growth. And the brain does not develop properly in utero without thyroid hormone. After birth, the effects of a deficit are apparent in sluggish thought processes or jitteriness resulting from excessive production. The amount of thyroid hormone secreted declines slightly from birth to puberty and then increases for an adolescent growth spurt. Parathyroid hormone is involved in maintaining calcium homeostasis by acting at three sites: the bones, the gastrointestinal (GI) tract, and the kidneys. This involvement continues throughout

TABLE 11–2

Hormonal Actions During Growth, Stress, and Aging

Hormone	Influence on Growth	Response to Stress	Effects of Aging
Growth hormone (GH)	Major postnatal growth stimulus Highest secretion in adolescence	Secretion increases	Secretion declines
Insulin	Stimulates fetal growth	Secretion declines	
Thyroid hormones	Needed for GH secretion in childhood and adolescence Needed for central nervous system development		Secretion declines Decreased target cell response
Estrogen	Increases GH at puberty Stimulates closure of epiphyses		Secretion declines, then ceases
Testosterone	Increases GH at puberty Stimulates eventual closure of epiphyses		Secretion declines
Cortisol	High concentrations inhibit growth Catabolizes protein		Levels maintained
Aldosterone		Secretion increases	Levels decline Adaptive response fails
Norepinephrine			Secretion increases
Epinephrine		Secretion increases	Unchanged in young-old Increased in old-old
Vasopressin (antidiuretic hormone)		Secretion increases	Increased sensitivity Decreased adaptive response with change in posture Decreased target cell response
Glucagon		Secretion increases	

Data from Davis PJ, Davis FB. Endocrine disorders. In Duthie EH, Katz PR (eds). *Practice of Geriatrics*. Philadelphia: WB Saunders, 1998, pp 563–578; Goodman CC, Boissannault WG. *Pathology: Implications for the Physical Therapist*. Philadelphia: WB Saunders, 1998; Purushothaman R, Morley JE. Endocrinology in the aged. In Gass GH, Kaplan HM (eds). *Handbook of Endocrinology*, 2nd ed. Boca Raton, FL: CRC Press, 1996, pp 241–260; Vander AF, Sherman JH, Luciano DS. *Human Psychology: The Mechanisms of Body Function*, 8th ed. New York: McGraw-Hill, 2001.

the life span. The thyroid hormones have an effect on dental development, so it is not surprising to find that skeletal maturity and dental maturity are usually correlated.

The earliest signs of puberty—the acquisition of axillary and pubic hair—are a result of increased secretion of androgens by the adrenal gland. The adrenal gland is directed to secrete androgens by corticotropin released from the pituitary. The adrenal androgens also play a major part in directing the course of the adolescent growth spurt in both sexes. The remaining changes that occur during puberty are the result of increased activity within the hypothalamic anterior pituitary system.

The hypothalamus produces increased amounts of gonadotropin-releasing hormone just before puberty. During childhood, only low levels of gonadotropin-releasing hormone, pituitary gonadotropins, and estrogen or testosterone are secreted. Gonadotropin-releasing hormone is released in rhythmic bursts during the night at 2-hour intervals, causing nocturnal release of gonadotropins, which in turn stimulate the cells of the ovary or testicle to secrete estrogen or testosterone. Testosterone and the adrenal androgens produce greater growth of muscle in the male. Female growth for the most part is dependent on the androgens of the adrenal cortex alone (Sinclair and Dangerfield, 1998).

The rise in estrogen triggers menarche, the first menstrual period. On average, the onset of menarche in the United States is 12 years (Vander et al, 2001). The advent of the first period is a late-stage phenomenon of puberty occurring after development of the breast and pubic hair and growth spurt. The onset of menses may be associated with the age-related change in body composition and body mass, such as the attainment of 17% body fat and a weight of 103 to 109 pounds (Santrock, 1998). This may explain the lack of onset of menarche or the cessation of menses in female athletes with low body fat and body mass. Rising estrogen levels also cause the epiphyses to close, thus terminating skeletal growth. Because girls go through puberty earlier than do boys, they attain peak height earlier and develop secondary sex characteristics sooner than do boys.

Testosterone is critical to the attainment of sexual maturity in males. Spermatogenesis begins at puberty under the direction of testosterone. It has negative-feedback effects on the hypothalamus and anterior pituitary. Testosterone also induces changes in the male reproductive organs and development of the secondary sex characteristics and sex drive. Testosterone stimulates growth during puberty through its effect on growth hormone secretion. It also causes the eventual closure of the epiphyses. Testosterone, unlike estrogen, has a strong anabolic effect on protein synthesis that can also account for the increased muscle mass of men compared with women. Anabolic steroids are synthetic agents that are converted into testosterone by the body. Some male and female athletes use anabolic steroids to build body mass and strength, but these drugs are potentially very dangerous and can have serious side effects such as liver damage.

Adulthood

During adulthood, our hormones are integrally associated with our normal physiological response to stress. The hypothalamus and anterior pituitary coordinate the release of corticotropin, which stimulates the adrenal cortex to secrete cortisol. The activity of the sympathetic nervous system is also increased during stress. The familiar fight-or-flight reaction is accompanied by an increased secretion of epinephrine, additionally readying the body for physical activity and for coping with new situations. The secretion of most other hormones also is affected by stress. Prolonged stress has been linked to increased susceptibility to disease by depressing the immune system (Vander et al, 2001).

Older Adulthood

As the body ages, it is less resilient to environmental stress. It becomes more difficult to maintain the status quo or homeostasis. There are four patterns of change in endocrine function during normal aging. The first pattern is related to endocrine gland failure, which is exemplified by the ovary. The universal female experience known as menopause is discussed later. The second pattern of change is associated with a decrease in sensitivity of target organs. Examples include the age-related decline in peripheral tissue response to insulin and the progressive resistance of the renal system to the effects of antidiuretic hormone. The third pattern is seen in the failure of an expected adaptive response, such as an insufficiency in the expected normal increase in blood pressure on standing from a supine or seated position caused by a lack of renin. The final pattern is marked by an increased sensitivity within the endocrine system as seen when there is a more aggressive response to an increase in antidiuretic hormone in older adults for a given level of osmolality. Older individuals tend to retain fluid more easily.

Menopause

Menopause is part of normal aging for a woman. On average, the menstrual cycles become less regular around the age of 50. The cessation of those cycles is known as *menopause*. Many changes occur during menopause. The failure of the ovaries to produce estrogen affects the genitourinary tract, the skeletal system, and body composition. A woman may experience an increased need to urinate and some urethral irritability. Loss of minerals from the bone puts a woman at risk for osteoporosis (see Chapter 6). Loss of estrogen also increases a woman's risk for cardiovascular disease.

Physiological changes associated with menopause include thinning of the walls of the vagina and decreased lubrication, vasomotor changes leading to hot flashes or flushes, less immediate responses to sexual arousal, and fewer contractions during orgasm (MacRae, 1999). There is a discernible decrease in function of the endocrine system in females at three levels. The decline at the organ level, the ovary, and effects of decline in circulating hormone levels have been briefly described. Last, target organs, the estrogen receptors in the body, also are affected. The breasts lose connective tissue, the skin becomes thin, and sweat glands and hair follicles become dry and less resilient due to the loss of estrogen (Smith, 1998).

Andropause

Men undergo less dramatic changes relative to a reduction in circulating testosterone levels. A gradual decline in the amount of testosterone in the circulation begins around the age of 60 but does not indicate a decrease in potency. Sperm continue to be produced but in smaller quantities. The decline in sperm production appears to be linked to connective tissue changes around the inside of the seminiferous tubules. This decline begins in the 40s and 50s with a decrease in motility noted after the age of 50.

The decline in testosterone with age does cause the libido to diminish but does not cause impotence. Impotence is typically related to vascular disease and present in half of men over the age of 70 (Purushothaman and Morley, 1996). The fact that the amount of gonadotropins in the serum increases with age supports the likelihood that the testes are less responsive to their effects. Some researchers prefer to use the term *androgen decline in the aging male* (ADAM) rather than *andropause* because they believe that the former is a clinical entity (Morales et al, 2000). There are hormonal changes in men with age; whether these are as universal as menopause is in women is not clear. Testosterone replacement therapy is not warranted based on the data (Davis and Davis, 1998).

Life-Span Changes of Vital Functions

BREATHING

Oxygen is needed by the body to convert organic carbon compounds into usable energy. Oxygen, however, cannot be stored in the body. The cardiovascular, pulmonary, musculoskeletal, and nervous systems work together to take in oxygen and to expel carbon dioxide in the act of *ventilation. Respiration,* the process of gas exchange, occurs at the cellular level within the alveoli. Ventilation and respiration involve the lungs, heart, thorax, diaphragm, central nervous system breathing centers, and central and peripheral chemoreceptors.

Control Mechanisms

Control of ventilation is achieved by two interacting systems, each with a specific purpose and affected by different stimuli. One system is neural and the other is chemical. Both systems are automatic but can be overridden by the need to talk, swallow, or perform other desired tasks such as swimming underwater.

The neural and chemical systems act on the muscular contraction of the diaphragm and intercostal muscles that are involved in the inspiratory phase of ventilation. During quiet breathing, expiration is usually passive. During forceful expiration, as in a cough, the abdominal muscles are activated.

Neural System

At least three brain stem centers coordinate the rhythmic ventilatory cycle and maintain the depth of ventilation. These sites are located in the medulla and the pons of the brain stem. The first site consists of several nuclei in the medulla. The inspiratory neurons provide the stimulus to fire the muscles of breathing. Voluntary control of breathing occurs through the corticospinal tract. The group of neurons in the medulla sends out repetitive bursts of inspiratory signals. The bursts of firing are cyclical and alternate with quiet periods.

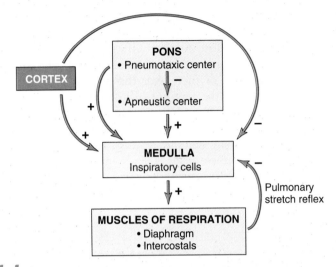

FIGURE 11–1

Schematic model of the body's control of breathing.

Two centers are located in the pons: the pneumotaxic center and the apneustic center. The apneustic center in the lower pons modulates the output of the medullary inspiratory neurons (Fig. 11–1). The pneumotaxic center in the upper pons controls the activity of the apneustic center. If the apneustic center goes unchecked, it produces apneustic breathing characterized by long inspiratory gasps. Pulmonary stretch receptors located in the smooth muscle of the airways can trigger cessation of inspiration through the Hering-Breuer reflex. This reflex sets the respiratory rhythm only during strenuous exercise when tidal volumes are large.

Chemical System

The chemical system regulates alveolar ventilation and monitors the blood gases. The central and peripheral chemoreceptors primarily control ventilation at rest. Central chemoreceptors located in the medulla respond to the composition of the extracellular fluid of the brain—specifically, to the hydrogen ion concentration in that fluid. Although hydrogen ions cannot pass through the blood-brain barrier, carbon dioxide in the extracellular fluid reacts with water to form hydrogen ions. Therefore, a rise in arterial P_{CO_2} causes an increase in hydrogen ion concentration and, consequently, an increase in ventilation. The neurons in the medullary inspiratory area are also very sensitive to chemicals, such as morphine and barbiturates, and can become so depressed that ventilation ceases.

Ventilation can be stimulated reflexively by a large decrease in arterial P_{O_2}. This mechanism uses the peripheral chemoreceptors: the aortic and carotid bodies. The chemoreceptors are directly influenced by the oxygen content of circulating arterial blood. A decrease in oxygen content excites the receptors to cause an increase in depth and rate of breathing. Peripheral receptors provide an accessory mechanism for controlling breathing activity. It is the central receptors, however, that account for approximately 70% of the increased ventilation due to chemical changes.

Breathing patterns can also be modified by sensory input from the lungs and chest wall, as in the case of a person who hyperventilates. By increasing the depth and rapidity of inspiration, alveolar and arterial carbon dioxide levels decrease and arterial oxygen levels increase. Swimmers may hyperventilate to increase the length of time they can hold their breath. Another example of altered breathing occurs when a person blows off too much carbon dioxide too quickly. The delay in the detection of the change in blood chemistry by the ventilatory centers causes periodic breathing (Fig. 11–2). This type of breathing is seen in patients with brain damage or chronic or severe cardiac failure.

Function Across the Life Span

Prenatal

The lungs develop early during gestation, but it is not until a pulmonary blood supply is established and adequate amounts of surfactant are produced that the lungs become capable of efficient gas exchange. The heart, although not a part of the pulmonary system per se, is needed to perfuse the lungs with blood to allow gas exchange to take place. For the fetus to receive an adequate supply of oxygen through the placenta, the fetal heart must pump a large volume of blood.

Although ventilation cannot occur during fetal life, respiratory movements do occur in utero. Respiratory movements are possible at the end of the first trimester, but because the amniotic fluid is very thick, the fetus "breathes" only a small amount. Fetal breathing movements, however, are a vital factor in the development of normal lungs (Goldstein, 1994). Fox and colleagues (1978) note that fetal breathing ceases for up to 1 hour after maternal ingestion of alcohol, which may be related to the developmental problems seen as a result of fetal alcohol syndrome.

The pattern of fetal breathing is used to diagnose labor and to predict the outcome of preterm delivery (Moore and Persaud, 1998). Breathing movements in utero appear to condition the respiratory muscles and may produce a pressure gradient between the lungs and the amniotic fluid. At birth, the lungs

FIGURE 11–2

Cheyne-Stokes breathing showing the changing P_{CO_2} in the pulmonary blood (solid line) and the delayed changes in P_{CO_2} of the fluids of the respiratory center (dashed line). (From Guyton AC, Hall JE. *Textbook of Medical Physiology*, 9th ed. Philadelphia: WB Saunders, 1996.)

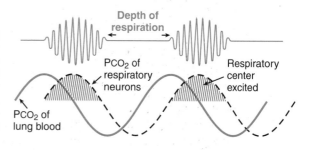

are half filled with fluid, so the first breath is possible only if the fluid is cleared from the lungs. This process is assisted by compression of the thorax during vaginal delivery.

Infancy and Childhood

The newborn infant must breath through its nose because the tongue takes up all of the space in the oral cavity. Babies efficiently use nasal breathing to bypass the impenetrable oral cavity. This anatomical arrangement provides a protective feature for the infant, because breathing is not yet coordinated with sucking and swallowing. However, when a baby has a cold, it is difficult to shift to breathing through the mouth, as occurs in older children and adults.

The depth and rate of ventilation change in relationship to the activity or work to be performed. The diaphragm is the major muscle of inspiration until around 5 to 7 years of age, after which the thoracic muscles play a larger role. Adult breathing patterns, according to Adkins (1968), are usually an equal combination of diaphragm and chest movements (diaphragm 2, chest 2), according to a 4-point scale that measures the four possible components of breathing: diaphragm, chest, neck accessory muscles, and abdominal muscles. Pathological changes in the musculoskeletal and cardiovascular systems can have a significant effect on the breathing pattern, as in scoliosis, spinal cord injury, or congenital heart defect. Major changes in lung volumes occur in childhood and correlate best with the height of the child. The relationship among work capacity, ventilation, and oxygen consumption is the same for a child as for an adult.

Older Adulthood

With normal aging, functional changes are seen in the volume of air moved, the rate of the airflow, and the amount of oxygen exchanged. Although the overall total lung volume remains constant, individual lung volumes change (for specific examples, see Chapter 8). Total lung capacity remains the same because the stiffness of the chest wall is balanced by the loss of elastic recoil of the lungs. Arterial oxygen tension (PaO_2) is the most often used measure of the amount of oxygen in the blood. There is a 4–mm Hg drop in PaO_2 per decade (Crapo et al, 1991). This decline has been attributed to increasing variability in ventilation-perfusion matching in different parts of the lung and premature airway closure. In addition, the amount of hemoglobin available for oxygen transport diminishes with age (Nilsson-Ehle et al, 1989). Despite these documented age-related changes in the cardiovascular and pulmonary systems, function can be improved with progressive endurance exercise (Cress et al, 1999).

SLEEP-WAKEFULNESS

Sleeping is a large part of our lives, but the exact benefits or purposes of sleep continue to be studied and elucidated. Sleep is a basic physiological drive like hunger or thirst. For most of us, sleep is a rhythmic, predictable process that occurs at night. It has always been said that a good night's sleep repairs the mind and the body. Anyone who has had difficulty sleeping knows the far-reaching effects of a lack of sleep. Research links sleep to time needed to allow the nervous system to reorganize and to promote memory and learning (Vander et al, 2001). Most of us have had the experience of going to bed trying to solve a problem and awaking in the morning to find the solution.

The sleep-wakefulness cycle consists of periods of sleep lasting from 6 to 10 hours and periods of wakefulness lasting from 14 to 18 hours a day. Timing of sleep and wakefulness is largely determined by internal factors, part of the so-called biological clock, and external factors such as the light in the environment. Physiologically, sleep is a state of unconsciousness from which a person can be aroused (Guyton and Hall, 1996). Human beings alternate between three states: wakefulness, non–rapid eye movement (NREM) sleep, and rapid eye movement (REM) sleep.

Wakefulness is associated with an increase in most physiological parameters from sleep levels; further increases in blood pressure and rate of breathing are associated with sympathetic nervous system activation. When we are awake, the brain wave pattern seen on an electroencephalogram is desynchronized (Fig. 11–3). An alpha rhythm is most likely to be recorded in an awake, relaxed adult whose eyes are closed. When attention is directed toward an external stimulus, the alpha rhythm is replaced by a beta rhythm. This change is termed *electroencephalographic arousal* (Vander et al, 2001). Arousal is the lowest level of attention. Once aroused, alertness is possible. When we are able to avoid distractions, it is termed *directed attention*. We can be so focused on a task that even a novel stimulus does not produce an orienting response.

There are two types of sleep: NREM sleep and REM sleep. Each involves

FIGURE 11–3

Progressive change in the characteristics of the brain waves during different stages of wakefulness and sleep. Stages of slow-wave sleep and corresponding electroencephalographic patterns. Stage 1: Very light sleep, low-voltage synchronized waves with sleep spindles. Stages 2 and 3: Light sleep characterized by low-voltage theta waves. Stage 4: Deep sleep characterized by high-voltage delta waves. (From Guyton AC, Hall JE. *Textbook of Medical Physiology*, 9th ed. Philadelphia: WB Saunders, 1996.)

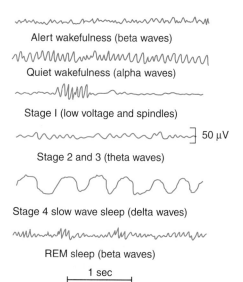

Alert wakefulness (beta waves)

Quiet wakefulness (alpha waves)

Stage I (low voltage and spindles)

Stage 2 and 3 (theta waves)   50 µV

Stage 4 slow wave sleep (delta waves)

REM sleep (beta waves)

1 sec

the brain, lungs, heart, and specific brain stem centers. NREM sleep is the initial phase of sleep and has four stages. The last stage is also known as *slow-wave sleep* because of its unique slow-wave sleep pattern on electroencephalography. All four stages of NREM sleep and REM sleep exhibit characteristic physiological functions and are further distinguished by different brain wave patterns (see Fig. 11–3).

NREM sleep occurs when decreased activity in the reticular activating system in the brain stem causes the brain waves to slow down. Slow-wave sleep is associated with a 10% to 30% decrease in blood pressure, rate of ventilation, and basal metabolic rate (Guyton and Hall, 1996). When we sleep, we go through the four stages of NREM sleep, with each stage showing a slower electroencephalographic wave pattern. Stage 1 is the lightest sleep, and stages 2, 3, and 4 are increasingly deeper. Each successive stage of NREM sleep exhibits a slower frequency and higher amplitude than the previous stage.

REM sleep occurs when the brain waves do not slow down but the person is asleep and exhibits rapid eye movements and muscle atonia. These incongruent characteristics explain why REM sleep is also called *paradoxical sleep*. Dreaming occurs in REM sleep, but the muscle atonia prevents us from acting out the dreams. An irregular heart rate and breathing rate and increased brain metabolism are characteristic of paradoxical sleep. Periods of paradoxical, or REM, sleep are interspersed between periods of NREM sleep and are characterized by low-voltage, asynchronous brain waves.

Sleep begins with stage 1 of NREM sleep and progresses to stage 4 in approximately 30 to 40 minutes. The cycle then reverses itself by going from stage 4 back to stage 1. At this point, the sleeper experiences an episode of REM sleep. Each period of REM sleep in adults can last from 5 to 40 minutes and usually happens every 90 minutes of sleep. Depending on how long we sleep, we may experience four or five episodes of REM sleep. When awakened while in REM sleep, we can recall our dreams.

Control Mechanisms

At least three endogenous pattern generators are responsible for the sleep-wake cycle. These centers are located in the brain stem. One group of mid-line nuclei, known as the *raphe nuclei*, secrete serotonin, a major neurotransmitter associated with sleep. Stimulation of this area causes sleep. Another collection of cells in the brain stem, called the *locus ceruleus*, secrete norepinephrine. According to one theory, the activity in the aminergic neurons, those that secrete serotonin and norepinephrine, is greater during wakefulness and cholinergic neurons are dominant during REM sleep. In this model, NREM sleep is an intermediate state. The third group of generators involved in sleep is located in the hypothalamus: the suprachiasmatic nucleus, preoptic area, and the posterior hypothalamus. The suprachiasmatic nucleus is the site of the biological clock in humans. The latter two areas produce sleep and arousal, respectively, through the use of γ-aminobutyric acid and histamine as neurotransmitters. Figure 11–4 illustrates this proposed model of consciousness.

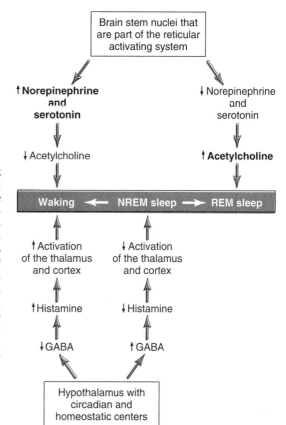

FIGURE 11-4

Proposed schema to explain differing states of consciousness. The change in neurotransmitters from norepinephrine and serotonin to acetylcholine is postulated to cause the shift from the waking state through non–rapid eye movement (NREM) sleep to rapid eye movement (REM) sleep. The rhythm of sleep-wake is also affected by the suprachiasmatic nucleus in the hypothalamus and other hypothalamic nuclei that use histamine and γ-aminobutyric acid (GABA) as neurotransmitters. (Redrawn from Vander AF, Sherman JH, Luciano DS. *Human Physiology: The Mechanisms of Body Function*, 8th ed. New York: McGraw-Hill, 2001, p 355. Copyright © 2001 by McGraw-Hill, Inc. Used by permission of McGraw-Hill Book Company.)

Sleep, then, is attributed to an active inhibitory process (Guyton and Hall, 1996).

Melatonin is produced by the pineal gland and exhibits a marked diurnal rhythm. More melatonin is produced at night than during the day. Sleep onset occurs with the onset of melatonin secretion. Melatonin production is controlled by the suprachiasmatic nucleus, and the timing of its secretion is capable of causing phase shifts in the sleep-wakefulness cycle. Light coming in through the retina can affect both the suprachiasmatic nucleus and pineal gland. When environmental stimuli adjust the function of the suprachiasmatic nucleus and other rhythm-generating systems of the brain, it is called *entrainment.*

A less well-defined group of cells, the reticular activating system, is responsible for arousing the cortex. If the reticular activating system is not inhibited by the sleep centers, the reticular nuclei spontaneously become active and continue to be aroused by the positive feedback from the cortex and the peripheral nervous system. Serotonin adjusts the body's general arousal level. Levels are high when alert, low in NREM sleep, and lowest in REM sleep.

When the reticular activating system tires or is inhibited, sleep occurs. Research continues on isolating additional transmitter substances and sleep factors. Although the first human gene that controls the sleep cycle has been discovered (Chicurel, 2001), there continues to be no complete explanation for the reciprocal, cyclical operation of the sleep-wake cycle.

Function Across the Life Span

Prenatal

Milani-Comparetti (1981) noted that the fetus had alternating periods of sleep and wakefulness at 29 weeks of gestation. Rosen and co-researchers (1973) distinguished REM, NREM, and wakefulness electroencephalographic patterns in the fetus during labor.

Infancy and Childhood

Preterm infants exhibit *ultradian rhythms,* which are rhythms with period lengths of less than 24 hours. This lack of circadian rhythm may reflect the effect of infant care schedules (Rivkees, 1997). A term newborn's 4-hour sleep-wake cycle appears to be related to cyclical variation in GI physiology and can be altered by changing the infant's feeding schedule. Newborns may spend as much as 16 hours sleeping each day. Half of that sleep will be REM sleep, which supports its speculated role in nervous system organization. A stable circadian rhythm is established between the second and fourth months after birth. Very little melatonin is produced until 3 months of age (Waldhauser et al, 1993). At that time, wakefulness is recognized as a stable state necessary for the infant to learn about the environment. Sleep reflects the infant's capability for self-regulation (Novosad et al, 1999). Gradually, the naps between wakeful periods at night lengthen until the infant sleeps through the night, at about 28 weeks after birth. The 3-month-old spends only 40% of sleeping time in REM sleep (Coons and Guilleminault, 1984). It is not until around 6 years of age, however, that children engage in the same amount of REM sleep as an average adult (Kohyama et al, 1997). This appears to be the result of functional maturation of the inhibitory systems active during REM sleep.

An infant's sleep begins with REM sleep and progresses to NREM, whereas an adult's sleep begins with NREM sleep. The quality of sleep within a state, changes in electroencephalographic activity, and percentage of time spent in different stages of sleep and wakefulness change during the first 2 years of life. NREM sleep is especially enhanced during early childhood and has been linked to an increase in protein synthesis and release of growth hormone. The ability of the nervous system to inhibit REM sleep, thus allowing more NREM sleep, may also be a result of central nervous system maturation (Challamel, 1988).

Sleep-wake states have traditionally been used to classify behavior. Prechtl (1977) first identified six behavioral states in newborns ranging from sleeping to crying. These states are taken into consideration when testing newborns. St. James-Roberts and Plewis (1996) reduced the six to four states (Table 11–3).

TABLE 11–3

Comparison of Infant Behavioral States

Prechtl	Infant State	St. James-Roberts and Plewis
Deep sleep, regular breathing, eyes closed	1	Alert inactivity—baby is calm, wide-eyed, and attentive to environment
Active rapid eye movement sleep, irregular breathing, eyes closed but movement can be detected	2	Waking activity—eyes open but unfocused, arm and leg thrusts
Drowsy, eyes open or closed, variable activity level	3	Crying—vigorous crying with agitated movements
Quiet alert, focused attention, minimal motor activity	4	Sleeping—still with regular breathing alternating with gentle movements with irregular breathing, and eyes closed
Active awake, eyes open, considerable motor activity	5	
Crying, jerky motor movements	6	

Data from Prechtl H. *The Neurological Examination of the Full-Term Newborn Infant,* 2nd ed. Clinics in Development Medicine, No. 63. Philadelphia: JB Lippincott, 1977; St James-Roberts I, Plewis I. Individual differences, daily fluctuations, and developmental changes in amounts of infant waking, fussing, crying, feeding, and sleeping. *Child Dev* 67:2527–2540, 1996.

Prechtl's states are related to physiology, whereas those of St. James-Roberts and Plewis are behaviorally defined. Prechtl's states are used to assess the newborn's ability to adjust to the extrauterine environment.

Unfortunately, sleep in infants is also linked to sudden death. Sudden infant death syndrome, or SIDS, is defined as the sudden death of an infant for no apparent reason due to a cessation of breathing. SIDS accounts for the largest percentage, approximately 13%, of all causes of death in the first year of life (Santrock, 1998). Because it has been related to sleeping in a prone position, the American Academy of Pediatrics has recommended since 1992 that infants sleep in positions other than prone. A "Back to Sleep" program was launched in 1994. These two preventive health measures resulted in a greater than 40% drop in the rate of SIDS in the United States (Gibson et al, 2000). The incidence of SIDS is higher in prematurely born infants and those of low birth weight. A study found that a disproportionate number of cases of SIDS, more than 20%, occur in child care settings (Moon et al, 2000). This finding was explained by a lack of instruction of caregivers regarding sleeping posture. Other potentially modifiable risk factors include maternal smoking, soft bedding, and covered airways (American Academy of Pediatrics, 2000).

Adolescence and Adulthood

Adolescents need about 10 hours of sleep a day, but many fall short of achieving the recommended amount. Loss of sleep has been shown to interfere with daytime functioning (Wolfson and Carskadon, 1998). Before puberty, the adolescent is an effective sleeper. However, after the onset of puberty, the adolescent's sleep and waking behavior changes. Levels of melatonin decline just before puberty (Cavallo, 1993). The adolescent stays up later but still has to get up early for school, and that dichotomy results in sleep deprivation (Keenan, 1999). By the age of 16, the average amount of sleep has dropped from 10 hours in middle childhood to less than 8 hours (Allen, 1992).

An adult generally spends about 8 hours sleeping, but there are great variations in adults' sleep needs. Some require as little as 5 hours, whereas others would prefer 10 hours for peak function. A normal range is from 3 to 12 hours (Keenan, 1999). An adult spends 75% of the time in NREM sleep and 25% in REM sleep. Decrements in the amount of stage 3 and 4 sleep are commonly seen in early adulthood; these are the deeper stages of NREM sleep. Work, family, and social demands can diminish total sleep time over the next several decades.

Older Adulthood

As we age, the length of time spent in deep, slow-wave (stage 4) sleep decreases, the quality of the sleep decreases, and the amount and relative proportion of REM to NREM sleep decrease (Fig. 11–5). Older adults take longer to fall asleep, wake up more frequently, and wake up earlier. Daily average sleep time decreases from a little over 7 hours at 25 years of age to less than 5 hours at 75 years of age (Atchley, 1991). Daytime napping often occurs as a means to maintain an adequate amount of total sleep time. Sleep efficiency as measured by the relative percentage of time spent in bed sleeping declines from 90% in young adults to 75% in older adults (Bundlie, 1998). The changes appear to be related to a decrease in both homeostatic drive for sleep and the strength of the circadian signal for early morning sleep (Dijk et al, 1999). Melatonin levels decline with advanced age, which also alters the sleep-wake cycle.

Circadian rhythms begin to shift with age. As we grow older, there is an advancement of the sleep phase, meaning that we become sleepy earlier in the evening. After 6 to 8 hours of sleep, we may awake even though it may be 4 or 5 AM. In addition, older adults may have other poor sleep habits such as remaining in bed when unable to sleep, which, when combined with the phase advancement, can lead to a decline in total nocturnal sleep time.

The likelihood of experiencing temporary cessation of breathing during sleep, or *sleep apnea*, increases with age. *Sleep-disordered breathing*, another name for sleep apnea, is a serious sleep disorder. A study in community-dwelling older adults found 24% of people 65 years or older had five or more apnea episodes per hour of sleep, and 81% had 10 or more episodes per hour (Ancoli-Israel et al, 1991). Research has shown that the quality of sleep in persons over 50 years of age can be improved by relying less on medication as a sleep aid, spending less time in bed when awake, and increasing exposure to bright light in the evening (Ancoli-Israel and Kripke, 1998).

Studies have indicated that changes in sleep patterns are not purely associated with age per se but rather with the level of activity that an individual is involved with on a daily basis. Older adults who exercise, such as walking or

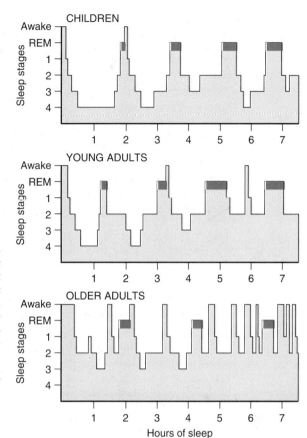

FIGURE 11–5

Comparison of sleep cycles across the life span. Note the dramatic changes in rapid eye movement sleep in the early years. As we get older, it takes us longer to fall asleep and we have less deep sleep, more awakenings, and less rapid eye movement sleep. (Redrawn from Kales A, Kales JD. Sleep disorders: Recent findings in the diagnosis and treatment of disturbed sleep. *N Engl J Med* 290: (9)487–499, 1974. Copyright © 1974 Massachusetts Medical Society. All rights reserved.)

swimming, for at least 30 minutes per day or spend greater than 50% of their day involved in functional activities have been shown to sleep for 6- to 7-hour periods, without experiencing difficulty falling or staying asleep (Guilleminault, 1994). Increased daytime activity and exercise, along with proper hydration and nutrition, and stress reduction, such as through biofeedback, meditation, and humor, have been shown to be effective in relieving the older adult's feelings of impaired nocturnal sleep (Guilleminault, 1994).

Deep sleep cycles are crucial for repair and healing for all age groups. It is during this time that all hormonal substances and their substrates needed for the efficient functioning of the neuroendocrine system are produced (Sapolsky et al, 1996). It has been demonstrated that submaximal activity and exercise levels stimulate the production of interleukin 1, a powerful component of immune system functioning. Interleukin 1 induces deep/slow-wave sleep and stimulates the production of growth hormone. Sleep can therefore be considered a nonspecific healing mechanism vital for the maintenance of health at all ages.

EATING AND DIGESTION

Eating involves taking in food to provide needed nutritional substrates that foster growth, maturation, and repair of all the body's systems (consult a basic nutrition text for the specific nutritional requirements for each system). Eating, a pleasurable experience for some people, is seen by others as merely something that must be done to keep the body fueled for movement. The initial act of ingesting food or taking in liquid continues in the acts of digestion, absorption, and elimination. Digestion and elimination are crucial to the smooth running of the human body and the maintenance of the internal chemical balance needed for homeostasis. The digestive and excretory systems function together to process all nutrients, except oxygen. The useful components of ingested food and liquids are extracted during the process of digestion and absorption. Waste products are removed and excreted via the GI or the genitourinary tract during elimination.

The act of eating is a skeletal motor activity that demands close coordination with breathing. Eating also requires neuromuscular coordination for mastication (chewing) and deglutition (swallowing), as well as the use of sensory input for motivation and feedback. The process of ingestion involves the mouth, teeth, tongue, pharynx, and esophagus. The process of digestion and absorption also requires the stomach, intestines, salivary glands, pancreas, liver, and gallbladder. The digestive tract consists of a hollow tube that begins at the mouth and ends at the anus. From the mid-esophagus to the anus, its wall contains two layers of smooth muscle cells: the inner layer is circular and can produce sphincter-like contractions, and the outer layer is longitudinal and can shorten the digestive tract when contracted.

There are four phases of swallowing: oral preparation, oral transport, pharyngeal transfer, and esophageal transport. Food is taken into the mouth during oral preparation and changed into a manageable bolus. During oral transport, the bolus is moved to the back of the pharynx by the tongue. In the third stage, the bolus moves past the throat arches to begin the swallow. The epiglottis folds over the trachea to direct the bolus into the esophagus. Last, the bolus is transported down the esophagus by a peristaltic wave toward the stomach (Fig. 11–6).

Control Mechanisms

The oral phase of swallowing is generally attributed to a reflex (Guyton and Hall, 1996). The presence of a bolus of food prevents the muscles of mastication from closing the jaw, allowing the lower jaw to drop and thus stretching the muscles of mastication, which in turn causes jaw closure. This chain of reflexes produces chewing. Although actual swallowing is also thought to be reflexive, the initial tongue tip elevation that occurs before the transfer of food to the pharynx is voluntary. The body of the tongue presses against the roof of the mouth, squeezing the food into the pharynx. The glottis is closed, preventing food from going into the trachea. Instead, the food is directed into the esophagus. As the food travels farther back in the pharynx, the epiglottis folds

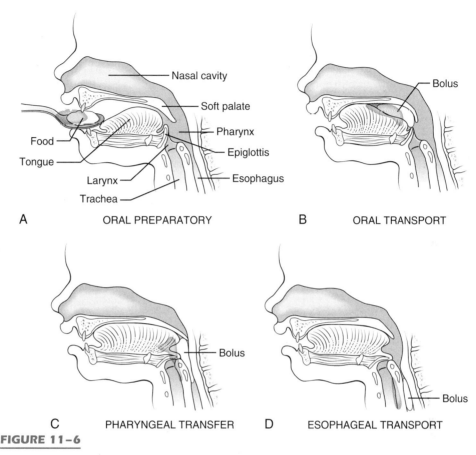

FIGURE 11-6

Four phases of swallowing. (Adapted from Batshaw ML. *Children with Disabilities*, 4th ed. Baltimore: Brookes Publishing, 1997, p 622.)

over the closed glottis. Touch receptors in the pharynx elicit the swallow, which propels the food into the esophagus. All of this occurs within seconds and is controlled by an area in the brain stem called the *swallowing center*.

The esophagus has two sphincters: the upper and lower. The esophageal phase of swallowing is marked by the relaxation of the upper sphincter. The size of the bolus dictates the amount the diameter of the upper sphincter increases. In the esophagus, the food is further conducted to the stomach by peristalsis. The lower esophageal sphincter opens at the end of the peristaltic wave to allow food into the stomach. The pharynx and the upper third of the esophagus are made up of skeletal muscle that is innervated by the glossopharyngeal (cranial nerve IX) and vagus (cranial nerve X) nerves. The remaining two thirds of the esophagus is made up of smooth muscle that is controlled by the myenteric plexus via the vagus nerve; thus, there is a back-up system for food to reach the stomach even if the swallowing reflex is paralyzed. The lower sphincter relaxes to allow food into the stomach and then closes. When the lower sphincter is inefficient, gastric contents can reflux into the esophagus, resulting in gastroesophageal reflux.

Although the reflex explanation for chewing and swallowing is plausible, there is another possible control mechanism that is more in keeping with the rhythmicity of this vital function. Broussard and Altshchuler's (2000) study of the timing of swallowing and respiration provides evidence that groups of premotor neurons function as pattern generators to initiate the repetitive rhythmic muscle activity seen in swallowing. Furthermore, these premotor neurons are involved in the phases of swallowing and are anatomically linked to integrate esophageal peristalsis with the pharyngeal phase of swallowing and airway protective reflexes. In fact, chewing is controlled by nuclei in the brain stem, which when stimulated near the center for taste produce continual, rhythmic chewing movements (Guyton and Hall, 1996).

The regulation and control of digestion take place within the GI tract itself. GI reflexes cause changes in muscle wall contractility and the secretion of digestive enzymes. Two major nerve plexuses control these reflexes: the myenteric plexus and the submucosal plexus. Together, they are called the enteric nervous system. The myenteric plexus lies within the intestinal wall between the two muscular layers. It controls the motor activity of the wall and the sphincters that separate the parts of the digestive tract and is needed for effective peristalsis. The submucosal plexus controls the local segmental responses such as secretion, absorption, and contraction. Endocrine cells scattered in the epithelial walls of the stomach and small intestine secrete the hormones that control the digestive system. Contractility of the wall of the digestive system is determined by the internal concentration of calcium ions in the smooth muscle cells of the lining (Hirst, 1999). Receptors for the two plexuses, along with the parasympathetic and sympathetic innervation, provide the neural support for the GI reflexes, which respond to the following conditions: stretch of the wall, concentration of the chyme, acidity of the chyme, and presence of specific organic digestive byproducts (Guyton and Hall, 1996). Secretions within the GI tract are therefore under hormonal, central, and local nervous system control.

Control of the GI tract can be divided into three phases: cephalic, gastric, and intestinal. These phases are named for where the initial stimulus occurs, not for where the reflex occurs. The first phase begins even before the food reaches the stomach, when the sight, smell, taste, and texture of the food and the emotional state of the person eating trigger the secretion of pepsinogen, the precursor of pepsin, an enzyme that digests protein. Next, gastrin is released in response to local vagal reflexes, which stimulates gastric acid secretion. The amount of acid secreted by the stomach is balanced by the absorptive and digestive abilities of the small intestines. Finally, secretin, cholecystokinin, and glucose-dependent insulinotropic peptide are secreted during the intestinal phase. The three phases occur in temporal order only at the beginning of a meal. Thereafter, the reflexes may occur simultaneously during ingestion and absorption.

Structural Changes Across the Life Span

The structures that support breathing, eating, and digestion grow over the course of the life span. These structural changes support the function of these three processes. For example, an infant goes from using one tube for both breathing and eating to using two tubes: the trachea for breathing and the esophagus for eating. The relationship between structure and function becomes apparent when examining the oropharyngeal and digestive systems.

The oropharyngeal anatomy of the newborn is significantly different from that of an adult. The infant's lower jaw is retracted and smaller (Fig. 11–7). The oral cavity is small, with the tongue occupying all of the space and being in proximity to the roof and floor. The chubby-cheeked appearance of the newborn is due to the presence of fat pads. These pads make sucking easier.

Up until 3 to 4 months, the child's epiglottis and soft palate are approximated. The larynx is elevated and in proximity to the base of the tongue. With growth, the posterior part of the tongue will descend with the larynx to become a segment of the front wall of the pharynx. The oral cavity enlarges with growth, and the elongation of the neck and pharynx changes the relationship of the tongue, larynx, and epiglottis.

The digestive system also begins in a more elevated location in the infant than the adult. The ends of the esophagus are two vertebral levels higher in the infant than in the adult. The capacity of the stomach increases from 30 mL

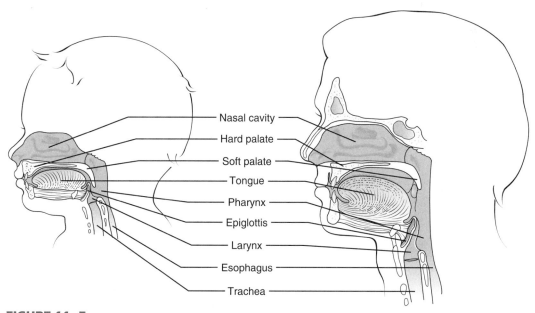

Nasal cavity
Hard palate
Soft palate
Tongue
Pharynx
Epiglottis
Larynx
Esophagus
Trachea

FIGURE 11–7

Comparison of oropharyngeal anatomy of an infant and an adult. (Adapted from Morris SE, Klein MD. *Pre-Feeding Skills.* Tucson, AZ: Therapy Skill Builders, 1987, p 8.)

at birth to 90 mL approximately 2 weeks later. At 1 year, the capacity increases further to 500 mL and finally to 1500 mL in adulthood (Sinclair and Dangerfield, 1998). The digestive system descends with growth like the respiratory system.

Length of the small intestines increases from infancy to puberty. Also because of the size of the infant pelvis, only a small amount of the intestines extend into the pelvis. In the adult, the majority of the small intestine and even some of the stomach may be in the pelvic region. Structurally, the wall of the intestines is thin and only with age develops the musculature needed for peristalsis. "Villi continue to form in the small intestine until puberty" (Sinclair and Dangerfield, 1998, p 94).

Five percent of the infant's body weight is due to the relatively large size of the liver, an organ of digestion. The liver has many important functions during intrauterine life, one of which is producing many types of blood cells. At adulthood, the liver will take up only 2.5% of the body's weight.

Function Across the Life Span

Prenatal

The earliest oral reflex in utero is the gag reflex, which is present at 17 weeks of gestation. Other oral reflexes, such as rooting and suck-swallow, are present by 28 weeks of gestation. The fetus has been shown to suck its thumb as well as to take in amniotic fluid. The oral reflexes are elicited by touch or pressure and can be considered survival reflexes because their purpose is to obtain nutrition and to protect the fetus from swallowing unwanted material.

Buchan and colleagues (1981) demonstrated the presence of regulatory gut peptides or hormones as early as 8 to 10 weeks after conception. These protein complexes regulate the activity of the digestive system. Aynsley-Green (1985) documented a large number of gut hormones and metabolites in the fetal and maternal circulations at 18 to 21 weeks of gestation and postulated that these circulating peptides facilitate the development of the fetal lung and GI tract. By the fifth month of gestation, the fetus shows peristaltic movements within the GI tract, and the liver is secreting bile. GI tract function approaches that of a normal newborn by 6 to 7 months of gestation (Guyton and Hall, 1996). Meconium, from the unabsorbed amniotic fluid and excretory byproducts, is continually formed and excreted in small amounts. All of these developments appear necessary to prepare the fetus to independently seek, find, and assimilate food efficiently after birth.

Infancy Through Childhood

The fetus uses glucose, which is primarily obtained from the mother's blood. Once the umbilical cord is cut, the infant must regulate her own blood glucose level. Because the infant has a very limited amount of stored glucose, the supply is quickly depleted. Because the infant's liver is not functionally adequate at birth, stored fats and proteins must be used as energy sources until feeding can begin.

The introduction of food produces changes in the digestive system and endocrine system that allow efficient utilization of food. Levels of blood glucose and plasma insulin increase after the first enteral or by-mouth feeding. Within days, the secretion of digestive hormones has fostered growth of the gastric mucosa. Their secretion also fosters the development of gastric motility and secretion, pancreatic endocrine function, and liver metabolism. Regulation of postnatal nutritional adaptation is schematically represented in Figure 11–8.

Aynsley-Green and colleagues (1997) described the patterns of metabolic adaptation in the newborn. Early nutrition has a long-term effect on metabolic homeostasis. Insulin secretion by the pancreas is not as well controlled in the newborn as it will be in the older child and adult. During the newborn period, insulin secretion may play a role in setting the stage for development of adult metabolic control.

Human milk is the optimal nutritional source of calcium during the first year of life (American Academy of Pediatrics, 1999a). Human milk also contributes trophic factors that aid digestive system maturation and immunoglobulins that reduce the risk of infection (Werk and Alpert, 1998). Evidence has been found that prolactin in maternal milk helps regulate the newborn's im-

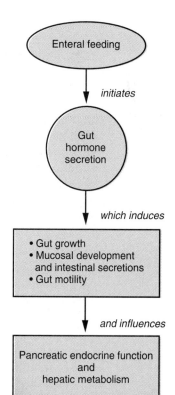

FIGURE 11–8

Hypothesis to explain regulation of postnatal nutritional adaptation. (Redrawn from Aynsley-Green A. Metabolic and endocrine interrelations in the human fetus and neonate. *Am J Clin Nutr* 41:399–417, 1985. Copyright *Am J Clin Nutr*, American Society for Clinical Nutrition.)

mune system, lending further support to the benefits of breast feeding (Ellis et al, 1997). The need for calcium to promote bone growth and metabolism in infants has led manufacturers of infant formulas to increase the concentration of calcium in their formulas to match the levels received in human milk.

Eating. Eating progresses from being reflexive at birth to being voluntary at 2 to 5 months of age. At this time, a voluntary sucking pattern is established that allows the tongue to stroke the food source. In the process of obtaining food, the tongue's shape is modified. This change also prepares the tongue for articulating specific speech sounds and is an example of feeding as preparation for speech. As oral control improves, the lips can close around a spoon to remove food and the infant learns to drink liquids from a cup. Again, this oral motor skill carries over into the ability to produce closed mouth sounds such as "p," "b," and "m."

The elevated position of the larynx and the space occupied by the tongue allow the infant to breath while feeding. Liquid flows down either side of the epiglottis and the uvula that are in contact while swallowing. Thus, the airway is protected anatomically during swallowing. When the one-tube system of eating and breathing is replaced with the adult two-tube system, the valving at the epiglottis is needed to protect the airway during swallowing.

Between 5 and 8 months of age, oral motor behavior shifts from sucking to chewing. This transition is supported by growth changes in the skull and mandible, peripheral afferent input, neural maturation, and motor learning (Green et al, 1997). "The basic chewing pattern of reciprocally activated antagonistic muscle groups is established by 12 months of age" (Green et al, 1997, p 2704). For further discussion of oral motor development, the reader is referred to Morris and Klein (1987) and Radliffe (1998).

The introduction of solid food should be based on the nutritional needs of the infant. At 6 months of age, an infant is no longer able to obtain sufficient amounts of iron from human or formula milk. Guidelines on solid feeding by Werk and Alpert (1998) recommend 4 to 6 months as a reasonable time to introduce solids. This age range is based on available scientific evidence. The digestive system seems unprepared for solid food until 4 to 6 months. The kidney also requires at least 4 months to mature to the point of being able to handle the higher osmolar load of solid foods. Adequate nutrition in the form of solid food allows infants to triple their birth weight by 1 year of age and quadruple it by age 2.

Dental Development. Dental development begins during gestation and continues through adolescence. The tooth buds of the deciduous or baby teeth form at 6 weeks of gestation. Some tooth buds of permanent teeth are formed before birth, whereas others are not developed until after birth. Healthy teeth are important to our nutrition, general health, and appearance. The timing of tooth eruption varies greatly among infants, although there is a set sequence. The average infant's first tooth appears at about 6 months; the remainder of the 20 baby teeth are in place by 2½ years of age. Typically, the first permanent tooth erupts at 6 years, with the third molars or wisdom teeth appearing last at 17 years. The replacement of the baby teeth by the 32 permanent ones is gradual and can span up to 11 years. Dental age can supplement bone age as a way to estimate skeletal maturity (Sinclair and Dangerfield, 1998).

Digestion. Digestion begins in the mouth, where the food is chewed and first exposed to saliva. In the absence of food, the mouth is kept moist by saliva. Salivation is triggered by chemoreceptors. The salivary glands are the most productive exocrine glands in the body given their size. After swallowing, digestion continues in the stomach, where chyme is produced. Chyme is partially digested food that is acidified by adding gastric acid. The amount of acid secreted into the stomach increases relative to the protein content of the meal. The final stage of digestion occurs in the small intestine, where food is maximally digested and absorbed. The pancreas and gallbladder supply organically specific digestive enzymes and bile to aid this process. The small intestine absorbs the nutrients, so that by the time material reaches the large intestine, the volume has been significantly reduced. Waste is stored temporarily until its bulk is sufficient for it to be moved on to the last segment of the GI tract, the rectum, where, after distension, defecation is initiated.

Motility in the small intestines initially takes place by segmentation that involves a stationary contraction and relaxation of segments of the intestinal wall. During this process, there is ongoing division and subdivision of the intestinal contents, allowing the mixing of the chyme. This mixing brings the chyme into contact with the intestinal wall. Motility is affected by the enteric nervous system, hormones, and our emotional state. After most of the meal is absorbed, segmentation is replaced by peristalsis. *Peristalsis* is a contraction of a segment of the digestive tract that moves undigested content to the large intestines. Slower contractions of the smooth muscle wall of the large intestine mean that content remains for a longer period of time until sufficient bulk is achieved. Mass movements occur three or four times a day in the large intestines. These intense contractions occur generally after a meal and spread to the rectum. If the time is not right for defecation, we inhibit the relaxation of the external sphincter, and reverse peristalsis sends the fecal mass back to the colon.

Older Adulthood

Dentition. Good oral hygiene and a regular schedule of preventive care will help us keep our teeth for our entire life span. However, oral tissues undergo substantial changes with age. Teeth can be lost because of deterioration in periodontal structures such as the gums, bones of the jaw, and membranes around the teeth. In the past, many older adults did not take proper care of their teeth, which resulted in tooth loss. One report states that 40% of those over 65 years of age lost all their teeth (Miller et al, 1987). Today, more older adults are retaining their teeth into advanced age (Shay, 1998; Ship, 1999); still, close to 2 million wear dentures. Although dentures can provide a more positive self-image, nutritional concerns should be of paramount importance.

Oral health and oropharyngeal function can be maintained into the 70s and 80s (Ship, 1999).

Digestion. Physiological changes in the digestive system related to aging are less obvious than in other systems. There are minor changes in all phases of digestion, but they appear to have a relatively small impact on function. A decrease in the amount of saliva produced was once thought to be a normal consequence of aging. Indeed, dry mouth is a common complaint by older adults, but it is not a normal change of aging (Shay, 1998). Rather, it is a common side effect of medication. Saliva is important for taste and maintenance of oral health. Although the amount of saliva produced by the parotid gland does not decline with age, there are conflicting reports about declines in the output from other salivary glands. Older adults need to chew their food more to achieve the desired degree of maceration before swallowing. The sequence of swallowing takes longer in the older adult but again with no apparent functional consequences.

Many community-dwelling older adults have a calorie intake below the recommended dietary allowance. Protein is less easily digested because of a decline in gastric acid production, an approximate 25% loss by the age of 60 (Whitbourne, 1996). Daily protein requirements for an older person are 0.8 g/kg body weight (Abbasi, 1998). Carbohydrates are also not as well metabolized as one ages. Normally aging individuals have minimal increases in fasting glucose concentration with age, and over age 45, there is a small decrease in insulin sensitivity (Davis and Davis, 1998). Blood glucose levels may rise to the point at which the older adult develops diabetes, but this is not a normal consequence of aging. Adult-onset diabetes is a disease related to genetics and obesity. Therefore, age-related changes in carbohydrate tolerance have been excluded in the National Diabetes Data Group's definition of impaired glucose tolerance because it is not considered normal aging (Davis and Davis, 1998).

Despite some structural changes in the villi of the small intestines with age, absorption remains functional for macronutrients such as sodium, potassium, and magnesium. The aging GI tract is less efficient in absorbing vitamin B-12, vitamin D, and calcium (Russell, 2000). Vitamin B-12 deficiency can cause memory impairment, dementia, and balance and gait problems (Abbasi, 1998). Vitamin D and calcium are important for bone integrity. Alterations in calcium absorption in the intestine are related to bone loss and osteoporosis (see Chapter 6). Based on the older adult's unique metabolic characteristics, new recommended dietary allowances for some of these vital nutrients have been proposed (Russell, 2000). Nutrition requirements in the aging population are likely to be updated as new research becomes available.

Fat is digested within the small intestines through the action of bile secreted by the liver. The liver shows definite anatomical changes with age, but because of its large margin of safety, none of these structural changes affects the production and secretion of bile; therefore, intestinal function, with regard to the digestion of fat, remains essentially unchanged.

ELIMINATION

The fourth vital function is elimination. Elimination includes defecation of solid waste, which is an extension of digestion, and micturition, which is the excretion of liquid waste from the urinary system.

Defecation

Control Mechanisms

Spinal level reflexes coordinate contraction of the colon and rectum to expel feces. These autonomic reflexes are mediated by the parasympathetic system and involve sacral cord segments S2-S4. These segments may be spared in a patient with an incomplete spinal cord lesion, allowing bowel control. The exit route for feces, the anus, is usually kept closed by contraction of the internal anal sphincter. This sphincter is made of smooth muscle, whereas the external anal sphincter is made of skeletal muscle and thus is under voluntary control. Mass movement of fecal material distends the rectal wall and initiates the defecation reflex. The defecation reflex consists of contraction of the rectum and external anal sphincter, relaxation of the internal sphincter, and increased peristalsis in the colon. After sufficient pressure builds up, the external sphincter reflexively relaxes and allows the stool to be passed.

Childhood. Children are usually ready to control defecation around the age of 2 years, but the age is highly variable. The following cues are helpful to determine a child's readiness to be toilet trained: regular bowel movements, the ability to sit alone well, the ability to recognize the need for a bowel movement, and the desire to cooperate with an adult, as seen when releasing an object on request. Guidelines for assessing toilet training readiness by the American Academy of Pediatrics recommend a child-oriented approach (1999b).

Older Adulthood. Despite what television commercials imply about an older adult's need for laxatives, there is no evidence for decreased motility in the large intestine. Autonomic nervous system responses to stress can aggravate GI function by decreasing salivary and gastric secretions. Other factors, such as decreased physical activity, decreased fluid or fiber intake, and living alone, often lead to, or compound, functional constipation. Unsound dietary practice, including decreased caloric and water intake, in addition to habitual use of laxatives, is far more likely to create constipation than any structural or physiological age-related change.

The Valsalva maneuver assists defecation but can be dangerous in older individuals with cardiovascular disease, especially if they are constipated. Along with the rise in abdominal pressure from bearing down, intrathoracic pressure rises, causing a rise in blood pressure and a decrease in the venous return to the heart.

Fecal continence requires good sphincter control. Although there is some evidence that sclerosis of the internal anal sphincter occurs with age, the majority of individuals with fecal incontinence do not demonstrate the associated decline in anal canal pressure. Rather, these individuals are likely to have some type of neurological disease.

Micturition

The process of micturition is far more complex than defecation. The urinary system is made up of two kidneys, two ureters, a bladder, and a urethra. The kidneys have been described as 1 million functional units held together by connective tissue. Normal function depends on circulatory, endocrine, and nervous system interaction. The kidneys are the filtering system for the body, and they produce urine as the byproduct of filtering the plasma. The purpose of the kidneys is to maintain water and electrolyte balance within the body and to regulate plasma concentration. Homeostasis of our internal environment is achieved via the multiple processes of filtration, absorption, and secretion.

Structural changes occur over the first year of life as the kidneys become fully functional. Their growth corresponds to that of the body as a whole during this period of development as evidenced by the organs' weight doubling in 6 months and tripling by the end of the first year (Sinclair and Dangerfield, 1998). Renal tubules continue to form and glomeruli enlarge. Most importantly, the epithelial layer of cells in the capsule of the glomeruli change from being cuboidal to flat, allowing better filtration after the first year. As with many structures in the body, work demand induces a change in the size of the kidneys.

The bladder is located in the abdominal cavity during infancy and moves into the pelvis only as that structure expands. The characteristic pyramidal shape of the bladder is achieved by the age of 6 years, at which time the bladder occupies its adult position. The ureters lengthen to accommodate the gradual change in position (Sinclair and Dangerfield, 1998). As with defecation, micturition depends on the physical control of sphincters, which is achieved somewhere between 18 and 24 months of age.

Control Mechanisms

Arterial blood pressure is controlled by regulation by the kidneys of the body fluid system, which is relatively simple. If there is too much fluid in the system, the pressure rises; if there is too little fluid, the pressure drops. The two determinants of arterial blood pressure are the volume of renal output and the amount of salt and water in the system. The kidneys control renal output by changing the extracellular fluid volume. An increase in extracellular fluid increases blood volume and ultimately cardiac output, which increases arterial pressure. This increase in arterial pressure is accomplished by controlling the amount of salt in the system, which is the main determinant of the amount of extracellular fluid.

The kidneys also are a part of the endocrine system, and as such, they have an additional means of controlling pressure: the renin-angiotensin system. This system is a more powerful mechanism than that already described for controlling arterial pressure, and it is also much more complex. After a drop in blood pressure, the kidneys release renin, which enzymatically causes the

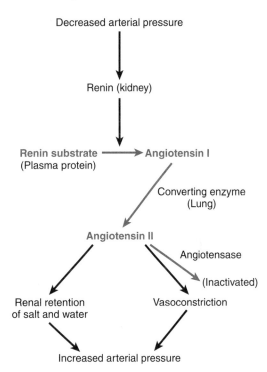

FIGURE 11–9

Renin-angiotensin vasoconstrictor mechanism for arterial pressure control. (From Guyton AC, Hall JE. *Textbook of Medical Physiology*, 9th ed. Philadelphia: WB Saunders, 1996.)

release of angiotensin I. Within seconds, angiotensin I is converted by an enzyme in the lungs to angiotensin II. The latter produces systemic vasoconstriction and decreased excretion of salt and water by the kidney. Angiotensin can secondarily cause fluid retention by stimulating the adrenal gland to secrete aldosterone (Fig. 11–9). The renin-angiotensin vasoconstriction system is important for the maintenance of normal arterial blood pressure despite wide fluctuations in salt intake. The system takes about 20 minutes to become fully active.

Function Across the Life Span

Prenatal

The human embryo develops three different sets of kidneys from mesoderm (Moore and Persaud, 1998). The first set is rudimentary and nonfunctional. The second set does function for a short time in utero but is replaced by a third and final set of permanent kidneys, which develop in the early part of the fifth week of gestation and are capable of producing urine 6 weeks later. The collecting tubules and ducts are of endodermal origin, as is the urinary bladder. Urine formation continues throughout fetal life and makes up a large part of the amniotic fluid. Because the placenta removes the waste products from the fetus, the kidneys do not need to function until after birth. However, because the mature fetus swallows amniotic fluid daily that is absorbed by the fetal intestines, the fetal kidneys do play a role in regulating amniotic fluid volume. The permanent kidneys ascend to their adult position around the ninth week of gestation (Moore and Persaud, 1998).

Infancy Through Childhood

The infant's kidney function is adequate but immature for the first few weeks of life. The rate of fluid intake and output in the infant is seven times that of the adult. The infant cannot readily adjust to large changes in fluid loads; any undue loss of water and solutes from fever, vomiting, and diarrhea can be life threatening. Renal function changes rapidly in response to increased blood flow at birth and steadily increasing metabolic demands. By 4 months of age, the kidneys have developed sufficiently to manage solid foods that create a higher osmolar demand than milk (Hendricks and Badruddin, 1992). Renal function improves greatly by 6 months; mature function of sphincters is possible between 18 months and 2 years of age. The kidneys enlarge after birth due to hypertrophy of the nephrons. In infants and children, the bladder occupies space within the abdomen. At 6 years, the bladder is still not fully contained in the pelvis; only after puberty is the bladder considered a pelvic organ.

Maturation of bladder function occurs by 4 years of age (Berk and Friman, 1990). During infancy, the bladder wall responds to a small amount of urine, contracting to expel its contents. Expulsion is automatic. From 18 months to 2½ years of age, the child develops an awareness of having to void and can retain urine for short periods before voiding. The daily urine volume gradually increases, and as a child gains control over the diaphragm and the abdominal and perineal muscles, she learns to initiate voiding. Bladder control continues to improve as he retains larger volumes of urine for longer periods. Mature bladder control is finally achieved between 2½ and 4½ years of age. A child may first sleep through the night dry when the bladder can retain about 10 to 12 ounces (300 to 360 mL) of urine. This is not quite double the amount normally voided during the day. There are gender differences in toileting. A boy's ability to gain bladder control appears to be related to maturation of sleep cycles, that is, being able to wake up in time to void (Brazelton et al, 1999). More boys are prone to nocturnal enuresis (bedwetting) (Howe and Walker, 1992). The fact that boys take longer to train than girls, by about 6 months, may be related to their anatomy and need to adopt a separate posture for elimination. Although bowel maturation precedes bladder maturation, bladder control is attained about 6 months before bowel control in toddlers. Brazelton and colleagues (1999) reported that most toddlers are completely trained at 2 to 3 years of age.

The kidneys contribute to homeostasis by expelling waste products in the form of urine and by regulating the balance of fluid and electrolytes in the body. One measure of kidney function and health status is how quickly certain substances, such as creatinine, are cleared from the body. Normal creatinine clearance averages 124 mL/min in men. The kidneys also secrete substances that are part of the hormonal system, including erythropoietin, renin, and active forms of vitamin D (Guyton and Hall, 1996). Renin is synthesized and stored in the kidneys and is important in the control of blood pressure.

Older Adulthood

Renal function declines with age; older adults have 40% of normal adult capacity to clear creatinine from the body (Rowe et al, 1976). Gross anatomical changes occur, with loss of nephrons and renal mass and thickening of membranes. Physiologically, the surface area for filtration decreases. Renal blood flow decreases with age, as does the glomerular filtration rate. The endocrine functions of the kidneys also change with age. The amount of renin declines, which may be why the ability to conserve salt and water diminishes with age. A decrease in erythropoietin, the hormone secreted by the kidney to stimulate red blood cell production, may contribute to anemia. The ability to concentrate urine is lessened and the diurnal rhythm of urine production is lost because of age-related changes in the renal tubules. These tubular changes may significantly affect the ability of older adults to benefit from medication. An adult dose may have an adverse rather than a beneficial effect because of the lower excretion rate in an individual.

The smooth muscular wall and elastic tissue of the bladder are replaced by noncontractile connective tissue as a result of aging. The person older than 65 years will experience the need to void earlier due to a reduction in the amount the bladder can store. Recognition of the need to void may occur closer to the bladder's capacity, failing to provide sufficient warning and necessitating a dash to the restroom. Weakening of the bladder and pelvic floor muscles prevents its complete emptying and may lead to *stress incontinence*, defined as a loss of urine associated with laughing, coughing, or lifting. Stress incontinence is primarily a problem of reduced urethral resistance. *Urge incontinence* is often related to prostate disease. The loss of self-esteem related to bladder dysfunction in the older adult is significant. The prevalence of urinary incontinence has been estimated at 15% to 30% in women. The prevalence is less in men. Many older women seem to expect some degree of incontinence to occur as a result of aging. Therefore, it is important to teach Kegel exercises to prevent stress incontinence. Urinary incontinence is not, however, inevitable (see Clinical Implications—Urinary Incontinence and Age).

Interrelationships Between Functions

BREATHING AND SLEEPING

The control of breathing becomes automatic during sleep. Communication between the sleep-wake and breathing brain stem centers would be expected, although this appears to occur more easily during NREM sleep than during REM sleep. During NREM sleep, the respiratory centers continue to regulate breathing in response to chemical feedback from chemoreceptors and input from upper airway receptors. During REM sleep, however, most respiratory

CLINICAL IMPLICATIONS
Urinary Incontinence and Age

Urinary incontinence is a condition that is not yet well understood, but it should not be viewed as an inevitable consequence of aging. When we are incontinent of urine, we involuntarily lose urine. The most common types of urinary incontinence are designated as stress and urge incontinence. Increased intraabdominal pressure is associated with stress incontinence, which may be caused by sneezing, laughing, or physical activity. Urge incontinence is linked to detrusor contractions and instability, and it is manifested by an abrupt, overwhelming need to void.

Urinary incontinence is both a social and a hygiene problem. Both men and women exhibit urinary incontinence, but women appear to be twice as likely to be affected. This may be related to the added stress of pregnancy on the efficacy of the pelvic floor muscles as well as to the loss of estrogen at menopause (for more information, see Pauls, 2000).

Urinary Incontinence

- Is a prevalent and costly health condition
- Significantly affects quality of life
- Affects both women and men
- Is not a natural consequence of aging
- Is more likely to be experienced by the oldest old

Risk Factors

- Increased age
- Higher-than-normal body mass index
- Presence of chronic disease such as diabetes or chronic obstructive pulmonary disease
- History of having had a hysterectomy

Prevention and Intervention

- Bladder training
- Timed voiding
- Kegel exercises
- Pelvic floor muscle exercises
- Use of anticipatory contraction of pelvic muscles before change of position, such as sit to stand

muscles are inactivated, and the ability of the respiratory system to respond to chemical changes is significantly decreased. The control of breathing must then rely on higher centers.

SLEEPING AND TEMPERAMENT

Novosad and colleagues (1999) related sleep and wake states to an infant's temperament at age 8 months. *Temperament* is the style or way in which an infant relates. Three types of temperaments have been identified in babies as a result of the classic research of Chess and Thomas (1977). Babies can be classified as difficult, easy, or slow-to-warmup. Temperament is stable during infancy but can be molded by experience. Inherent in that experience is the match or mismatch between the infant's temperament and that of her parents.

BREATHING AND EATING

The relationship between breathing and eating is also one of coordination and, by necessity, is established early in development. For the first 6 months of life, the infant is protected from choking by the anatomical proportions of the oral structures and their relationship during swallowing. The movements of the tongue allow the mouth to be separated from the trachea, so, as noted previously, sucking and breathing can occur simultaneously. The infant loses this ability as the oral cavity grows. Once voluntary control of oral motor function is established at 6 to 8 months, the infant interrupts sucking and swallowing to breathe.

Older adults have a longer duration of swallowing, but there has been no reported increase in the incidence of aspiration. In the presence of neuromuscular disease, however, aspiration must always be considered a risk.

FUNCTIONAL IMPLICATIONS

The functional implications of vital functions are listed in Table 11–4 and are fairly obvious. Without the ability to provide oxygen and food substrates to the body, the body would be incapable of sustaining life. There are many age-related functional implications of disturbances of vital functions.

Breathing

Breathing difficulties in the form of apnea plague the young and the old. Premature and full-term infants can experience periods of not breathing. Older adults are more prone to sleep-disordered breathing, of which one form is sleep apnea.

Eating and Digestion

During the prenatal period, loss of the ability to receive nutrition from the mother may lead to intrauterine growth restriction. Before enteral feeding, the

TABLE 11–4

Age-Related Vital Function Concerns

Age Period	Vital Function Concern
Prenatal	Intrauterine growth restrictions Cretinism
Newborn	Apnea Failure to thrive Sudden Infant Death Syndrome Gastroesophageal reflux
Childhood	Obesity Encopresis Enuresis
Adolescence	Obesity Anorexia Bulimia
Adulthood	Obesity Sleep apnea
Older adulthood	Urinary incontinence Constipation Fecal incontinence Dehydration

placenta is the link between the mother's intake and availability of nutrients to the growing fetus. Postnatally, failure to thrive in an infant can have developmental consequences in several domains. At the opposite extreme, obesity is an increasing problem in children and adults. Also, during adolescence, eating disorders such as anorexia and bulimia can be life threatening. For the older adult, nutritional intake can be compromised by lack of dentition, poorly fitting dentures, or an inability to shop and prepare meals.

Elimination

Toilet training can be a stressful time for both toddler and parents. Enuresis and encopresis do not occur in the majority of children, but the loss of bladder and bowel control can be disturbing to child and parent. Seeking the advice of the pediatrician in these cases is always a good idea.

An older adult may also have to deal with urinary incontinence, constipation, or fecal incontinence. In a population-based study in Sweden, 26% of women aged 18 to 70 years experienced urinary incontinence, with a surprising 12% of these women between the ages of 18 and 30 (Hagglund et al, 1999). Nygaard and colleagues (1996) documented that incontinence in community-dwelling women was not a static problem but one in which there can be fluctuations between periods of continence and incontinence.

Summary

All of the vital functions depend on an adequate blood supply to deliver the necessary nutrients for the organs involved. The skeletal system provides the frame on which the muscles of mastication, respiration, digestion, and elimination work. The autonomic nervous system and the endocrine system play a significant role in maintaining homeostasis. Breathing, sleeping, and eating are cyclical activities that conform to neural control mechanisms based on oscillations. Developmentally, intrinsic pacemakers for these repetitive functions buy time until other structures and the systems they serve mature. Vital functions that do not appear to have such neural control, such as digestion and elimination, do exhibit cyclical function and require precise neural coordination demonstrated by the GI nervous system, which has as many neurons as the spinal cord. The ability to maintain a fixed level of performance allows each of us to adapt to a fluctuating environment.

The environment can and does influence the adaptation of vital functions to changing internal and external demands. Humans are motivated to preserve life and to satisfy the basic drives for air, food, and water. Possibly because these functions are vital, the age-related changes in them do not often result in significant or life-threatening effects. No one system of the body works entirely without the other. If one system malfunctions, it will affect all the others, in some way, at some time, and eventually lead to either adaptation or failure.

References

Abbasi A. Nutrition. In Duthie EH, Katz PR (eds). *Practice of Geriatrics*. Philadelphia: WB Saunders, 1998, pp 145–158.

Adkins HV. Improvement of breathing ability in children with respiratory muscle paralysis. *Phys Ther* 48:577–581, 1968.

Allen R. Social factors associated with the amount of school week sleep lag for seniors in an early starting suburban high school. *Sleep Res* 21:114–119, 1992.

American Academy of Pediatrics. Calcium requirements of infants, children, and adolescents. *Pediatrics* 104:1152–1157, 1999a.

American Academy of Pediatrics. Toilet training guidelines: Parents—The role of the parents in toilet training. *Pediatrics* 103(6 Pt 2):1362–1363, 1999b.

American Academy of Pediatrics Task Force on Infant Sleep Position and Sudden Infant Death Syndrome. Changing concepts of sudden infant death syndrome: Implications for infant sleeping environment and sleep position. *Pediatrics* 105(3 Pt 1):650–656, 2000.

Ancoli-Israel S, Kripke DF. Sleep and aging. In Duthie EH, Katz PR (eds). *Practice of Geriatrics*. Philadelphia: WB Saunders, 1998, pp 237–243.

Ancoli-Israel S, Kripke DF, Klauber MR, et al. Sleep disordered breathing in community-dwelling elderly. *Sleep* 14:486–495, 1991.

Atchley RC. Physical aging. In Atchley RC (ed). *Social Forces and Aging*. Belmont, CA: Wadsworth, 1991, pp 69–81.

Aynsley-Green A. Metabolic and endocrine interrelations in the human fetus and neonate. *Am J Clin Nutr* 41:399–417, 1985.

Aynsley-Green A, Hawdon JM, Deshpande S, et al. Neonatal insulin secretion: Implications for the programming of metabolic homeostasis. *Acta Paediatr Jpn* 39(suppl 1):S21–S25, 1997.

Berk LB, Friman PC. Epidemiologic aspects of toilet training. *Clin Pediatr* 29:278–281, 1990.

Brazelton TB, Christophersen ER, Frauman AC, et al. Instruction, timelines, and medical influences affecting toilet training. *Pediatrics* 103(6 Pt 2):1353–1358, 1999.

Broussard DL, Altshchuler SM. Central integration of swallow and airway-protective reflexes. *Am J Med* 108(suppl 4a):62S–67S, 2000.

Buchan AMF, Bryant MG, Polak JM, et al. Development of regulatory peptides in the human fetal intestine. In Bloom SR, Polak JM (eds). *Gut Hormones*. London: Churchill Livingstone, 1981, pp 119–126.

Bundlie SR. Sleep in aging. *Geriatrics* 53(suppl 1):S41–S43, 1998.

Cavallo A. Melatonin and human puberty: Current perspectives. *J Pineal Res* 15:115–121, 1993.

Challamel MBJ. Development of sleep and wakefulness. In Meisami E, Timiras PS (eds). *Handbook of Human Growth and Developmental Biology*, vol I, part B. Boca Raton, FL: CRC Press, 1988, pp 269–284.

Chess S, Thomas A. Temperamental individuality from childhood to adolescence. *J Am Acad Child Psychiatry* 16:218–226, 1977.

Chicurel M. Mutant gene speeds up the human clock. *Science* 291:226–227, 2001.

Coons S, Guilleminault C. Development of consolidated sleep and wakeful periods in relation to the day/night cycle in infancy. *Dev Med Child Neurol* 26:169–176, 1984.

Crapo RO, Jensen RL, Berlin SL. PaO$_2$ in healthy subjects at 1500m altitude are well predicted by meta analysis. *Chest* 100:96S, 1991.

Cress ME, Buchner DM, Questad KA, et al. Exercise: Effects on physical functional performance in independent older adults. *J Gerontol* 54:M241–M248, 1999.

Davis PJ, Davis FB. Endocrine disorders. In Duthie EH, Katz PR (eds). *Practice of Geriatrics*. Philadelphia: WB Saunders, 1998, pp 563–578.

Dijk DF, Duffy JF, Riel E, et al. Ageing and the circadian and homeostatic regulation of human sleep during forced desynchrony of rest, melatonin and temperature rhythms. *J Physiol* 516(Pt 2):611–627, 1999.

Ellis LA, Mastro AM, Picciano MF. Do milk-borne cytokines and hormones influence neonatal immune cell function? *J Nutr* 127:985S–988S, 1997.

Fox HE, Steinbrecher M, Pessel D, et al. Maternal ethanol ingestion and the occurrence of human fetal breathing movements. *Am J Obstet Gynecol* 132:354–358, 1978.

Gibson E, Dembofsky CA, Rubin S, Greenspan JS. Infant sleep position practices 2 years into the "back to sleep" campaign. *Clin Pediatr (Phila)* 39:285–289, 2000.

Goldstein RB. Ultrasound evaluation of the fetal thorax. In Callen PW (ed). *Ultrasonography in Obstetrics and Gynecology*, 3rd ed. Philadelphia: WB Saunders, 1994, pp 426–455.

Green JR, Moore CA, Ruark JL, et al. Development of chewing in children from 12 to 48 months: Longitudinal study of EMG patterns. *J Neurophysiol* 777:2704–2716, 1997.

Guilleminault C. Sleep and sleep disorders in the elderly. In Cassel S, Walsh B (eds). *Geriatric Medicine*. New York: Springer-Verlag, 1994, pp 342–351.

Guyton AC, Hall JE. *Textbook of Medical Physiology*, 9th ed. Philadelphia: WB Saunders, 1996.

Hagglund D, Olsson H, Leppert J. Urinary incontinence: An unexpected large problem among young females. Results from a population-based study. *Fam Pract* 16:506–509, 1999.

Hendricks KM, Badruddin SH. Weaning recommendations: The scientific basis. *Nutr Rev* 50:125–133, 1992.

Hirst GDS. A calcium window to the gut. *Nature* 399:16–17, 1999.

Howe AC, Walker CE. Behavioral management of toilet training, enuresis, and encopresis. *Pediatr Clin North Am* 39:413–432, 1992.

Iverson S, Iverson L, Saper CB. The autonomic nervous system and the hypothalamus. In Kandel ER, Schwartz JH, Jessell TM (eds). *Principles of Neuroscience*, 4th ed. New York: McGraw-Hill, 2000, pp 960–981.

Keenan SA. Normal human sleep. *Respir Care Clin North Am* 5:319–331, 1999.

Kohyama J, Shimohira M, Iwakawa Y. Maturation of motility and motor inhibition in rapid-eye-movement sleep. *J Pediatr* 130:117–122, 1997.

MacRae N. Sexuality and aging. In Chop WC, Robnett RH (eds). *Gerontology for the Health Care Professional*. Philadelphia: FA Davis, 1999, pp 203–225.

Milani-Comparetti A. The neurophysiological and clinical implications of studies on fetal motor behavior. *Semin Perinatol* 5:183–189, 1981.

Miller AJ, Brunelle JA, Carlos JP, et al. *Oral Health of United States Adults.* Washington, DC: US Department of Health and Human Services, National Institutes of Health, Public Health Service, 1987. NIH publication No. 87-2868.

Moon RY, Patel KM, Shaefer SJ. Sudden infant death syndrome in child care settings. *Pediatrics* 106(2 Pt 1):295–300, 2000.

Moore KL, Persaud TVN. *Before We Are Born: Essentials of Embryology and Birth Defects.* Philadelphia: WB Saunders, 1998.

Moore RY. A clock for all ages. *Science* 284:2102–2103, 1999.

Morales A, Heaton JP, Carson CC. Andropause: A misnomer for a true clinical entity. *J Urol* 163: 705–712, 2000.

Morris SE, Klein MD. *Pre-Feeding Skills.* Tucson, AZ: Therapy Skill Builders, 1987.

Nilsson-Ehle H, Jagenburg RJ, Landahl S, et al. Decline of blood hemoglobin in the aged: A longitudinal study of an urban Swedish population from age 70–81. *Br J Haematol* 71:437–442, 1989.

Novosad C, Freudigman K, Thoman EB. Sleep patterns in newborns and temperament at eight months: A preliminary study. *J Dev Behav Pediatr* 20:99–105, 1999.

Nygaard IE, Kreder KJ, Lepic MM, et al. Efficacy of pelvic floor muscle exercises in women with stress, urge, and mixed urinary incontinence. Part 1. *Am J Obstet Gynecol* 174:120–125, 1996.

Pauls J. Urinary incontinence and impairment of the pelvic floor in the older adult. In Guiccione AA (ed). *Geriatric Physical Therapy*, 2nd ed. St. Louis: Mosby, 2000, pp 340–350.

Prechtl H. *The Neurological Examination of the Full-Term Newborn Infant*, 2nd ed. Clinics in Developmental Medicine, No. 63. Philadelphia: JB Lippincott, 1977.

Purushothaman R, Morley JE. Endocrinology in the aged. In Gass GH, Kaplan HM (eds). *Handbook of Endocrinology*, 2nd ed. Boca Raton, FL: CRC Press, 1996, pp 241–260.

Radliffe KT. *Clinical Pediatric Physical Therapy.* Philadelphia: WB Saunders, 1998.

Rivkees SA. Developing circadian rhythmicity: Basic and clinical aspects. *Pediatr Endocrinol* 44:467–487, 1997.

Rosen MG, Scibetta JJ, Chik L, Borgstedt AD. An approach to the study of brain damage: The principles of fetal EEG. *Am J Obstet Gynecol* 115:37–47, 1973.

Rowe JW, Andres RA, Tobin JD, et al. The effect of age on creatinine clearance in man. *J Gerontol* 31:155–163, 1976.

Russell RM. The aging process as a modifier of metabolism. *Am J Clin Nutr* 72(2 suppl):529S–532S, 2000.

Santrock JW. *Child Development*, 4th ed. New York: McGraw-Hill, 1998.

Sapolsky RM, Krey LC, McEwen BS. The neuroendocrinology of stress and aging: The glucocorticoid cascade hypothesis. *Endocrine Rev* 17:284–289, 1996.

Shay K. Dental and oral disorders. In Duthie EH, Katz PR (eds). *Practice of Geriatrics.* Philadelphia: WB Saunders, 1998, pp 481–493.

Ship JA. The influence of aging on oral health and consequences for taste and smell. *Physiol Behav* 66:209–215, 1999.

Sinclair D, Dangerfield P. *Human Growth After Birth*, 6th ed. New York: Oxford University Press, 1998.

Smith M. Gynecologic disorders. In Duthie EH, Katz PR (eds). *Practice of Geriatrics.* Philadelphia: WB Saunders, 1998, pp 524–534.

St. James-Roberts I, Plewis I. Individual differences, daily fluctuations, and developmental changes in amounts of infant waking, fussing, crying, feeding, and sleeping. *Child Dev* 67:2527–2540, 1996.

Vander AF, Sherman JH, Luciano DS. *Human Psychology: The Mechanisms of Body Function*, 8th ed. New York: McGraw-Hill, 2001.

Waldhauser F, Ehrhart B, Forster E. Clinical aspects of the melatonin action: Impact of development, aging and puberty, involvement of melatonin in psychiatric disease and importance of neuroimmunoendocrine interactions. *Experientia* 49:671–681, 1993.

Werk LN, Alpert JJ. Solid feeding guidelines. *Lancet* 352:1569–1570, 1998.

Whitbourne SK. *The Aging Individual: Physical and Psychological Perspectives*. New York: Springer, 1996.

Wolfson AR, Carskadon MA. Sleep schedules and daytime functioning in adolescents. *Child Dev* 69:875–887, 1998.

12 Posture and Balance

OBJECTIVES

After studying this chapter, the reader will be able to:

1 Define posture, balance, righting, and equilibrium.

2 Discuss the theoretical approaches to the study of posture and balance.

3 Differentiate between static and dynamic balance and between reactive and anticipatory postural control.

4 Describe posture and balance across the life span.

Posture is defined as the attitude or position of the body (Thomas, 1997). As such, being in a prone position and in a sitting position are both postures. When talking about someone's posture, most of us think of the alignment of body segments with respect to each other as well as with respect to the outside world. Posture has three functions. First, posture must maintain alignment of the body's segments in any position: supine, prone, sitting, quadruped, and standing. Second, posture must anticipate change to allow our engagement in voluntary, goal-directed movements. When reaching or stepping, our body must be able to make postural adjustments before, during, and after the movement. Third, posture must react to unexpected perturbations or disturbances in balance. This last function requires quick adaptation. Thus, posture is more than just maintaining a position of the body such as standing. Posture is active, whether it is in sustaining an existing posture or moving from one posture to another.

Posture is determined and maintained by coordination of the various muscles that move the limbs, by proprioception, and by the sense of *balance*. Control of posture is balance. The term *postural control* is often used by physical therapists to describe balance; in this chapter, it is synonymous with balance. The goal of the postural control system is to attain a stable vertical posture of the head and trunk against the force of gravity. When this is accomplished, a base is provided for adequate reaching, sitting, standing, and walking (Forssberg, 1999).

Models of Postural Organization

Posture is organized at two different levels (Massion, 1998). The first level is that of the body scheme. The body scheme includes posture as a reference to gravity, its anatomical relationships, and the concept of support. The postural body scheme represents the body's structures such as the head, trunk, and feet and the sensory receptors that provide information about gravity and the external environment.

The second level organizes postural control on the basis of the information from the representational level to form postural networks. The internal representation of the body segments involved in a posture makes up the representational level. The ways in which the various segments of the body relate to one another and how the relationships change based on sensory information are also represented within the postural networks. Posture is represented as a whole entity rather than as just its component parts.

Postural networks are formed during development. For example, as a child experiences sitting, postural muscles are activated. The large numbers of muscle combinations that are initially available are eventually narrowed to those combinations that are most functional. The process of selection forms networks and is illustrated in Figure 3–7. The neural basis for the development of these postural networks is discussed in Chapter 3.

Assaiante and Amblard (1995) proposed an ontogenetic model for the sensorimotor organization of balance control. Their model is based on two functional principles. One principle assumes that the organization of balance depends on which frame of reference is used by the body. The two possible frames of reference are the support surface and gravity. If the support surface is the frame of reference, balance control is organized in an ascending direction from the feet to the head (as seen in a quiet standing posture) or from the hip to the head (as seen in locomotion). If the vertical line of gravity is the frame of reference, balance control is organized in a descending direction from head to feet. A second functional principle is that children learn to control increasing degrees of freedom during a movement. The linkage between the head and trunk can be "en bloc" or articulated. When the head and trunk are en bloc, they move as a unit so that the head is stable on the trunk. When the linkage between the head and neck is articulated, the head is stable in space.

The model of Assaiante and Amblard is based on typical, natural movement activities of children when balance is not disturbed. Four periods of development of postural control have been identified across the life span (Fig. 12–1). In the figure, the direction of the organization is listed across the top along with the organization of the head and trunk linkage. From birth to the achievement of upright stance, a cephalocaudal or descending type of organization is predominant. Control appears first in the muscles of the neck, then in the trunk, and finally in the legs. The second period lasts from the achievement of upright bipedal posture up to 6 years of age.

During this second period, control is ascending from the support surface, that is, from the feet during standing, or ascending from the hips up during locomotion.

At age 7, there is a return to a descending organization with an articulated linkage between the head and trunk. This is not a return to the original condition found in the first period but rather a progression to establishment of

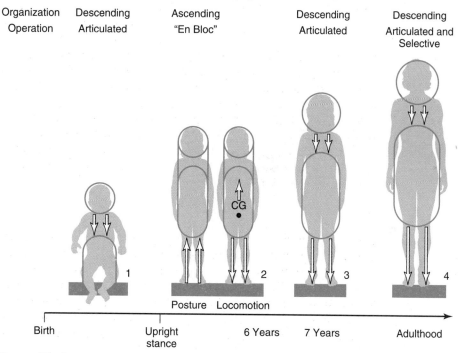

Organization	Descending	Ascending	Descending	Descending
Operation	Articulated	"En Bloc"	Articulated	Articulated and Selective

Birth   Upright stance   6 Years   7 Years   Adulthood

Posture   Locomotion

CG

Figure 12–1

Ontogenetic scheme of the organization of posturokinetic activities. (Adapted and reprinted from *Human Movement Science,* vol 14, 1995, pages 13–43, Assaiante C, Amblard B. An ontogentic model of the sensorimotor organization of balance control in humans, p. 13, copyright (1995), with permission from Elsevier Science.

head stabilization in space strategy (HSSS). HSSS is a basic means of organizing descending temporal control of balance. By being able to master the degrees of freedom allowed by the neck joint, the child improves the accuracy of the visual and vestibular messages received relative to balance or postural control. The final period of postural development adds a measure of selectivity to the articulated operation of the head and trunk unit. This selective control of the degrees of freedom is presumed to be task dependent. The fourth period is present in adulthood.

Types of Postural Control and Balance

There are four types of postural control: static, reactive, anticipatory, and adaptive. *Static postural control* ensures stability by maintaining the body's center of mass (COM) within its base of support (BOS). All of the forces acting on the body are balanced when the COM is within its limits of stability, that is, within the boundaries of the BOS. When static posture is controlled, we are said to have good static balance in a particular position. Although balance in quiet standing is considered static, there is movement occurring during quiet

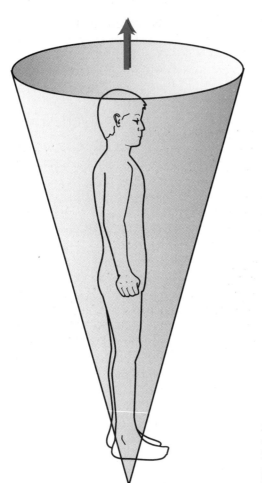

Figure 12–2

Cone of stability. (From Martin ST, Kessler M. *Neurologic Intervention for Physical Therapist Assistants*. Philadelphia: WB Saunders, 2000, p 37.)

standing. Static posture is also termed *steady-state posture*, exemplified when we gently sway over our ankles. The area circumscribed by the sway represents a cone of stability (Fig. 12–2). The cone represents the limits of stability for that posture.

Reactive postural control governs the unexpected movement of the COM within or outside the BOS. Various balance responses are possible given the speed of the displacement and whether the displacement results in the COM exceeding the BOS. Righting or equilibrium reactions are produced in response to weight shifts within the BOS. When the COM moves out of the BOS, as in a slip or fall, additional automatic postural responses occur. An unexpected perturbation on a force platform is an example of reactive postural control or balance. In this case, the BOS is moved to shift the COM.

Postural adjustments made before a movement are classified as *anticipatory*. We typically make such postural adjustments before reaching, lifting, and walking. Anticipatory postural adjustments require that the nervous system feed information forward to postural muscles to prepare for the movement to follow. Think of being a water skier in the water, waiting for the first pull of the rope. You may hear the acceleration of the boat before you feel the pull, but you had better be ready to successfully achieve your goal of being lifted to an upright position. When you prepare to lift a box of heavy books, you expect the load and you prepare your posture accordingly. Experience is important in acquiring *anticipatory postural control*.

Last, *adaptive postural control* is demonstrated when we modify a motor response due to a change in environmental conditions or task demands. Most individuals change their speed and step width when walking on slippery ground. Aspects of cognition, such as attention, motivation, and intention, influence anticipatory and adaptive postural control. When attention is directed away from the balance task, it may be more difficult to adapt.

Postural control is the process by which the central nervous system, sensory system, and musculoskeletal system produce muscular strategies to regulate the relationship between the COM and BOS (Maki and McIlroy, 1996). Stability involves the use of two mechanisms: (1) development of torques at the joints of the supporting leg or legs and trunk to control COM motion and (2) stepping or grasping movements of the limbs to alter the BOS when a person's balance is disturbed. If the source of the destabilization is recognized, it can be anticipated. Sensory information about the body's orientation and motion is also needed and may not be available ahead of an unexpected disturbance in balance. In that case, the sensory information of the instability can either be fed forward or fed back for postural correction. The way in which the postural system may operate is shown in Figure 12–3.

There are three types of perturbations possible: physiological, mechanical, and informational. Physiological events can disrupt the operation of the nervous system control by changing the set point and blocking incoming sensory information. Examples of mechanical disturbances of balance are changes in the forces acting on the body such as a push or shove, slip, or trip. Another example could come from a change in range of motion at the ankle that could change the available BOS in standing. A change in the ambient light, as when walking into a dark room, is an example of an informational perturbation. Changes in sensory information coming in from the environment can affect the set point or reactive balance.

Components of a Postural Control System

During the 1990s, posture has come to be recognized as a complex interaction of biological, mechanical, and movement components. A conceptual model of the systems involved in postural control is depicted in Figure 12–4. Seven components have been identified: limits of stability, sensory organization, eye-head stabilization, the musculoskeletal system, motor coordination, predictive central set, and environmental adaptation.

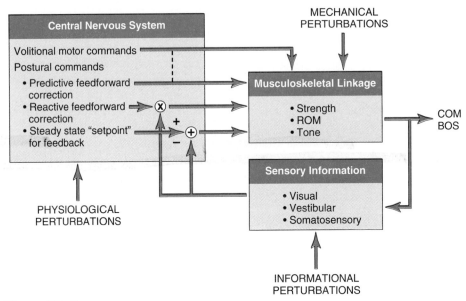

Figure 12-3

A conceptual model of the postural control system. In feedback control, sensory information is used to continuously update the corrective changes to the center of mass (COM) or base of support (BOS). In feedforward control, preprogrammed stabilizing reactions are released, either predictively (anticipatory postural adjustments) or in reaction to sensory information pertaining to the state of instability (triggered postural reactions). Mechanical perturbations involve change in the forces acting on the body (due to movement of the body or interaction with the environment). Informational perturbations pertain to transient change in the nature of the orientational information available from the environment. Physiological perturbations refer to transient internal events that disrupt the operation of the neural control system. ROM, range of motion. (Adapted from Maki BE, McIlroy WE. Postural control in the older adult. *Clin Geriatr Med* 12(4):635–658, 1996, p. 637.)

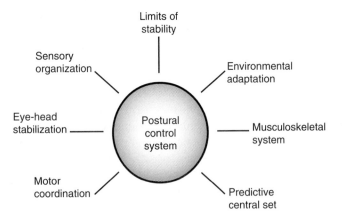

Figure 12-4

Components of normal postural control. (Adapted from Duncan P. *Balance. Proceedings of the APTA Forum*. Alexandria, VA: American Physical Therapy Association, 1990, with permission of the American Physical Therapy Association.)

LIMITS OF STABILITY

Every posture has a BOS. The BOS is that area of the body in contact with the support surface. The perimeter of the BOS is the typical limit of stability. When the mass of the body is maintained within the limits of the BOS, the posture is maintained. Developmental postures such as sitting, quadruped, and standing all have a different BOS. Keeping the COM of body within the BOS constitutes balance. During quiet stance, as the body sways, the limits of stability depend on the interaction of the position and velocity of movement of the COM. We are more likely to lose balance if the velocity of the COM is high and at the limits of the BOS. The body perceives changes in the COM in a posture by detecting amplitude of center of pressure (COP) motion. The COP is the point on the BOS at which muscular reaction forces are produced. In standing, there would be a COP under each foot. Feel how the COP changes as you shift weight forward and back while standing.

SENSORY ORGANIZATION

The visual, vestibular, and somatosensory systems provide the body with information about movement and cue postural responses.

Somatosensation is the combined input from touch and proprioception. Sensory input appears to be needed for the development of postural control. Vision is very important for the development of head control. Newborns are sensitive to the flow of visual information and can even make postural adjustments in response to this information (Jouen, 1992). Input from the visual system is mapped to neck movement initially and then to trunk movement as head and trunk control is established. The production of spatial maps of the position of various body parts appears to be linked to muscular action. The linking of posture at the neck to vision forms before somatosensation is mapped to neck muscles (Shumway-Cook and Woollacott, 2001). Vestibular information is also mapped to neck muscles at the same time as somatosensation is mapped. Eventually, mapping of combinations of sensory input such as visual-vestibular information is done (Jouen, 1984). This bimodal mapping allows for comparisons to be made between previous and present postures. The mapping of sensory information from each individual sense proceeds from the neck to the trunk and on to the lower extremities (Shumway-Cook and Woollacott, 2001). The visual system dominates postural response decisions for the first 3 years of life. Information from vision acts as feedback when the body moves and as an anticipatory cue in a feedforward manner before movement. As the child learns to make use of somatosensory information from the lower extremities, somatosensory input emerges as the primary sensory input on which postural response decisions are made. Adults use somatosensation as their primary source for postural response. When there is a sensory conflict, the vestibular system acts as a tiebreaker in making the postural response decision. If somatosensation says you are moving and vision says you are not, the vestibular input should be able to resolve the conflict to maintain balance.

EYE-HEAD STABILIZATION

The head carries two of the most influential sensory receptors for posture and balance: the eyes and labyrinths. These two sensory systems provide ongoing sensory input about the movement of the surroundings and head, respectively. The eyes and labyrinths provide orientation of the head in space. The eyes must be able to maintain a stable visual image even when the head is moving, and the eyes have to be able to move with the head as the body moves. The labyrinths relay information about head movement to ocular nuclei and about position, allowing the mover to differentiate between *egocentric* (head relative to the body) and *exocentric* (head relative to objects in the environment) motion. Lateral flexion of the head is an egocentric motion. The movement of the head in space while walking or riding in an elevator is an example of exocentric motion.

The HSSS involves an anticipatory stabilization of the head in space before body movement. A child first displays this strategy at 3 years of age while walking on level ground (Assaiante and Amblard, 1993). By maintaining the angular position of the head with regard to the spatial environment, vestibular inputs can be better interpreted. Older adults have been shown to adopt this strategy when faced with distorted or incongruent somatosensory and visual information (DiFabio and Emasithi, 1997).

MUSCULOSKELETAL SYSTEM

The body is a mechanically linked structure that supports posture and provides a postural response. The viscoelastic properties of the muscles, joints, tendons, and ligaments can act as inherent constraints to posture and movement. The flexibility of body segments such as the neck, thorax, pelvis, hip, knee, and ankle contribute to attaining and maintaining a posture or making a postural response. Each body segment has mass and grows at a different rate. Each way in which a joint can move represents a degree of freedom. Because the body has so many individual joints and muscles with many possible ways in which to move, certain muscles work together in synergies to control the degrees of freedom.

Normal muscle tone is needed to sustain a posture and to support normal movement. *Muscle tone* has been defined as the resting tension in the muscle (Lundy-Ekman, 1998) and the stiffness in the muscle as it resists being lengthened (Basmajian and DeLuca, 1985). Muscle tone is determined by assessing the resistance felt during passive movement of a limb. Resistance is due mainly to the viscoelastic properties of the muscle. On activating the stretch reflex, the muscle proprioceptors, the muscle spindles, and Golgi tendon organs contribute to muscle tone or stiffness. The background level of activity in antigravity muscles during stance is described as postural tone by Shumway-Cook and Woollacott (2001). Others also describe patterns of muscular tension in groups of muscles as postural tone (Bobath, 1978). Together, the viscoelastic properties of muscle, the spindles, Golgi tendon organs, and descending motor commands regulate muscle tone.

MOTOR COORDINATION

Motor coordination is the ability to coordinate muscle activation in a sequence that preserves posture. The use of muscle synergies in postural reactions and sway strategies in standing are examples of this coordination and are described in the upcoming section on neural control. Determination of the muscles to be used in a synergy is based on the task to be done and the environment in which the task takes place.

Strength and muscle tone are prerequisites for movement against gravity and motor coordination. Head and trunk control require sufficient strength to extend the head, neck, and trunk against gravity in prone; to flex the head, neck, and trunk against gravity in supine; and to laterally flex the head, neck, and trunk against gravity in side-lying.

PREDICTIVE CENTRAL SET

Predictive central set can best be thought of as postural readiness. This ability to anticipate the need for a change in posture is part of anticipatory postural control. Recognizing the consequence of a movement would allow an individual to prepare for the movement. Think of how you prepare for the act of catching a ball. Sensation and cognition are used as anticipatory cues before movement. Anticipatory postural adjustments serve three purposes (Massion, 1998). One purpose is to keep postural disturbance to a minimum. A second purpose is to prepare for movement as initiating gait. A third purpose is to assist a movement in terms of force or velocity such as throwing a ball. It appears that an internal representation of the dynamics of movements is built up during development that allows for anticipatory postural control to guide movement under similar task conditions.

ENVIRONMENTAL ADAPTATION

Postural responses are made in reaction to internally and externally perceived needs. Movement performance is changed when we encounter ice on a sidewalk. A young child may change the manner in which stairs are descended based on perception of safety. Developmentally, the sensorimotor system of an infant must adapt to gravity. The nervous system generates movement solutions to the problems the infant encounters during the attainment of an upright erect posture. The sensory systems also signal the need for automatic postural reactions to preserve posture. With development of postural networks, anticipatory postural control develops and is used to preserve posture (see Chapter 4). Adaptive postural control allows changes to be made to movement performance in response to internally or externally perceived needs.

Neural Basis for Postural Control and Balance

There are two ways to view the neural basis of postural control. One is the traditional reflex and hierarchical model of postural control already discussed in Chapter 3. The development of postural control does appear to follow a hierarchy and to proceed in a cephalocaudal sequence. Head control is developed before trunk control. Once an erect posture is achieved, however, it is more beneficial to use a systems approach to analyzing postural control.

HIERARCHICAL MODEL

Postural Reflexes

Reflexes and reactions help to restore stability before the activation of voluntary systems. As described in Chapter 3, the hierarchical view of motor control attributes certain reflexes and reactions to specific levels of the nervous system. Figure 3–4 depicts specific reflexes and reactions at each anatomical level. Cervicospinal and vestibulospinal reflexes assist in maintaining postural stability. Vestibular responses are used primarily to stabilize the head in space. Therefore, the brainstem is involved in postural control. It coordinates information from the spinal cord, cerebellum, cerebrum, and special senses. "Brainstem nuclei react reflexively to stimuli and in response to commands issued by other motor centers" (Iyer et al, 1999, p 234). The reticular formation within the brainstem contributes to postural tone by balancing activation of flexor and extensor muscles to allow us to express these reflexes. Posture and proximal movement emanate from brainstem centers (Lundy-Ekman, 1998).

Automatic Postural Adjustments

The act of bringing or moving body segments into alignment with one another has traditionally been referred to as *righting* the head or the body. Righting means to bring the body into "normal" alignment. For humans, normal alignment is considered erect bipedal stance. Newborn infants cannot stand up by themselves or balance. During the first year of life, infants acquire righting and balance abilities that enable them to move from lying to standing position and to balance in the transitional postures they might assume while rising: sitting, quadruped, and kneeling. Righting functions enable an individual to move from one stable posture, such as lying supine, to another stable posture, such as lying prone. The essence of righting is movement from one stable posture to another while seeking a more upright posture. When we can stand without assistance, we move out of the period of infancy and enter childhood. Thus, the postural function of rising is so important to our development that it has been used as a marker of transition to childhood.

Postural reactions are the basis of voluntary movement in a reflex/hierarchical model of postural control. The postural reactions of protective extension, head- and trunk-righting, and equilibrium responses are seen as providing a basis for posture/balance, locomotion, and prehension. These postural reactions occur in response to changes in the body's orientation to gravity and in the pattern of weight distribution within the BOS. Automatic postural reactions maintain or regain balance and make it safe to move voluntarily. There are three kinds of automatic postural reactions: protective, righting, and equilibrium.

The earliest *protective reactions* are seen in response to quick lowering of the body toward a support surface. A protective reaction is an extremity response to a quick displacement of the center of gravity out of the BOS. A downward response of the legs is seen at 4 months. Protective extension of the upper extremities becomes evident when the infant begins to sit with support. Displacement in sitting results in his brisk extension of the arm to catch and protect against falling. The infant can prop forward on extended arms if placed around the same time. Upper extremity protective reactions begin at 6 months in sitting and develop sequentially forward, sideways, and backward. Haley (1986) found that this order of acquisition is not always followed. Protective reactions are generally completely developed by 10 months of age. These reactions become our backup system if we fail to regain our balance by the use of an equilibrium reaction. Unfortunately, the use of these automatic responses can result in unintentional injury, as when an older adult sustains a Colles fracture from falling on an outstretched arm.

Righting reactions begin at birth and exhibit peak occurrence at 10 to 12 months. These reactions can be elicited by any one of a number of sensory stimuli: vestibular, proprioceptive, visual, or tactile. Righting reactions become incorporated into equilibrium reactions and therefore persist as part of our automatic balance mechanism (Table 12–1).

Righting is defined as maintenance or restoration of the proper alignment of the head or trunk in space. One category of righting reactions produces movement in one plane; these movements are described as anterior, posterior, or lateral head-righting or trunk-righting. When held upright in vertical and tilted in any direction, the head and trunk right or tilt in the opposite direction. Likewise, when we are in side-lying position, the somatosensory cue of the trunk on the supporting surface cues lateral head-lifting (righting). Head-righting develops during the first several months in response to gravity's effect on the vestibular system and through the body's contact (somatosensation) with the supporting surface.

A second category of righting reactions produces rotation around the body axis, as in rolling to maintain alignment of body segments. These righting reactions of the head and trunk function to produce rotation around the long axis of the body and are an integral part of producing a smooth movement transition from one posture to another. Mature neck- and body-righting allow for the developmental change from log rolling to segmental rolling seen in the 4- to 6-month-old infant.

Equilibrium reactions are more sophisticated than righting reactions and involve a total body response to a slow shift of the center of gravity outside the BOS. In a lateral sitting equilibrium reaction, the head and trunk right, and the arm and leg abduct opposite the weight shift, followed by head and trunk rotation toward the abducted extremities (Fig. 12–5). Equilibrium reactions begin to appear at 6 months of age in the prone position, even as the infant is experiencing supported sitting. The remaining equilibrium reactions appear in an orderly sequence: prone, supine, sitting, quadruped, and standing. The maturation of the reactions in these postures lags behind the attainment of movement in the next higher developmental posture. For example, equilibrium

TABLE 12–1

Automatic Postural Reactions

Reaction	Age at Onset	Age at Integration
Head-Righting		
Neck (immature)	34 weeks of gestation	4–6 months
Labyrinthine	Birth–2 months	Persists
Optical	Birth–2 months	Persists
Neck (mature)	4–6 months	5 years
Trunk-Righting		
Body (immature)	34 weeks of gestation	4–6 months
Body (mature)	4–6 months	5 years
Landau	3–4 months	1–2 years
Protective		
Downward lower extremity	4 months	Persists
Forward upper extremity	6–7 months	Persists
Sideways upper extremity	7–8 months	Persists
Backward upper extremity	9 months	Persists
Stepping lower extremity	15–17 months	Persists
Equilibrium		
Prone	6 months	Persists
Supine	7–8 months	Persists
Sitting	7–8 months	Persists
Quadruped	9–12 months	Persists
Standing	12–24 months	Persists

Data from Barnes MR, Crutchfield CA, Heriza CB. *The Neurophysiological Basis of Patient Treatment*, vol 2. Atlanta: Stokesville Publishing, 1982.

reactions mature in the sitting position when the child is creeping and mature in the quadruped position when the child is walking.

The various protective, righting, and equilibrium reactions are triggered by sensory cues such as visual recognition of a changing horizon. Vestibular or somatosensory cues are also used to perceive that a postural response is needed. Head-righting occurs before trunk-righting. Postural control is mastered in developmental positions sequentially but with some overlap. For example, equilibrium reactions may mature in a lower developmental position such as sitting as the child moves around in quadruped. In summary, the common concept of posture has two facets: the idea of balance, or preserving alignment, and the function of righting, or moving from one posture to another to attain erect standing posture.

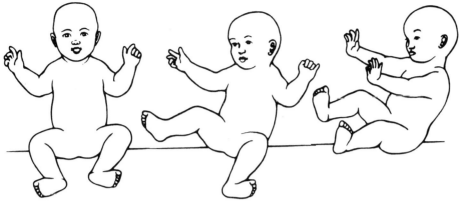

Figure 12–5

Sitting equilibrium reaction in response to lateral weight shift. Equilibrium reactions in sitting mature when the infant begins creeping.

SYSTEMS MODEL

A fundamental concept in the systems perspective is that postural adjustments precede most functional movement. That is, posture is adjusted before the performance of an overt action or movement. For example, if we stand flush against a wall, it is impossible to lean forward and pick up an object on the floor directly in front of our feet. We will fall. To lean forward, weight must be shifted back onto the heels. In the latter description, this shift is prevented from occurring because the wall is in the way. Lee and colleagues (1995) looked at the postural adjustments required to abduct one leg while in a standing position. The COP moves over the leg to be stood on even before the ankle rises. In fact, the shoulder and hip movements that counteract the change in COP also occur before the rise of the ankle.

Anticipatory responses depend on feedforward or proactive control (defined in Chapter 4). These responses change over time and appear to depend on age, musculoskeletal maturity, context, and cognitive abilities. Anticipatory control develops along with reactive postural control (Shumway-Cook and Woollacott, 2001). The ability to anticipate changes in COP before movement comes from experiences in responding to perturbations of the COP within and out of the BOS. Sensory-motor information about position of the head precedes that of the trunk. The COM is higher in children because of their larger heads and shorter legs, resulting in a greater rate of postural sway. As strategies are acquired, picking the most favorable one within a given context becomes more challenging. Within the context of a task, posture supports movement. The standing posture we would assume while stirring a pot on the stove is different from the standing posture we would assume while playing tennis.

Postural control can be changed through learning and experience. One of the most basic premises of a systems perspective is that with practice and repetition, motor behavior can change. The more a pattern of movement, in this case, a postural adjustment, is repeated, the more adaptable it becomes. Practice and experience allow the organization of postural responses to accomplish a functional end such as support of movement. Learning requires that all perceptual systems contribute useful information to the control of posture. Infants are capable of using perceptual information from many different senses after 6 months of age. Therefore, the development of postural control as viewed within a systems model is also suggestive of mapping or associating sensory input from a sensory systems to a particular action, such as head lifting. ". . . The CNS [central nervous system] appears to map the relationship between body movements in space and the motor strategies used to control those movements" (Shumway-Cook and Woollacott, 2001, p 179). When learning is compromised, as in persons with mental disabilities, it may be possible to make postural adjustments but not in a timely manner. The implementation of the muscular response is slower due to nervous system immaturity. Also, anticipatory postural control, which requires experiential learning, appears to be inadequate or delayed in children with Down syndrome (Sugden and Keogh, 1990).

Although the reflex/hierarchical model of postural control is central nervous system dependent and focused on reactive balance, the systems model encompasses the maturation of the musculoskeletal system as well as the central nervous system and focuses on all aspects of balance: reactive, anticipatory, and adaptive. Two systems models of the control of standing balance have been proposed.

Nashner's Model of Postural Control of Stance

Nashner formulated a model for the control of standing balance over the course of some 20 years (Nashner, 1990). His model describes three common sway strategies seen in steady-state standing: the ankle strategy, the hip strategy, and the stepping strategy. Depending on the characteristics of the support surface, the speed of perturbation, and the degree of displacement, different strategies emerge.

An adult sways about the ankle when the foot is fully supported during quiet stance (Fig. 12–6A). This strategy depends on solid contact under the foot to provide a resistive force, enabling the ankle muscles to exert their effect through "reverse action." With the foot fixed on the ground, either the plantar flexors or the dorsiflexors contract to pull the leg backward and forward with respect to the foot, keeping the COM within the BOS. If we sway backward, the anterior tibialis fires to bring us forward; if we sway forward, the gastrocnemius fires to bring us back to midline. This strategy depends on having a solid surface under the feet and intact vision, vestibular system, and somatosensation. The ankle strategy is used when the perturbations or disturbances to balance are small.

An adult sways about the hip when standing crosswise on a narrow balance beam, as shown in Figure 12–6B. An ankle strategy cannot be used in this situation because there is no support under the toes and heels to provide

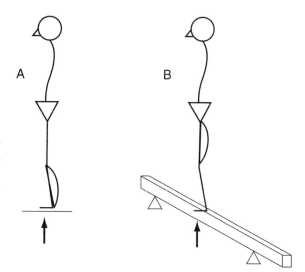

Figure 12–6

Sway strategies. *A,* Postural sway about the ankle in quiet standing, with the foot fully supported. *B,* Postural sway about the hip in standing on a balance beam, with the foot partially supported. (From Martin ST, Kessler M. *Neurologic Intervention for Physical Therapist Assistants.* Philadelphia: WB Saunders, 2000, p 38.)

a reactive force to the ankle motion. Therefore, the only successful strategy is the hip strategy, in which hip flexion and extension combine with knee extension and flexion to ensure balance. Larger perturbations elicit a hip strategy if the feet are supported, as when performing a postural stress test.

The last sway strategy, that of stepping, occurs when the speed and strength of the balance disturbance are sufficient to produce a protective step. By taking a step, the BOS is widened and balance is regained because the COM is once again within the BOS. It had been thought that the COM had to exceed the BOS for stepping to occur, but such is not the case (Brown et al, 1999). Some researchers have found that the directions given to subjects during a balance task may constrain them from stepping (McIlroy and Maki, 1993).

Children 18 months old are able to demonstrate an ankle strategy in quiet standing when balance is disturbed (Forssberg and Nashner, 1982). Their response time is longer than that for adults. According to Shumway-Cook and Woollacott (1985), children 4 to 6 years old displayed varying strategies to the same type of perturbations in standing; sometimes a hip strategy was used, and sometimes an ankle strategy was used. A consistent ankle strategy performed in a timely manner was not evident until 7 to 10 years of age. This coincides with the maturation of nervous system myelination of major tracts by age 10. Adult sway strategies are present in 7- to 10-year-old children.

Winter's Stiffness Model of Postural Control of Stance

Research has looked at how the body's COM is controlled during quiet stance. Winter and colleagues (1998) proposed a straightforward model that gives an almost immediate corrective response. "The model assumes that muscles act as springs to cause the center-of-pressure (COP) to move in phase with the center-of-mass (COM) as the body sways about some desired position" (Winter et al, 1998, p 1211). The stiffness control in the sagittal plane comes from the torque produced by the ankle plantar flexors/dorsiflexors. In the frontal plane, the stiffness comes from the hip abductor/adductor torque. The model of Winter and colleagues is also an inverted pendulum. Movement of the COP under the feet regulates the body COM. The difference between the body COM and the COP are proportional to the acceleration of body COM. The researchers showed that the torque needed to restore posture was set by the joint stiffness.

Rietdyk and coworkers (1999) measured joint moments during balance recovery from a mediolateral perturbation at the trunk or pelvis. Their results validated the model of Winter and colleagues (1998) and showed that the first response to the perturbation was provided by muscle stiffness, not reflex-activated muscle activity. The joint moments detected were sufficient to move the COP in appropriate directions to control the lateral collapse of the trunk. The moments at the hip and spine accounted for 85% of the recovery response, whereas the ankles contributed 15%.

In a review of proprioceptive control of posture, Allum and colleagues (1998) questioned whether the proprioceptive cues from the ankles do trigger balance responses in standing and during locomotion. The research reviewed supports the idea that postural strategies other than sway strategies are possible. Input to the trunk and hip may be more important than input to the ankle in triggering balance correction in standing. This may reflect the fact that the hip is the joint in the lower extremity that is used to recover stability when posture/balance is disturbed in a mediolateral direction. Hip muscles are activated before ankle muscles when balance is disturbed mediolaterally (Horak and Moore, 1989). Responses to mediolateral postural disturbances activate muscles in a proximal-to-distal order.

Assessment of Posture and Balance

There are many ways in which to assess balance (see Clinical Implications—Assessment of Balance for an overview). Testing of the sensory systems that support balance can be done using the Clinical Test of Sensory Integration on Balance (CTSIB) or the Sensory Organization Test (SOT) (Fig. 12–7A, B). Essentially, these are the same test. The examiner measures how long a client can stand in six different sensory conditions; those conditions are shown (Fig. 12–7A). The clinical test uses dense foam support to provide inaccurate somatosensory input and a Japanese lantern to provide inaccurate visual input. A force platform is not used. In the SOT (Fig. 12–7B), a force platform is used. Measurement of standing balance under changing sensory conditions is dynamic *posturography*. The client stands on a force platform in each of the six conditions. The platform is perturbated to provide inaccurate somatosensory input in three conditions. The apparatus moves to provide inaccurate visual information in two conditions.

Postural sway with eyes open and eyes closed can be observed under different stance configurations, such as those used in the Romberg and sharpened Romberg. The Postural Stress Test is a way to quantify the effect of nudging or pushing someone by using a defined force to displace them back-

VISUAL CONDITIONS

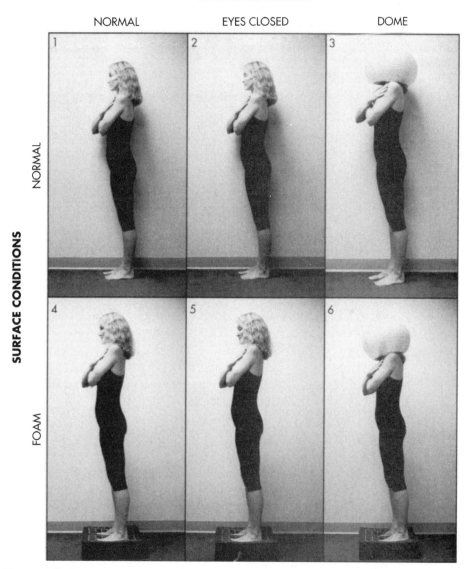

Figure 12–7

Assessment of balance using tests of sensory reception and organization. *A,* The Clinical Test of Sensory Integration on Balance (CTSIB) uses foam and a Japanese lantern to replicate six sensory conditions. (From Umphred DA. *Neurological Rehabilitation,* 4th ed. St. Louis: Mosby, 2001, p 631.)

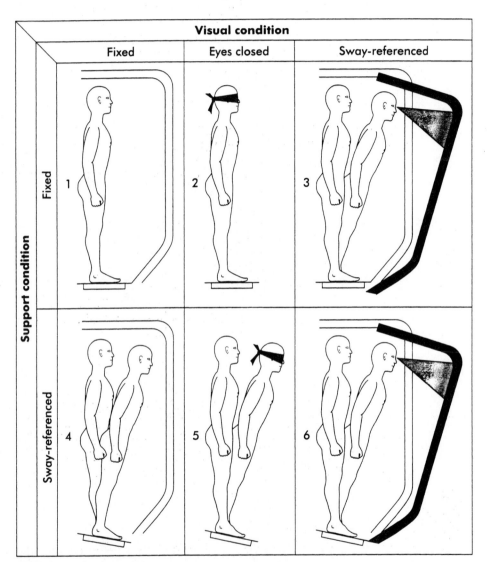

Figure 12-7 *Continued*

B, The six conditions used in the sensory organization test (SOT). (From Hasson S. Clinical Exercise Physiology. St. Louis: Mosby, 1994, p 216.)

ward (Whipple and Wolfson, 1990). Functional reach (Duncan et al, 1990) is a quick measure of balance in standing. The subject stands with an arm outstretched and reaches as far forward as possible without losing balance (Fig. 12–8). The test measures the limits of stability while performing a forward

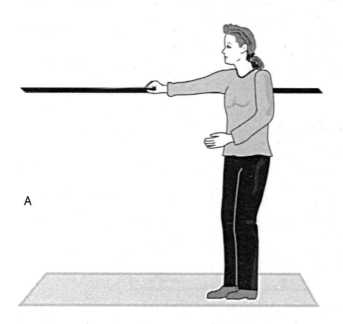

A

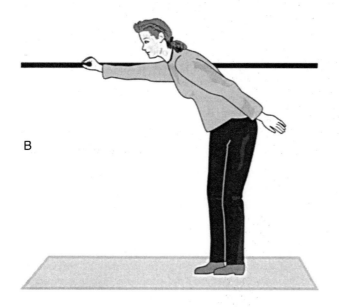

B

Figure 12–8

During the functional reach test, the client is asked to reach forward as far as possible from a comfortable standing posture. The excursion of the arm from start to finish is measured via a yardstick affixed to the wall at shoulder height. *A*, Functional reach—starting position. *B*, Functional reach—ending position. (From Umphred DA. *Neurological Rehabilitation,* 4th ed. St. Louis: Mosby, 2001, p 629.)

maximal reach. The test assesses dynamic balance and anticipatory control. Even though the test was originally devised for a geriatric population, norms have been established for children.

Functional scales of balance are used mainly with the older population to screen for risk of falls and include the Berg Balance Scale (Berg, 1993), the Get Up and Go (Mathias et al, 1986) or Timed Up and Go test (Podsiadlo and Richardson, 1991), and the Tinetti Performance Oriented Mobility Assessment (Tinetti, 1986) that includes balance and gait (see Clinical Implications—Assessment of Balance).

Posture and Balance Across the Life Span

For physical therapists, the study of posture and balance development is an integral part of the study of motor development. Posture, like movement, varies characteristically with age. *Balance* is a developmental characteristic related to posture. In this chapter, the specific changes in human postural function are examined from a life-span perspective. A real constraint to a broad and systematic study of posture is the lack of information about posture during large periods of the human life span. Typically, research and collections of literature regarding posture, even when claiming a life-span perspective, skip important life periods. We know most about the very young infant and child and older adults. Less is known about postural development in later childhood, adolescence, and young and middle adulthood.

INFANCY AND CHILDHOOD

Postural control develops in a cephalocaudal and proximal-distal sequence in infants. Head control is achieved before trunk control, shoulder control before finger control, and pelvic control before foot control. Once erect stance is achieved, the relationship with the support surface initiates a caudocephalic sequence of responses or distal to proximal as described by Nashner (1990). Postural control is essential to developing skilled actions such as locomotion and manipulation. Bertenthal and Von Hofsten (1998) stated that eye, head, and trunk control are the foundation for reaching and manipulation.

Development of Spinal Curves

Static postural alignment is dependent to some extent on the spinal curves seen when viewing upright posture from the side. Everyone is familiar with the anatomical landmarks used to determine alignment. Spinal curves develop over the life span. Although the adult spine has sagittal curves in the cervical, thoracic, lumbar, and pelvic regions, the infant has only two curves. The flexed posture of the newborn is the result of physiological flexor tone and the need to conform to the mother's uterus. The infant's two curves are concave forward: one in the thoracic region and the other in the pelvic region. The latter

CLINICAL IMPLICATIONS
Assessment of Balance

There are many ways to assess postural control and balance. Thus, it is important to understand the types of assessment to differentiate the components and types of postural control. Some tests are specific to the component or type of control, whereas others are more general measures of balance. Functional scales are also available. A brief description of some of these tests is provided in the text, but an in-depth discussion of balance assessment is beyond the scope of this chapter.

Component of Postural Control	Test
▪ Sensory reception and organization	▪ Clinical Test of Sensory Integration on Balance (CTSIB) ▪ Sensory Organization Test (SOT)
▪ Musculoskeletal system	▪ Manual muscle test ▪ Range of motion

Type of Postural Control	Test
▪ Quiet standing	▪ Posturography ▪ Postural sway ▪ Romberg
▪ Reactive	▪ Righting and equilibrium reactions postural stress test (nudge/pull test)
▪ Anticipatory	▪ Functional reach

Functional Scales of Balance	Test
▪ Berg Balance Scale	▪ Fourteen tasks from everyday life test static and dynamic balance skills. Items use mainly steady-state and anticipatory balance. The test is able to discriminate older adults at risk for falls.
▪ Get Up and Go/Timed Up and Go	▪ A quick measure of mobility and balance. Timed version is a good indicator of fall status in community-dwelling older adults.
▪ Tinetti Performance Oriented Mobility Assessment (POMA)	▪ Scale rates performance on 16 items involving balance and gait. Static and dynamic tasks use reactive, steady-state, and anticipatory balance. The score can be used to determine risk for falls.

is formed by the curve of the sacrum that is composed of separate vertebral components at this stage of development.

As the infant grows and develops sufficient strength to lift the head, the cervical curve develops and is convex forward. This curve becomes more noticeable as the infant holds the head up at 3 to 4 months. The lumbar curve is also convex forward and develops when the baby begins to sit up. The curves could fail to develop if the child is unable to develop head control and sitting.

Development of Postural Control

Postural development proceeds from head control to trunk control. The infant assumes a prone on elbows posture around 3 months when the head and upper back are extended sufficiently to allow the freeing of the arms from under the infant. Weight bearing in the posture is important for developing proximal shoulder girdle stabilization. The prone progression of developmental postures consists of achieving a prone on elbows position and then moving to prone on extended arms and finally moving up to quadruped or all fours. From a hands and knees posture, the infant pulls to stand and achieves upright posture. Initially, support of hands or tummy may be required.

With the achievement of upright stance, erect posture is precarious. Because the newly erect infant's center of gravity is relatively high (T12 compared with L5-S1 in an adult), the BOS is widened. The center of gravity is also forward due to a large liver. For the upper trunk to achieve vertical, the lumbar lordosis is increased and the arms are brought into high guard (see Fig. 3–11F).

Standing Posture in Childhood

Children 2 to 3 years of age exhibit a characteristic lumbar lordosis that ranges between 30 and 40 degrees (Asher, 1975). When infants begin to stand and walk, their feet are flat and they begin to exhibit a longitudinal arch only as the fat pad in the foot diminishes. Changes in lower extremity alignment in the stance posture occur over a 6-year period. The 18-month-old child stands with bow legs (genu varum), but by 3 years of age the legs may exhibit genu valgus or knock knees. The legs straighten out by 6 years (Staheli, 1998).

Balance on two feet increases as independent locomotion is achieved (see Chapter 13). Once double limb support is mastered in standing, the next challenge is to develop balance while standing on one foot. Unilateral support begins momentarily at age 3 years and progresses sequentially to 10+ seconds at 6 years (Table 12–2). Momentary one foot standing balance is needed to ascend a step or to step over an object. Longer unilateral standing balance is a prerequisite for motor skills such as hopping, galloping, and skipping.

TABLE 12–2

Age-Related Expectations for One-Foot Standing Balance

Age (yr)	Time
3	Momentary
4	4–6 seconds
5	8–10 seconds
6	10+ seconds eyes open and eyes closed

Balance Strategies in Sitting and Standing

Infants develop directionally specific postural responses before being able to sit (Hadders-Algra et al, 1996a, 1996b). These responses appear to be innate and are guided by an internal representation of the limits of stability such as orientation of the vertical axis and relationship of COM to BOS. This is consistent with the hypothesis of a central pattern generator being the source of initial postural responses (Hirschfeld and Forssberg, 1994). This circuitry determines the spatial characteristics of muscle activation that is triggered by afferent information. During this period of time, the infant demonstrates a large number of responses. With further development, the circuitry at the first level matures, and with experience, the initial variability is reduced. The temporal and spatial features of responses are fine-tuned to match task-specific demands. The second level of control is supported by the neuronal group selection theory in which experience shapes connections by changing the synaptic strength of intergroup and intragroup connections (Allum et al, 1998). Multisensory afferent input is used to shape these adaptive responses.

Sensory Contributions to Balance

Vision appears to be a dominant influence on the development of posture and balance during the first 3 years of life (Butterworth and Hicks, 1977). Spontaneous head control is noted in infants at 10 weeks of age when electromyographic responses can be recorded in reaction to being tilted (Prechtl and Hopkins, 1986). Jouen (1992) showed that 3-day-old infants made postural adjustments of the head in response to optical flow patterns. These are patterns of light associated with movement. The brain uses this information to know where the head and the body are relative to the surrounding environment. Bertenthal and associates (1997) investigated the developmental changes in postural control of 5-, 7-, 9-, and 13-month-old infants in response to optical flow. The infants were able to scale their postural responses to the visual information. The scaling was even possible in pre-sitters but improved with practice and the development of sitting. The ability to use visual information for postural responses increased from 5 to 9 months of age. Vestibular and somatosensory systems can also trigger balance responses in infants and toddlers in sitting (Hirschfeld and Forssberg, 1994).

Sitting Strategies

Sitting is a new posture in which the COM is suspended above the BOS. Fairly rapid postural adjustments are needed to resist or to compensate for sudden losses of balance. Even infants who were unable to sit alone were able to integrate visual information and make a motor response (postural adjustment) without having the strength and coordination to maintain a sitting posture independently. Improvement in muscle activation patterns is a function of experience with perceptual modulation of posture (Hadders-Algra et al, 1996b).

Studies of the development of anticipatory postural control have been conducted in sitting using reaching as the task. Postural activity in the trunk was measured while an infant reached from a seated posture (Riach and Hayes, 1990). Trunk muscles were activated before muscles used for reaching. Researchers concluded that anticipatory postural control occurs before voluntary movements and is present in infants by 9 months of age (Hadders-Algra et al, 1996a). Children appear to tolerate more imbalance as they grow up (Hay and Redon, 1999). Anticipatory control of posture increase from 3 to 8 years of age, with older children demonstrating more refined scaling of responses.

Sit to Stand Transition

Moving from sitting to standing is an everyday occurrence and a necessary prerequisite for walking. Cahill and colleagues (1999) studied three age groups of children on a sit to stand task. The children were grouped as follows: 12 to 18 months, 4 to 5 years, and 9 to 10 years. The movement became more coordinated as measured by the smoothness of phase-plane plots. The youngest group could perform the movement but could not cease moving once a standing posture was attained and either took steps or raised onto their toes. The oldest group generated a pattern of vertical ground reaction force like that of adults when coming to stand but could not do so consistently. Differences in performance were attributed to developmental differences in the children's ability to control horizontal momentum of the body mass, use sensory input for balance, and understand the task.

Sensory Contributions to Standing

The ability of the infant to use visual information shifts during motor development. Vision is important during behavioral transitions such as learning to sit, stand, and walk independently (Foster et al, 1996; Sundermier and Woollacott, 1998). Vision is needed for postural control during these transitions (Sveistrup and Woollacott, 1996). Sundermier and Woollacott (1998) report that postural sway of early walking infants is highly influenced by visual flow information inaccurately signaling self-movement. With age, the importance of vision as a cue for postural response declines.

As children master independent walking, the primacy of vision for postural control wanes. Postural sway in standing on a moveable platform under normal vestibular and somatosensory conditions is greater for children 4 to 6 years of age than for children 7 to 10 years of age (Shumway-Cook and Woollacott, 1985). Within this 4- to 6-year-old age range, vision is still important for balance, but proprioception and touch are being used more. By 7 to 10 years of age, an adult sway strategy is demonstrated wherein the child depends primarily on somatosensory information. Interestingly, children with visual impairments are not able to minimize postural sway to the same extent as nonvisually impaired children (Portfors-Yeomans and Riach, 1995).

By 7 years of age, children are able to make effective use of HSSS that depends on dynamic vestibular cues (Assaiante and Amblard, 1995). These researchers further postulate that this may be a prelude to adult postural responses where vestibular input acts as a deciding factor when conflicting sensory information regarding balance is received. Vision dominates in the first two developmental periods, discussed earlier in this chapter, before development of the HSSS. Vision reaches its maximum importance around the age of 6 years according to Assaiante and Amblard (1995). Vestibular input becomes important in the third period. Somatosensation may be at work during all periods according to these authors.

Standing balance responses in 4- to 6-year-olds are marked by a great deal of variability when testing postural responses using a force platform perturbation paradigm. Multiple sway strategies such as a hip, ankle, or stepping strategy can be elicited when the child's balance is disturbed. According to Shumway-Cook and Woollacott (1985), the child increases use of proprioceptive and vestibular input during this period of time and is less dependent on vision for postural responses. Foudriat and associates (1993) studied the effect of altered sensory environments on balance in healthy children between 3 and 6 years of age. Their data suggest that visuovestibular control of balance shifts to a somatosensory-vestibular dependence by age 3. Although the 6-year-olds generally demonstrated better postural control than other age groups, they did not achieve adult-like balance responses for all sensory conditions.

Nougier and colleagues (1998) studied the contribution of central and peripheral vision to the regulation of stance in 6-, 8-, and 10-year-old children under four visual conditions. For each visual condition, two conditions of support (normal and altered ankle somatosensory input) were used. Children were more stable with vision and under normal support conditions. There was no effect of age. Children used central and peripheral visual input equally well for postural stability at ages 6 and 10. For 8-year-olds, central vision produced greater postural stability than peripheral vision. It is generally accepted that visual, vestibular, and somatosensory information must be integrated to control posture.

In summary, visual input dominates posture and balance during the first 3 years of life. The 4- to 6-year-old child is able to make more use of proprioceptive information, but the balance responses in standing are highly variable. By 7 to 10 years of age, he is able to demonstrate adult strategies in response to perturbations in standing, such as swaying over the ankles like an inverted pendulum.

ANTICIPATORY CONTROL

Donahoe and associates (1994) tested children between 5 and 15 years of age using the functional reach test. Balance was seen to improve with age up to the 11- to 12-year-old age category and then appeared to stabilize. The ability to anticipate the postural adjustments needed to allow for reaching forward is used on a daily basis in childhood activities. The task is an example of feedforward control of balance and is a test of anticipatory control.

ADOLESCENCE AND TRANSITIONAL MOVEMENTS

Lebiedowska and Syczewska (2000) looked at the relationship between body size and its effect on postural sway in children 7 to 18 years of age. They wanted to know if the structural changes in body height and mass affected spontaneous sway parameters. They found no significant correlations between the parameter and developmental factors of age, body height, and body mass. However, there was a decrease in sway parameter when values were normalized to body height that indicated a small improvement in static equilibrium with taller children. COP was used as a measure of the movement of the center of gravity. As such, COP motion did not change in the children studied.

A study of rising movements in teenagers revealed what appears to be a peak in incidence of symmetrical movement patterns around the age of 15 years (Sabourin, 1989). Younger and older teens were found to exhibit more asymmetry while rising than did middle teens. This is particularly true for lower limb movements. It may be that peak performance in a task occurs when most individuals demonstrate the greatest ability to control force within this task. Although children seem to have difficulty controlling force production in this task, and as a result demonstrate asymmetry in their rising actions, teens exhibit a refined competence in simultaneously controlling the upper limb, trunk, and lower limb movements. They move from recumbency by flexing the trunk and moving the feet directly in front of their buttocks while balancing in sitting position, and then they transfer weight from the buttocks to the feet with ease. Control of the force and direction of movement in the righting task is impressive at this age.

ADULTHOOD AND TRANSITIONAL MOVEMENTS

The mid-teen peak in symmetrical performance is diminished slightly during the late-teen period and in the early 20s. Although symmetrical performance is the most common form of rising, it is the mode of action of approximately one fourth of young adults. The remainder demonstrate asymmetry in at least one component of body action, be it the upper limbs, the trunk, or the lower limbs. This is when individuals are making the transition from high school to college or the work force. Compared with the high school years, young adulthood presents fewer formalized opportunities to participate in physical activity. Green and Williams (1992) found that activity level is related to performance in the rising task during the middle adult years. More active adults are more likely to use symmetrical patterns. Another study demonstrated that body size is also a significant factor among adult women performing the righting task (VanSant et al, 1989). Taller and more slender women are more likely to demonstrate symmetrical patterns than were shorter and heavier women.

Patterns of movement change with age, and movement patterns used by older adults are highly variable (Ford-Smith and VanSant, 1993; Thomas et al, 1998; VanSant, 1988a, 1988b). Figure 12–9 depicts three common ways in which older adults rise from the floor. Posture and balance may decline as an individual ages due to changes in static posture, loss of flexibility and muscle strength, vestibular impairments affecting postural awareness and head stabilization, tone changes resulting from medications or pathologies, changes in sensorimotor input and integration, and visual changes. Many of the changes

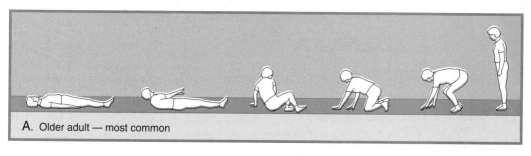

A. Older adult — most common

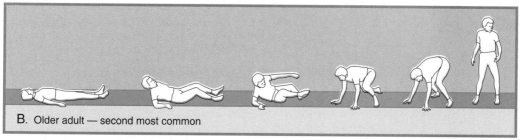

B. Older adult — second most common

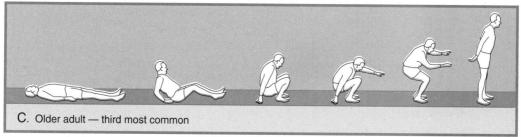

C. Older adult — third most common

Figure 12–9

Common patterns of rising from the floor in older adults aged 65 to 88 years. (Adapted from Thomas RL Jr, Williams AK, Lundy-Ekman L. Supine to stand in elderly persons: Relationship to age, activity level, strength, and range of motion. *Issues Aging* 21:3–18, 1998, pp 12–14.)

in movement patterns seen in an older adult are the result of inactivity and the lack of motor practice (Woollacott and Tang, 1997).

BALANCE IN OLDER ADULTS

Posture

The ability to maintain an erect aligned posture decreases with advanced age. Figure 12–10 depicts the general postural differences that can be anticipated to occur as a result of typical aging. The secondary spinal curves that developed in infancy begin to be modified. The cervical curve decreases. The lumbar curve usually flattens. Decreased movement can accentuate age-related pos-

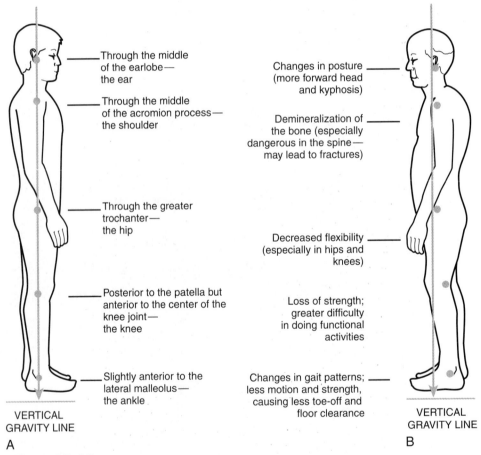

Through the middle of the earlobe— the ear

Through the middle of the acromion process— the shoulder

Through the greater trochanter— the hip

Posterior to the patella but anterior to the center of the knee joint— the knee

Slightly anterior to the lateral malleolus— the ankle

VERTICAL GRAVITY LINE

A

Changes in posture (more forward head and kyphosis)

Demineralization of the bone (especially dangerous in the spine— may lead to fractures)

Decreased flexibility (especially in hips and knees)

Loss of strength; greater difficulty in doing functional activities

Changes in gait patterns; less motion and strength, causing less toe-off and floor clearance

VERTICAL GRAVITY LINE

B

Figure 12–10

Comparison of standing posture: Changes associated with age. *A,* Young adult. *B,* Older adult. (Adapted from Lewis C [ed]. *Aging: The Health Care Challenge,* 2nd ed. Philadelphia: FA Davis, 1990.)

tural changes. The older adult who sits most of the day may be at greater risk for a flattened lumbar area. The thoracic spine becomes more kyphotic. Aging alters the properties and relative amount of connective tissue in the interior of the disk (Moncur, 2000). The disks lose water, and initially flexible connective tissue stiffens, causing older adults to lose spinal flexibility. In general, there is a decrease in connective tissue flexibility. The strength of the muscles declines with age and could contribute to a decline in the ability of the older adult to maintain postural alignment. Figure 12–11 presents a comparison of posture in women from 10 to 60 years of age.

Postural changes seen with aging can include forward head, kyphosis of the thoracic spine, loss of lumbar lordosis, loss of hip and knee flexion, and loss of ankle mobility. All of these changes shift the center of gravity forward and create instability during standing and walking. A loss of flexibility and diminished postural responses lead to less-organized motor patterns, further leading to destabilization and diminished motor coordination. Postural, somatosensory, and vestibular changes diminish an older adult's ability to accom-

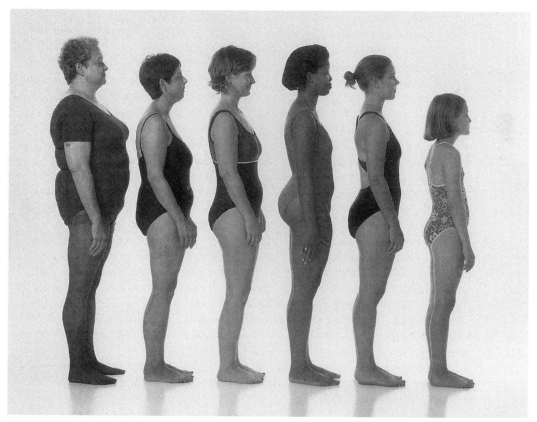

Figure 12–11

Comparison of posture in females from 10 to 60 years of age.

modate to loss of balance, to environmental changes, and to other concurrent tasks often involved in functional activities.

Effect of Sensory Changes with Age

Sensory input for balance changes with advancing age. The three sensory systems (visual, vestibular, and somatosensory) responsible for posture undergo age-related changes. The visual system is less able to pick up contours and depth cues due to a decline in contrast sensitivity. Both of these losses can impair postural control. If there are cataracts or macular degeneration, the problems can be intensified. The vestibular system loses hair cells that detect changes in direction of flow of the endolymph within the semicircular canals and saccule and utricle. The eighth cranial nerve may show a reduction of nerve fibers. Both of these changes can affect otolith function and result in positional vertigo. Vibratory sense in the lower extremities declines and could contribute to a decrease in somatosensory input from the support surface and awareness of the degree of postural sway. Older adults exhibit an increased postural sway when standing on a foam surface. The researchers associated the increased sway with a decline in visual contrast sensitivity and visual acuity in older adults because they could not compensate for decreased somatosensation with vision (Lord et al, 1991). These and other findings demonstrate the importance of vision for maintaining balance under challenging conditions (Lord and Menz, 2000).

Older adults appear to have more difficulty using the built-in redundancy of the sensory systems linked to postural responsiveness (Hay et al, 1996). Under typical circumstances, an adult will use vestibular input to resolve a conflict situation in which somatosensory cues indicate the body is moving and the visual cues do not indicate movement or vice versa. The vestibular system acts as the deciding vote as to whether we need to respond. Hay and colleagues (1996) found that older adults were less stable in standing than were younger adults when visual cues were removed. Both groups had difficulty when a vibratory stimulus was applied at the ankle, thus altering proprioceptive input. However, the older adults responded less well to having normal proprioceptive input restored than did the younger adults. It appears that in addition to age-related changes in sensory receptors producing peripheral deficits, there also may be a slowing of central control mechanisms responsible for postural regulation. Conflicting sensory inputs were presented to the older adults to test the hypothesis that central processing is also involved in age-related changes of postural responsiveness. The older adults were much more affected by a combined conflicting situation that involved proprioceptive and visual information than were young adults.

Four age groups were tested using the SOT. The young, middle-aged, old, and older old showed a decline in overall scores with age and changes in movement strategies (Cohen et al, 1996). Age-related declines in those parts of the vestibular system that deal with posture and balance were evident into the 80s. When Chaput and Proteau (1996) studied younger and older adults performing aiming movements, they found that older subjects processed the available sources of sensory information separately rather than together. Each source of sensory information (visual, vestibular, and somatosensory) was used, but an integrated sensory reference such as linking visual and vestibular information was not produced, as it was in young adults.

Standing Balance

Postural sway has been shown to increase in older adults (Tanaka et al, 1995). Individuals aged 50 to 80 years showed significantly more postural sway in quiet stance than did young adults (Woollacott et al, 1988). Several factors contribute to the increase in sway. One factor is the increased time it takes to respond when a platform moves and causes a posterior sway. Older adults are slower to respond. Latency of leg muscle reflex responses to stance perturbations increase significantly after age 50 (Nardone et al, 1995). Second, the organization of the muscular response may be lacking. In one group of older adults, 50% showed occasional disorganized responses. Older adults used more of a coactivation pattern of muscles compared with the orderly sequence of distal to proximal activation seen in younger adults. Last, older adults are more likely to use a hip strategy or proximal-to-distal activation of muscles rather than the typical adult strategy to control postural sway (Woollacott et al, 1986). This may be related to decreased strength and flexibility at the ankle.

Musculoskeletal System

Aging affects the musculoskeletal system that is responsible for generating sufficient strength to move, ensuring sufficient range of motion to move through, and providing sufficient endurance to continue to move as long as a response is needed. Strength is needed in muscles that stabilize proximal body parts, whereas quick contractions of more distal muscles may be needed to counteract rapid perturbations. As discussed in Chapter 6, strength declines, especially in the lower extremities, with age. Lower extremity strength is needed to maintain postural stability in standing (Wolfson et al, 1995). Concentric contractions occur less quickly in older adults. Change in fiber type, especially type II, have been linked to a dramatic decline in the generation of high-frequency postural muscle contractions (Huang et al, 1999).

Postural changes in stance, especially the position of the hips, knees, or ankles in quiet stance, can hinder an effective postural response. Excessive flexion at these joints may make it more difficult to respond safely to posterior perturbations. Decreased ankle muscle strength was associated with stair climbing ability in older individuals (Duncan et al, 1993).

Attention and Postural Control

Attention to task is required to exhibit adaptive or anticipatory postural control. In addition to declines in sensory reception and central sensory processing, the older adult's ability to attend to more than one task is reduced. For example, it may be difficult for an older adult to perform a cognitive task, such as carrying on a conversation, at the same time as preparing for a motor task, like stepping onto an escalator, that requires anticipatory postural response.

Brown and colleagues (1999) found that older adults needed to focus more attention on their balance than younger adults when recovering a stable posture after external perturbation. There was a hierarchy of increasing attentional demands between the use of the ankle strategy and the stepping strategy in the older adults. A further study looking at a choice reaction time auditory task during quiet standing under six different sensory conditions found that as sensory information decreases, attentional demands for postural control increase as a factor of age (Shumway-Cook and Woollacott, 2000).

Maylor and Wing (1996) reported on a study of postural stability of two groups with mean ages of 57 and 77. Subjects had to perform five cognitive tasks while standing on a force platform. There was no cognitive task in the control condition. Postural stability was negatively affected by age in all conditions. The age differences in postural stability were increased for those tasks involving visual and spatial manipulation such as a spatial memory task or backward digit recall.

Adaptive Control

Adapting to changing situations within the environment also depends on processing sensory data and being able to initiate a response. Hay and colleagues (1996) further suggested that because older adults were more affected by an absence of visual input than young adults, perhaps older adults rely more heavily on visual input. Another plausible explanation for the overdependence of older adults on vision might be because the proprioceptive or vestibular systems are less efficient in detecting or transmitting information to make postural response decisions. When older adults were deprived of sensory input and then the input was reinstated, it took them longer than young adults to overcome the destabilizing effects of the deprivation after the reinstatement. Both adapted well to enriched sensory inputs.

Anticipatory Postural Control

Inglin and Woollacott (1988) looked at the ability of two groups to activate postural muscle responses before engaging in either pushing or pulling a handle after a visual cue. The older adults (mean age of 71 years) were much slower to respond. They had longer muscle onset latencies than the young adults (mean age 26 years) performing the same task. The pattern of muscle activation used to counteract the destabilization effects of the voluntary movement was different in the two groups. These differences may be attributable to many causes. Differences could be due to nervous system deficits, such as vestibular pathology, or other constraints within the musculoskeletal system, such as lack of strength.

Functional reach, a measure of anticipatory control, was shown to predict recurrent fallers (Duncan et al, 1992) and to indicate frailty in older adults (Weiner et al, 1992). However, Franzen and associates (1998) found that functional reach scores could not differentiate between fallers and non-fallers in a group of community-dwelling elders. Functional reach correlates positively with height: the taller the individual, the further is the reach. Functional reach was found to differ by gender because men were taller than the women studied. When the functional reach scores where normalized to body height, no significant gender differences remained (Hageman et al, 1995). Functional reach negatively correlates with age from adulthood to older adulthood. The older you are, the less you are able to reach.

Summary

Posture and balance rely on the sensory and motor subsystems of the central nervous system and the musculoskeletal system to influence age-related changes in the various types of postural control. In addition, the somatosensory, visual, and vestibular systems play a pivotal role in organizing responses to external disturbances of posture. It is important to recognize that many types of balance (static, dynamic, and reactive), as well as anticipatory and adaptive postural control, can be exhibited within a task-specific context. The ability to maintain a posture whether standing still or while moving is an ongoing challenge. Balance requires reacting to challenges appropriately as well as generating an anticipatory posture before the onset of overt movement. Last, adaptive postural control allows us to adapt to changing task and environmental conditions, including gravity, which protects us from losing balance.

Postural networks evolve during the course of early development. Changes in synaptic strength within the nervous system based on use occur at a relatively rapid rate early and later in the human life span. These changes contribute to both the acquisition of postural abilities and their decline. The neural control of posture varies with age.

The effects of the musculoskeletal system on posture are related to physical growth. We grow when we are young. We get bigger and taller, and our body proportions change. These physical changes challenge the postural systems across the growing years. The anatomical structures of bone and muscle also change with age. These changes contribute to our ability to generate force, to be flexible, and to attain a certain stature. The acquisition and loss of spinal curves provide a perfect example of age-related change.

During adulthood, activity level influences our weight and body dimensions, which influence postural alignment and righting abilities. Physical dimensions vary with age, not only because of internally mediated growth processes but also because of psychological and sociocultural factors related to work, lifestyle, mental status, and activity level.

The factors that contribute to age-related change in posture and balance are widely and richly varied. Understanding these various factors and their relationships leads to increased understanding not only of postural development but also of all motor development throughout the human life span.

References

Allum JH, Bloem BR, Carpenter MG, et al. Proprioceptive control of posture: A review of new concepts. *Gait Posture* 8:214–242, 1998.

Asher C. *Postural Variations in Childhood.* Boston: Butterworths, 1975.

Assaiante C, Amblard B. Ontogenesis of head stabilization in space during locomotion in children: Influence of visual cues. *Exp Brain Res* 93:499–515, 1993.

Assaiante C, Amblard B. An ontogenetic model of the sensorimotor organization of balance control in humans. *Hum Move Sci* 14:13–43, 1995.

Basmajian JV, DeLuca CJ. *Muscles Alive: Their Function Revealed by Electromyography,* 5th ed. Baltimore: William & Wilkins, 1985.

Berg K. *Measuring Balance in the Elderly: Validation of an Instrument.* Dissertation. Montreal: McGill University, 1993.

Bertenthal B, Rose JL, Bai DL. Perception-action coupling in the development of visual control of posture. *J Exp Psychol Hum Percept Perform* 23:1631–1643, 1997.

Bertenthal B, Von Hofsten C. Eye, head and trunk control: The foundation for manual development. *Neurosci Biobehav Rev* 22:515–520, 1998.

Bobath B. *Adult Hemiplegia: Evaluation and Treatment.* London: Wm Heineman Medical Books, 1978.

Brown AL, Shumway-Cook A, Woollacott MH. Attentional demands and postural recovery: The effects of aging. *J Gerontol A Biol Sci Med Sci* 54:M165–M171, 1999.

Butterworth G, Hicks L. Visual proprioception and postural stability in infancy: A developmental study. *Perception* 6:255–262, 1977.

Cahill BM, Carr JH, Adams R. Inter-segmental co-ordination in sit-to-stand: An age cross-sectional study. *Physiother Res Int* 4:12–27, 1999.

Chaput S, Proteau L. Modifications with aging in the role played by vision and proprioception for movement control. *Exp Aging Res* 22:1–21, 1996.

Cohen H, Heaton LG, Congdon SL, Jenkins HA. Changes in sensory organization test scores with age. *Age Ageing* 25:39–44, 1996.

DiFabio RP, Emasithi A. Aging and the mechanisms underlying head and postural control during voluntary action. *Phys Ther* 77:458–475, 1997.

Donahoe B, Turner D, Worrell T. The use of functional reach as a measurement of balance in boys and girls without disabilities ages 5–15 years. *Pediatr Phys Ther* 6:189–193, 1994.

Duncan PW, Chandler J, Studenski S, et al. How do physiological components of balance affect mobility in elderly men? *Arch Phys Med Rehabil* 74:1343–1349, 1993.

Duncan PW, Studenski S, Chandler J, Prescott B. Functional reach: Predictive validity in a sample of elderly male veterans. *J Gerontol* 47:M93–M98, 1992.

Duncan PW, Weiner DK, Chandler J, Studenski S. Functional reach: A new clinical measure of balance. *J Gerontol* 45:M192–M197, 1990.

Ford-Smith CD, VanSant AF. Age differences in movement patterns used to rise from bed in subjects in the third through fifth decades of age. *Phys Ther* 73:(5): 300–309, 1993.

Forssberg H. Neural control of human motor development. *Curr Opin Neurobiol* 9:676–682, 1999.

Forssberg H, Nashner LM. Ontogenic development of postural control in man: Adaptation to altered support and visual conditions during stance. *J Neurosci* 2:545–552, 1982.

Foster E, Sveistrup H, Woollacott MH. Transitions in visual proprioception: A cross-sectional developmental study of the effect of visual flow on postural control. *J Mot Behav* 28:101–112, 1996.

Foudriat BA, DiFabio RP, Anderson JH. Sensory organization of balance responses in children 3–6 years of age: A normative study with diagnostic implications. *Int J Pediatr Otorhinolaryngol* 27: 255–271, 1993.

Franzen H, Hunter H, Landreth C, et al. Comparison of functional reach in fallers and nonfallers in an independent retirement community. *Phys Occup Ther Geriatr* 15:33–40, 1998.

Green LN, Williams K. Differences in developmental movement patterns used by active versus sedentary middle aged adults coming from a supine position to erect stance. *Phys Ther* 72: 560B–568B, 1992.

Hadders-Algra M, Brogren E, Forssberg H. Ontogeny of postural adjustments during sitting in infancy: Variation, selection and modulation. *J Physiol* 493:287–288, 1996a.

Hadders-Algra M, Brogren E, Forssberg H. Training affects the development of postural adjustments in sitting infants. *J Physiol* 493:289–298, 1996b.

Hageman PA, Leibowitz JM, Blanke D. Age and gender effects on postural control measures. *Arch Phys Med Rehabil* 76:961–965, 1995.

Haley SM. Sequential analysis of postural reactions in non-handicapped infants. *Phys Ther* 66:531–536, 1986.

Hay L, Bard C, Fleury M, Teasdale N. Availability of visual and proprioceptive afferent messages and postural control in elderly adults. *Exp Brain Res* 108:129–139, 1996.

Hay L, Redon C. Feedforward versus feedback control in children and adults subjected to a postural disturbance. *Exp Brain Res* 125:153–162, 1999.

Hirschfeld H, Forssberg H. Epigenetic development of postural responses for sitting during infancy. *Exp Brain Res* 97:528–540, 1994.

Horak FB, Moore S. Lateral postural responses: The effect of stance width and perturbation amplitude. *Phys Ther* 69:363, 1989.

Huang RP, Rubin CT, McLeod KJ. Changes in postural muscle dynamics as a function of age. *J Gerontol A Biol Sci Med Sci* 54A:B352–B357, 1999.

Inglin B, Woollacott MH. Age-related changes in anticipatory postural adjustments associated with arm movements. *J Gerontol* 43:M109–M110, 1998.

Iyer MB, Mitz AR, Winstein C. Motor 1: Lower centers. In Cohen H (ed). *Neuroscience for Rehabilitation*, 2nd ed. Philadelphia: Lippincott Williams & Wilkins, 1999, pp 209–242.

Jouen F. Visual-vestibular interactions in infancy. *Infant Behav Dev* 7:135–145, 1984.

Jouen F. Head position and posture in newborn infants. In Berthoz A, Graf W, Vidal PP (eds). *The Head-Neck Sensory-Motor System*. New York: Oxford University Press, 1992, pp 118–120.

Lebiedowska MK, Szczazewska M. Invariant sway properties in children. *Gait Posture* 12:200–204, 2000.

Lee RG, Tonolli E, Viallet F, et al. Preparatory postural adjustments in parkinsonism patients with postural instability. *Can J Neurol Sci* 22:126–135, 1995.

Lord SR, Clark RD, Webster IW. Visual acuity and contrast sensitivity in relation to falls in an elderly population. *Age Ageing* 20:175–181, 1991.

Lord SR, Menz HB. Visual contributions to postural stability in older adults. *Gerontology* 46:302–310, 2000.

Lundy-Ekman L. *Neuroscience: Fundamentals for Rehabilitation*. Philadelphia: WB Saunders, 1998.

Maki BE, McIlroy WE. Postural control in the older adult. *Clin Geriatr Med* 12:635–658, 1996.

Maki BE, Perry SD, Norrie RG, McIlroy WE. Effect of facilitation of sensation from plantar foot-surface boundaries on postural stabilization in young and older adults. *J Gerontol A Biol Sci Med Sci* 54:M281–M287, 1999.

Massion J. Postural control systems in developmental perspective. *Neurosci Biobehav Rev* 22:465–472, 1998.

Mathias S, Nayak U, Isaacs B. Balance and elderly patients: The "get up and go" test. *Arch Phys Med Rehabil* 67:387–389, 1986.

Maylor EA, Wing AM. Age differences in postural stability are increased by additional cognitive demands. *J Gerontol B Psychol Sci Soc Sci* 51:P143–P154, 1996.

McIlroy WE, Maki BE. Changes in early 'automatic' postural responses associate with the prior-planning and execution of a compensatory step. *Brain Res* 63:203–211, 1993.

Moncur C. Posture in the older adult. In Guccione AA (ed). *Geriatric Physical Therapy*, 2nd ed. Philadelphia: Mosby, 2000, pp 265–279.

Nardone A, Siliotto R, Grasso M, Schieppati M. Influence of aging on leg muscle reflex responses to stance perturbation. *Arch Phys Med Rehabil* 76:158–165, 1995.

Nashner LM. Sensory, neuromuscular and biomechanical contributions to human balance. In Duncan P (ed). *Balance: Proceedings of the APTA Forum*. Alexandria, VA: American Physical Therapy Association, 1990, pp 5–12.

Nougier V, Bard C, Fleury M, Teasdale N. Contribution of central and peripheral vision to the regulation of stance: Developmental aspects. *J Exp Child Psychol* 68:202–215, 1998.

Podsiadlo D, Richardson S. The timed "Up & Go": A test of basic functional mobility for frail elderly persons. *J Am Geriatr Soc* 39:142–148, 1991.

Portfors-Yeomans CV, Riach CL. Frequency characteristics of postural control of children with and without visual impairment. *Dev Med Child Neurol* 37:456–463, 1995.

Prechtl HFR, Hopkins B. Developmental transformations of spontaneous movements in early infancy. *Early Hum Dev* 14:233–238, 1986.

Riach CL, Hayes KC. Anticipatory control in children. *J Mot Behav* 22:25–26, 1990.

Rietdyk S, Patla AR, Winter DA, et al. NACOB presentation CSB New Investigator Award. Balance recovery from medio-lateral perturbations of the upper body during standing. North American Congress on Biomechanics. *J Biomech* 32:1149–1158, 1999.

Sabourin P. *Rising from Supine to Standing: A Study of Adolescents.* Thesis, Virginia Commonwealth University, 1989.

Shumway-Cook A, Woollacott MH. The growth of stability: Postural control from a developmental perspective. *J Mot Behav* 17:131–147, 1985.

Shumway-Cook A, Woollacott MH. Attentional demands and postural control: The effect of sensory context. *J Gerontol A Biol Sci Med Sci* 55:M10–M16, 2000.

Shumway-Cook A, Woollacott MH. *Motor Control: Theory and Practical Applications*, 2nd ed. Lippincott Williams & Wilkins, 2001.

Staheli L. *Pediatric Orthopedic Secrets.* Philadelphia: Hanley and Belfus, 1998.

Sugden DA, Keogh JF. *Problems in Movement Skill Development.* Columbia: University of South Carolina Press, 1990.

Sundermier L, Woollacott MH. The influence of vision on the automatic postural muscle responses of newly standing and newly walking infants. *Exp Brain Res* 120:537–540, 1998.

Sveistrup H, Woollacott MH. Longitudinal development of automatic postural response in infants associated with developmental transitions in balance abilities. *J Mot Behav* 28:58–70, 1996.

Tanaka T, Hashimoto N, Noriyasu S, et al. Aging and postural stability: Change in sensorimotor function. *Phys Occup Ther Geriatr* 13:1–16, 1995.

Thomas CL (ed). *Taber's Cyclopedic Medical Dictionary*, 18th ed. Philadelphia: FA Davis, 1997.

Thomas RL Jr, Williams AK, Lundy-Ekman L. Supine to stand in elderly persons: Relationship to age, activity level, strength, and range of motion. *Issues Aging* 21:9–18, 1998.

Tinetti ME. Performance-oriented assessment of mobility problems in elderly patients. *J Am Geriatr Soc* 34:119–126, 1986.

VanSant AF. Rising from a supine position to erect stance: Description of adult movement and a developmental hypothesis. *Phys Ther* 68:185–192, 1988a.

VanSant AF. Age differences in movement patterns used by children to rise from a supine position to erect stance. *Phys Ther* 68:1130B–1138B, 1988b.

VanSant AF, Cromwell S, Deo A, et al. Relationships among body dimensions, age, gender, and movement patterns in a righting task. Poster Presentation at the 64th Annual Conference of the American Physical Therapy Association, Nashville, TN, June 12, 1989.

Weiner DK, Duncan PW, Chandler J, Studenski SA. Functional reach: A marker of physical frailty. *J Am Geriatr Soc* 40:203–207, 1992.

Whipple R, Wolfson LI. Abnormalities of balance, gait and sensorimotor function in the elderly population. In Duncan P (ed). *Balance: Proceedings of the APTA Forum.* Alexandria, VA: American Physical Therapy Association, 1990.

Winter DA, Patla AE, Prince F, et al. Stiffness control of balance in quiet standing. *J Neurophysiol* 80:2111–2121, 1998.

Wolfson L, Judge J, Whipple R, King M. Strength is a major factor in balance, gait and the occurrence of falls. *J Gerontol A Biol Sci Med Sci* 50A(special issue):64–67, 1995.

Woollacott MH, Inglin B, Manchester D. Response preparation and posture control. Neuromuscular changes in the older adult. *Ann NY Acad Sci* 515:42–53, 1988.

Woollacott MH, Shumway-Cook A, Nashner LM. Aging and posture control: Changes in sensory organization and muscular coordination. *Int J Aging Hum Dev* 23:97B–114B, 1986.

Woollacott MH, Tang PF. Balance control during walking in the older adult: Research and its implications. *Phys Ther* 77:646–660, 1997.

Donna J. Cech
Patricia A. Wilder

Chapter

13 Locomotion

OBJECTIVES

After studying this chapter, the reader will be able to:

1 Describe the importance of clinical research to the development of locomotion across the life span.

2 Describe the acquisition of locomotion across the life span.

3 Define several locomotion patterns and describe how each pattern evolves across the life span, including rolling, crawling and creeping, erect walking, running, galloping, hopping, and skipping.

4 Explain how our body systems, the environment, and the exact task to be accomplished interact to produce locomotion from one point to another.

Locomotion is defined as the process of moving from one place to another (American Physical Therapy Association, 2001). It is a task critical to independent function, reflecting our ability to move safely and efficiently from one place to another. The essential elements of locomotion include progression, stability, and adaptation. We must have the strength and control necessary to progress toward a location, sufficient dynamic balance to maintain our posture and to overcome the force of gravity or other external forces, and we must have the ability to adapt the locomotor pattern to meet our needs and the demands of the environment (Shumway-Cook and Woollacott, 2001).

Exactly how we accomplish the task of getting from point A to point B depends on many factors: the exact task to be done, the interaction of our body systems that will perform the task, and the environment in which the task is to take place. For example, walking uphill, walking downhill, and walking in water are very different tasks than walking on a level, firm surface. Children, young adults, and older adults will all perform these tasks differently, depending on their size, strength, and balance. We will discuss the development of locomotion across the life span, including its various forms—rolling, crawling, skipping, and walking. Further, we will examine the interrelationships between the body systems of the organism, the environment, and the specific task. All three are equally important to an individual's ability to accomplish the desired movement.

Clinical Research on Locomotion

The task of independently moving from one place to another can be accomplished using any one of a variety of motor patterns: rolling, crawling, creeping, walking, running, galloping, hopping, and skipping. The work of Shirley (1931), McGraw (1945), and Whitall (1989) reveals that independent locomotion progresses from birth to childhood and develops from rolling to crawling to creeping to walking, the first form of erect locomotion. After walking, the locomotion patterns that develop are the upright patterns of running, galloping, hopping, and skipping.

Researchers, such as McGraw (1945), studied motor development by dividing the development of a particular pattern into phases (e.g., the four phases of rolling, the nine phases of prone progression, and the seven phases of erect locomotion). McGraw also studied transitional patterns—those patterns used to move between postures, such as moving from supine to sitting position or moving from sitting to standing position.

Another way in which researchers of motor development used descriptive analysis to study locomotion patterns was to divide a particular pattern into its component parts, that is, movement of the head and neck, the trunk, the upper extremities, and the lower extremities. The research of Roberton and Halverson (1984, 1988) was instrumental in this concept. These researchers identified a developmental progression for the hopping patterns of children.

Exactly how a researcher investigating motor pattern development decided to study a particular motor pattern depended most often on the underlying theory chosen by the researcher. McGraw (1945) was guided in her thinking by the neuromaturational theory that posits the motor patterns of infants and young children are the results of the developing central nervous system (see Chapters 2, 3, and 4). Roberton and Halverson thought that the changes in motor patterns over time were partly due to physical development (Getchell and Roberton, 1989).

Another way of studying developing motor patterns has been to describe the pattern and the changes that occur over time by using some type of biomechanical analysis. Inman and colleagues (1981), Murray (1967), Sutherland and coworkers (1988), and Winter (1991) have given the most comprehensive biomechanical analyses of the locomotion patterns for upright walking. There is little biomechanical information available on most other locomotion patterns, except for running.

A biomechanical analysis of a movement pattern usually includes a description of the kinematics and the kinetics of the movement pattern—the dynamics of the movement pattern. *Kinematics* refers to the relationships between the segments that produce the motion: displacements, velocities, and accelerations in translational or rotational motion. *Kinetics* refers to the moving bodies and the forces that produce the motion. Forces involved include both internal and external forces: internal forces are referred to as the *stresses* that are needed to produce the motion or that result from the motion (i.e., joint forces), and external forces are referred to as the *loads* that are necessary to produce the motion or that result from the motion (i.e., ground reaction forces).

Many variables are used in a biomechanical analysis of a locomotion pattern. Walking, the most common of locomotion patterns, is usually described by the variables of step length, step width, stride length, cycle time, velocity, and cadence—variables that involve distance or time.

Most forms of locomotion involve some aspect of reciprocal movements of the extremities. Reciprocal movements of the extremities were once linked conceptually by describing stance time and swing time of a particular limb. Now the extremities are linked through the ideas of interlimb and intralimb phasing. Phasing relationships are used to describe the coordination of the movement pattern (Clark et al, 1988). *Temporal phasing* refers to the proportion of time of the stride of one limb before the contralateral limb starts its stride. *Distance* or *amplitude phasing* is defined as the proportion of the distance covered in the stride of one limb when the contralateral limb starts its stride. A *stride* is defined as the time or distance from the heel strike of one foot to the next heel strike of that same foot. In the locomotion pattern of erect walking, temporal and distance phasing are considered to be at 50%, that is, the contralateral limb starts its cycle when the other limb has completed 50% of its cycle.

The traditional method used to describe the development of locomotion patterns has been to divide the particular pattern into specific phases or component parts. Although the descriptive method of analysis has been beneficial, biomechanical analysis has provided a more in-depth and objective method for analyzing movements.

Locomotion Patterns Across the Life Span

ROLLING

Rolling is the earliest pattern used for locomotion. *Rolling* is defined as moving from supine to prone or from prone to supine position, and it involves some aspect of axial rotation.

Rotation has been described as a righting reaction because, as the head rotates, the remainder of the body twists or rotates to become realigned with the head. The earliest spontaneous axial rotation is seen in the fetus at about 10 weeks of gestation (deVries et al, 1984). Rotation around the longitudinal axis can result from rotation of the head followed by trunk rotation or from rotation of the leg or lower extremity followed by trunk rotation. In either instance, one part of the body initiates the movement, and the other parts of the body follow, which is called *segmental rotation*. Researchers believe that the functional significance of these movements is for the fetus to become repositioned from time to time to prevent adhesions and stasis (Prechtl, 1986).

McGraw (1945) provided the most detailed account of how rolling progresses from infancy to the toddler stage. Figure 13–1 provides a modified version of those four phases of rolling. The first phase is the *newborn phase*, phase A. In this phase, the newborn infant is predominantly in a posture of

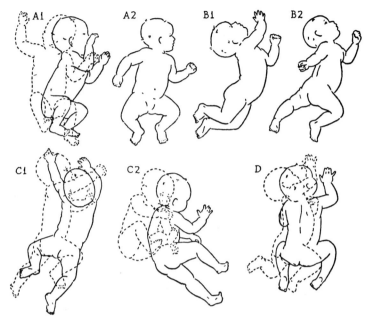

Figure 13–1

Four positions (*A–D*) in the pattern of an infant rolling from supine to prone position. (From McGraw MB. *The Neuromuscular Maturation of the Human Infant.* 1945, © Columbia University Press, New York. Reprinted by permission of the publisher.)

flexion and is unable to produce the movements that would create the activity of rolling. Infants first begin to roll spontaneously. The first pattern of rolling is from side-lying posture to supine position; this pattern, phase B, *spinal extension,* is seen at about 1 to 2 months of age. Rolling from side-lying to prone position is observed at about 4 to 5 months of age. These movements are initially performed with the body moving as a unit; the movement is described as "log rolling," a movement performed without segmental rotation.

Why is the infant unable to roll segmentally at 1 to 2 months of age when the infant was capable of segmental rotations in utero? The answer to this question is best sought from a biomechanical perspective. The infant at 1 to 2 months of age does not have the necessary strength to overcome gravity for rolling supine to prone or for rolling segmentally. Muscle strength was not as critical in utero to produce movement, because gravity for the most part was eliminated in the fluid-filled environment. According to McGraw (1945), infantile rolling is complete but has no purpose—that is, the movement is not performed to accomplish some other function, such as to obtain a toy or to achieve a sitting posture.

At about 4 months of age, infants begin to roll from prone to supine position more deliberately; by 6 to 8 months, such deliberate action involves segmental rotations of the body. This pattern is referred to as phase C, or

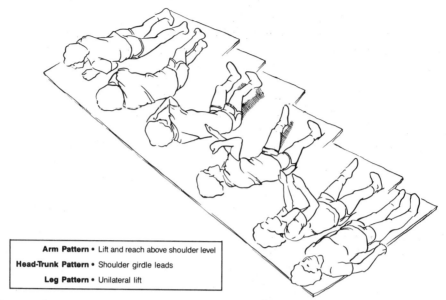

Arm Pattern • Lift and reach above shoulder level	
Head-Trunk Pattern • Shoulder girdle leads	
Leg Pattern • Unilateral lift	

Figure 13–2

A common form of rolling in adults, as shown from the lower right-hand corner to the left-hand corner. (From Richter RR, VanSant AF, Newton RA. Description of adult rolling movements and hypotheses of developmental sequence. *Phys Ther* 69:67, 1989.)

automatic rolling. It is most often initiated by the upper extremities, followed by the trunk and lower extremities; the pattern can also be initiated by the lower extremities, followed by the trunk and the upper extremities. Performance of the movement with more segmentation and with more deliberation is described by McGraw as phase D, *deliberation.* Rolling from supine to prone is also seen at 6 to 8 months of age.

Adult rolling patterns have been described by Richter and colleagues (1989), who studied young adults, aged 20 to 29 (Figs. 13–2 and 13–3). The most important finding was that normal adults used a variety of movement patterns to roll. Most likely, the variety of the patterns was related to flexibility and muscle strength of the individual performing the movement.

CRAWLING AND CREEPING

Crawling is defined as prone progression in which the belly remains on the supporting surface as the arms and legs move in a reciprocal pattern to propel the body forward or backward. *Creeping* is defined as a prone progression in which the abdomen is lifted off the supporting surface while the arms and legs move reciprocally to propel the body forward or backward.

According to McGraw (1945), the prone progression of crawling and creeping is a nine-phase sequence (see Fig. 2–6). McGraw further indicated

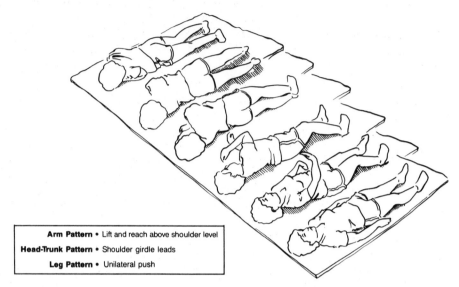

Arm Pattern •	Lift and reach above shoulder level
Head-Trunk Pattern •	Shoulder girdle leads
Leg Pattern •	Unilateral push

Figure 13–3

A second common pattern of rolling in adults, as shown from the lower right-hand corner to the left-hand corner. (From Richter RR, VanSant AF, Newton RA. Description of adult rolling movements and hypotheses of developmental sequence. *Phys Ther* 69:67, 1989.)

that she had not observed a movement sequence with more individual variation than this progression. The majority of infants are able to perform a reciprocal creeping pattern (belly off the floor) by 10 months of age.

McGraw (1945) attributed the progression to cortical maturation, which results in effective inhibition of earlier components of reflexive control of the movement. From a biomechanical perspective, muscle strength is important in getting the belly up off the ground and propelling the body forward or backward. Most likely, the truth behind this or any motor pattern progression is a combination of cortical development, musculoskeletal development, and the environment in which the progression is taking place.

According to McGraw (1945), the newborn phase of the prone progression (the first phase) describes the general posture of the infant, which is flexion. The weight is forward on the head, making head lifting in prone position difficult for the newborn. In phase B, *spinal extension*, the center of mass (COM) has moved inferiorly, and the extensor muscles actively promote head lifting in prone position. Phase C, *advanced spinal extension*, shows spinal extension is even more evident, and the infant can maintain the head and trunk in an elevated position for some time. In phase D, *incipient propulsion in superior region*, the infant attempts to move the superior region of the body, but the inferior region of the body remains unorganized, and propulsion of the body is inhibited. In phase E, *incipient propulsion in inferior region*, the inferior region becomes organized but the two regions remain mostly unsynchronized, and the infant still cannot move the body as a unit. Phase F, *assumption of creeping posture,* represents some coordination between the regions of the body, but the infant does not make deliberate attempts to progress. Often in this phase, the infant lifts the abdomen from the surface but loses balance and falls. In this phase, the infant spends time rocking back and forth on hands and knees, but again without any progression. In phase G, *deliberate but unorganized progression,* the infant may raise one arm forward and then the other, but the legs move as a unit. The infant moves across the floor by pulling with the arms and pushing with the toes. When the infant has a definite creeping pattern seen in phase H, *organized progression,* the abdomen is up off the floor with contralateral movements of the extremities propelling the infant forward. McGraw describes the movement pattern as "staccato" and somewhat uncoordinated. Finally, in phase I, *integrated progression,* the progression is smoothly integrated.

Adult patterns of crawling and creeping have not been studied extensively. The literature indicates that the reciprocal pattern used in early childhood is the adult pattern of this movement behavior. How this pattern of locomotion evolves with aging has not yet been studied. We can assume, however, that the patterns of creeping and crawling for older adults remain very similar to the patterns that young adults display. The parameters that would change the progression of creeping in older adults most likely are biomechanical, such as muscle strength and joint flexibility.

ERECT WALKING

Walking is the act of moving on foot. *Ambulation* is another term that is used synonymously with walking. A third term, *gait,* refers to the manner in which a person walks (American Physical Therapy Association, 2001). Gait can be described by several parameters of time and distance, including stride length, step length, cadence, and velocity. A complete *gait cycle* is defined as one complete stride of one limb. *Stride length* is the time or distance from heel strike of one foot to heel strike of that same foot. *Step length* is the distance from heel strike of one foot to heel strike of the other foot. *Cadence* or step frequency refers to the number of steps taken per a unit of time and is usually reported as number of steps per minute. *Velocity of gait* is the speed with which the body moves through space. This is usually measured over several strides and is reported in meters per second.

Walking is a complex task, where we must use all parts of the body in a coordinated manner. The muscular and skeletal systems provide the support and mechanical mechanisms to move, whereas the nervous system assists in controlling the walking pattern. Sensory information from the visual, proprioceptive, and vestibular systems allows us to navigate through their environment.

The erect walking pattern is defined as a two-phase pattern of movement in the upright position: the *stance phase,* which is approximately 60% of a complete gait cycle, and the *swing phase,* which is approximately 40% of a complete gait cycle. The stance phase provides stability, maintaining the body in an upright position against the force of gravity, whereas the swing phase is responsible for progressing the body forward through space. At the beginning and end of the stance phase, both lower extremities are in contact with the floor, referred to as *double limb support*. In a mature gait pattern, double limb support occurs in the first and last 10% of the stance phase (Shumway-Cook and Woollacott, 2001). The percent of time spent in double limb support varies as we walk slowly or quickly and at various times across the life span.

The upper and lower extremities move in a reciprocal, contralateral pattern during walking and help to propel the body forward or backward in space. A 50% temporal and distance phasing relationship exists between the lower limbs. As stated earlier, 50% phasing between the limbs indicates that when one limb is 50% completed with its cycle, the contralateral limb starts its cycle. According to Clark and Whitall (1989), newly walking infants coordinate their limbs in a 50% temporal phasing relationship, just like adults. These researchers revealed, however, that the young walkers exhibited significantly increased variability compared with infants who had been walking for 3 to 6 months.

Body System Communication Impact on Walking Control

How do we control the act of walking? Arm, leg, trunk, and head movements all work together to maintain balance as our center of gravity moves outside of the base of support (BOS), but how do we organize and control this finely coordinated movement?

The nervous system plays a key role in the control of walking. Early stepping movements and locomotor patterns are controlled by pattern generators in the spinal cord or the brainstem (Connelly and Forssberg, 1997; Grillner, 1981). Initially stepping, controlled only by these pattern generators, is stereotypic. The early stepping pattern that is produced is related to the pattern seen in reflex stepping and kicking in the infant (Thelen et al, 1989). Descending nervous system influences from the cerebellum contribute to modulation of the gait pattern and error correction. This level of control helps fine-tune the gait pattern and assists us in walking over uneven terrain. The cortex also assists in the development of spatially directed movement. The visual cortex processes information from the environment so that perception and action can be linked (Shumway-Cook and Woollacott, 2001).

Sensory information is also critical to control of locomotion, assisting in the adaptation of the gait pattern to the environment in which it is occurring. Visual information is an important stimulus for locomotion. The infant is first enticed to move and to explore by seeing something or someone to move toward. Visual orientation also is important as we align ourselves with the support surface. Visual flow information helps us align the body in reference to the environment and helps in assessment of the speed of walking.

The somatosensory system contributes to the control of walking. Information from the muscle spindles and joint receptors contribute to the rhythm of walking, whereas the Golgi tendon organ influences timing of the transition from stance to swing phase of the gait cycle. Information from cutaneous receptors may also contribute to the ability to negotiate over obstacles. The vestibular system assists in alignment of the head in relationship to gravity, and the vestibulo-ocular reflex is important for head stabilization in space. The vestibular system does not appear to contribute to head stabilization during walking until age 7 years. Children up to age 6 depend primarily on visual and somatosensory information to organize and control walking. This sensory information allows them to use an ascending temporal organization of balance control (feet/pelvis to head). As the visual and vestibular systems become more functional in modulating ambulation, descending temporal organization of balance control (from head to toe) is seen in the walking child (Assaiante, 1998). Temporal organization of balance control is described in more detail in Chapter 12.

Developmental Stages

Infants and Toddlers

Independent ambulation is attained by 11.5 months of age in 50% of infants (Piper and Darrah, 1994). Until this point, the infant does not have sufficient strength or balance control of the head and trunk for independent walking. Extensor muscle strength is thought to be the critical variable in the development of independent locomotion (Thelen et al, 1989). The initial gait pattern is characterized by a wide BOS, arms held in a high guard position, short swing phase, lack of heel strike or push-off, and a need for the infant to propel themselves forward by leaning forward at the trunk. As the new walker gains balance and control of the upright position during movement, the gait pattern changes slowly into the mature gait pattern of the adult by approximately 3 to 4 years of age. As described, the child uses somatosensory sensory information and an ascending temporal organization of balance control during walking.

McGraw (1945) defined seven phases for the development of erect locomotion, which are illustrated in Figure 13–4. In phase A, *the newborn* or *reflex stepping,* the infant is in a flexed posture when held upright, and attempts to step are the result of elicitation of the stepping reflex, a primitive reflex movement pattern. In phase B, *inhibition,* or the *static phase,* elicitation of the stepping reflex is not readily observed. As seen in the development of creeping, the infant can maintain a supported upright posture that includes active cervical and spinal extension. The infant moves the body up and down, holding the feet in position, in phase C, *transition.* The infant may stand in position and stamp the feet, but there is no progression forward. In phase D, *deliberate stepping,* the infant attempts to step when held upright. Although in phase E, *independent stepping,* the infant takes steps independently. During this phase, the early walker uses a wide BOS; feet are flat, and the upper extremities are maintained in a high regard position (arms held high with the shoulders in external rotation and abducted, with the elbows flexed and the wrist and fingers extended). The early walker maintains hips and knees in slight flexion, to bring the COM closer to the ground. At about 12 to 13 months of age, infants are learning to walk alone.

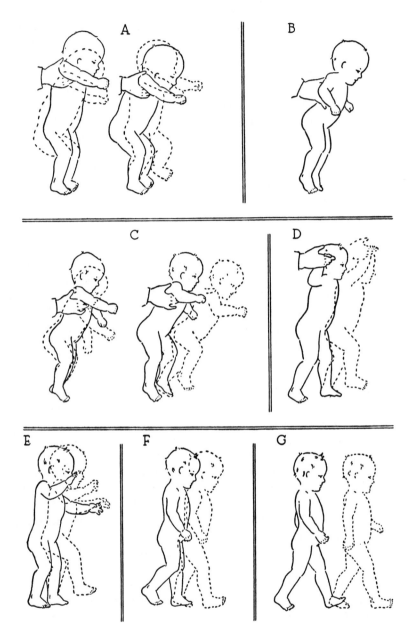

Figure 13–4

The seven phases (A–G) of the assumption of the upright position. (From McGraw MB. *The Neuromuscular Maturation of the Human Infant.* 1945, © Columbia University Press, New York. Reprinted by permission of the publisher.)

The later, more mature walker ambulates with a narrower BOS. Feet are closer together and show a heel-toe progression. The upper extremities are in "low regard" (shoulders in more of a neutral position with the elbows in extension), and the hips and knees are extended more. McGraw (1945) called this pattern phase F, or *heel-toe progression*. Phase G, *integration,* or *maturity of erect locomotion,* finds the arms down and moving reciprocally, synchronous with the movements of the lower extremities; out-toeing has been reduced, and pelvic rotation is present, along with the double knee lock pattern. In the double knee lock pattern, there is knee extension just before heel contact, but at the moment of heel contact, there is knee flexion to help absorb impact shock; then, as the body moves forward over the foot, the knee returns to extension for weight bearing during the stance cycle. These characteristics indicate a mature gait pattern and usually have developed by age 3 or 4. According to Sutherland and coworkers (1988), 98% of toddlers have mature gait pattern by age 4. The gait pattern continues to be refined through 7 years of age.

Several other factors contribute to the development of walking in the infant and toddler. Biomechanical factors influence the infant's acquisition of upright locomotion. Reflex stepping is limited by the increased weight of the 2- to 3-month-old infant and relative lack of muscle strength to move the legs in a stepping pattern against the force of gravity. Because of the physical dimensions of the beginning walker, the COM is at the lower thoracic level, which makes balance control more difficult. By 18 to 24 months, the COM has descended, and as the COM moves closer to the BOS, the body becomes more stable. The new walker attempts to improve balance control by using a wide BOS with the hips abducted and externally rotated. This provides medial lateral stability, but if the new walker's head moves out of the BOS in an anteroposterior direction, loss of balance occurs. There is more mediolateral movement than anteroposterior movement in the gait pattern of new walkers. With experience, the walker's BOS narrows and forward progression over a planted foot is possible. The new walker also stabilizes himself in upright by using coactivation of muscles to decrease the degrees of freedom that have to be controlled. The gait pattern becomes more fluid and reciprocal as this muscle coactivation is released. Reciprocal muscle action begins at approximately 18 months of age.

The gait parameters of time and distance—step length and width, stride length, cadence, and walking velocity—all change as the physical characteristics of the child change. Step length increases as there is growth in stature and leg length. The taller and longer-legged a person, the bigger is the step length. Cadence of the infant is much greater than that of the adult. The number of steps taken per minute decreases gradually throughout childhood, with the biggest reduction seen during the first year of walking. Walking velocity increases with age in a linear manner from 1 to 3 years of age. From age 4 to 7, the rate of change of walking velocity diminishes, but the relationship to age remains linear (Sutherland et al, 1988). The gait patterns of toddlers is depicted in Figure 13–5 and compared with those of children, adults, and older adults.

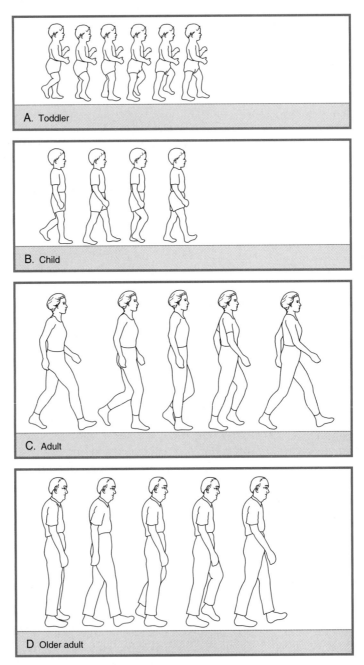

Figure 13–5

Comparison of gait pattern in the toddler, child, adult, and older adult. (Data from Gallahue DL. *Understanding Motor Development: Infants, Children, Adolescents.* Indianapolis: Benchmark, 1989, p 237; Perry J. Gait Analysis: *Normal and Pathological Function.* Thorofare NJ: Slack, 1992; Shumway-Cook A, Woollacott MH. *Motor Control: Theory and Practical Application,* 2nd ed. Philadelphia: Lippincott Williams and Wilkins, 2001; Winter DA. Biomechanical motor patterns in normal walking. *J Mot Behav* 15:302–330, 1983.)

Children

A child demonstrates a mature gait pattern between 3 to 4 years of age and continues to use an ascending organization of postural control with somatosensory information. On level surfaces, some influence of vestibular control is noted as the child begins to use a head stabilization in space strategy (Assaiante and Amblard, 1993). Consistent heel strike and knee flexion in early stance are present. A mature muscle activation pattern is also exhibited on electromyography. Further refinements in the temporal and spatial aspects of the gait pattern occur between 5 and 6 years of age. Step speed and step length are greater in the 6-year-old than the 5-year-old. The 5-year-old also spends more time in double limb support. Ground reaction forces generated during gait may also continue to increase into the sixth year (Pellico et al, 1995).

By 7 years of age, the child's COM has descended to the level of L3 vertebrae (Palmer, 1944). Head stabilization in space strategy is used in a variety of walking environments by age 7 years (Assiante and Amblard, 1993). The gain of the vestibular ocular reflex does not reach adult levels until at least 7 years of age (Assiante and Amblard, 1996). With this level of visual and vestibular maturation, the child is now able to stabilize himself using a descending temporal organization of postural control.

Adults

The gait pattern of the adult was presented earlier in this chapter when erect walking was introduced. The adult can efficiently use walking as a primary means of locomotion to carry out daily tasks. An adult is able to vary gait velocity as he dashes across a busy street, adjusts to the need to walk up or down hill, and walks for long distances. While maintaining an erect posture and when normal muscle strength and endurance are present, the adult easily performs walking. In adulthood, the COM has descended to the sacral level, improving the stability of gait. The adult easily changes pace, starts and stops, and changes direction.

Older Adults

Does the gait pattern change as we age? It is commonly considered that the gait pattern of older adults differs from that of younger individuals in several areas. Some of these common changes are listed in Table 13–1. Are similar gait pattern changes seen in all older adults? Although many of the body systems that support walking change with age (see Chapters 6 to 10), it should also be noted that psychosocial factors such as ageism can also contribute to changes in gait pattern. Stereotypical concepts of aging can influence an older individual's self-perception, alter gait speed, and increase time spent in the double limb support phase of gait (Hausdorff et al, 1999).

It must be understood that within the older adult population, much variation exists. Healthy, active older adults in their 60s to 70s may walk using the same pattern as a younger population. Other older adults who present with

TABLE 13–1

Gait Pattern Changes in the Older Adult

Gait Changes	Characteristics
Associated with normal aging	Decreased gait velocity
	Decreased stride length
	Decreased peak knee extension range of motion
	Decreased peak knee flexion in swing
	Slightly increased ankle dorsiflexion
	Decreased ankle plantar flexion power
Associated with decreased strength	Increased pelvic tilt, may be related to decreased abdominal muscle strength
	Decreased vertical displacement of body during gait
	Decreased gait velocity
	Decreased cadence, may be related to decreased dorsiflexion strength
Associated with decreased balance	Increased base of support
	Decreased gait velocity
	Increased time in double limb support
	Increased use of visual scanning

Data from Ostrosky KM, VanSwearingen JM, Burdett RG, et al. A comparison of gait characteristics in young and old subjects. *Phys Ther* 74:637–646, 1994; Judge JO, Ounpuu S, Davis RB. Effects of age on the biomechanics and physiology of gait. *Clinc Geriatr Med* 12:659–678, 1996; and Bohannon RW. Comfortable and maximum walking speed of adults aged 20–79 years: Reference values and determinants. *Age Ageing* 26:15–19, 1997.

chronic illness, such as arthritis, diabetes, or heart disease, may demonstrate pathological gait deviations or exaggerated gait changes. The pain of arthritis, the sensory loss accompanying diabetes, and the lack of endurance seen in patients with cardiac disease will all affect our gait pattern. Falling becomes more of a problem as adults continue to age, becoming a health problem for the older adult population (see Clinical Implications—Falling: A Preventable Problem for Older Adults?). Attempts to clarify the relationship between aging and walking date back to at least the early 1940s and continue today. Research provides conflicting information about exactly how the gait of older adults changes with age. It is necessary to carefully study healthy older adults and to try to separate out the gait pattern changes that are related solely to increasing age.

Older adults have been reported to have a slower walking velocity, shorter step length, longer stance phase, and shorter swing time than younger adults (Crowinshield et al, 1978; Hageman and Blanke, 1986; Lord et al, 1996a; Murray, 1970). When comparing younger adults (age of 25 years) and older adults (age of 75 years) walking at a slow speed, a fast speed, and a self-selected walking speed, differences in step and stride length were seen primarily at higher walking speeds (Larish et al, 1988). Younger subjects took longer strides at the faster speeds. There was an age-related decrease in stride length for the faster condition but not for the slower condition. In the self-selected speed condition, the stride of the older adults was shorter than that of the younger adults. As a result of their shorter stride length in the faster condition, older adults compensated by increasing their stride frequency to a greater degree than younger adults. It has been confirmed that gait velocity appears to decline per decade. Gait velocity at comfortable walking speeds begins to change slightly when adults are in their 60s and 70s, whereas maximum walking speed more steadily and dramatically declines throughout adulthood (Bohannon, 1997). The difficulty with maintaining maximum walking speed appears to be related to an older adult's inability to generate as great a peak ankle plantar flexor moment as a younger adult. Older adults tend to rely instead on increasing hip flexion power to increase speed (Judge et al, 1996)

Changes in ankle range of motion and pelvic obliquity have also been noted in older adults (Hageman and Blanke, 1986). Ankle plantar flexion at terminal stance can be decreased and the anterior pelvic tilt increased (Judge et al, 1996). Peak knee extension range of motion is also significantly decreased in the older adult compared with the younger adult (Judge et al, 1996; Ostrosky et al, 1994).

Ostrosky and colleagues (1994) confirmed that some differences do exist in the gait pattern of older adults, regardless of activity level and health. In other words, certain age-related differences in gait may surface but only when the functional capacity of the older adult becomes stressed. Functionally, the impacts of these changes are seen when an older adult is unable to cross the street quickly enough before the light changes. Older adults with arthritis or other chronic medical conditions in particular may not have the endurance and muscle strength to walk for long distances or navigate difficult terrain. The full impact of the aging process on gait may be realized only when researchers begin to examine gait patterns across a variety of walking speeds and in a variety of environmental conditions.

RUNNING, GALLOPING, HOPPING, AND SKIPPING

The locomotion patterns that evolve after upright walking are the patterns of running, galloping, hopping, and skipping (Clark and Whitall, 1989). Most literature on the development of these patterns has been descriptive research focusing on the head and neck, the trunk, and the extremities and on how these components relate to each other as a particular pattern evolves. Accomplishment of these locomotor skills is a good indicator of the development of balance (Shumway-Cook and Woollacott, 2001)

The contemporary theory of dynamic systems explains these subsequent patterns of locomotion as examples of different coordinative structures. A *coordinative structure* is defined as the coordination of the movement—how the muscles within a limb (intralimb) and between limbs (interlimb) are constrained to act as a unit. Dynamic action theory defines *coordination of a movement pattern* as the distance and temporal phasing relationships of the limbs, the stance swing relationships of the limbs, or some combination of time, distance, and velocity, which are collective variables that distinguish among different patterns of upright locomotion.

CLINICAL IMPLICATIONS
Falling: A Preventable Problem for Older Adults?

Falling is a common problem in older adults, often resulting in injury and hospitalization. Several factors associated with changes in the older adults' gait pattern may contribute to falls. The problem is then exacerbated because after a fall, the older adult may become less active, fearing and trying to prevent another fall. Further changes in the gait pattern may be made in an attempt to increase safety during ambulation. Decreased activity levels may eventually lead to decreased levels of functional independence, and limited mobility may negatively affect quality of life.

Several factors have been identified that contribute to the increased incidence of falling in older adults, some of which are summarized here. There are also several strategies that can help in the prevention of falls in the older adult, improving functional independence and health status.

Characteristics of Gait Pattern in Older Adults Who Have Fallen

- Decreased stride length compared with non-fallers (Wolfson et al, 1995)
- Walking speed decreased compared with non-fallers (Wolfson et al, 1995)
- Wider step width compared with non-fallers (Heitman et al, 1989)
- Mediolateral instability in standing (more predictive of falls than anteroposterior instability) (Maki et al, 1999)

Possible Factors Contributing to Falls in Older Adults

- Ability to regain balance decreased
  - Older adults need at least two steps to prepare for the avoidance of an obstacle, whereas younger adults can adequately respond in one step (Shumway-Cook and Woollacott, 2001).
  - Older adults have difficulty shortening step length quickly enough to avoid an obstacle (Patla et al, 1992).
  - The ability to take a protective step to maintain stance declines (Medell and Alexander, 2000).
  - Speed and length of the step are less than they are in younger adults (Medell and Alexander, 2000).
- Increased fall risk if a task has time-critical components or high strength demands (Shultz et al, 1997)
- Increased difficulty performing another task while walking (i.e., talking to a friend while crossing a street) (Shumway-Cook and Woollacott, 2001)
- Slower rate of ankle torque development in response to a trip, making it more difficult to regain balance (Thelen et al, 1996)
- Decreased strength of lower extremity musculature, especially ankle plantar flexors and dorsiflexors

- Sufficient plantar cutaneous sensation needed for postural stability in standing to recognize when the center of pressure approaches the limits of stability (Maki et al, 1999)
- Risk of falls greater when descending stairs than when ascending stairs (Shumway-Cook and Woollacott, 2001; Svanstrom, 1974)

Intervention Strategies for Fall Prevention

- Visual scanning of the environment used more by older adults than by younger adults (Patla et al, 1992)
- Lower extremity strength training programs to increase functional ambulation, walking speed, and stride length (Lord et at, 1996b; Sauvage et al, 1992)
- Participation in a strengthening and balance exercise home program to improve balance and reduce incidence of falls (Campbell et al, 1997)
- Therapeutic exercise and balance training for positive outcomes of increased balance, increased lower extremity strength and balance, increased safety, increased physical and functional capacity, and increased ability to perform instrumental and basic activities of daily living (American Physical Therapy Association, 2001).

Running

Running is defined as a pattern of movement that has a stance phase and a swing phase but, more importantly, a flight phase, a period of nonsupport. The stance phase of running is 40% of the gait cycle, whereas the swing phase is 60%. When running, a longer time is spent in swing phase than in walking when 60% of the gait cycle was spent in stance phase and 40% was spent in swing phase. As with walking, the temporal phasing of running is such that halfway through the cycle of one limb, the other limb begins its cycle—50% phasing (Clark and Whitall, 1989).

In the transition from walking to running, we have to produce sufficient force to project the body into the air for the flight phase of running. The toddler, for instance, can run only when there are sufficient vertical ground reaction forces. These forces most likely result from increases in muscle mass, changes in anthropometric measurements, improved motor neuron recruitment, improved postural system, or some combination of these parameters and others not yet defined. Footwork of the beginning runner recalls the early foot-flat pattern of walking. The early runner returns the arms to a high regard position. Initially, there is no reciprocal arm swing or the forward-and-back driving swing of the arms. The arms are thought to be used more for balance. Until approximately 2 years of age, the runner does not exhibit a flight stage in the running pattern (Shumway-Cook and Woollacott, 2001). Stride length of the more advanced runner is longer because more force can be generated in the lower extremity during push-off. This ability to increase force also allows for a longer flight phase and heel strike. The more advanced runner demonstrates an increase in trunk rotation and arm swing. These patterns have been documented by descriptive studies of children aged 18 months to 10 years (Woodward, 1986). The developmental levels of running are outlined below; these levels are adapted from the developmental levels of running defined by Roberton and Halverson (1984).

Level 1:

Upper Extremities—the arms are held in high regard to assist balance control and are otherwise not active.

Lower Extremities—the feet are flat, there is minimal flight, and the swing leg is slightly abducted.

Level 2:

Upper Extremities—the arms begin to swing as spinal rotation counterbalances the rotation of the pelvis; the arms may give the appearance of "flailing."

Lower Extremities—the feet may remain flat and may support knee flexes more during weight transfer; there is more flight time.

Level 3:

Upper Extremities—the arm swing increases because of the spinal rotation.

Lower Extremities—heel contact is made at foot strike; the swing leg is in the sagittal plane; and at toe-off, the support leg reaches full extension.

Level 4:

Upper Extremities—the arm swing becomes independent of spinal rotation; the arms move in opposition to each other and contralateral to the leg swing.

Lower Extremities—the level is similar to that of level 3.

Running in the older adult is defined according to the abilities of the adult being assessed. Many older adults who have remained active show no changes in their overall running patterns compared with a younger group of adults. The assumption is that the qualities of the running pattern change when our physical characteristics such as muscular strength, balance, and range of motion change. Although not substantiated, the logical conclusion is that as individual characteristics show the effects of aging, the running pattern returns to that of the early infant runner. More research is needed to confirm or reject this notion.

Galloping

Galloping is defined as the first asymmetric gait mode in the young child—a walk on the leading leg followed by a running step on the rear leg. There is an asymmetrical phasing of approximately 65/35% (Whitall and Clark, 1986). Clark and Whitall (1989) state that galloping can be seen 20 months after a toddler begins to walk; by 4 years of age, 43% of children can gallop; and by 6.5 years, children are proficient at galloping. The phasing modes are variable but predominantly consist of two distance phasing modes: 66/33% and 75/25%. The variability of temporal phasing was also found to be low across subjects who ranged in age from 2 years to adulthood.

In early attempts at galloping, the arms are stiff and rarely become involved in projecting the body off the floor. They are usually held in the high regard position or out to the side to assist in balance, as was seen in the early form of running. During the early experiences of galloping, the stride is short, landings are flat-footed, and there is little trunk rotation. In addition, the tailing limb may land ahead of the lead limb. In contrast, the more advanced gallop appears more rhythmic and relaxed. The arms are no longer needed for balance and come into a low regard position or swing rhythmically in opposition to the movements of the lower extremities. These changes are accompanied by an increase in trunk rotation, which allows for more reciprocal arm movements. Research related to older adults and galloping is not available.

Hopping

Hopping (one-footed hopping) is an asymmetric pattern of locomotion. Clark and Whitall (1989) found that 33% of 4-year-old children could hop and that by 6.5 years of age, children were proficient at hopping. Halverson and Williams (1985) studied a group of children longitudinally and presented developmental levels for the upper and lower extremities for the hop. The developmental levels of hopping as defined by Roberton and Halverson (1984) are outlined here.

Level 1:

Upper Extremities—the arms are held in high regard, out to the side, and not very active.

Lower Extremities—hip and knee quickly flex, pulling the body toward the floor more than lifting the body off the floor; the flight is momentary, only one or two hops; and the swing leg is inactive.

Level 2:

Upper Extremities—the arms swing upward together, perhaps to assist in balance.

Lower Extremities—body lean allows extension of the knee and ankle to lift the body off the floor; there are repeated hops, but the swing leg is mostly inactive.

Level 3:

Upper Extremities—the arms are active together, pumping the body to help lift the body.

Lower Extremities—there is better coordination among the hip, knee, and ankle for functional takeoff and landing, and the swing leg now assists in the movement by pumping up and down; however, the swing leg remains down and behind the support leg.

Level 4:

Upper Extremities—the arm in opposition to the swing leg is moving forward with the swing leg, assisting in the movement (to a minimal degree); the other arm is in the front or to the side.

Lower Extremities—the ball of the foot is now used for the landing; the support leg has good extension at takeoff; the swing leg helps in the upward and forward movement at takeoff; and the increase in the swing leg's range of movement assists with the movement.

Level 5:

Upper Extremities—the arms work in coordination with the swing leg to assist the movement.

Lower Extremities—the level is similar to that of level 4.

The swing leg is inactive in the earliest form of the one-leg hop. It is not until about 4 years of age that the swing leg begins to move in the hop, helping to propel the body forward. Ultimately, it is the swing leg that pumps up and down to assist in projection; the range of the swing leg increases so that it passes behind the support leg when viewed from the side. The arms follow a similar pattern. Initially, the arms are inactive, held in high regard. As the pattern progresses, the arms become more active, swinging in opposition to the legs. Specifically, the arm opposite the swing leg moves forward and upward in a pumping action to assist the propulsion of the body forward; the other arm moves in the direction opposite the action of the swing leg. In the adult form of hopping, the arms and legs are active, swinging in opposition as just described. The interlimb phasing patterns are probably 50% temporal and distance phasing. What should be remembered for this pattern of locomotion, as with all such patterns, is that children progress at different rates; the rate of progression can be attributed to many different parameters, including muscle strength and balance.

No studies on the hopping patterns of older adults have been published. It might be appropriate to assume, as with the other patterns of locomotion, that the hopping patterns of older adults would resemble the patterns of the early hoppers; as muscle strength and balance decrease in the older adult hoppers, their hopping patterns resemble those of the young toddlers or children hopping at levels 1, 2, or 3.

Skipping

Skipping is defined as an alternating gait, a step, then a hop on one leg, followed by a step, then a hop on the other leg. Clark and Whitall (1989) found that only 14% of children could skip at 4 years of age. The developmental levels for skipping as defined by Roberton and Halverson are outlined here.

Level 1:

Upper Extremities—the arms move bilaterally to assist as the weight is transferred from foot to foot.

Lower Extremities—One foot completes the step-and-hop sequence before weight is transferred to the other foot.

Level 2:

Upper Extremities—the arms begin to oppose each other, but they mostly work together.

Lower Extremities—the child continues to complete one step-and-hop sequence before transferring the weight; the feet are flat during the movement.

Level 3:

Upper Extremities—the arms are in opposition to each other.
Lower Extremities—action is completely on the ball of the foot; weight transfer is more smooth between the hop-and-step sequences.

Again, the literature yields little information on skipping. The arms are initially held in high regard. The advanced pattern ultimately involves a swinging of the arms in opposition to the moving lower extremities. It has been suggested that interlimb phasing of this locomotion pattern is most likely 50% (Clark and Whitall, 1989). Although research on older adults and skipping was not found, it is assumed that older adults demonstrate patterns similar to the early patterns of skipping, depending on the characteristics of the older population being studied.

Body System Interactions Related to Locomotion

Structural and functional changes occur in all of the body systems with aging (see Chapters 6 to 10). The musculoskeletal, cardiovascular and pulmonary, and neurologic and sensory systems contribute most to walking. Changes in these systems seen from infancy through older adulthood affect the development and refinement of the gait pattern.

MUSCULOSKELETAL SYSTEM

Infants cannot support themselves in a standing position or walk because of insufficient strength to support the body against gravity and insufficient range of motion to fully extend their hips in the standing position. Through infancy, muscle mass increases and the child gains controlled mobility through a full range of motion to allow standing and then walking. Postural changes from lower extremity varus in the beginning walker to a more valgus posture in the 3-year-old influence heel and foot position during gait. In children, the gait pattern changes with increasing length of the limbs and increasing muscle strength. With increasing lower extremity length, the stride length increases. Increasing strength allows the child to exert greater forces when pushing off from the support surface. Running cannot occur until the child can generate sufficient force to push into a flight phase.

Changes in the musculoskeletal system with aging are described in detail in Chapter 6. Some of the most specific changes within muscle tissue that may have an impact on walking include a decrease in type II muscle fibers, a decrease in the number of functional motor units, and changes in the muscle tissue with increased fat content and fibrin within the muscle fibers. Muscle strength loss is one of the main causes of a decline in activities of daily living in the older adult population (Aniansson et al, 1978). It has been suggested that the changes observed in the locomotion patterns and reduced gait velocity of older adults are most likely the result of decreases in muscular strength. Wilder (1992) identified that 64% of the variation seen in the gait characteristics such as step length and time in double support of older adults was accounted for by the variable of muscle strength. Small differences in ankle muscle strength and significant differences in hip muscle strength resulted in significant differences in certain gait pattern parameters of older adult women (Wilder, 1992). Strengthening exercise programs have been shown to increase walking speed, cadence, and stride length of older adults. Increased cadence was found to be related to increased ankle dorsiflexion strength, whereas increased stride was found to be related to increased hip extension strength (Lord et al, 1996b). Decreased plantar flexion strength has also been thought to reduce step length and increase time in double limb support (Winter, 1991). Decreased knee extension strength affects maximum walking speed, whereas hip abductor strength affects comfortable walking speed (Bohannon, 1997).

Changes in the skeletal system may also contribute to changes in gait pattern because of the postural changes that occur. With increasing age, bone density decreases, vertebral disk height decreases, and changes occur at the articular surface, such as thinning of the cartilage. These factors, in association with loss of strength of postural muscles, may result in a more kyphotic posture and a shift of the body's COM. As the COM shifts, adjustments to posture may be necessary to maintain balance.

CARDIOVASCULAR AND PULMONARY SYSTEMS

The cardiovascular and pulmonary systems are important for providing fuel to the body tissues active in walking. Under normal conditions, cardiovascular and pulmonary function should be adequate to support walking. Maximal walking speed has been associated with cardiac output and levels of fitness in older men. In general, physically active and fit individuals of any age should be able to easily walk and complete their daily activities. In deconditioned individuals, walking uses a much higher proportion of the energy reserve than when we are conditioned, and everyday functional activities and walking may become too strenuous for someone with severe deconditioning.

NERVOUS SYSTEM

The nervous system is important in the process of motor control and provision of sensory information needed for walking. Children begin to walk at approximately 1 year of age, but their gait pattern becomes more refined and coordinated over the next 6 years. Factors such as myelination of the nervous system, dendritic formation, and the number of functional motor units contribute to the development and quality of walking. Through infancy and young childhood, these factors develop and increase in number. In older adulthood, the number of dendrites and functional motor units decreases, as does nerve conduction velocity due to changes in myelination and the motor unit itself. These changes with age can contribute to increased reaction time and changes in the gait pattern.

The ability to perceive and use sensory input is critical to functional gait. In older adults, cutaneous receptors are not as efficient as in younger adults.

Diminished proprioception is seen, especially at the ankles. Visual and vestibular function also decreases. It may also be more difficult for older adults to integrate multiple sources of sensory input because of changes in central processing ability. These factors are thought to contribute to decreased gait velocity and increased balance difficulty.

Summary

Locomotion is a functional necessity of our lifestyle as humans. Parents celebrate and remember the first time their baby rolls, crawls, creeps, and takes a step marking this function as a sociocultural milestone. The ability to move independently from one place to another is important to our independence and identity. In a rehabilitation setting, the first question a patient or his family often asks is, "When will I [he] walk again?" For some, the answer is that the important function of locomotion will be is achieved using a wheelchair.

Locomotion develops across the life span from rolling to crawling and creeping to erect walking to running, galloping, hopping, and skipping. The transition from one form of locomotion to another depends on a number of factors: the interactions of the tasks to be accomplished, body systems function, and the environment in which the behavior is to be produced. The change in locomotor patterns across the life span charts a bell curve, first becoming more efficient and then potentially becoming less efficient and safe. The challenges to locomotion for the older adult may include falling, which presents health risk and negatively impacts quality of life. We, as therapists, can better help our patients improve their functional independence and quality of life when we appreciate factors that contribute to efficient ambulation.

References

American Physical Therapy Association. Guide to Physical Therapist Practice, 2nd ed. *Phys Ther* 81: 9–744, 2001.

Aniansson A, Grimby G, Hedberg M, et al. Muscle function of old age. *Scand J Rehabil Med* 43(suppl 6):43–49, 1978.

Assaiante C. Development of locomotor balance control in healthy children. *Neurosci Biobehav Rev* 22:527–532, 1998.

Assaiante C, Amblard B. Ontogenesis of head stabilization in space during locomotion in children: Influence of visual cues. *Exp Brain Res* 93:499–515, 1993.

Assaiante C, Amblard B. Visual factors in the child's gait: Effects on locomotor skills. *Percept Mot Skills* 83:1019–1041, 1996.

Bohannon RW. Comfortable and maximum walking speed of adults aged 20–79 years: Reference values and determinants. *Age Ageing* 26:15–19, 1997.

Campbell AJ, Robertson MC, Gardner MM, et al. Randomized controlled trial of a general practice programme of home based exercise to prevent falls in elderly women. *BMJ* 315:1065–1069, 1997.

Clark JE, Whitall J. Changing patterns of locomotion: From walking to skipping. In Woollacott M, Shumway-Cook A (eds). *Development of Posture and Gait Across the Life Span*. Columbia, SC: University of South Carolina Press, 1989, pp 128–151.

Clark JE, Whitall J, Phillips SJ. Human inter-limb coordination and control: The first 6 months of independent walking. *Dev Psychobiol* 21:445–456, 1988.

Connolly KJ, Forssberg H. *Neurophysiology and Neuropsychology of Motor Development*. London: MacKeith Press, 1997.

Crowinshield RD, Brand RA, Johnston RC. The effects of walking velocity and age on hip kinematics and kinetics. *Clin Orthop* 132:140–144, 1978.

deVries JIP, Visser GHA, Prechtl HFR. Fetal motility in the first half of pregnancy. In Prechtl HFR (ed). *Continuity of Neural Functions From Prenatal to Postnatal Life*. Philadelphia: JB Lippincott, 1984, pp 46–64.

Getchell N, Roberton MA: Whole body stiffness as a function of developmental level in children's hopping. *Dev Psychol* 25:920–928, 1989.

Grillner S. Control of locomotion in bipeds, tetrapods, and fish. In Geiger SR (ed). *Handbook of Physiology*, vol 2. Bethesda, MD: American Psychological society, 1981, pp 1179–1236.

Hageman PA, Blanke DJ. Comparison of gait of young women and elderly women. *Phys Ther* 66: 1382–1387, 1986.

Halverson LE, Williams K. Developmental sequences for hopping over distance: A prelongitudinal screening. *Res Q Exer Sport* 56:37–44, 1985.

Hausdorff JM, Levy BR, Wei JY. The power of ageism on physical function of older persons: Reversibility of age-related gait changes. *JAGS* 47:1346–1349, 1999.

Heitmann DK, Gossman MR, Shaddeau SA, Jackson JR. Balance performance and step width in non-institutionalized elderly female fallers and nonfallers. *Phys Ther* 69:923–931, 1989.

Inman VT, Ralston HJ, Todd F. *Human Walking*. Baltimore: Williams and Wilkins, 1981.

Judge JO, Ounpuu S, Davis RB. Effects of Age on the Biomechanics and Physiology of Gait. *Clin Geriatr Med* 12:659–678, 1996.

Larish DD, Martin PE, Mungiole M. Characteristic patterns of gait in the healthy old. *Ann N Y Acad Sci* 515:18–33, 1988.

Lord, SR, Lloyd DG, Li SK. Sensori-motor function, gait patterns and falls in community-dwelling women. *Age and Ageing* 25:292–299, 1996a.

Lord SR, Lloyd DG, Nirui M, et al. The effect of exercise on gait patterns in older women: A randomized controlled trial. *J Gerontol A Biol Sci Med Sci* 51:M64–M70. 1996b.

Maki BE, Perry SD, Norrie RG, McIlroy WE. Effect of facilitation of sensation from plantar foot-surface boundaries on postural stabilization in young and older adults. *J Gerontol A Biol Sci Med Sci* 54:M281–M287, 1999.

McGraw MB. *The Neuromuscular Maturation of the Human Infant*. New York: Hafner Press, 1945.

Medell JS, Alexander NB. A clinical measure of maximal and rapid stepping of older women. *J Gerontol A Biol Sci Med Sci* 55:M429–M433, 2000.

Murray MP. Gait as a total pattern of movement. *Am J Phys Med* 46:290–333, 1967.

Murray MP, Kory RC, Sepic SB. Walking patterns of normal women. *Arch Phys Med Rehabil* 51: 637–650, 1970.

Ostrosky KM, VanSwearingen JM, Burdett RG, Gee Z. A comparison of gait characteristics in young and old subjects. *Phys Ther* 74:637–646, 1994.

Palmer CE. Studies of the center of gravity in the human body. *Child Dev* 15:99–180, 1944.

Patla AE, Prentice SD, Martin C, Rietdyk S. The bases of selection of alternate foot placement during locomotion in humans. In Woollacott MH, Horak F (eds). *Posture and Gait: Control Mechanisms*. Eugene, OR: University of Oregon Press, 1992, pp 226–229.

Pellico LG, Torres RR, Mora CD. Changes in walking pattern between five and six years of age. *Dev Med Child Neurol* 37:800–806, 1995.

Perry J. *Gait Analysis: Normal and Pathological Function*. Thorofare, NJ: Slack, 1992.

Piper MC, Darrah J. *Motor Assessment of the Developing Infant*. Philadelphia: WB Saunders, 1994.

Prechtl HFR. Prenatal motor development. In Wade MG, Whiting HTA (eds). *Motor Development in Children: Aspects of Coordination and Control*. Dordecht: Martinus Nijhoff, 1986.

Richter R, VanSant AF, Newton RA. Description of adult rolling movements and hypothesis of developmental sequences. *Phys Ther* 69:63–71, 1989.

Roberton MA, Halverson LE. *Developing Children—Their Changing Movement: A Guide for Teachers*. Philadelphia: Lea & Febiger, 1984.

Roberton MA, Halverson LE. The development of locomotor coordination: Longitudinal change and invariance. *J Mot Behav* 20:197–241, 1988.

Sauvage LR, Muklebust BM, Crow Pan J, et al. A clinical trial of strengthening and aerobic exercise to improve gait and balance in elderly male nursing home residents. *Am J Phys Med Rehabil* 71:333–342, 1992.

Schultz AB, Ashton-Miller JA, Alexander NB. What leads to age and gender differences in balance maintenance and recovery? *Muscle Nerve Suppl* 5:S60–S64, 1997.

Shirley MM. *The First Two Years: A Study of Twenty-Five Babies, vol 1: Postural and Locomotor Development.* Minneapolis: University of Minnesota Press, 1931.

Shumway-Cook A, Woollacott MH. *Motor Control: Theory and Practical Applications,* 2nd ed. Philadelphia: Lippincott Williams & Wilkins, 2001.

Sutherland DH, Olshen RA, Biden EN, Wyatt MP. The development of mature walking. *Clin Dev Med* 104–105, 1988.

Svanstrom L. Falls on stairs: An epidemiological study. *Scand J Soc Med* 2:113–120, 1974.

Thelen DG, Ashton Miller JA, Schultz AB, Alexander ND. Do neural factors underlie age differences in rapid ankle torque development? *J Am Geriatr Soc* 44:804–808, 1996.

Thelen E, Ulrich BD, Jensen JL. The developmental origins of locomotion. In: Woollacott MH, Shumway-Cook A (eds). *Development of Posture and Gait Across the Life Span.* Columbia: University of South Carolina, 1989, pp 25–47.

Whitall J. A developmental study of the inter-limb coordination in running and galloping. *J Mot Behav* 21:409–428, 1989.

Whitall J, Clark JE. The development of interlimb coordination in galloping: Theory and data. Presented at the North American Society for the Psychology of Sport and Physical Activity, June 1986, Scottsdale, AZ.

Wilder PA. Developmental changes in the gait patterns of women: A search for control parameters. PhD Thesis, University of Wisconsin, 1992.

Winter DA. *The Biomechanics and Motor Control of Human Gait: Normal, Elderly, and Pathological,* 2nd ed. Waterloo, Canada: Waterloo Press, 1991.

Winter DA. Biomechanical motor patterns in normal walking. *J Mot Behav* 15:302–330, 1983;

Wolfson L, Judge J, Whipple R, King M. Strength is a major factor in balance, gait and the occurrence of falls. *J Gerontol* 50A:64–67, 1995.

Woodward KM. *Life Span Motor Development.* Champaign, IL: Human Kinetics, 1986.

Susan V. Duff

Chapter

14 Prehension

OBJECTIVES

After studying this chapter, the reader will be able to:

1 Delineate the components and systems involved in a prehensile act.

2 Identify classic prehension patterns observed in a typical adult.

3 Describe prehensile skill as it develops and changes across the life span.

4 Demonstrate an awareness of the functional adaptations needed for prehension when underlying systems have been altered.

The human hand enhances our life through its dexterity and serves to express our intelligence, as well as our emotions, through gesture. *Prehension*, or the ability to use our hands and upper limbs effectively, can be a strong determinant of functional independence. Upper limb dysfunction limits the degree to which we use our prehensile skills even during simple tasks. To understand dysfunction, it is important to first review normal capabilities and explore prehension at different phases of the life span.

Components of Prehension

Imagine yourself supported in a chair, gazing at a cup of tea resting in front of you. Reach for the cup and secure the handle. As you drink the tea, adjust the handle within your hand. Now set the cup down on the table and let go of the handle. This simple task of drinking tea exemplifies the primary components of prehension: visual regard, reach, grasp, manipulation, and release. *Regard* is the visual attention held on an object; you perceive the location of the cup of tea. *Reach,* or transport, incorporates directing and grading arm position and preshaping the hand to match the location, size, and shape of an object, such as the handle of the cup. *Grasp* involves the act of closing and stabilizing the hand on an object; you secure the cup handle in your hand. *Manipulation* incorporates movement of an object while it is being held, as noted by the adjustment of the handle within your hand. *Release* is the manner in which an object leaves the hand; you let go of the cup handle. If necessary, you may also lift and carry an object, such as the cup, with both hands. The cooperative effort of both hands is termed *bimanual coordination*. The act of drinking a cup of tea, like other prehensile tasks, reflects the interaction between goal-directed movement and environmental constraints. Prehension uses proactive and reactive postural control (Patla, 1995), allowing us to prepare the body for intended movement or to respond to perturbations. Postural control and biomechanics are inherent features of prehension.

POSTURAL CONTROL

Visual exploration and functional reaching are closely linked to postural control. Under *proactive control* (Patla, 1995), stabilizing muscle contractions or anticipatory postural adjustments (APAs) are elicited in anticipation of upcoming disturbances in equilibrium. APAs prevent undesired movement and allow for adjustment in our center of gravity before the upper limb moves in space. Under *reactive control* (Patla, 1995), muscle responses are also elicited after disturbances or perturbations induced by a prehensile act such as reaching to a distant target.

Historically, it was believed that proximal stability was a prerequisite for distal mobility or fine-motor control. Although we have learned from neurophysiological studies that the nerves to the proximal joint musculature myelinate approximately 1 month ahead of the small hand muscles (McBryde and Ziviani, 1990), it is possible to have good fine-motor control despite having poor proximal stability. Clinically, we find that children who have sustained injuries to the brachial plexus at birth (Erb's palsy) often have proximal weakness and instability yet have good distal function.

The motor responses of the proximal and distal musculature are considered to be task dependent (Case-Smith et al, 1989; Schieppati et al, 1996). In general, the joint to be stabilized is determined by the goal of the activity. Proximal trunk activation stabilizes the body during reach to grasp movements. Sustained pinch or grip can be viewed as a form of distal stabilization that frees the proximal joints to move. For example, when we hold a toothbrush, the wrist, forearm, and elbow are free to move while the fingers and thumb stabilize the toothbrush for use. Thus, postural control prepares us for movement or provides stability for the completion of a task. The stabilizing muscles vary depending on the goal and constraints of the task.

BIOMECHANICS

Flexible postural control that adheres to select biomechanical principles allows us to use prehensile skill effectively. Select biomechanical principles dictate efficient function, including length-tension relationships and related active and passive insufficiency of muscle-tendon units. The length-tension curve compares the tension produced in a muscle with its resting length at the time of contraction (Fig. 14–1). *Resting muscle length* is the length of the resting muscle when it is measured from attachment to attachment. Peak tension, which is necessary for a strong contraction, can be developed when the muscle is within 70% to 105% of its resting length, termed the *useful range* (Smith at al, 1996). A contracting muscle or agonist demonstrates active insufficiency when

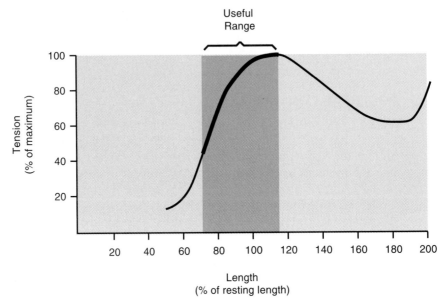

Figure 14–1

Length-tension diagram for isometrically stimulated muscle fiber, including extreme shortened and stretched states of fiber. (Redrawn from Smith LK, Weiss EL, Lehmkuhl LD. *Brunnstrom's Clinical Kinesiology*, 5th ed. Philadelphia: FA Davis, 1996, p 140, and modified from Ramsey RW, Street SF. Isometric length-tension diagram of isolated muscle fibers of the frog. *J Cell Comp Physiol* 15:11, 1940. Reprinted by permission of John Wiley & Sons, Inc.)

its attachments are too close together, limiting tension development. Passive insufficiency results when the attachments of the antagonist are too far apart for the muscle to generate adequate tension for effective contraction.

Based on these principles, many manipulative tasks are best performed with the wrist stabilized in approximately 20 to 30 degrees of extension and 10 degrees of ulnar deviation (O'Driscoll et al, 1992). Wrist extension keeps the finger flexors within the useful range of the length-tension curve, allowing for adequate tension development during grip and pinch activities. When the wrist is extended, the thumb can move into a plane of opposition in relation to the other digits, and the fingers can achieve full flexion. These and other biomechanical principles play a significant role in manual acts.

VISUAL REGARD

Visual regard and perception prompt us to reach for and grasp objects. These functions depend on the strength of our attention, visual acuity, and ocular control, including accommodation and convergence (see Chapter 10). *Visual perception* is the ability to use visual information to recognize, recall, discriminate, and understand what we see. As infants and children gain experience through play involving various systems, perceptual constructs are developed.

Visual memory is established and complex processes develop with exposure to and interaction with different environments. Visual regard and perception also guide reach and refine manipulation skills in terms of accuracy and control. Selected visuoperceptual constructs such as depth perception, figure ground, and visuoconstruction play key roles in reach, grasp, and manipulation. Depth perception allows us to localize objects in space and to estimate size and distance. For example, we can discriminate how far a cup is out of reach before retrieving it. Figure-ground refers to the ability to visually focus on specific details in the foreground by selectively screening out competing background stimuli. And visuoconstruction is related to the spatial planning process involved in building up and breaking down two- and three-dimensional objects. This skill is used in putting together a puzzle or copying a three-dimensional design.

Visual-motor control, or *eye-hand coordination,* is the ability of an individual to use visual information for precise guidance of movement. Visual information is used to amend an internal representation or model of an object's physical properties and location before reaching for it and to enhance accuracy before object contact during an unfolding reach. It has been postulated that *peripheral* vision aids reaching because it provides cues about object distance and direction along with object or limb motion (Abahnini et al, 1997). Conversely, *central* vision supports grasp and manipulation because it provides information about object size and shape required for grip calibration and dexterous hand movement. Sighted individuals use vision to guide reaching in many everyday tasks, such as retrieving a specific shirt hanging in the closet. When our vision is compromised, we rely on proprioceptive and tactile cues or visual memory to guide reach to grasp movements.

REACH AND GRIP FORMATION

The entire upper extremity is involved in the act of reaching and grasping an object. During reach to grasp movements, the shoulder moves the hand in space over a wide area and the elbow places it closer to or further away from the body. The forearm and wrist position the hand before grasp of an object or receipt of a weight-bearing surface. The fingers and thumb adjust their position to accommodate the perceived spatial properties of an object during grip formation, such as its size and shape. Therefore, when reaching for a cup visualized at chest level, the shoulder may flex to about 80 degrees, while the scapula rotates up and protracts, and the elbow extends. As the cup handle is approached, the wrist may extend and the forearm may rotate into neutral. As the handle is approximated, the fingers may extend and the thumb may abduct in preparation. The fingers may close in on the handle by flexing, and the thumb may adduct. When the reach requires greater than 90 degrees of shoulder flexion, the trunk and neck may rotate (Kaminski et al, 1995) or laterally flex and the ipsilateral pelvis may elevate.

The *trajectory* of a reaching movement can be defined by the extent, orientation, and speed of the hand path as it moves the hand to a new position

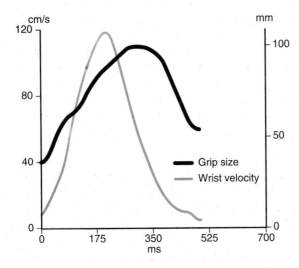

Figure 14–2

Sample velocity profile with imbedded grip aperture. (Redrawn from Paulignan Y, Jeannerod M. Visuomotor channels in prehension. In Wing AM, Haggard P, Flanagan JR [eds]. *Hand and Brain: The Neurophysiology and Psychology of Hand Movements*. New York: Academic Press, 1996, p 268.)

(Abend et al, 1982). In adults, reaching behaviors include smooth velocity profiles and relatively continuous, straight hand paths with and without visual feedback (Jeannerod, 1984) (Fig. 14–2). Studies examining differences between the dominant and nondominant arm reveal distinct neural control mechanisms for each limb for reaching (Sainburg and Kalakanis, 2000).

Reach and grasp are associated with two hypothesized visuomotor channels activated in parallel (Jeannerod, 1981). One channel pertains to an object's extrinsic properties, such as location, and activates proximal shoulder musculature used in the reach. The second channel is related to preshaping the grip and provides intrinsic information about the object such as its location and contour. This information activates distal finger musculature. The preshaping of the hand, termed *grip formation,* can be divided into finger opening and finger closure or aperture. Maximum finger opening adjusts in anticipation of the size and shape of an object, based on an internal representation of the object's physical properties. As a reach to grasp movement unfolds, this representation is updated via current sensory information. In typical adults, peak aperture occurs within 70% to 75% of total movement time at the point of peak deceleration (Jakobson and Goodale, 1991; Jeannerod, 1984) (see Fig. 14–2). Inadequate timing between reach and grasp may extend the movement time and alter the path of the reach, compromising appropriate grip formation. In essence, the timing and size of peak aperture within a reach to grasp movement indicate whether it is planned for the expected target object's location and spatial properties. Impairments in central vision clearly impede grip formation. Studies of transport and grasp have reported maximal finger aperture and velocity of finger aperture to be greater when the vision of healthy subjects was restricted (Chieffi and Gentilucci, 1993). Without a clear idea of the size or shape of an object, individuals overestimated grip aperture to ensure successful grasp. From his work on transport and grasp, Jeannerod

(1986) provided evidence that grip accuracy improved given visual feedback and degraded in those with visual impairment.

GRASP

Classification of Adult Grasp Patterns

Once an object is approached, one of a variety of grip patterns will be used to secure it. The location, size, and shape of an object determine the type of grasp pattern used. Traditionally, adult prehension patterns have been classified according to the work of Napier (1956) and Landsmeer (1962). Napier (1956) described two types of grip: power and precision. *Power grips* are defined as forcible activities of the fingers and thumb that act against the palm to transmit a force to an object. Examples include the cylindrical, spherical, and hook grip (Fig. 14–3). During *precision grip* and *pinch* activities, forces are directed between the thumb and fingers, not against the palm. Examples of precision grip or pinch include pad-to-pad prehension, tip-to-tip prehension, and pad-to-side, or lateral, prehension (Fig. 14–4). Sustained hold of power and precision grips require isometric muscular contractions. Landsmeer (1962) kept the expression power grip in his classification scheme but used the phrase "precision

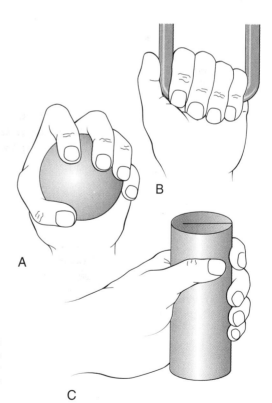

Figure 14–3

Three varieties of power grip. *A*, Spheric grip. *B*, Hook grip. *C*, Cylindric grip. (Redrawn from Norkin CC, Levangie PK. *Joint Structure and Function: A Comprehensive Analysis.* Philadelphia: FA Davis, 1983.)

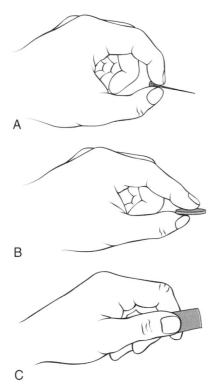

Figure 14-4

Three varieties of precision pinch and handling. *A,* Tip-to-tip. *B,* Pad-to-pad. *C,* Pad-to-side (lateral). (Redrawn from Norkin CC, Levangie PK. *Joint Structure and Function: A Comprehensive Analysis.* Philadelphia: FA Davis, 1983.)

handling" to describe the manipulative quality of prehensile function. *Precision handling* requires changes in position of the handled object, either in space or about its own axes, as well as exact control of finger and thumb position. Muscular contractions will vary between isometric and isotonic. Typical grip and pinch patterns and the joints and muscles involved are listed in Table 14–1. Despite their wide acceptance, the classic prehension patterns continue to be challenged.

After an extensive survey of the literature, Casanova and Grunert (1989) introduced a new classification system based on anatomical nomenclature and contact surfaces. They proposed the use of the terms "static" and "dynamic prehension." *Static prehension* refers to any form of prehension in which the object does not move within the hand, although proximal joint movement may occur. An example of static prehension is isometrically holding a key using a lateral pinch. *Dynamic prehension* is associated with object manipulation within the hand. The positional changes of the object occur within the hand rather than at the proximal joints, as when we roll a needle between the fingers to visualize its eye before threading it. The force used during static or dynamic prehension may be strong or light in magnitude. For example, during precise static prehension, as in turning a key in a tough lock, a strong steady force is used, but a light force is sufficient to secure an empty soda can.

We usually grade the force used during prehension. This ability to grade

TABLE 14-1

Classification of Prehension Patterns

Patterns	Joint Motion	Muscles Used	Function
Cylindrical grasp	Thumb opposition, finger adduction and flexion	FPL and thenar group, AdP, select interossei (task dependent), fourth lumbrical and FDP (FDS for more power)	Holding onto a cylindrically shaped object such as a soda can
Spherical grasp	Thumb opposition, finger flexion and abduction	FPL and thenar group, AdP, FDP (FDS for more power), fourth lumbrical interossei (except second)	Holding onto a round object such as a baseball
Hook grasp	MCPs neutral, finger flexion at PIPs and DIPs, thumb extension	Finger FDS and FDP, thumb, EPL and EPB, EDC, fourth lumbrical and fourth dorsal interossei	Holding onto a briefcase handle
Pad-to-pad prehension	Thumb opposition and slight flexion of all thumb joints; finger flexion at MCP and PIP; flexion or extension of DIP of involved fingers	Thenar group, FPL, select interossei and FDS of involved fingers (FDP if DIP flexion is present)	Holding onto a coin
Tip-to-tip prehension	As in pad-to-pad prehension, with greater thumb and finger flexion, including DIP flexion	As in pad-to-pad prehension, with greater FDP force FDP secondary to DIP flexion, interossei of involved fingers	Holding a needle
Pad-to-pad prehension (lateral)	Thumb adduction with IP flexion, index finger flexion, and abduction	Thumb, FPL, FPB and AdP; involved fingers; FDS and FDP; reduced interossei and lumbricals except first dorsal interossei	Holding a key

FPL, flexor pollicis longus; AdP, adductor pollicis; FDP, flexor digitorum profundus; FDS, flexor digitorum superficialis; MCP, metacarpophalangeal; PIP, proximal interphalangeal; DIP, distal interphalangeal; EPL, extensor pollicis longus; EPB, extensor pollicis brevis; EDC, extensor digitorum communis; IP, interphalangeal.

Data from Landsmeer JMF. Power grip and precision handling. *Ann Rheum Dis* 21:164–169, 1962; Long C, Conrad PW, Hall EA, Furler SL. Intrinsic-extrinsic muscle control of the hand in power grip and precision handling. *J Bone Joint Surg* 52(5):853–867, 1970; Napier JR. The prehensile movement of the human hand. *J Bone Joint Surg* 38:902–913, 1956; Napier JR, Function of the hand. In Napier JR (ed). *Hands.* New York: Pantheon Books, 1980, pp 68–83.

forces is based on previous learning and memory of the weight, texture, and other properties of the object. Sensorimotor memories help form internal representations of the physical properties of objects and are used to scale the grip (squeeze) and load (vertical) forces in advance. This ability to scale fingertip forces in advance of object contact is called *anticipatory control.*

Significance of Thumb Opposition

Although prehension is evident in many forms of animal life, it attains maximum function in humans given the addition of thumb opposition. *Opposition* involves rotation at the carpometacarpal joint of the thumb to place the thumb pad diametrically opposite to the pad of one or all of the other digits (see Fig. 14–4). The thumb, because of its unique ability to oppose, is a common feature in most grip classifications, contributing 40% to 70% of total hand function (Flatt, 1977). The comparative length of the index finger to the thumb is a major factor when attempting opposition or pad-to-pad contact. A reduction in thumb length, seen in an individual whose distal thumb phalanx has been amputated, limits the ability to fully rotate the thumb to the index pad. Thumb opposition in conjunction with movement at other digits is used to execute functional prehension such as turning a doorknob or buttoning a shirt.

Significance of Other Digits

The index finger is considered the most important digit after the thumb because of its mobility and independent musculature attachments. It has been found to be the most dominant of the four fingers (Raj and Marquis, 1999) and accounts for 20% of lateral pinch, 20% of power grip from a supinated position of the forearm, and 50% of power grip from a pronated forearm position (Tubiana, 1984). The long finger is the longest and strongest and also has significant functional value. In some individuals, it replaces the index finger as the dominant finger and is used for pointing and manipulating small objects (Raj and Marquis, 1999). The index and long fingers are considered the prehensile digits and are the most anatomically stable. The small and ring fingers are recruited for power grip prehension. Although they are considered the most anatomically mobile, they also are the weakest digits (Tubiana, 1984). Both the index and small fingers can produce isolated extension via the extensor indicis and the extensor digiti minimi. All of the digits are important in prehension, and the loss of any one of them will limit prehensile ability to some degree.

MANIPULATION

Once we pick up an object through grasp, we may either sustain a hold on it or manipulate it with one or both hands to accomplish a task. All forms of manipulation demand the use of the small intrinsic and extrinsic muscles of the fingers or thumb.

Sustained Grip and Pinch

Manipulation involves a series of tasks used to achieve a specific goal. Once the index finger and thumb contact a target object with a stable grip, the goal is to generate sufficient fingertip forces to lift it. Sustaining a grip or pinch on an object or tool is done primarily with isometric contractions and intermittent isotonic contractions, as when writing with a pencil over a long period.

During object manipulation, a dynamic lift is generally combined with static hold and release of an object. The sequential tasks involved in grasping and lifting an object are triggered by discrete mechanical events that relay information from somatosensory receptors (Johansson and Cole, 1992). Experience aids in the development of internal representations of an object's properties. This information is used for anticipatory control or planning before lifting and manipulating an object. Without anticipatory control or scaling of finger-tip forces, objects may slip from grasp or be squeezed too tight because the feedback mechanisms are too slow to upgrade or to downgrade forces quickly.

In-Hand Manipulation

The ability to move objects within one hand, termed *in-hand manipulation*, is divided into three categories, called shift, rotation, and translation (Exner, 1990). Shift refers to the movement of an object on the finger pads or among the fingers. Rotation is the movement of an object around its axis using the fingers. Translation is the movement of an object from fingers to palm or from palm to fingers.

To translate objects such as a raisin from the palm to the fingertips, finger flexion and extension are used. Shift incorporates the pads of the fingers with thumb opposition as when turning thin pages in a book. *Simple rotation* involves turning an object on its axis 90 degrees, such as when turning a pencil to write. *Complex rotation* is defined as 180 to 360 degrees of object rotation, as when using the pencil eraser (Fig. 14–5A). In-hand manipulation skills can also incorporate stabilization of one object or part of an object within the hand while another object or object part is simultaneously being manipulated within the same hand (Exner, 1990). Typically, if two objects are held in the same hand, the ring and small (ulnar) fingers stabilize one object while the index and long (radial) fingers manipulate the other object or part. Shift with stabilization is used to separate a group of keys from a single key when opening a lock (Fig. 14–5B). All three forms of in-hand manipulation can be exemplified with the use of a penny. For example, a penny can be translated from the palm up to the fingertips and then shifted across the finger pads to end with a hold between the index finger and the thumb. If you turned the penny

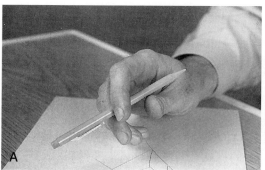
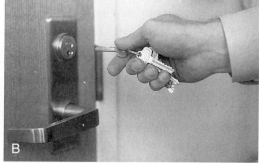

Figure 14–5

Examples of in-hand manipulation: *A*, Rotation component used to access the eraser of a pencil. *B*, Shift component with ulnar stabilization used to manipulate a key when opening a lock.

over from heads to tails with your fingertips, that would be considered a rotation.

Stereognosis

Haptic perceptual exploration, or *stereognosis,* is the ability to recognize the names and properties of objects without vision through sensory cues and in-hand manipulation. Manipulation abilities, as well as sensibility, foster object identification, yet it is the memory of an object that makes it recognizable. Reach into your purse or pocket and retrieve a quarter. How did you know it was a quarter and not a nickel? You probably used tactile cues and proprioceptive-kinesthetic input to judge the size and weight of the coin, based on memory of a previous visual or other sensory experience. Although visual memory is a strong component of stereognosis, individuals without sight can develop this ability once they are taught, demonstrating that memory based on haptic exploration also plays a significant role in object recognition.

The vast number of receptors in our fingertips, muscles, joints, and skin provide the tactile and proprioceptive cues used to identify characteristics of an object. The slow and fast adapting mechanoreceptors in the fat pads and ridges of our fingers supply varied tactile information (Vallbo and Johansson, 1984). Proprioception conveys information regarding muscle force, limb movement, and changes in limb position. Afferent input contributing to proprioception includes information from muscle spindles, Golgi tendon organs, joint receptors, and cutaneous mechanoreceptors (Edin and Abbs, 1991). All of the receptors contribute to stereognosis. Without sensory input, the ability of humans to identify objects without vision is significantly impaired.

RELEASE

Release is the process of letting go of a held object or taking pressure off an object. Release can be crude, as when we drop the hot handle of a frying pan, or it can be graded and controlled, as when we set a crystal glass onto a counter. Graded release is mastered and refined individually through the practice of specific tasks. Playing a musical instrument is a beautiful demonstration of how graded release is achieved. A master jazz pianist is able to hold and release pressure on the keys in such a controlled and graded fashion that the end result is a varied sound combination of loud or soft, sustained or short-lasting tones. A novice player may not exhibit the same degree of finesse with regard to holding or releasing the pressure on the piano keys, perhaps making all the tones loud and sustained. Tool use also demonstrates graded release. When using a screwdriver to drive in screws, a series of quick, graded grasps and releases are used to turn the handle effectively without engaging the whole shoulder girdle. Imagine a 5-year-old performing the same task. He would probably display an alternating lateral trunk tilt or engage the shoulder girdle. This may be due to weakness, reduced ability to supinate the forearm, or insufficiently graded grasp and release. As control of release improves, our repertoire of fine-motor activities enlarges.

BIMANUAL COORDINATION

Bimanual coordination requires the spatial and temporal cooperation of both hands. Bimanual skills can be separated into *symmetrical* tasks in which there is a strong coupling between limbs, as when we throw a ball with two hands, and *asymmetrical* tasks or differentiation, as when our hand stabilizes an object while the other manipulates it. Examples of asymmetrical bimanual tasks include opening small containers (Fig. 14–6) or playing musical instruments such as the guitar. The neural organization associated with these two types of bimanual tasks varies depending on task goals and constraints.

Wiesendanger and colleagues (1996) described motor control principles that affect bimanual coordination: (1) the assimilation effect, (2) neural division of labor, and (3) hierarchical organization. The *assimilation effect* refers to the temporal coupling and synchronization of two hands during movement initiation. It is possible that coupling of bimanual actions occurs at the level of bilaterally linked central pattern generators or neuronal ensembles. The *neural division of labor* refers to the asymmetric roles taken by the two hands, which reflects a specialization of brain function. For example, in right-handed individuals, the left or dominant hemisphere may strongly influence the roles assumed by each hand during asymmetrical bimanual tasks. *Hierarchical organization* incorporates the concepts of goal invariance and motor equivalence in which the goal of a task remains intact yet can be accomplished by variable means. Research has shown that even when the task conditions were altered (visual occluded, unilateral pull load varied, anesthetized unilateral thumb and index), the goal of a task remained intact, thus maintaining a motor equivalence (Perrig et al, 1999). Any or all of the three principles described may be

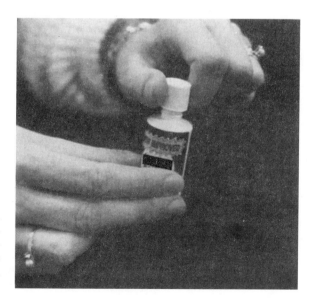

Figure 14–6

Asymmetrical bimanual coordination demonstrating two prehension patterns: three-fingered palmar pinch (three-jaw chuck) to hold the base, and dynamic lateral pinch to turn off the top.

involved in specific bimanual activities depending on individual capabilities, task goals, and environmental and task conditions.

Prehension Development Across the Life Span

PRENATAL PERIOD

Growth of the Upper Limb

The limb buds, which represent the earliest form of the upper limb, begin to appear between the 26th and 27th days of gestation. By the end of the seventh week, the fingers are defined and the upper limb has rotated medially to its typical position at birth. Table 14–2 describes and illustrates upper limb growth until the seventh week of gestation. The dermatomes of the skin, which influence both the tactile and proprioceptive systems, begin to develop as early as 7 weeks of gestation. The classic proprioceptive system also begins to develop in utero with the differentiation of the articular skeleton and muscular systems around the seventh week of gestation (Moore and Persaud, 1998). The prenatal period ends with full development of the upper limbs.

Prenatal Action Development

Upper limb actions do not develop in isolation from the environment in which they occur. Therefore, the uterine environment plays a significant role in early prehension development. Sparling and colleagues (1999) used ultrasound imaging to examine fetal movements and found that although limb movements are variable, they are not random. Instead, they found that movements were directed toward specific targets, as seen in the thumb-to-mouth activity of an 18-week-old fetus. This thumb-to-mouth action may have been facilitated by the ease of movement available within the amniotic fluid and sac. McCartney and Hepper (1999) provided evidence for the expression of preferred hand use prenatally, reporting that in utero 83% of arm movements were with the right versus the left arm. They hypothesized that lateralized motor behavior may play a causative role in later asymmetric brain development and eventual lateralized behavior postnatally.

INFANCY

Upper limb and hand movements are present at birth, yet continued development is strongly influenced by neuromaturation, task goals, and the ever-changing interaction between the environment and the characteristics of an individual infant (Thelen, 1995). All components of prehension undergo a great deal of development during infancy.

Visual Regard

At birth, vision is limited. Newborns seem to have 20/800 vision, a fixed gaze of 7.8 inches (20 cm), and little accommodation (Coren et al, 1999). Because vision needs the stimulation of light to develop, it is not until the second

TABLE 14–2

Development of the Upper Limb in the Embryonic Period

Age of Embryo	Upper Limb Development	Illustration
28–30 days	Upper limb buds "flipper-like" Lower limb buds appear	
31–32 days	Upper limb buds "paddle-like"	
33–36 days	Hard plates formed	
41–43 days	Digital or finger rays appear	
44–46 days	Elbow region visible, notches appear between finger rays	
47–48 days	All limb buds extend ventrally	
49–51 days	Upper limb longer and bent at elbow Fingers distinct but webbed	
52–53 days	Hands and feet approach each other Fingers are free and longer	
7th week	Upper limb rotates 90° laterally in longitudinal axis (elbows face posterior) Lower limb rotates 90° medially (knees face anterior) Tissue breaks down between digits from the circumference inward, producing fingers and toes	

Adapted from Moore KL, Persund TVN. *The Developing Human:* Clinically Oriented Embryology, 6th ed. Philadelphia: WB Saunders, 1998.

month of life that the structures associated with accommodation, occulomotor function, and convergence are established. Despite having low vision, newborns can fixate or sustain their gaze for brief periods and follow or track a moving target through a small range. As the newborn follows moving visual information (visual flow) from birth to 1 month of age, his gaze typically lags behind a moving stimulus. Rosander and von Hofsten (2000) have provided evidence that vestibular control over smooth gaze stabilization and adjustment, while the head and body are moving, functions earlier than visual control. This is not surprising, because ocular movements induced by vestibular input in the fetus occur several months earlier than do ocular movements stimulated by light postnatally. By 2 to 3 months of age, visual control improves as convergence and accommodation enable the infant to fixate for sustained periods and to follow a moving target through a wider range (Rosander and von Hofsten, 2000). Around 3 months of age, the initial visual lag to a moving stimulus is diminished, and by about 5 months of age, the infant begins to demonstrate anticipatory tracking and can project his gaze ahead of the moving object (von Hofsten and Rosander, 1997). By 4 to 5 months of age, the infant often can reach for objects in his visual field. As visual memory develops, between 6 and 7 months, the infant may realize that an object still exists even if it falls out of the visual field, and by 8 months, she will search for it. Binocular vision, accommodation, and acuity progress over an infant's second year of life, strengthening eye-hand coordination. It is not until 2 years of age that the infant can attend to stimuli presented in two visual fields, simultaneously demonstrating interhemispheric coordination (Liegeois et al, 2000).

Reaching

Although reaching behaviors in young infants are quite variable, they become more refined and consistent with age and experience. *Early reaching* is described as a fling or thrust and is considered a ballistic, preprogrammed, and inaccurate movement. Visually guided, anticipatory reaching behaviors begin to emerge around 4 months of age. von Hofsten and Lindhagen (1979) confirmed that 18-week-old (4-month-old) infants could visually catch a ball moving at 15.4 inches/sec (39 cm/sec). Thus, they could *predict* the future position of the moving ball and direct the reach toward the point of contact between the hand and the moving object. Although vision provides a stimulus to reach forward, Clifton and colleagues (1993) found infants as young as 15 weeks were able to reach for glowing or sounding objects without the use of guided vision. Despite the ability of infants to reach by 3 or 4 months of age, it is not until 2 years of age that more stereotypic adult-like reaching patterns are displayed (Konczak and Dichgans, 1997) (see Fig. 4–1). With experience and gains in motor control, reaching behaviors become less variable.

Factors that are likely to influence the type of reach an infant performs include the degree of postural control, the location of the target object, and task goals, motivation, and cognition. Rochat (1992) reported that when infants initially began to reach, even if they could not sit independently, they tended to do so with two hands. Older infants who sit independently often display unimanual reaches. Halverson (1931, 1932) documented that practically all reaches in the 9-month-old infant were unilateral and directed straight at the target. These findings infer a strong connection between postural control and reaching. Changing coordination in other behaviors, however, may also influence how reaching movements are executed. Corbetta and Thelen (1996) found unimanual and bimanual reaching to fluctuate during the first year. During periods of strong bimanual reach, nonreaching interlimb activity tended to be synchronous. Yet, no specific form of interlimb coordination was observed during periods of unimanual reach. The authors postulated that changing coordination tendencies seems to influence the organization of goal-oriented reaching behaviors during the first year of life.

Grip Formation

As reviewed earlier, we preshape our hand to the contour and size of target objects during reaching. Crude preshaping of the hand or anticipatory grip formation has been documented in infants as young as 18 weeks (von Hofsten and Fazel-Zandy, 1984). von Hofsten and Ronnqvist (1988) later examined grip formation during reaching in older infants 5 to 6, 9, and 13 months of age. They found that although the 5- to 9-month-old infants began to close the hand near the time of target contact, the 13-month-old infants began to close the hand well before object contact. Opening aperture was adjusted to target size in the 9- to 13-month-old infants but not in the 5- to 6-month-old infants. In addition, finger opening was initiated earlier in the reach in 13-month-olds than in 9-month-olds, yet the timing did not vary for different-sized objects. Adults showed an earlier onset of opening for larger objects, thus showing greater anticipatory grip formation. The progression in anticipatory grip formation or preshaping of the grasp develops in infancy yet does not become adult-like until late childhood (Kuhtz-Buschbeck et al, 1998).

Grasp and Manipulation

Within the first 6 months of life, early random responses and reflexes become voluntary prehension. In the first few months, tactile and proprioceptive reflexes control closure via palmar stimulation and opening of the fingers via dorsal stimulation (Table 14–3). Mass movement patterns are exemplified by a traction response, in which stretching of the flexor muscle groups induces flexion of the upper limb.

When the newborn enters infancy, the hand reflexes are gradually integrated and progress into voluntary prehensile patterns. As the motor cortex develops, prenatally and postnatally, independent finger movements or fractionation emerge. Initial grasp patterns typically involve the fingers only, leaving the thumb passive. Thumb function, including opposition, usually develops between 3 and 12 months and is responsible for the progression in prehensile patterns. Index isolation typically begins around 10 months of age, and by the end of the first year, the infant is able to isolate the index finger as a dominant pointer. Sometime around 11 months of age, the infant demonstrates pad-to-pad opposition of the thumb to the index finger to grasp small

TABLE 14–3

Hand Reflexes

Reflex	Appears	Disappears	Stimulus	Response
Grasp	2 weeks	4–5 months	Tactile stimulus initially; later, proprioceptive input also is needed to elicit grasp	Flexion of fingers, adduction and flexion of the thumb
Traction response	Week 28 of gestation	2–5 months	Stretch to shoulder flexors and adductors with traction	Flexion of the wrist and fingers with synergistic flexion of elbow and shoulder
Avoidance response	Neonatal period	5–6 months; fully integrated by 6–7 years	Light tactile stimulus along dorsum of hand to fingertips	Extension and abduction of fingers and wrist (withdraw from stimulus)
Instinctive grasp reaction	4–5 months	Remnants persist into adult life	Stationary or moving light touch; radial palm contact; ulnar palm contact	Orienting reaction; slight supination; slight pronation
	6–7 months		Ulnar or radial palm contact	Orienting and groping to find the object
	8–10 months		Moving stimulus withdrawn from any part of the palm	Orienting, groping, and grasping of stimulus
Asymmetrical tonic neck reflex	Week 28 of gestation	4–5 months	Passive rotation of head	Elbow flexion on skull side, with elbow extension on face side

Data from Ammon JE, Etzel ME. Sensorimotor organization in reach and prehension: A developmental model. *Phys Ther* 57(1):7–14, 1974; Fiorentino MR. *Normal and Abnormal Development: The Influence of Primitive Reflexes on Motor Development.* Springfield, IL: Charles C Thomas, 1972; Twitchell TE. Reflex mechanisms and the development of prehension. In Connelly K (ed). *Mechanisms of Motor Skill Development.* London: Academic Press, 1970, pp 25–59.

objects. Prehension patterns become more adult-like as the infant approaches 1 year of age. Further development and experience with objects allow the infant's repertoire of grasp patterns to expand, and adapt to functional need.

Table 14–4 depicts a historical sequence of prehension development. Some researchers have begun to view this sequence as conservative and inflexible because it does not accurately reflect the functionally adaptive prehension seen in infants given various task constraints (Hohlstein, 1982; Lantz et al, 1996; Newell et al, 1989). For example, Halverson's work (1932) on prehension indicated that an ulnar grasp, elicited by tactile cues to the ulnar side of the

TABLE 14–4

Historical Sequence of Prehension Development from Birth to 1 Year

Description	Age	Illustration	Stimulation
Recognizes hands	8 wk (2 mo)		Hand enters visual field assisted by the ATNR
Reflexive ulnar group	12 wk (3 mo)		Ulnar placement of objects encourages grasp; hanging toys may promote visual tracking
Retains objects placed in hand: Midline fingering; mouthing of fingers; swiping in visual field	16 wk (4 mo)		Placing objects anywhere in hand will encourage grasp; hanging toys will encourage swiping if they are within visual field and reach
Primitive squeeze grasp (wrist flexed); raking	20 wk (5 mo)		Introduction of toys of varied textures, sizes, and shapes will promote voluntary grasp and raking
Palmar grasp (no thumb participation, wrist moving into neutral)	24 wk (6 mo)		Placing toys in different positions will encourage eyes and hands to search prior to reach and grasp
Radial palmar grasp (thumb adduction begins); mouthing of objects	28 wk (7 mo)		Ideal toys are washable and those that can be picked up and transferred easily from one hand to the other
Scissors grasp (thumb adduction stronger)	32 wk (8 mo)		Introduction of toys with a thin circumference will strengthen thumb adductor
Radial-digital grasp (beginning opposition)	36 wk (9 mo)		Pliable materials such as clay or finger food will encourage opposition of thumb
Inferior pincer grasp (volar hold vs. pad to pad; hand supported prior to grasping); isolated index pointing	36–52 wk (9–12 mo)		Small objects varied in shape will promote exploration via poking, feeling, and manipulation
Pincer grasp—pad to pad (some support before grasping)	38–52 wk (10–12 mo)		Tiny objects, such as raisins, to pick up and drop will encourage development
Superior pincer grasp—tip to tip (hand unsupported prior to grasping)	52–56 wk (1 y)		Thin yet safe objects the size of a pin will encourage development
Three-jaw chuck (wrist extended and ulnarly deviated); maturing release	52–56 wk (1 y)		Toys requiring a strong radial finger hold and blocks and containers providing repeated motions will encourage strong grasp and release

hand, preceded a radial grasp. Frossberg and colleagues (Lantz et al, 1996), however, found that following palm contact, infants may reach for and grasp a dumbbell-like object, without consistently using an ulnar grip. Even the young infant uses the index finger to contact and initiate the grasp first; the index finger exhibits a stronger grip force than the other fingers. Although inconsistency in the prehensile responses of normal infants makes it difficult to accurately label patterns, their prehensile responses can be grouped into three phases. During phase 1, infants use their whole hands in a gross or unspecialized manner. In phase 2, infants use parts of their hands as they begin to develop specialization. By phase 3, infants use the pads of their distal phalanges in a precise, specialized manner (Hohlstein, 1982).

The ability to use anticipatory control to coordinate fingertip forces during grasp and manipulation of objects is not innate (Forssberg at al, 1995; Pare and Dugas, 1999). It develops gradually over the first 2 years of life, as the young child interacts with various objects. Observing the ability to grasp and lift before 2 years of age, Forssberg and colleagues (1995) found that infants and toddlers increase grip and load forces sequentially, using a feedback strategy. After the second year, grip and load forces begin to be generated in parallel, demonstrating a transition to anticipatory (proactive) control. Such coordination of fingertip forces is important to smooth prehension and development of in-hand manipulation and stereognosis.

In-hand manipulation skills develop gradually from infancy to childhood. The easiest skills are those of finger to palm translation and simple rotation, seen before 2 years of age. Complex rotation is still being refined in the 6- to 7-year-old child. Stereognosis also develops gradually after birth. In early infancy, the mouth and hands are used to gain information about objects. Intramodal and intermodal exploration and integration begin to develop in infancy and continue through adolescence. Intramodal integration is the ability to recognize objects by one modality (touch) after learning about the object using the same modality (touch). This ability appears first in infants as young as 2 to 3 months of age (Streri, 1987). Intermodal integration develops next and is the ability to recognize an object by a different modality (vision) from which it was first explored (touch). Infants as young as 6 months can visually recognize a shape after only tactile contact with it (Rose et al, 1978). Recognition of common objects through haptic exploration is relatively good by 2 to 3 years of age and seems to mature around 5 years of age (Stilwell and Cermak, 1995).

Release

The ability to release objects progresses in early infancy, as voluntary control over wrist, finger, and thumb extensors emerges. Release develops off a point of stability. For example, mutual fingering in midline by the 4-month-old and transferring of objects from hand to hand in the 5- to 6-month-old infant is possible because one hand can release off the stability provided by the other hand. Voluntary release typically emerges around 7 to 9 months of age. It is initially achieved through stabilization provided by an external surface, such as the tray of a highchair or from the stable hand of someone attempting to take an object from the infant. Once a child is able to accurately release an object into a container, without external support, she is on the way to developing graded release patterns. An infant can usually release a block into a small container by 12 months and release a pellet into a small container by 15 months (Hirschel et al, 1990). Ball throwing is an example of release that improves in control and accuracy as the infant moves into childhood.

Bimanual Coordination

The development of bilateral arm and hand use combines the components of prehensile function. Initially, asymmetry predominates, as seen in the 2-month-old, and antigravity control is limited. The 3-month-old displays greater symmetry, as seen during bilateral hand play on the chest in midline. The 4-month-old often displays a bilateral, or two-handed, approach to reach objects visible in midline. After 5 months of age, object presentation and size determine whether the reach will be unilateral or bilateral. The 5-month-old is able to crudely transfer objects from one hand to the other. Midline hand play away from the chest becomes more extensive as shoulder girdle strength improves. At this age, the infant can hold the bottle with two hands and displays more active object manipulation, such as banging and shaking toys. The 6- to 7-month-old displays a stronger unilateral reach and a mature hand-to-hand transfer.

Differentiated bimanual movements begin at 8 to 10 months, when the two hands begin to have different roles or functions. For instance, one hand can hold the bottle while the other reaches to grasp a new toy. By 12 to 18 months of age, differentiated movements are advancing; each hand assumes either the active or stabilizing role. For example, the *active* hand may operate the dial of a toy telephone with the index finger, and the *stabilizing* hand may hold the edge of the telephone. After 2 years of age, the complexity of bimanual, or two-handed, tasks, increases significantly.

Gross Motor Development and Prehension

Advances in manual performance, visuoperceptual skill, and cognition coincide with exploration of objects and the environment made available through gross motor skill development. When making gross motor transitions from one position to another, the infant strengthens and stretches various muscle groups that are later used in numerous prehensile tasks. For instance, weight bearing on extended arms in quadruped recruits shoulder and trunk musculature for stability, and weight shifting alternates pressure from the ulnar to the radial side of the hand, stretching out the intrinsic muscles.

As gross motor skill and postural control improve, the infant becomes capable of executing visuomotor acts with greater ease. Although strength and early prehensile skills naturally develop through activities executed in prone, supine, and quadruped, once postural control in sitting develops, prehensile ability improves dramatically. As trunk and upper limb strength and motor control expand, the infant is able to reach unilaterally and bilaterally with graded control. Studies examining the development of postural control in sitting reveal basic, direction-specific synergies, including anticipatory postural adjustments, adapted to task-specific conditions. von Hofsten and Woollacott (1990) reported that some 9-month-old infants demonstrated proactive control by activating proximal trunk muscles before reaching.

PRESCHOOL CHILD

During the preschool years, prehensile patterns and eye-hand coordination skills are refined and practiced. Prehensile tasks are learned through trial and error and rehearsal from a model in collaboration with developing perceptual and cognitive processes. Often, a young child is unable to demonstrate a particular skill independently, yet can do so in the presence of an adult or more capable peer. A 3-year-old child may be unable to cut paper with scissors independently, yet may be successful in the presence of another capable 3-year-old, by internalizing the perceptual and cognitive strategies provided. Skilled hand function and the use of implements develop rapidly during this period.

Reach and Grip Formation

Adult-like reaching patterns are assumed by 2 years of age, yet continue to be refined through late childhood. Consistent temporal coordination across arm segments for multijoint reaches improves up until 3 years of age (Konczak and Dichgans, 1997). In other work, Kuhtz-Buschbeck and colleagues (1998) compared reach and grip formation (hand preshaping) in children 4 to 12 years of age against adult behaviors. They found younger children opened their hand wider before object contact than did the older children or adults, suggesting that they grasp using a higher safety margin of error to prevent missing the target. The younger group also seemed to be more dependent on vision to scale their grip aperture to the target. With increasing age, the dependence on vision decreased and reaching trajectories became straighter. In general, anticipatory reach to grasp behaviors continue to develop through the preschool years and are refined into late childhood.

Grasp and Manipulation

Preschool children gradually become more socialized and begin to engage in activities that require grasp and manipulation of various implements. Implements commonly used at this age include utensils, such as eating devices and banging instruments; tools, such as scissors or writing implements; and self-care items, such as fasteners, shoelaces, or hairbrushes.

The use of implements requires the employment of one or all three forms of manipulation: sustained grip or pinch force, in-hand manipulation, and bimanual coordination. As strength of the intrinsic muscles develops, the child usually can demonstrate *sustained pinch force* on items such as a crayon when coloring. Young children improve in the ability to coordinate fingertip forces with practice but still demonstrate inefficient control. For example, they may crush fragile objects such as paper cups or potato chips or lift light objects too quickly. This lack of anticipatory control may be due in part to insufficient internal representations for the properties of the lifted objects.

TABLE 14–5

Sequential Acquisition of Pencil Grip

Pencil Grip	Age	Description	Illustration
Palmar-supinate	1–2 y	Pencil or crayon is held by fisted hand; forearm slightly supinated; wrist slightly flexed; shoulder motion produces movement of pencil	
Digital-pronate	2–3 y	Pencil or crayon is held by fingers and thumb; forearm pronated, wrist ulnarly deviated; pencil controlled by shoulder movement	
Static-tripod	3+ y	Pencil held proximally between thumb and radial two fingers; minimal wrist mobility; pencil controlled by shoulder movement	
Dynamic-tripod	4+ y	Pencil is held distally through thumb opposition to the index and long fingers, with the ring and small fingers stabilizing in flexion; small movements at the metacarpophalangeal and interphalangeal joints control the pencil; stabilization occurs at the shoulder, elbow, forearm, and wrist	

Data from Erhardt RP. *Developmental Hand Dysfunction: Theory, Assessment, and Treatment.* Laurel, MD: RAMSCO, 1982, pp 9–3; Knobloch H, Stevens F, Malone AF. *Manual of Developmental Diagnosis: The Administration and Interpretation of the Revised Gesell and Amatruda's Developmental and Neurological Exam.* Houston, TX: Developmental Evaluation Materials, 1987, pp 24–260; Rosenbloom L, Horton ME. The maturation of fine prehension in young children. *Dev Med Child Neurol* 13:3–8, 1971.

As distal control improves, crayon and pencil grips are modified. A typical sequence of pencil grip development is outlined in Table 14–5. Before in-hand manipulation skill advances, the child often adjusts the crayon position in one hand with the contralateral hand. Once fingertip force coordination improves and in-hand manipulation develops, the crayon can be translated, rotated, or shifted ipsilaterally without assistance from the opposite hand.

Bimanual coordination for symmetrical and asymmetrical tasks expands through the preschool years as children begin to incorporate anticipatory prehensile behaviors as needed for such tasks as catching a ball (Fig. 14–7). Many skills develop as each hand begins to refine coordinated, asymmetrical roles. Initially, the child may need to stabilize the paper she is coloring with both elbows, but eventually just the opposite hand is needed. Other examples of bimanual skills a preschooler typically engages in are cutting paper with scissors, buttoning clothing, zipping zippers, and tying shoelaces. Motor planning, the ability to execute novel motor acts, and task-specific practice play significant roles in the acquisition of new fine-motor tasks such as those described above. Through trial and error, modeling, and practice, the preschooler expands and refines sustained pinch ability, in-hand manipulation, and bilateral hand use. By the end of this period, hand preference for specific tasks such as coloring and cutting with scissors may be demonstrated.

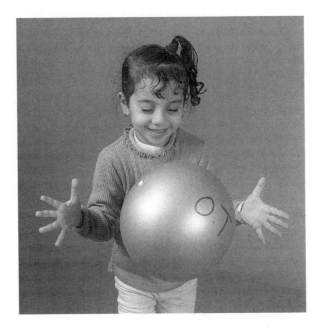

Figure 14–7

Bimanual anticipatory reach and grip formation exhibited by a 4-year-old when catching a ball.

Hand Preference

Hand preference and hand dominance are often confused in definition. *Hand preference* refers to a *tendency* to use one hand for prehension instead of the other. *Hand dominance* is the *consistent use* of one hand over the other for such tasks as throwing a ball, writing with a pencil, and eating with a fork. Hand preference can be verified through interview and observation of performance during select tasks. Although some researchers have reported that hand preference for swiping objects can be noted within days after birth, it remains controversial (Korczyn et al, 1978). The preschooler develops a hand preference as she practices skilled tasks such as eating with utensils, coloring, and throwing a ball. By 4 to 6 years, hand preference is well established. Lateralization of the brain, the process by which the hemispheres become specialized for particular functions, is generally thought to be the driving force behind hand dominance. Consistent use of one hand also promotes lateralization. Some children may not demonstrate a hand preference during the preschool years because the preferred hand is not yet sufficiently influenced by the contralateral motor cortex. However, by 6 to 7 years of age, laterality is demonstrated through the consistent and superior use of one hand to hold a pencil during writing tasks. Most agree that the dominant hand performs better than the nondominant during fine, dexterous activities. However, for some manual tasks, it is possible that by altering the context requirements such as speed and accuracy of the task, performance between hands may become more similar (Lewis et al, in press).

SCHOOL-AGED CHILD

Mastery

During this period, children often demonstrate mastery of many components of prehension. A child's knowledge and abilities for an activity are considered domain or task specific, which allows for rapid encoding and response to certain fine-motor situations. The degree to which a particular skill is mastered depends on the amount of time spent practicing specific tasks and the strength of the supporting systems.

Reach to grasp behaviors expand in the school-aged child. For instance, 6-year-olds display an exaggerated grip aperture during reaching, whereas 12-year-olds can scale the grip aperture more closely to object size (Kuhtz-Buschbeck, 1998). Although some children between 6 and 8 years of age may demonstrate adult-like fingertip force coordination when grasping and lifting objects, some do not achieve this capacity until 11 years of age or later (Forssberg et al, 1995). Reportedly by 6 years of age, most children can demonstrate relatively good in-hand manipulation, which allows for expansion of prehensile activities in which they can engage. Complex asymmetrical bimanual coordination progresses during the school-aged period. For example, building model airplanes is a complex task that requires one hand to stabilize the base and the other hand to glue small parts onto that stable base. Children of the same age demonstrate very different levels of skill at building models. As a child matures into adolescence, interest and experience further guide the refinement of prehensile skills.

School-aged children often spend a large amount of their time involved in task-specific practice. For example, the demands for written work increase by 8 to 9 years of age, necessitating skill in holding and sustaining a pencil grip while completing the complex task of handwriting. Writing requires selective attention and other cognitive processes and is affected by the state of arousal.

Handwriting

Many of the components of prehension play a role in handwriting. Visual regard of the paper and pencil and accurate perception of the workspace are needed. When copying from a chalkboard, we must shift visual gaze from the board to the paper without losing our place. The spatial relationships among the desk, the paper, and the blackboard need to be accurately perceived, as do the spatial relationships among the letters, words, and sentences on a page. Position in space and form constancy will guide recognition of letters and numbers. Grasp and manipulation, sustained grip and pinch, in-hand manipulation, and bimanual coordination contribute to handwriting and can be analyzed separately for clarity.

Pencil grip is an example of sustained pinch. Examples are shown by order of frequency in Figure 14–8. The most frequently used pencil grip is the dynamic tripod, which is demonstrated when a pencil is held between the pads of the index and thumb while it rests against the long finger. This position is considered the most efficient in terms of speed and dexterity,

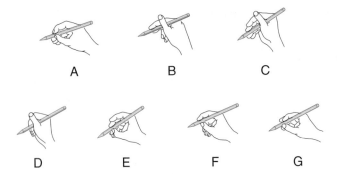

Figure 14–8

Pencil grips. *A*, Dynamic tripod. *B*, Lateral tripod. *C*, Transpalmar interdigital. *D*, Cross-thumb. *E*, Dynamic bipod. *F*, Dynamic bipod with omitted third digit. *G*, Static tripod. (Redrawn from Bergmann KP. Incidence of atypical pencil grasps among nondysfunctional adults. *Am J Occup Ther* 44:736–740, 1990.)

because pencil movement is controlled distally by the fingers and thumb. Alternative pencil grips are considered efficient if the thumb and index form a circle or open web space, allowing for skillful distal manipulation. Inefficient grips limit the range, speed, and fluidity of distal movement and demand greater proximal movements of the wrist and elbow to control the pencil, reducing precision. The lateral tripod, considered a functional yet inefficient grip because the web space is closed, is used by up to 25% of nondysfunctional children and up to 10% of adults (Schneck and Henderson, 1990). With adequate strength and somatosensory feedback, a child can sustain a hold on a pencil without the need for excess pressure. Endurance for sustained pinch required during prolonged handwriting tasks is gained with practice.

Gains in grip and pinch strength increase throughout childhood and contribute to all prehensile abilities. Mathiowetz and colleagues (1986) collected normative data on grip and pinch strength for children and adolescents 6 to 19 years of age, comparing males to females. Figure 14–9*A* illustrates the increasing grip strength exhibited by these children. Pencil grip strength may be best inferred from palmar pinch and key pinch strength.

In-hand manipulation is frequently used for pencil writing. If a demand is made for quick writing and erasing, a child learns to adjust the pencil in one hand and rotate it longitudinally to use the eraser. Bimanual coordination is required for writing, because one hand must stabilize the writing surface and the other hand must actively use the pencil.

ADOLESCENCE

During this phase of development, primary occupations include schoolwork, socialization, part-time employment, and prereadiness for later employment or career. The prehensile demands resemble those of the school-age child, except that the skill level is often higher. Less time is spent in trial and error and more time is spent in perfecting skill. Skills performed with the dominant hand continue to advance beyond those of the nondominant hand. Bimanual skills, including the use of a computer keyboard or sports-related activities, do play a strong role at this stage of development. Adolescents often are cognitively aware of their strengths and weaknesses in terms of coordination and skill with manipulative tasks. Success heightens interest and helps boost self-esteem; thus, motivation for a task and practice are strongly correlated. A comparison between male and female grip strength in adolescents is shown in Figure 14–9. Young adults demonstrate a significant increase in grip and pinch strength, which may reflect functional gains seen in prehensile tasks.

By the time we reach adolescence, adult-like coordination of fingertip forces is demonstrated. This ability allows an individual to fine-tune manual skill related to specific areas of interest.

ADULTHOOD

Occupational Choices

Early in adulthood, most vocational and avocational choices are made. Some occupations require fine dexterity and skilled hand use. Dental hygiene, sur-

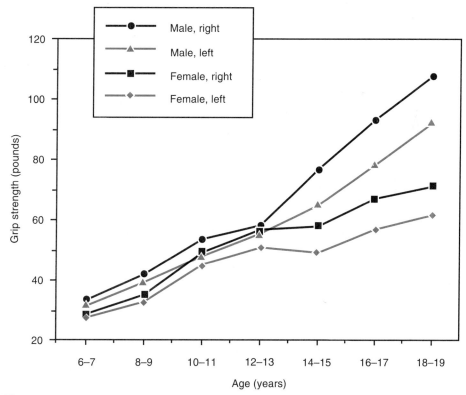

Figure 14–9

A, Grip strength of males and females from 6 to 19 years old. (Data from Mathiowetz V, Wiemer DM, Federman SM. Grip and pinch norms for 6 to 19 year olds. *Am J Occup Ther* 40:705–711, 1986.) *Figure continued on following page.*

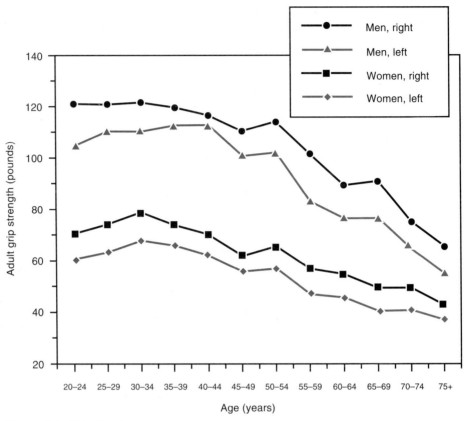

Figure 14–9 *Continued*

B, Grip strength of men and women. Note the downward trend from 20 to 75 years of age. (Data from Mathiowetz V, Kashman N, Volland G, et al. Grip and pinch strength: Normative data for adults. *Arch Phys Med Rehabil* 66:16–21, 1985.)

gery, and stained glass artistry all require skill in precision handling and a strong pinch for sustained tool use. Pickleman and Schueneman (1987) devised a rating form for testing proficiency in surgery and a neuropsychological test battery for assessing psychomotor, perceptual, and perceptual-motor abilities in surgical residents. They found that those with demonstrated strength in the area of complex visuospatial problem-solving and manual dexterity displayed superior surgical technique. Not all researchers agree with these results. Graham and Dreary (1991) discussed that although spatial ability tests correlate with surgical skill ratings, manual dexterity tests do not. Harris and colleagues (1994) assessed manual dexterity, eye-hand coordination, and visuospatial ability. They found that although surgical trainees performed quicker than other trainees on tests of eye-hand coordination, there were no differences between specialties or sex in terms of visuospatial ability. In all specialties, women were significantly more accurate than men on eye-hand coordination tests. They concluded that self-selection of a surgical specialty based on skill is unlikely. Technical proficiency does improve over time, which probably correlates with motivation and task-specific practice.

Although not measured, other components play a role in the fine manual dexterity needed for such occupations as dentistry and surgery, including endurance, efficiency, and accuracy. When we enter early adulthood with strong prehensile skill, those other components may require nurturing before the achievement of true mastery. Motivation, patience, and task-specific practice help most prehensile skills improve. If skills do not improve, the individual may need to choose a profession in which strong prehension is not required.

Strength

The magnitude of grip and pinch strength needed to perform most activities of daily living tasks and job duties varies. Available grip and pinch strength may influence our career choice. Conversely, grip and pinch strength increase as our occupational tasks require greater hand use (Josty et al, 1997). For example, office workers have the weakest grips and heavy manual workers have the strongest.

Reportedly, if the right hand is dominant, the strength of the right hand is approximately 10% greater than that of the left hand, and if the left hand is dominant, the strengths of the two hands are usually equal (Peterson et al, 1989). However, other studies have found the grip strengths of the dominant and nondominant hands to be relatively equal (Armstrong and Oldman, 1999; Mathiowetz et al, 1985). Interestingly, grip and pinch strength can vary between 14% and 24% when tested over a 2-week period (Young et al, 1989). Therefore, improvements in grip strength documented as progress in rehabilitation settings may in fact just represent the day-to-day variability and should be interpreted with caution.

Mathiowetz and colleagues (1985) outlined normative data on people older than 20 years of age in terms of grip strength (see Fig. 14–9B). The 25- to 39-year-old age group exhibited the highest grip strength values. Although the values varied little between 20 to 59 years of age, a gradual decline was noted between 60 to 75+ years of age, especially among men.

Maintenance of Prehensile Skill and Function

In middle adulthood, most of the systems involved with prehension continue to function well, as long as they are maintained and not overextended. Performance in most activities of daily living is maintained easily because such activities are practiced repeatedly over the years and are generally nonstrenuous. When dysfunction does occur, it is commonly caused by congenital or traumatic limb loss, learned nonuse, peripheral neuropathy, or cumulative trauma disorders. We discuss strategies to improve function in Clinical Implications—Prehensile Dysfunction Across the Life Span.

Maintenance of skill during the period of middle adulthood is differentiated from early adulthood in terms of performance; that is, the amount of

CLINICAL IMPLICATIONS
Prehensile Dysfunction Across the Life Span

Skilled prehension helps us perform many everyday activities. Throughout the life span, however, individuals may be faced with the challenge of completing prehensile tasks despite injury or illness. Some of the common causes of prehensile dysfunction are described here, as well as strategies that are available to enhance prehensile function.

Common Causes of Prehensile Dysfunction

- Congenital and Traumatic Upper Extremity Limb Loss

Limb deficiencies may develop in response to abnormal constraints (i.e., amniotic bands) placed on the developing upper extremity. For example, amniotic bands present in a growing hand or upper limb may result in partial amputations or other tissue damage in response to band-induced compression and ischemia (Light and Ogden, 1993). Trauma can result in amputations or neuromuscular damage leading to a loss in upper limb function. Injury to the brachial plexus at birth or injury to cervical spinal nerves secondary to an accident can result in paralysis of one or more muscles of the upper limb. Prehensile capabilities present after injury depend on the muscles that remain innervated.

- Learned nonuse

Learned nonuse (Taub et al, 1975) occurs when voluntary movement of a limb is suppressed, as seen in individuals with congenital limb deficiencies, unilateral brachial plexus injury, or hemiplegia secondary to cerebral palsy or stroke. In cases of unilateral nonuse, one limb does not develop efficient prehension secondary to neuromuscular or musculoskeletal impairments and thus is ignored while tasks are primarily performed with the intact extremity.

- Peripheral neuropathy

Carpal tunnel syndrome, diabetes mellitus, Raynaud's disease, and other peripheral neuropathies are pathological conditions that can reduce sensibility and function (Casanova et al, 1991; Lowe and Freivalds, 1999; Patri and Gatto, 1986). Studies reveal that tactile deficits alone lead to errors when reaching and pointing (Gentilucci et al, 1997) and impair fingertip force coordination during object manipulation (Westling and Johansson, 1984). Individuals with proprioceptive deficits due to large fiber sensory neuropathy exhibit large errors in reaching movements (Gordon et al, 1995) and interjoint coordination (Sainburg et al, 1993). In the presence of tactile and proprioceptive deficits, visual cues have been found to greatly improve prehensile performance (Ghez et al, 1995).

- Cumulative trauma disorders

Cumulative trauma disorders, such as tendinitis, can result from sustained pinch or prehensile activities performed repetitively without adequate endurance and subsequent rest to refuel energies (Duff, 1997).

Cumulative trauma disorders are the most frequent cause of lost work and workers' compensation claims in certain industries. For example, as many as 30% of professional musicians will develop cumulative trauma disorders (Markison, 1990). The presence of tendinitis can lead to compensatory prehension patterns, which are often less efficient than those typically used.

Strategies to Improve Prehensile Function

Those with limited prehension have options. They can use adaptive devices, take advantage of surgical reconstruction, or use a standard or neuroprosthetic device. Before intervention, however, it is important to evaluate individual needs and long-range plans based on the current functional level.

▪ Adaptive devices

Most individuals adapt quite easily to subtle deficits in prehension. If the deficits make simple tasks difficult, the use of adaptive devices may be required. Self-care items commonly used to maximize prehensile capabilities include universal cuffs to hold various implements (e.g., an eating utensil) and button hooks to button clothing with one hand. Writing devices that place the fingers and thumb in a position resembling a tripod or lateral grip can be fabricated or obtained commercially. While adaptive devices can increase independent function, they are not always accepted.

▪ Surgical reconstruction

An example of surgical intervention is fetal upper limb surgery, which has been introduced to reduce the negative effects of congenital anomalies on limb development. For example, there has been reported success with the release of amniotic bands, which constrict limb development and growth (Quintero et al, 1997). If these circumferential bands are released in utero, they may prevent amputations or other limb deficits.

Tendon transfers are an option available to individuals with peripheral nerve damage. The transfer of intact muscles to nonfunctional muscle-tendon units can improve shoulder motion in the case of brachial plexus birth injury (Erb's palsy) (Waters, 1997) and provide opposition to those with median nerve injury (Brand, 1985) and lateral pinch prehension or elbow extension for reach in those with tetraplegia secondary to cervical spinal cord injury (James, 1996; Kutz et al, 1999; Weiss, 1996). Research indicates that tendon transfers improve independence in everyday activities and may allow individuals to resume life roles with greater satisfaction (Mulcahey et al, 1999).

Pollicization is a procedure used to reconstruct an opposable digit, which may be an option for those born without a thumb or those who have sustained a traumatic loss of a thumb. Typically, the index finger is rotated to oppose the remaining digits (Kozin et al, 1992; Manske et al, 1992). Transplantation of the great or second toe to replace a lost thumb can also be performed successfully. Although function after transplantation is generally good, the resultant sensibility seems to vary between adults and children and among surgical techniques performed (Cheng et al, 1998; Songcharoen et al, 1995).

▪ Prostheses

Prosthetic devices provide an alternative means of prehension to those with nonfunctional hands or upper limb amputation, whether congenital or traumatic. The addition of a prosthesis has the potential to enhance unilateral as well as bilateral function. Passive prostheses without active control can be used as a first prosthesis in infants who sit independently, or as a cosmetic prosthesis. The key to acceptance of an upper limb prosthesis in cases of congenital absence is fitting before the age of 2 years and promoting parental involvement in the process (Datta and Ibbotson, 1998; Postema et al, 1999).

Prosthetic devices include the standard hook and harness unit, myoelectric devices, and implanted electrical stimulation, termed a *neuroprosthesis*. Standard prosthetic devices use a terminal device that resembles a hand or consists of a hook to provide a strong pinch force. Terminal devices are activated through a harness via shoulder movement. Myoelectric units use remaining arm musculature to activate the terminal device through the use of electrodes strategically placed in the socket to lie over the most active site of the muscle belly. A neuroprosthesis, or Freehand system, has been implanted in those with high-level cervical spinal cord injuries without adequate transfer muscles. This system can provide lateral pinch and palmar grasp function. Research has indicated that implantation of the Freehand system in adolescents with tetraplegia improves their independence in activities of daily living (Kilgore et al, 1997; Mulcahey et al, 1997). New methods for controlling the hand are being developed, including the use of implanted intracortical electrodes (Lauer et al, 1999).

- Strategies for learned nonuse

Individuals with learned nonuse can be encouraged to use the involved extremity through constraint-induced or forced-use therapy. This approach has been used successfully in adults poststroke (Ostendorf and Wolf, 1981; Taub et al, 1993) and in children with hemiplegic cerebral palsy (Charles et al, 2001; Crocker et al, 1997). Impairments in anticipatory control found in children with cerebral palsy when they manipulate objects (Eliasson et al, 1992, 1995) also can be addressed with extended practice. Gordon and Duff (1999) found that extended practice in grasping and lifting novel objects, without constraining the limb, was an effective means of promoting anticipatory scaling of fingertip forces in children with hemiplegic cerebral palsy. Improvements in anticipatory control may contribute to greater prehensile skill.

- Strategies to prevent cumulative trauma disorder

For adults, the best methods for maintaining prehensile skill without causing undue harm to neuromuscular structures require (1) the use of correct postural alignment for tasks, (2) frequent breaks during sustained pinch or grip tasks, (3) use of tools to simplify tasks, and (4) use of ergonomically redesigned tools and musical instruments to prevent undue stress on anatomic structures (Blair and Bear-Lehman, 1987; Markison, 1990; Meagher, 1987). Given the prevalence of cumulative trauma disorders, it may be important to implement these strategies to a greater degree within recreational and work-related activities.

domain-specific practice, motivation, and efficiency of performance. When interest in and motivation for activities drop, so does practice time. We may have been an expert at the piano at the age of 25 years, but by age 50, we may spend too little time at the keyboard to maintain and preserve our former skill. Conversely, concert pianists, who continue to demonstrate fine technique well into their older adult years, may be able to maintain their skills because of continued practice. Sustained practice time promotes greater endurance, yet it is demanding. It requires us to maintain a high tolerance for aerobic work to avoid fatigue of associated structures.

OLDER ADULTHOOD

Manual performance and psychomotor behaviors decline as adults age (Hughes et al, 1997; Weir et al, 1998). Shiffman (1992) found that hand strength, performance time, and the frequency with which prehension patterns are used are affected by age. These changes seem to reflect functional adaptation to changes in the visual, nervous, somatosensory, and musculoskeletal systems associated with aging.

Sensory Changes

Sensory changes have been documented through the visual and somatosensory systems. Visual acuity, imaging power of the retina, and the transparency of the lens are all reduced during older adulthood. It also takes older individuals 33% longer to process visual information than it does younger people (Kline et al, 1983). In addition, there is a sharp decrease in depth perception from 60 to 75 years. Loss in sensibility through the arms and hands may be due to a decrease in sensory nerve conduction, alterations in mechanoreceptors, or a decline in spatial acuity of touch (Stevens and Cruz, 1996). Cole and colleagues (1998) reported that there is an increased threshold to touch pressure and a decreased sensitivity to vibration sense.

Musculoskeletal Changes

Musculoskeletal changes are seen in both muscle performance and skeletal integrity. The decline in muscle strength with aging may be attributed to a notable loss in muscle mass as well to as a decrease in motor nerve conduction velocity. A general decrease in the number of muscle fibers affects muscle strength and mass. Functionally, there is a decrease in the speed of muscle contraction and in the ability to sustain a contraction. Within the skeletal system, degeneration of the articular cartilage reduces the efficiency of movement at the joints and reduces shock absorption. This may also result in pain and altered use of the hands during manipulation.

During complex hand movements, an increase in planning time in older adults was most frequently noted (Williams, 1990). The time needed to plan for precise movements of the distal extremities increases linearly from 50 to 90 years of age. Thus, an older adult often cannot easily achieve the quick reaction time needed to count out change in checkout line at a grocery store.

Adaptations to System Changes

What are some of the adaptations that older adults make in response to system changes, and what are the resultant alterations in hand function? Due to changes in mechanoreceptors, there may be a greater dependency on muscular feedback to maximize tactile awareness and proprioception. If somatosensory feedback is reduced, a tighter grip may be used to provide the needed sensory input. A tighter grip may not only strain joints but also recruit more muscle fibers to sustain a contraction. This extra effort may put the muscle at even greater risk for fatigue, because the muscles already have a reported reduction in strength and speed of contraction. If the speed of muscular contractions is reduced, quick dexterous hand function will be affected. This system change combined with reduced sensibility and increased time to plan precise distal movements may expand time to perform select tasks. For example, older adults may need more time to count out change at the checkout line.

Despite the system changes that occur with aging, overall eye-hand coordination and manipulative skills may be relatively maintained in older adults as long as task-specific practice is continued and the systems involved remain generally intact. For example, although a reduction in sensibility typically affects fine-motor function, it may not reduce function in all tasks (Cole et al, 1998). Furthermore, studies have indicated that with significant practice, older adults can decrease their overall response time for select motor tasks (Falduto and Baron, 1960). This is beneficial because improving the speed of performance can enhance movement consistency and safety (Light, 1990). In general, motivation and arousal for specific tasks do not decline with age. Therefore, unless there are specific system deficits, prehensile skills can continue to be useful into older adulthood.

Summary

During many everyday activities, the primary components of prehension are engaged: visual regard, reach, grasp, manipulation, and release. Depending on the task goal and constraints, bimanual coordination may also be used. The development and maintenance of prehensile skill incorporate many interdependent systems. Indeed, strong relationships exist among prehension, postural control, cognition, and visuoperceptual skill.

Flexible prehensile skills allow us to mold actions to constraints and environmental demands while meeting task goals. When prehension is viewed across the life span, we can only marvel at its highly developed features. The prehensile abilities of someone at any age with hand dysfunction are even more amazing. Simple tasks become ambitious acts of adaptation enhanced with a touch of creativity.

ACKNOWLEDGMENTS

I would like to thank Jeanne Charles, MSW, PT, and Ann-Christian Elliason, PhD, OT, for their throughtful reviews of this chapter.

References

Abahnini K, Proteau L. Evidence supporting the importance of peripheral visual information for the directional control of aiming movements. *J Mot Behav* 29:230–242, 1997.

Abend W, Bizzi E, Morasso P. Human arm trajectory formation. *Brain* 105:331–348, 1982.

Ammon JE, Etzel ME. Sensorimotor organization in reach and prehension: A developmental model. *Phys Ther* 57:7–14, 1974.

Armstrong CA, Oldman JA. A comparison of dominant and non-dominant hand strengths. *J Hand Surg* 24:421–425, 1999.

Blair SJ, Bear-Lehman J. Editorial comment: Prevention of upper extremity occupational disorders. *J Hand Surg* 12:821–822, 1987.

Brand PW. *Drag in Clinical Mechanics of the Hand.* St. Louis: Mosby, 1985, pp 166–191.

Casanova JE, Casanova JS, Young MJ. Hand function in patients with diabetes mellitus. *South Med J* 84:1111–1113, 1991.

Casanova JS, Grunert BK. Adult prehension: Patterns and nomenclature for pinches. *J Hand Ther* 2: 231–244, 1989.

Case-Smith J, Fisher AG, Bauer D. An analysis of the relationship between proximal and distal motor control. *Am J Occup Ther* 43:657–662, 1989.

Charles J, Lavinder G, Gordon AM. Constraint-induced therapy in children with hemiplegic CP. *Ped Phys Ther* 13(2):68–76, 2001.

Cheng GL, Pan DD, Zhang NP, Fang GR. Digital replantation in children: A long term follow-up study. *J Hand Surg* 23:635–646, 1998.

Chieffi S, Gentilucci M. Coordination between the transport and the grasp component during prehension movements. *Exp Brain Res* 94:471–477, 1993.

Clifton RK, Muir DW, Ashmead DH, Clarkson MG. Is visually guided reaching in early infancy a myth? *Child Dev* 64:1099–1110, 1993.

Cole KJ, Rotella DL, Harper JG. Tactile impairments cannot explain the effect of age on a grasp and lift task. *Exp Brain Res* 121:263–269, 1998.

Corbetta D, Thelen E. The developmental origins of bimanual coordination: A dynamic perspective. *J Exp Psychol Hum Percept Perform* 22:502–522, 1996.

Coren S, Ward LM, Enns JT. *Sensation and Perception*, 5th ed. Orlando: Harcourt Brace and Company, 1999.

Crocker MD, MacKay-Lyons M, McDonnell E. Forced use of the upper extremity in cerebral palsy: A single-case design. *Am J Occup Ther* 51:824–833, 1997.

Datta D, Ibbotson V. Powered prosthetic hands in very young children. *Prosthet Ortho Int* 22:150–154, 1998.

Duff SV. Neuromuscular conditions. In Sanders MJ (ed). *Management of Cumulative Trauma Disorders.* Boston: Butterworth-Heinemann, 1997, pp 41–103.

Edin BB, Abbs JH. Finger movement responses of cutaneous mechanoreceptors in the dorsal skin of the human hand. *J Neurophysiol* 65:657–670, 1991.

Eliasson AC, Gordon AM, Forssberg H. Impaired anticipatory control of isometric forces during grasping by children with cerebral palsy. *Dev Med Child Neurol* 34:216–225, 1992.

Eliasson AC, Gordon AM, Forssberg H. Tactile control of isometric fingertip forces during grasping in children with cerebral palsy. *Dev Med Child Neurol* 37:72–84, 1995.

Exner C. The zone of proximal development in in-hand manipulation skills of nondysfunctional 3 and 4 year old children. *Am J Occup Ther* 44:884–891, 1990.

Falduto L, Baron A. Age-related changes and effects of practice and task complexity on card sorting. *J Gerontol* 41:659–661, 1960.

Fiorentino MR. *Normal and Abnormal Development: The Influence of Primitive Reflexes on Motor Development.* Springfield, IL: Charles C Thomas, 1972.

Flatt A. The absent thumb. In Flatt A (ed). *The Care of Congenital Hand Anomalies.* St. Louis: Mosby, 1977.

Forssberg H, Eliasson AC, Kinoshita H, et al. Development of human precision grip. IV: Tactile adaptation of isometric finger forces to the frictional condition. *Exp Brain Res* 104:323–330, 1995.

Gentilucci M, Toni I, Daprati E, Gangitano M. Tactile input of the hand and the control of reaching to grasp movements. *Exp Brain Res* 114:130–137, 1997.

Ghez C, Gordon J, Ghilardi MF. Impairments of reaching in patients without proprioception. II. Effects of visual information on accuracy. *J Neurophysiol* 73:361–372, 1995.

Gordon AM, Duff SV. Fingertip forces during object manipulation in children with hemiplegic cerebral palsy. I. Anticipatory scaling. *Dev Med Child Neurol* 41:166–175, 1999.

Gordon J, Ghilardi MF, Ghez C. Impairments of reaching movements in patients without proprioception. I. Spatial errors. *J Neurophysiol* 73:347–360, 1995.

Graham KS, Deary IJ. A role for aptitude testing in surgery? *J R Coll Surg Edinb* 36:70–74, 1991.

Halverson HM. An experimental study of prehension in infants by means of systematic cinema recording. *Genet Psychol Monogr* 19:107–285, 1931.

Halverson HM. A further study of grasping. *J Gen Psychol* 7:34–64, 1932.

Harris CJ, Herbert M, Steele RJ. Psychomotor skills of surgical trainees compared with those of different medical specialists. *Br J Surg* 81:382–383, 1994.

Hirschel A, Pehoski C, Coryell J. Environmental support and the development of grasp in infants. *Am J Occup Ther* 44:721–727, 1990.

Hohlstein RR. The development of prehension in normal infants. *Am J Occup Ther* 36:170–175, 1982.

Hughes S, Gibbs H, Dunlop D, et al. Predictors of decline in manual performance in older adults. *J Am Geriatr Soc* 45:905–910, 1997.

Jakobson LS, Goodale MA. Factors affecting higher-order movement planning: A kinematic analysis of human prehension. *Exp Brain Res* 86:199–208, 1991.

James MA. Surgical treatment of the upper extremity: indications, patient assessment, and procedures. In Betz RR, Mulcahey MJ (eds). *The Child With a Spinal Cord Injury*. Rosemont, IL: American Academy of Orthopaedic Surgeons, 1996, pp 393–404.

Jeannerod M. Intersegmental coordination during reaching at natural visual objects. In Long J, Baddeley A (eds). *Attention and Performance IX*. Hillsdale, NJ: Lawrence Earlbaum, 1981.

Jeannerod M. The timing of natural prehension movements. *J Mot Behav* 16:235–254, 1984.

Jeannerod M. Mechanisms of visuomotor coordination: A study in normal and brain-damaged subjects. *Neuropsychologia* 24:41–78, 1986.

Johansson RS, Cole KJ. Sensory-motor coordination during grasping and manipulative actions. *Curr Opin Neurobiol* 2:815–823, 1992.

Josty IC, Tyler MP, Shewell PC, Roberts AH. Grip and pinch strength variations in different types of workers. *J Hand Surg* 22:266–269, 1997.

Kaminski TR, Bock C, Gentile AM. The coordination between trunk and arm motion during pointing movements. *Exp Brain Res* 106:457–466, 1995.

Kilgore KL, Peckham PH, Keith MW, et al. An implanted upper-extremity neuroprosthesis: Follow-up of five patients. *J Bone Joint Surg* 79:533–541, 1997

Kline D, Schieber F, Coyne A. Aging, the eye and visual channels: Contrast sensitivity and response speed. *J Gerontol* 33:211–216, 1983.

Konczak J, Dichgans J. The development toward stereotypic arm kinematics during reaching in the first 3 years of life. *Exp Brain Res* 117:346–354, 1997.

Korczyn AD, Sage JI, Karplus M. Lack of limb motor asymmetry in the neonate. *J Neurobiol* 9:483–488, 1978.

Kozin SH, Weiss AA, Webber JB, et al. Index finger pollicization for congenital aplasia or hypoplasia of the thumb. *J Hand Surg [Am]* 17:880–884, 1992.

Kuhtz-Buschbeck JP, Stolze H, Joehnk M, Boczek-Funcke A. Development of prehension movements in children. *Exp Brain Res* 122:424–432, 1998.

Kutz JE, Van Heest AE, House JH. Biceps-to-triceps transfer in tetraplegic patients: Report of the medial routing technique and follow-up of three cases. *J Hand Surg* 24:161–172, 1999.

Landsmeer JMF. Power grip and precision handling. *Ann Rheum Dis* 21:164–169, 1962.

Lantz C, Melen, K, Forssberg H. Early infant grasping involves radial fingers. *Dev Med Child Neurol* 38:668–674, 1996.

Lauer RT, Peckham PH, Kilgore KL. EEG-based control of a hand grasp neuroprosthesis. *Neuroreport* 10:1767–1771, 1999.

Lewis S, Duff SV, Gordon AM. *Handedness and the Coordination of Movement and Fingertip Forces during Object Release in Children. Am J Occup Ther* (in press).

Liegeois F, Bentejec L, de Schonen S. When does inter-hemispheric integration of visual events emerge in infancy? A developmental study on 19- to 28- month-old infants. *Neuropsychologia* 38:1382–1389, 2000.

Light KE. Information processing for motor performance in aging adults. *Phys Ther* 70:820–826, 1990.

Light TR, Ogden JA. Congenital constriction band syndrome: Pathophysiology and treatment. *Yale J Biol Med* 66:143–155, 1993.

Long C, Conrad PW, Hall EA, Furler SL. Intrinsic-extrinsic muscle control of the hand in power grip and precision handling. *J Bone Joint Surg* 52:853–867, 1970.

Lowe BD, Freivalds A. Effect of carpal tunnel syndrome on grip force coordination on hand tools. *Ergonomics* 42:550–564, 1999.

Manske PR, Rotman MB, Dailey LA. Long-term functional results after pollicization for the congenitally deficient thumb. *J Hand Surg* 17:1064–1072, 1992.

Markison RE. Treatment of musical hands: Redesign the interface in hand injuries. *Sports Performing Arts Hand Clin* 6:525–544, 1990.

Mathiowetz V, Kashman N, Volland G, et al. Grip and pinch strength: Normative data for adults. *Arch Phys Med Rehabil* 66:16–21, 1985.

Mathiowetz V, Wiemer DM, Federman SM. Grip and pinch strength norms for 6 to 19 year olds. *Am J Occup Ther* 40:705–711, 1986.

McBryde C, Zivani J. Proximal and distal upper limb motor development in 24 week old infants. *Can J Occup Ther* 57:147–154, 1990.

McCartney G, Hepper P. Development of lateralized behaviour in the human fetus from 12 to 27 weeks' gestation. *Dev Med Child Neurol* 41:83–86, 1999.

Meagher SW. Tool design for prevention of hand and wrist injuries. *J Hand Surg* 12:855–857, 1987.

Moore KL, Persaud TVN. *The Developing Human: Clinically Oriented Embryology*, 6th ed. Philadelphia: WB Saunders, 1998.

Mulcahey MJ, Betz RR, Smith BT, Weiss AA. A prospective evaluation of upper extremity tendon transfers in children with cervical spinal cord injury. *J Pediatr Ortho* 19:319–326, 1999.

Mulcahey MJ, Betz RR, Smith BT, et al. Implanted functional electrical stimulation hand system in adolescents with spinal cord injuries: An evaluation. *Arch Phys Med Rehabil* 78:597–607, 1997.

Napier JR. The prehensile movement of the human hand. *J Bone Joint Surg* 38:902–913, 1956.

Napier JR. Function of the hand. In Napier JR (ed). *Hands*. New York: Pantheon Books, 1980, pp 68–83.

Newell KM, Scully DM, McDonald PV, Baillargeon R. Task constraints and infant grip configurations. *Dev Psychobiol* 22:817–831, 1989.

O'Driscoll SW, Horil E, Ness R, Richards RR. The relationship between wrist position, grasp size, and grip strength. *J Hand Surg* 17:169–177, 1992.

Ostendorf CG, Wolf SL. Effect of forced use of the upper extremity of a hemiplegic patient on changes in function. *Phys Ther* 61:1022–1027, 1981.

Pare M, Dugas C. Developmental changes in prehension during childhood. *Exp Brain Res* 125:239–247, 1999.

Patla AE. A framework for understanding mobility problems in the elderly. In Craik RL, Oatis CA (eds). *Gait Analysis: Theory and Application*. St. Louis: Mosby, 1995, pp 436–449.

Patri B, Gatto A. Raynaud's syndrome, Dupuytren's disease, force of prehension and sensitivity of the hand: Study of age-related changes. *Ann Chir Main* 5:144–147, 1986.

Perrig S, Kazennikov O, Wiesendanger M. Time structure of a goal-directed bimanual skill and its dependence on task constraints. *Behav Brain Res* 103:95–104, 1999.

Peterson P, Petrick M, Connor H, Conklin D. Grip strength and hand dominance: Challenging the 10% rule. *Am J Occup Ther* 43:444–447, 1989.

Pickleman J, Schueneman AL. The use and abuse of neuropsychological tests to predict operative performance. *Am Coll Surg Bull* 72:7–11, 1987.

Postema K, van der Donk V, van Limbeek J, et al. Prosthesis rejection in children with unilateral congenital arm defect. *Clin Rehabil* 13:243–249, 1999.

Quintero RA, Morales WJ, Phillips J, et al. In utero lysis of amniotic bands. *Ultrasound Obstet Gynecol* 10:316–320, 1997.

Raj R, Marquis C. Finger dominance. *J Hand Surg* 24:430, 1999.

Rochat P. Self-sitting and reaching in 5- to 8-month-old infants: The impact of posture and its development on eye-hand coordination. *J Mot Behav* 24:210–220, 1992.

Rosander K, von Hofsten C. Visual-vestibular interaction in early infancy. *Exp Brain Res* 133:321–333, 2000.

Rose SA, Gottfried A, Bridger W. Cross-modal transfer in infants: Relationship to prematurity and socioeconomic background. *Dev Psychol* 14:643–652, 1978.

Sainburg RL, Kalakanis D. Differences in control of limb dynamics during dominant and nondominant reaching. *J Neurophysiol* 83:2661–2675, 2000.

Sainburg RL, Poizner H, Ghez C. Loss of proprioception produces deficits in interjoint coordination. *J Neurophysiol* 70:2136–2147, 1993.

Schieppati M, Trompetto C, Abbruzzese G. Selective facilitation of responses to cortical stimulation of proximal and distal arm muscles by precision tasks in man. *J Physiol* 491(Pt 2):551–562, 1996.

Schneck CM, Henderson A. Descriptive analysis of the developmental progression of grip position for pencil and crayon control in nondysfunctional children. *Am J Occup Ther* 44:893–900, 1990.

Shiffman LM. Effects of aging on adult hand function. *Am J Occup Ther* 46:785–792, 1992.

Smith LK, Weiss EL, Lehmkuhl LD. *Brunnstrom's Clinical Kinesiology,* 5th ed. Philadelphia: FA Davis, 1996.

Songcharoen P, Thanapipatsiri S, Mahaisavariya B, Chotigavanich C. Thumb reconstruction with a big toe microvascular wrap-around flap: A report of fifteen cases. *Ann Acad Med Singapore* 24(4 suppl):46–50, 1995.

Sparling JW, Van Tol J, Chescheir NC. Fetal and neonatal hand movement. *Phys Ther* 79:24–39, 1999.

Stevens JC, Cruz LA. Spatial acuity of touch: Ubiquitous decline with aging revealed by repeated threshold testing. *Somatosens Mot Res* 13:1–10, 1996.

Streri A. Tactile discrimination of shape and intermodel transfer in 2- to 3-month-old infants. *Br J Dev Psychol* 5:213–220, 1987.

Stilwell JM, Cermak SA. Perceptual functions of the hand. In Henderson A, Pehoski C (eds). *Hand Function in the Child: Foundations for Remediation.* Philadelphia: Mosby, 1995, pp 55–80.

Taub E, Goldberg IA, Taub P. Deafferentation in monkeys: Pointing at a target without visual feedback. *Exp Neurol* 46:176–186, 1975.

Taub E, Miller NE, Novack TA, et al. Technique to improve chronic motor deficit after stroke. *Arch Phys Med Rehabil* 74:347–354, 1993.

Thelen E. Motor development: A new synthesis. *Am Psychol* 50:79–95, 1995.

Tubiana R. Architecture and functions of the hand. In Tubiana R, Thomine JM, Mackin EJ (eds). *Examination of the Hand and Upper Limb.* Philadelphia: WB Saunders, 1984, pp 1–98.

Twitchell TE. Reflex mechanisms and the development of prehension. In Connelly K (ed). *Mechanisms of Motor Skill Development.* London: Academic Press, 1970, pp 25–59.

Vallbo AB, Johansson RS. Properties of cutaneous mechanoreceptors in the human hand related to touch sensation. *Hum Neurobiol* 3:3–14, 1984.

von Hofsten C, Fazel-Zandy S. Development of visually guided hand orientation in reaching. *J Exp Child Psychol* 38:208–219, 1984.

von Hofsten C, Lindhagen K. Observation on the development of reaching for moving objects. *J Exp Child Psychol* 28:158–173, 1979.

von Hofsten C, Ronnqvist L. Preparation for grasping an object: A developmental study. *J Exp Psychol Hum Percept Perform* 14:610–621, 1988.

von Hofsten C, Rosander K. Development of smooth pursuit tracking in young infants. *Vision Res* 37:1799–1810, 1997.

von Hofsten C, Woollacott HM. Postural preparations for reaching in 9-month-old infants. Unpublished manuscript, 1990.

Waters PM. Obstetric brachial plexus injuries: Evaluation and management. *J Acad Ortho Surg* 5:205–214, 1997.

Weir PL, MacDonald JR, Mallat BJ, et al. Age-related differences in prehension the influence of task goals. *J Mot Behav* 30:79–80, 1998.

Weiss AA. Tendon transfers in tetraplegia: Surgical technique. In Betz RR, Mucahey MJ (eds). *The Child With a Spinal Cord Injury.* Rosemont, IL: American Academy of Orthopaedic Surgeons, 1996, pp 405–418.

Westling G, Johansson RS. Factors influencing the force control during precision grip. *Exp Brain Res* 53:277–284, 1984.

Wiesendanger M, Kazennikov O, Perrig S, Kaluzny P. Two hands-one action: The problem of bimanual coordination. In Wing AM, Haggard P, Flanagan JR (eds). *Hand and Brain: The Neurophysiology and Psychology of Hand Movements.* San Diego: Academic Press, 1996.

Williams HG. Aging and eye-hand coordination. In Bard C, Fleury M, Hay L (eds). *Development of Eye Hand Coordination Across the Life Span.* Columbia, SC: University of South Carolina Press, 1990, pp 327–357.

Young VL, Pin P, Kraemer BA, et al. Fluctuation in grip and pinch strength among normal subjects. *J Hand Surg* 14:125–129, 1989.

15 Health and Fitness

OBJECTIVES

After studying this chapter, the reader will be able to:

1 Discuss the relationships among health, fitness, and physical activity.

2 Understand the integrated role of all body systems in the development and maintenance of fitness.

3 Identify the effects of exercise and training on the body systems.

4 Identify age-related considerations in developing exercise, training, and fitness programs.

We discussed the theories, mechanics, and roles of our various body systems in relation to functional physical activity. The ability to function at our best in all activities throughout the life span is a goal shared by everyone. What is functioning at our best? Is it health? What role does fitness play? More important, how can we be proactive and ensure an optimal level of functioning throughout the life span?

We discuss the issues of health and fitness and encourage readers to incorporate concepts for healthy lifestyles into their own life plans. As health care providers, we are uniquely qualified to assist clients in reaching the goal of lifelong fitness.

Health and Fitness

HEALTH

General definitions of *health* describe a state of physical, mental, and social well-being (McArdle et al, 1991; World Health Organization, 1958). These definitions discuss freedom from defect, pain, and disease, while emphasizing that health is not merely the absence of these entities. In reality, health is a condition of the human body and mind. As a condition, health is represented on a continuum from good health to poor health.

Bouchard and colleagues (1990) defined health as a human condition with physical, social, and psychological dimensions within positive and negative poles. Positive health reflects the ability to enjoy life and to withstand challenges, not merely the absence of disease. It has also been referred to as the highest level of functional capability (McArdle et al, 1991). Negative health

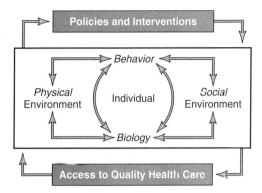

Figure 15–1

Schematic model of determinants of health. (Redrawn from U.S. Department of Health and Human Services. *Healthy People 2010: Understanding and Improving Health*, 2nd ed. Washington, DC: U.S. Government Printing Office, 2000.)

reflects morbidity and ultimately mortality. Diseases such as arthritis, heart disease, and diabetes have the potential to diminish functional capacity. These limitations in physical function can also interfere with the ability to actively meet social demands and to enjoy leisure-time activities. The term *wellness*, which comprises biological and psychological well-being, is also used to denote a state of positive health (Bouchard et al, 1990). This term reflects a holistic concept of health.

Each of us along with society contribute to our health (Fig. 15–1). Society contributes to the health of a community through policies such as laws mandating the use of seat belts, childhood immunization policies, and clean air regulations. Access to health care is also important, and social policies can assist in making health care available to all individuals. Communities sponsor health promotion efforts aimed at the prevention of smoking or drug abuse, hoping to improve the health of their citizens. Each individual, however, has an individual biological makeup that includes both genetic and medical profiles. These profiles may indicate an increased risk for specific diseases such as diabetes or heart disease. We also make choices about our level of physical activity, smoking habits, and diet. The social and physical environment in which we live contributes to the choices we make about following healthy lifestyles (U.S. Department of Health and Human Services, 2000).

FITNESS

There is no universally accepted definition of fitness (O'Toole and Douglas, 1988). Some general definitions describe *fitness* as a state of optimal well-being and the capacity to successfully meet the present and potential physical challenges of life. To be fit is to be adapted, adjusted, qualified, or suited to some purpose, function, or aim. The term *fit* is also used to describe a person who is in good physical condition, someone who is healthy. Physical fitness allows us to carry out daily tasks with vigor and alertness, without undue fatigue, and with ample energy to enjoy leisure and to meet unusual circumstances and unforeseen emergencies (Biegel, 1984).

More specifically, from an exercise perspective, *physical fitness* is related to our ability to perform physical activity (McArdle et al, 1991). And as defined by the World Health Organization, it is our ability to perform muscular work satisfactorily. Cardiovascular and respiratory endurance, muscular strength, and flexibility contribute to fitness, but physical fitness is determined by habitual activity level, diet, and heredity (Bouchard et al, 1990). Therefore, fitness equals the capacity for physical work and varies with activity level (O'Toole and Douglas, 1988). Exercise scientists differentiate physical from physiological fitness. *Physiological fitness* is the fitness of the biological systems and is influenced by physical activity. Blood pressure, glucose tolerance, blood lipid levels, and body composition are markers of physiological fitness (Bouchard et al, 1990).

Components of Fitness

The components of fitness are cardiovascular and respiratory endurance, muscular strength and endurance, flexibility, and body composition. They contribute to one's agility, power, balance, coordination, and speed during physical activity.

Cardiovascular and *respiratory endurance* reflect the ability of the heart, vasculature, and lungs to provide oxygen to working muscle during physical activity. *Muscular strength* is the force that can be generated in a muscle, whereas *muscular endurance* reflects the ability of the muscle to complete many repetitions of muscle contraction before fatiguing. *Flexibility,* the ability to move without restriction, depends on adequate muscle length and appropriate mobility within the joints of the body. Good flexibility improves efficiency of movement and decreases the potential for injury. *Body composition* refers to the amount of lean body mass and fat mass. Lean body mass includes muscle, bone, other nonfat substances (e.g., water, minerals), and a small amount of fat stored in the nervous system and bone marrow (McArdle et al, 1991). Because in most physical activity we must support and carry the body weight, our active lean body mass should preferably be greater than nonactive fat mass (O'Toole and Douglas, 1988).

Factors Influencing Health and Fitness

Individual factors such as heredity, age, sex, physical activity, lifestyle, and environment contribute to one's level of physical and physiological fitness. A model of the interactions among exercise, health, and fitness was developed by Bouchard and colleagues in 1990 (Fig. 15–2). Personal attributes as defined for this diagram are age, sex, socioeconomic status, personality, and motivation.

PHYSICAL FACTORS

Age, growth, and sex can influence fitness. The ability to perform physical activities with physiological efficiency improves through childhood, adoles-

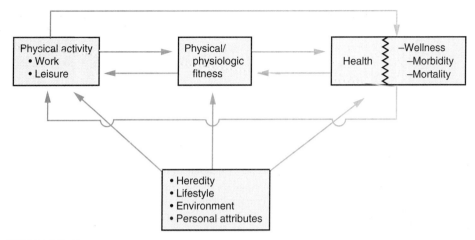

Figure 15–2

Schematic model of the complex relationships among habitual physical activity, fitness, and health. (Redrawn from Bouchard C, Shepard RJ, Stephens T, et al. *Exercise, Fitness and Health: A Consensus of Current Knowledge.* Champaign, IL: Human Kinetics. Copyright 1990 by Human Kinetics Publishers, Inc.)

cence, and young adulthood but then declines. Some of this decline may be related to physical changes, but social and environmental factors also are influential. Functional losses in physical fitness may be due to decreased activity level rather than to aging. An active lifestyle appears to minimize physical changes within the various body systems and to contribute to overall fitness (Frontera and Evans, 1986; Jackson et al, 1996; Lemura et al, 2000; McArdle et al, 1991; Sarkisian et al, 2000). Physiological improvements through training occur at a similar rate and magnitude in all individuals, regardless of age (Green and Crouse, 1995; McArdle et al, 1991).

Growth leads to changes in height and weight. The developmental pattern of aerobic capacity, muscular strength and endurance, and power is similar to that of growth (Malina, 1990). Increase in stature gradually slows and ceases after adolescence, whereas weight increases into the mid 20s (Malina, 1990). After age 35, body weight continues to slowly increase, reflecting an increase in body fat. After age 60, the percentage of lean body mass decreases further because of age-related decreases in muscle and bone mass (McArdle et al, 1991). Physical activity appears to minimize increases in fat mass of older individuals, but even in older adults who participate in moderate- to high-intensity exercise, fat mass increases 2% to 2.5% per decade (McArdle et al, 1991; Pollack et al, 1997).

Before puberty, gender does not appear to greatly affect fitness. Maximal aerobic capacity is slightly higher in boys than in girls through childhood (Armstrong and Welsman, 2000). After puberty, differences in maximal aerobic capacity between males and females become more dramatic. This change reflects the increased percentage of body fat in females, increased oxygen carrying capacity in males compared with females due to increased levels of blood hemoglobin, and larger muscle fiber area in males compared with females (Armstrong and Welsman, 2000).

HEREDITY

Heredity influences several factors that contribute to fitness, such as body size and muscle fiber composition. Whether we are tall or short is determined by heredity. The percentage of slow-twitch and fast-twitch muscle fibers found in skeletal muscle also is determined genetically (Faulkner and White, 1990; McArdle et al, 1991). Twin studies have shown genetics to be a factor in determining maximal aerobic capacity and heart rate (Cunningham et al, 1984). Inherited factors may influence our selection of physical activities, such as choosing to be a sprinter rather than a marathon runner, or impose limits on the possible level of fitness we may achieve.

ENVIRONMENTAL FACTORS

Environmental factors such as climate, oxygen pressure, and air quality can affect exercise performance. Extreme hot or cold climates stress the exercising individual trying to maintain internal body temperature. This is especially true for children and older adults. Children have a high ratio of surface area to body weight, allowing a greater rate of heat exchange with the environment. Children are also less able to sweat, making it more difficult to dissipate heat (Bar-Or, 1984). People who live and exercise in regions of high altitude must adjust to low oxygen pressures. Indoor air contaminants such as cigarette smoke, radon, and wood smoke may diminish air quality. Environmental air quality is compromised by byproducts of industry and engine exhaust. Specific pollutants such as ozone and sulfur dioxide affect lung function (Folinsbee, 1990).

PHYSICAL ACTIVITY

Participation in regular physical activity contributes positively to both health and fitness. Physical activity has been demonstrated to improve muscle strength, cardiorespiratory endurance, and physical function in older adults (Cress et al, 1999; Lemura et al, 2000). Through adulthood, levels of fitness are influenced by exercise habits and body composition (Jackson et al, 1996). Regular physical activity and increased fitness diminish the risk for cardiovascular disease, non–insulin-dependent diabetes mellitus, and osteoporosis decrease. In fact, research has suggested that if adults participate in regular physical activity, the mortality rate related to coronary heart disease, colon cancer, and diabetes decreases (Powell and Blair, 1994).

SOCIAL FACTORS

Social factors play a role in determining an individual's involvement in physical activity and fitness. Within our society, sedentary leisure-time activities such as watching television, playing video games, and computer-based activity are becoming prevalent. As individuals of all ages spend more time in these sedentary activities, the amount of leisure time spent in physical activity is reduced.

Toddlers and preschoolers are very active. Their "job" is to learn new skills and to explore their environment through movement. Parents may influence this level of activity by guiding the child's choice of movement experiences and minimizing more sedentary activities such as television watching. By school age, children become more competitive, and achieving an adequate level of skill in sports and games is important for the child's social acceptance. Children who function well motorically are encouraged to continue with physical activities, whereas children who are less skilled may become frustrated and less active. Successful motor performance is a positive reinforcer for increasing levels of physical activity. Physical activity decreases for both boys and girls in late adolescence. Especially through high school, significant decreases in the number of individuals participating in vigorous physical activity have been reported (Francis, 1999). This reduction may be influenced by social models, peer pressure, and the need to enter the work force (Malina, 1990). Adults report that job and family demands frequently do not allow time for exercise programs (Buskirk, 1990). Other lifestyle changes, such as smoking and alcohol consumption, may affect fitness in adolescence and adulthood (Malina, 1990).

Society influences the awareness of and participation in fitness programs. With increased public awareness of the benefits of fitness, fitness centers and aerobic exercise programs have become more available in the United States. Community agencies sponsor fitness-related activities for individuals of all ages. Corporations also provide fitness programs for their employees, seeking to improve health and productivity. As the communities we live and work in provide social and physical environments that foster increased levels of physical activity, individuals are encouraged to make positive choices regarding physical activity and fitness.

Perception—How Fit Are We?

Fitness has been associated with increased health and well-being. Improved quality of life and preventive health maintenance are valuable benefits of fitness. In recognition of these benefits, the U.S. Department of Health and Human Services included physical activity and fitness objectives in their Year 2010 objectives for the nation (U.S. Department of Health and Human Services, 2000). The goals of these fitness and exercise objectives are to increase public awareness of appropriate levels of exercise, promote cardiovascular fitness, and

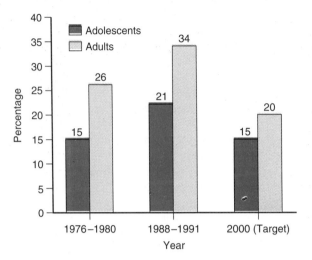

Figure 15-3

Percentage of adults (aged 20 years and older) and adolescents (aged 12 to 19 years) who are overweight. (Redrawn from Francis KT. Status of the year 2000 health goals for physical activity and fitness. *Phys Ther* 1999, 79: 405–414, with permission of the American Physical Therapy Association.)

increase participation in physical activity programs. Low levels of physical activity and overweight/obesity are leading health concerns in the United States and are among areas targeted by Healthy People 2010 (U.S. Department of Health and Human Services, 2000). The number of adolescents and adults in the United States who were reported to be overweight continues to increase according to the progress reports on Healthy People 2000 (Francis, 1999) (Fig. 15–3).

Public awareness of the importance of fitness may be increasing, but even though many individuals start exercise programs, often they will stop within a short period of time. The number of adults who participate in moderate to vigorous levels of physical activity remains well below targeted levels (Fig. 15–4). Most studies reflect that only 10% to 20% of adults in the United States exercise regularly and vigorously enough to benefit health and fitness (Francis, 1999; U.S. Department of Health and Human Services, 2000).

A progressive and predictable decline in regular physical activity participation with age has been reported (Brooks, 1987; Buskirk, 1990; Caspersen et al, 1986; Katch and Katch, 1988; McArdle et al, 1991; Talbot et al, 2000). Activity rates decline from childhood to adolescence and then through adulthood. Regular physical activity by adults also has been reported to decrease as education and income levels decrease (Caspersen et al, 1986). As levels of education and income increase, we are better able to engage in health promotion activities and to understand health promotion information.

Physical fitness of the nation's children is a concern because 20% of children fail one or more standards on fitness tests (Pate and Shepard, 1989). In 1988, Malina reviewed studies of the activity level of adolescent girls and reported that they do not get enough regular exercise to maintain high aerobic fitness. In response to the Healthy People 2000 initiative, public education programs have incorporated fitness programs into physical education and are

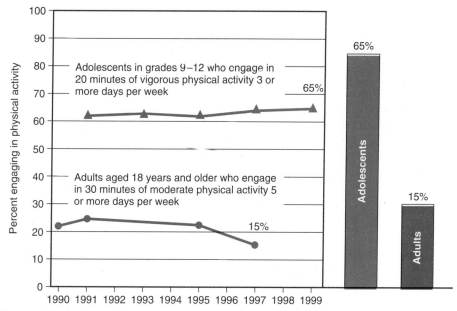

Figure 15-4

Regular physical activity throughout life is important for maintaining a healthy body, enhancing psychological well-being, and preventing premature death. This graph shows the percentage of adolescents and adults who participated in regular physical activity in the United States during the period of 1990 to 1999. (Redrawn from U.S. Department of Health and Human Services. *Healthy People 2010: Understanding and Improving Health*, 2nd ed. Washington, DC: U.S. Government Printing Office, 2000.)

increasing the time spent in promoting lifetime physical activities (U.S. Dept. of Health & Human Services, 1990). Some schools, with local grants and support, are providing fitness equipment in their playgrounds (Fig. 15–5).

In a longitudinal study of 18- to 94-year-olds, leisure-time physical activities decreased with age, especially those involving high-intensity activity (Talbot et al, 2000). To meet the needs of adults, increasing numbers of employers are providing workplace fitness programs. These programs benefit both the employee and the employer because there are fewer employee absences and less sick time. Community agencies also strive to provide physical activity programs for older adults. Older adults living in senior communities also take advantage of multiple opportunities for activities such as tennis, swimming, and fitness club facilities (Fig. 15–6).

While individuals in any age group participate in leisure-time physical activity to varying degrees, the most active tend to be the most fit. Significant efforts are being made to increase the public's awareness of the importance of physical activity and fitness.

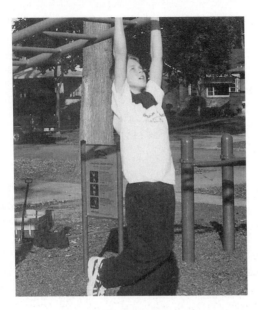

Figure 15–5

Schools and communities work together to provide fitness equipment and programs for children. This fitness court was designed to be used with six individualized activity stations at an elementary school. A local community hospital donated the funds to build the court, which is enhanced by signs that describe the preferred regimens to be used for each activity.

Body Systems Involved in Fitness

Fitness results when several body systems—the cardiovascular, pulmonary, musculoskeletal, nervous, and endocrine systems—interact optimally and efficiently. In the course of development, changes in these systems affect the way in which the body delivers fuel and produces energy for movement. Levels of

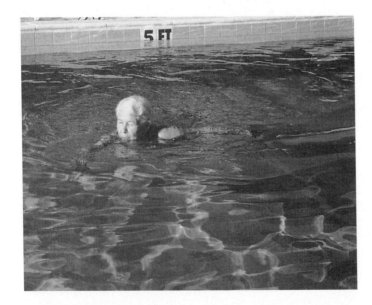

Figure 15–6

Older adults can stay active by taking advantage of community facilities such as swimming pools.

fitness and capacity for physical activity may vary throughout development as a result.

Exercise and training have been found to improve body system function and levels of fitness. *Exercise* is defined as leisure-time physical activity (Bouchard et al, 1990) that is planned, repetitive, and purposeful (McArdle et al, 1991). *Training* is regular and repeated exercise, carried out over several weeks or months, with the intention of developing physical or physiological fitness (Bouchard et al, 1990). *Trainability* reflects the ability of different body systems to adapt to repeated exercise stimuli (Bar-Or, 1988).

Exercise and training affect an adult's body systems in different ways, and the endocrine system plays a special role in exercise and training. For additional information, the reader is referred to the specific system chapters in Unit 2.

EFFECTS OF EXERCISE AND TRAINING ON THE CARDIOVASCULAR SYSTEM

During exercise, the cardiovascular system must carry large amounts of oxygen to the muscle tissue and remove waste products associated with energy production.

Cardiovascular responses to exercise and training are summarized in Table 15–1.

Short-Term Adaptation

During aerobic exercise, skeletal muscle demand for oxygen increases, resulting in increased cardiac output. Heart rate increases in proportion to the intensity of the exercise for 3 to 5 minutes. A steady state is then attained and maintained for short periods of exercise. After 15 to 30 minutes, heart rate again begins to rise due to fatigue and increased body temperature. Vasodilation occurs, helping shunt blood flow away from the viscera to the working

TABLE 15–1

Cardiovascular Adaptation to Exercise and Training

Exercise	Training
Increased cardiac output	Increased heart weight
Increased heart rate	Increased heart volume
Increased blood flow to working muscles	Increased plasma volume
Increased systolic blood pressure	Increased hemoglobin
Increased cardiac contractility	Decreased resting heart rate
Decreased peripheral resistance	Increased maximum cardiac output and stroke volume
Increased venous return	Increased arterial-to-venous oxygen difference
	Decreased systolic and diastolic blood pressure

skeletal and heart muscles. Muscle contraction squeezes nearby veins, facilitating venous return. Systolic blood pressure increases in proportion to exercise intensity and theoretically is related to the increased cardiac output. Diastolic blood pressure increases only slightly. In general, dynamic, aerobic exercise results in increased cardiac contractility, decreased peripheral resistance, and increased venous return (Noble, 1986).

Long-Term Adaptation

Heart weight and volume, plasma volume, and hemoglobin levels increase with training (Green, 1990; McArdle et al, 1991; Zernicke et al, 1991). Ventricular filling, stroke volume, and cardiac output also increase (Saltin, 1990). Therefore, more blood can be pumped per heartbeat, and necessary circulation is delivered to body tissues at a lower heart rate. Increased blood volume improves removal of waste products and heat, dilution of hormones, and perfusion of the kidneys while decreasing resistance to capillary flow.

Resting heart rate decreases, an effect that appears to be related to decreased sympathetic input. Maximum heart rate remains relatively stable, whereas maximum cardiac output and stroke volume increase (Noble, 1986). Stroke volume increases because of greater end-diastolic volume of the left ventricle and more forceful contraction of strengthened cardiac muscle (McArdle et al, 1991; Noble, 1986).

Both systolic and diastolic blood pressures decrease with training (McArdle et al, 1991; Noble, 1986; Zernicke et al, 1991). Decreases in blood pressure may be related to reduced sympathetic input, which decreases peripheral resistance to blood flow (McArdle et al, 1991).

When our body is physiologically trained, we are better able to extract oxygen from the blood, as reflected by a widening of the arterial-to-venous oxygen difference (A-$\dot{V}O_2$ difference) (McArdle et al, 1991; Noble, 1986). Increased capillary and mitochondrial capacities are seen in working muscle, improving the ability of the muscle to extract oxygen from the capillaries (Noble, 1986; Zernicke et al, 1991).

EFFECTS OF EXERCISE AND TRAINING ON THE PULMONARY SYSTEM

During exercise, greater airflow is required to meet the demands of the body. Airflow is increased by taking deeper breaths and increasing the respiratory rate.

Adaptations of the pulmonary system to exercise and training are summarized in Table 15–2.

Short-Term Adaptation

At the onset of exercise, ventilation increases rapidly and reaches a steady state within 3 to 4 minutes (Noble, 1986). The amount of air exchanged with the atmosphere per minute (*minute ventilation*) is increased as more air is moved in each breath (*tidal volume*) and as breathing frequency increases. At

TABLE 15–2

Pulmonary Adaptation to Exercise and Training

Exercise	Training
Increased minute ventilation	Increased vital capacity
Increased tidal volume	Increased tidal volume
Increased breathing frequency	Decreased respiratory rate at submaximal exercise
Decreased inspiratory/expiratory reserve	

low-intensity exercise, changes in tidal volume are sufficient to maintain adequate minute ventilation. Greater tidal volume allows inspired air to perfuse more lung tissue, opening more alveoli and maximizing the ability for gas exchange between the capillaries and the alveoli (Shepard, 1987). As exercise intensity becomes greater and tidal volume is 50% to 60% of vital capacity, breathing rate increases (Frontera and Evans, 1986).

The breathing rate at rest is approximately 14 breaths per minute. During exercise, the respiratory rate may rise up to 40 breaths per minute. Even at these higher rates, there is enough time for alveolar gas exchange to occur because alveolar ventilation increases more than does pulmonary capillary blood flow. This process works until fatigue or cardiac function limits the exercise (Noble, 1986).

In light to moderate exercise, ventilation increases linearly with levels of oxygen consumption and carbon dioxide production. At higher exercise levels, ventilation increases in relation to increased carbon dioxide concentrations produced by anaerobic metabolism. For example, blood lactate levels increase during anaerobic metabolism and must be buffered to prevent acidosis. The end product of this buffering is carbon dioxide. As the carbon dioxide levels in the blood increase, chemoreceptors in the aortic and carotid bodies, as well as in the medulla, cue the system to increase ventilation (McArdle et al, 1991; Noble, 1986).

Long-Term Adaptation

After training, resting lung volumes show little change. Slight increases in vital capacity may occur as respiratory muscle strength is improved (Shepard, 1987). During submaximal exercise, respiratory rate decreases and tidal volume increases. Air stays in the lungs longer, allowing more oxygen to be extracted (McArdle et al, 1991; Shepard, 1987). The amount of air that must be breathed in to deliver adequate oxygen to the tissues is decreased, requiring less work by the respiratory system. Studies of endurance athletes have demonstrated increased vital capacity and increased total lung capacity (Nobel, 1986). With training, the efficiency of the ventilatory system increases in adolescents, young adults, and older adults (McArdle et al, 1991). Conclusive studies of the effects of training on the ventilatory system of children have not been done (Mahon and Vaccaro, 1989).

EFFECTS OF EXERCISE AND TRAINING ON THE MUSCULOSKELETAL SYSTEM

The muscular and skeletal systems form the mechanical basis for human movement. Muscle cells also contain energy stores necessary for movement. Within skeletal muscle, three types of muscle fibers (type I, type IIa, and type IIb) are found, and they are used differently to produce energy. Oxygen provided during respiration activates metabolic pathways that convert carbohydrates, fats, and proteins into stored energy sources in muscle. Type I and type IIa muscle fibers effectively work in these aerobic metabolic pathways. Type IIb muscle fibers assist in the production of energy via anaerobic pathways.

At the onset of exercise, energy is produced anaerobically as the high-energy phosphate bonds of adenosine triphosphate (ATP) and creatinine phosphate stored within the muscle are broken. Only small amounts of these substances are stored; this source of energy can be used only for short periods. ATP stores in muscle can be replenished through anaerobic and aerobic pathways utilizing carbohydrates, fats, and proteins. In light to moderate exercise, oxidative pathways can successfully meet the energy demands. In more strenuous exercise, carbohydrate stores in the form of glycogen can be broken down anaerobically to release energy. Lactic acid is formed as an end product and is transferred from muscle to the blood. As blood levels of lactic acid increase, fatigue results. This may be due to the increased acidity produced as attempts are made to buffer the lactic acid. Anaerobic threshold is reached when the lactate buildup limits continued activity (McArdle et al, 1991).

Adaptations of the musculoskeletal system to exercise and training are summarized in Table 15–3. Depending on the type of activity, type I, type IIa, and type IIb muscle fibers are affected differently.

TABLE 15–3

Musculoskeletal Adaptation to Exercise and Training

Exercise	Training
Increased blood flow to working muscle	Increased bone density
	Increased strength, flexibility, and thickness of ligaments
	Increased thickness of articular cartilage
	Increased muscle strength
	Increased glucose tolerance
	Increased oxidative capacity
	Increase number of type I fibers
	Increase oxidative enzymes
	Increase mitochondria
	Onset of blood lactate accumulation at higher percent of maximum oxygen uptake

Short-Term Adaptation

At the onset of exercise, blood flow to exercising muscle increases. Increased blood flow delivers more oxygen to the muscle and helps to dissipate heat, which results from muscular work. With exercise at less than 60% to 70% of maximum aerobic power, first type I and then type IIa muscle fibers are recruited.

Long-Term Adaptation

Training affects all components of the musculoskeletal system. Exercise increases the bone density (Kemper, 2000) and strengthens the bone architecture. Ligaments become stronger, thicker, and more flexible. Articular cartilage also becomes thicker and more resistant to compression (Shepard, 1987). Muscle tissue undergoes significant change, which varies with the type of exercise performed.

Resistance training increases muscle strength via hypertrophy of muscle fibers or neural recruitment of motor units. Children and older adults increase strength primarily via increased neural recruitment. In older adults, increases in strength also have been related to reversal of fast-twitch fiber atrophy (Knortz, 1987). Muscle hypertrophy is seen in adults when high levels of resistance are used. Anaerobic metabolic pathways are used primarily in this type of exercise, resulting in increased anaerobic enzyme levels in type II muscle fibers.

With endurance training, oxidative capacity of the muscle is maximized, increasing the number of type I muscle fibers (Van Praagh, 2000). Levels of enzymes used by oxidative metabolic pathways increase, especially in oxidative type I and type IIa muscle fibers. The size and number of mitochondria increase with training (Knortz, 1987; Zernicke et al, 1991), as does capillarization (Green, 1990; Noble, 1986; Shepard, 1987) and myoglobin content (Zernicke et al, 1991). These changes all contribute to the efficient utilization of oxygen by muscle tissue, fueling the oxidative metabolic pathway. Aerobic exercise also improves the ability of the skeletal muscle to utilize glucose, improving glucose tolerance (Thompson, 2000)

High-intensity training increases the number of type II fibers, active in anaerobic metabolism (Van Praagh, 2000). Anaerobic threshold increases during submaximal exercise as a result of increased mechanical efficiency and muscle strengthening (Shepard, 1987). Blood lactate accumulation begins at 55% to 65% of maximal oxygen uptake in the untrained individual and at approximately 80% of maximal oxygen uptake in the trained individual (McArdle et al, 1991).

ENDOCRINE SYSTEM AND HORMONAL CONTRIBUTIONS TO FITNESS AND TRAINING

The endocrine system (see Chapter 11) allows the body to adapt to vigorous physical activity and ensures that fuel is delivered to working muscles (Shep-

TABLE 15–4

Hormonal Activity Related to Physical Activity

Hormone	Secreted by	During Exercise
Growth hormone	Anterior pituitary gland	Decreased carbohydrate utilization Increased fat utilization
Corticotropin	Anterior pituitary gland	Increased fat utilization Increased protein utilization; stimulates secretion of cortisol
Antidiuretic hormone	Posterior pituitary gland	Increased water retention
Norepinephrine/epinephrine	Adrenal medulla	Affects cardiac contractability and distribution of blood in vascular system Fat → fatty acid, Glycogen → glucose
Cortisol	Adrenal cortex	Protein → glucose Fatty acid → glucose
Insulin	Pancreas	Decreased secretion during exercise; inhibits epinephrine and glucagon
Glucagon	Pancreas	Increased secretion during exercise; forms glucose from liver, glycogen, and amino acids; breaks down fat

ard, 1987). Several endocrine organs are activated during exercise. The hormones they secrete play a role in the utilization of carbohydrates and fatty acids, maintenance of fluid volume, contractility of the heart, and distribution of blood within the vascular system (Table 15–4). Certain hormones make specific contributions to fitness and wellness.

Growth hormone, secreted by the anterior pituitary gland, decreases the use of carbohydrates and increases the use of fat metabolism for energy production. By maintaining glucose levels, growth hormone increases endurance. Growth hormone also promotes protein synthesis, cartilage formation, and skeletal growth. Intensity and duration of exercise affect the secretion of growth hormone. The mechanism for control of growth hormone secretion during exercise is not known, but it is probably related to neural mechanisms. There does not appear to be a training effect on the levels of growth hormone in adults (McArdle et al, 1991).

Corticotropin (ACTH), also secreted by the anterior pituitary gland, improves the mobilization of fat as an energy source, increases the rate of glucose formation, and stimulates the breakdown of proteins. ACTH also controls the secretion of hormones from the adrenal cortex, including cortisol, which is important during intense exercise. After training, ACTH levels are slightly elevated during exercise (McArdle et al, 1991).

Antidiuretic hormone secretion is controlled by the posterior pituitary gland. During exercise, this gland increases water retention by the kidneys, maintaining fluid volume (McArdle et al, 1991).

Norepinephrine and epinephrine secretion, by the adrenal medulla, is stimulated by exercise and increases as the intensity of the exercise increases. A greater response to exercise is seen in older than in younger individuals and in men than in women. Also known as catecholamines, these hormones are related to activity of the sympathetic branch of the autonomic nervous system. They increase cardiac contractility, heart rate, distribution of blood within the vascular system, and so forth. They are also active in the breakdown of stored fat into free fatty acids and of glycogen into glucose (McArdle et al, 1991; Noble, 1986). After training, levels of norepinephrine and epinephrine are decreased at rest and during submaximal work.

Cortisol is secreted by the adrenal cortex. It promotes the formation of glucose from proteins and fatty acids during intense exercise. ACTH stimulates the release of cortisol. After training, levels of cortisol are slightly increased with exercise.

Insulin is secreted by the pancreas when blood glucose levels are too high. It inhibits the effects of epinephrine and glucagon on fat metabolism and facilitates glucose uptake by the muscle cells. Insulin secretion is usually decreased during prolonged exercise (McArdle et al, 1991; Noble, 1986; Sutton et al, 1990). After training, levels of insulin are maintained at closer to resting levels during exercise (McArdle et al, 1991).

Glucagon also is secreted by the pancreas when blood glucose falls below a threshold. It stimulates the formation of glucose from liver glycogen stores and amino acids. It can also stimulate the breakdown of fat stores. Glucagon acts in opposition to insulin; its secretion is increased during exercise (McArdle et al, 1991; Noble, 1986). Similar to insulin, after training, glucagon levels remain closer to resting level during exercise.

MAXIMAL AEROBIC CAPACITY AND MAXIMAL OXYGEN UPTAKE

All of the systems discussed here work together to allow our bodies to efficiently use their energy stores and to produce the mechanical work necessary for physical activity. A measure of how efficiently the body can perform this task is the *maximal aerobic capacity,* or *maximal oxygen uptake* ($\dot{V}O_2max$), which reflects the maximal rate at which oxygen can be utilized by the tissues during exercise. Both how well the cardiovascular and pulmonary systems deliver oxygen to the tissues and the ability of the tissues to utilize the oxygen contribute to $\dot{V}O_2max$. Maximal aerobic capacity measures the maximum level of work an individual can perform. It is a major determinant of overall functional ability and a good measure of aerobic fitness. Aerobic fitness has also been related to levels of health risk.

Maximal aerobic capacity appears to be closely related to our level of activity and body composition. This measure improves as our level of fitness improves and decreases with inactivity. Aerobic capacity decreases as percent of body fat increases and is improved in individuals with lower percentages of body fat. Indeed, our habitual level of physical activity is thought to be more of a determinant of aerobic capacity than chronological age.

Age does affect maximal aerobic capacity. Maximal aerobic capacity appears to be lower in children than in adults, but it increases through childhood, as size increases. Through adulthood, maximal aerobic capacity again decreases. The cause of this decrease is not thought to be totally age related.

There is some controversy as to the ability to measure maximal aerobic capacity ($\dot{V}O_2max$) in children because it is difficult to ensure that they work to full capacity of the cardiovascular and pulmonary systems. Instead, for a child, measurement of peak $\dot{V}O_2$ may be used to reflect the point to which the child will work before his efforts plateau or he stops because he is tired. Through childhood, peak $\dot{V}O_2$ of boys is slightly greater than that of girls, with the difference increasing even more in puberty. The increased muscle mass of boys compared with girls contributes to this difference (Armstrong and Welsman, 2000; Stout, 2000). Peak $\dot{V}O_2$ increases by 150% in boys and 80% in girls between the ages of 8 and 16 years. Much of this increase seems to be related to increased left ventricular size and stroke volume (Armstrong and Welsman, 2000).

Longitudinal and cross-sectional studies of adults and older adults have demonstrated that aerobic capacity decreases through adulthood (Jackson et al, 1996; Lemura et al, 2000; Pollock et al, 1997; Talbot et al, 2000). When considering the previously discussed cardiovascular, pulmonary, and musculoskeletal system changes with age, it is understandable that the ability to transport and utilize oxygen at the tissue level would also change with age. More specifically, the maximum heart rate does decrease with age regardless of training (Pollock et al, 1997). Muscle mass also decreases with age, affecting the amount of oxygen that can be utilized. Not all of the changes in aerobic capacity of adults can be attributed to changes in the body systems. Lifestyle factors such as an increase in percent body fat and decreased levels of physical activity are major contributors to the diminishing aerobic capacity in adults (Jackson et al, 1995). The age-associated decrease in peak $\dot{V}O_2$ has been estimated to be approximately 7% per decade (Talbot et al, 2000).

Developmental Changes Produced by Exercise and Fitness

CARDIOVASCULAR, PULMONARY, AND AEROBIC CAPACITY

Childhood

Body size and especially body height are predictive of cardiovascular system capacity in childhood (Cunningham et al, 1984). Cardiac size and pulmonary capacity increase through childhood and limit the child's aerobic capacity. The child's higher heart rate does not appear to totally compensate for decreased stroke volume, because the cardiac output of children is smaller than that of adults (Payne and Isaacs, 1987). Other differences in the cardiovascular system of children compared with adults are seen. Blood volume and hemoglobin levels increase through childhood and are correlated with the peak $\dot{V}O_2$ that can be attained (Armstrong and Welsman, 2000). Because children have less hemoglobin than adults, they have less oxygen-carrying capacity than adults. Their ability to extract oxygen from the blood at the tissue level (A-$\dot{V}O_2$ difference) has been reported to increase slightly with age, especially after puberty, and reaches adult levels by late adolescence. This change may be related to the growing child's increased muscle mass, changes in muscle enzyme perfusion, and changes in the ratio of capillary to muscle fiber (Armstrong and Welsman, 2000; Cunningham et al, 1984).

The pulmonary system development also affects aerobic power. The growth of the lungs also parallels the general growth of the child. Children's airways are small in diameter, resulting in higher resistance to airflow and increased work of breathing. Because children demonstrate poorer ventilatory efficiency than adults in both submaximal and maximal exercise, they must maintain a higher breathing frequency when performing similar tasks.

Training effects, specifically improvements in maximal aerobic power, in prepubescent children have not been conclusively demonstrated. High levels of habitual activity, mechanical inefficiency in performing physical activity, and body size limitations affect the maximal aerobic capacity of children (Bar-Or, 1983). A running child must move her short legs more frequently and faster than an adult, who can sprint with a long stride. This inefficient pattern results in higher energy cost in a child than in an adult. As the child grows, mechanical efficiency increases and endurance improves. Through childhood and adolescence, a child's level of physical activity is slightly to moderately related to their aerobic fitness (Morrow and Freedson, 1994).

Slight improvements of less than a 10% increase in aerobic capacity have been reported after endurance exercise in 8- to 14-year-old children (Krakenbuhl et al, 1985; Rowland and Boyajian, 1995). Holman and colleagues (1988) reported significant effects of endurance training on aerobic capacity and "athlete's heart" (increased heart volume, increased left ventricular wall diameter, increased end diastolic diameter) in prepubescent swimmers. In 1984, Cunningham and coworkers reported that physical activity can help improve cardiorespiratory function in the year before peak height increases and thereafter. Other reviews of the effectiveness of training with adolescents report inconsistent results (Bailey and Mirwald, 1988; Malina, 1988).

Adulthood

Once adult levels of cardiovascular performance have been reached, some sex-related differences surface. The stroke volume of women is approximately 25% less than that of men. Men have 15 to 16 g Hb/100 mL blood, whereas women have 14 g Hb/100 mL blood; this gives men a greater oxygen-carrying capacity. Teenage and adult women have a 5% to 10% higher cardiac output during submaximal exercise than do men, possibly to compensate for their decreased oxygen-carrying capacity (McArdle et al, 1991).

Older Adulthood

Oxygen consumption and heart rate changes with submaximal exercise in older adults are similar to those seen in younger adults. Maximum heart rate decreases with age. Decreased pacemaker activity and sensitivity to catecholamines may contribute to decreased peak heart rate (Peel, 1990). Blood pressure increases are seen in older adults during submaximal and maximal exercise and are due to decreased arterial compliance (Noble, 1986). During maximal exercise, the older adult's cardiac output, cardiac contractility, and A-VO$_2$ difference are decreased. Diminished cardiac compliance, valvular thickening, higher vascular resistance, poor myocardial perfusion, and poor contractility contribute to reduced stroke volume. At high workloads, older adults experience a 10% to 20% decrease in maximum stroke volume compared with younger adults (Shephard, 1987). Lower arterial oxygen saturation, less hemoglobin, and poor peripheral vascular distribution may decrease maximal A-VO$_2$ difference (Shepard, 1987; Wei, 1986).

Aerobic capacity and oxygen consumption can be increased two ways. The first way is to increase blood flow to the muscles by increasing cardiac output. The second way is to extract more oxygen at the tissue level by increasing the capillarization of the trained muscle tissue, number of mitochondria, and levels of enzymes necessary for aerobic metabolism (Knortz, 1987; McArdle et al, 1991; Noble, 1986; Shepard, 1987; Zernicke et al, 1991). In older adults, maximal oxygen uptake is limited by the inability to increase cardiac output (O'Toole and Douglas, 1988; Saltin, 1990), but older adults in exercise programs demonstrate improved maximal aerobic power (Cunningham and Paterson, 1990; Green and Crouse, 1995; Lemura et al, 2000).

Structural pulmonary system changes such as a stiffer bony thorax increase the work of breathing for the older adult. Decreased compliance of the lungs and airways also increases resistance to airflow. As a result of structural and functional changes, the older adult's residual lung capacity is increased with age. Vital capacity, inspiratory reserve, and expiratory reserve volumes are decreased in both resting and dynamic states. The surface area available for gas exchange also is decreased because of changes within the alveoli and a decrease in the number of pulmonary capillaries (Peel, 1990; Shepard, 1987). Ventilatory responses to increased carbon dioxide or decreased oxygen levels in the blood also decrease with age, possibly because of receptor, neuronal, or muscular changes (Peel, 1990).

Older adults require increased ventilation during activity compared with young adults, but considering the changes discussed here, they may not be able to breathe fast enough. For this reason, the pulmonary system, rather than the cardiovascular system, of older adults often limits the amount of exercise performed (Peel, 1990; Shepard, 1987). Some evidence shows that training can counter the changes in lung function attributed to age (McArdle et al, 1991).

MUSCLE STRENGTH AND ENDURANCE

Childhood and Adolescence

Muscle strength and endurance increase proportionally with growth, through childhood. With exercise, prepubescent children demonstrate increased strength, but this seems to be related to improved neural control and recruitment of motor units. Potential for aerobic and anaerobic muscle metabolism is smaller in children than in adults. Aerobic capacity is related to the available muscle mass and increases with growth. Children have smaller muscles and therefore less aerobic capacity. Anaerobic capacity is also limited in children because of lower glycolytic capacity and a smaller percentage of type II muscle fibers compared with an adult. Because of the limited glycolytic capacity, high-intensity or heavy resistance exercise would be difficult for the prepubescent child. Once the child reaches puberty, increased muscle mass and metabolism contribute to muscle strength and endurance improvement with training. Anaerobic capacity improves in adolescence and appears to be related to hormonal changes at puberty (Van Praagh, 2000).

Older Adulthood

Muscle changes with aging are reported. Decreases in strength, which appear to be related to decreased muscle mass, are reported. Muscle fibers are lost through denervation and selective atrophy of type II muscle fibers. Type I fibers are used in activities of daily living and remain more stable (Knortz, 1987). It is difficult to determine whether these changes are due to inactivity or to aging (McArdle et al, 1991). Increases in muscle mass and strength have been demonstrated with training (Cress et al, 1999; Pollock et al, 1997; Thompson, 2000).

FLEXIBILITY AND BODY COMPOSITION

Childhood and Adolescence

Especially after periods of skeletal growth, flexibility is an issue for children. Because bone growth precedes muscle growth, children should be reminded to stretch before exercising. Throughout childhood, girls are more flexible than boys.

Body composition is related to a person's amount of lean body mass versus fat mass. Through infancy, the amount of fat mass increases, but then it decreases once children start increasing muscle mass. Girls' fat mass is slightly higher than that of boys in early childhood, and the difference increases with puberty. The incidence of obesity in children continues to increase and presents a health risk for children. Exercise and diet are important to control increased fat mass, and with strength training, increased bone density and muscle mass contribute to increase fat-free body mass.

Adulthood

Flexibility and body composition change through adulthood. Body fat increases 2% to 2.5% per decade even in individuals who participate regularly in moderate- to high-intensity exercise (Pollock et al, 1997). Both longitudinal and cross-sectional studies have also found fat weight to increase per decade, even when fat-free body mass remains stable (Jackson et al, 1996). Activities to increase muscle strength and mass and to sustain or improve bone density assist in the maintenance of fat-free body mass.

EXERCISE AND TRAINING CONSIDERATIONS ACROSS THE LIFE SPAN

As body systems mature and develop across the life span and an individual's work and leisure habits are formed, regular participation in physical activity is important. Because of differences in the aerobic capacity and the ability of muscle tissue to respond to exercise, exercise programs must be designed for each individual based on his or her lifestyle and age. General recommendations regarding appropriate exercise for individuals of different ages are listed in Clinical Implications—Components of Beneficial Exercise Prescriptions.

Childhood

It is difficult to define optimal intensity, duration, and frequency of endurance training for children. Regular physical activity should be encouraged to promote optimal physiological fitness and to establish health behavior patterns for the child to carry into adulthood. Children are learning and perfecting motor skills that promote agility, balance, coordination, speed, and power. Fitness evaluations and programs for children should include a motor skills component (Malina, 1990). Endurance activities that require anaerobic metabolism should be thoroughly evaluated for appropriateness. Events such as long distance running may be inappropriate for prepubescent children (Smith, 1988).

Older Adulthood

Older adults are generally happy with their level of fitness but underestimate their ability to exercise (Buskirk, 1990). As maximal exercise capacity decreases with age, it begins to affect the intensity of exercise that can be considered submaximal work. For example, activities of daily living are considered submaximal work. The energy required to perform these activities remains constant, but the percentage of maximal capacity they require increases as the maximal exercise capacity decreases. In older adults, activities such as walking or housework may be considered high-intensity exercise; in younger adults, these same activities offer a low-intensity exercise. For the older adult, these activities may become more stressful. If the individual can no longer complete activities of daily living because of the level of physiological stress, functional independence is decreased (Peel, 1990). Therefore, it is very important for older adults to maintain aerobic capacity and to maximize their functional

---

CLINICAL IMPLICATIONS
Components of Beneficial Exercise Prescriptions

In general, we all benefit from maintaining a physically active lifestyle with regular exercise. Regardless of age, physical activity assists in increasing fat-free body mass and in improving cardiovascular and pulmonary endurance. Not only does this reduce the incidence of obesity, but it also decreases the risk for heart disease and osteoporosis. Exercise can increase our functional capacity and minimize the decrease often experienced in older individuals. Our capacity to participate in physical activity is influenced by the development of the body systems and their level of fitness. Exercise considerations that affect this capacity include the following for children (American College of Sports Medicine, 2000), adults (American College of Sports Medicine, 2000), and older adults (Green and Crouse, 1995).

Children

- Encourage young children to participate in physically active play.
- Structure 30 minutes of moderate physical activity for children older than 6 years, preferably 7 days per week.
- Include the following in moderate physical activity:
    1. *Activities that use all muscle groups*
    2. *Activities that will go through the full range of motion*
    3. *Multijoint exercises*
- Structure weight training with the following provisions:
    1. *Limits that allow the child to complete eight or more repetitions before fatigue*
    2. *To be limited to twice weekly*
    3. *To avoid power lifting*
    4. *To avoid maximum weights until at least adolescence*
    5. *To use proper technique*
    6. *To maintain controlled speed*
- Build in precautions that include the following:
    1. *Avoidance of stress to growth plates of bones and growth plate injuries*
    2. *Use of appropriate protective equipment*
    3. *Use caution when exercising in temperature extremes*

Adults

- Include warm-up, endurance activities, cool down, and recreational physical activity in the exercise routine.
- Include endurance activities with 20 to 60 minutes of physical activity that will raise the heart rate to 70% to 85% of the maximum heart rate,* 3 to 5 days per week.
- Include important flexibility and strength training at least twice weekly.
- Structure endurance exercise to include large muscle groups (i.e., walking, running, swimming, dancing).

- Know that 30 minutes of moderate-intensity exercise, on most days of the week, will benefit health but not always increase aerobic capacity.
- Build in precautions that include the following:

  1. Awareness of the effects of medication (i.e., it may influence cardiovascular response to exercise)

  2. Awareness that high-intensity exercise increases the risk of musculoskeletal and cardiovascular injuries

Older Adults

- Structure 30 minutes of moderate activity, preferably three times per week.
- Understand that benefits are also seen with three short 10-minute exercise sessions per day.
- Structure training to increase $\dot{V}O_2$max with intensity at 50% to 85% of $\dot{V}O_2$max.
- Know that improvement in submaximal exercise response is seen at an exercise intensity of less than 50% $\dot{V}O_2$max.
- Include a strength training component to minimize loss of muscle strength and endurance often seen with aging.
- Know that activities such as walking, aquatics, and cycle ergometry minimize musculoskeletal stress.
- Avoid injury in a progressive exercise program by increasing the duration of the exercise session, not the intensity of exercise.
- Build in precautions to include the following:

  1. Use of conservative exercise prescriptions and progression for older adults due to their varied health and fitness levels

  2. Use of a percentage of measured peak heart rate, because it is more accurate than an age-predicted maximum heart rate

  3. Consideration of the prescription medications a client is taking, because medication may influence exercise response

  *There are many ways to calculate maximum heart rate. An exercise physiology textbook will provide additional information about several possible methods. If an "age-predicted" maximum heart rate is used to recommend an exercise prescription, recognize that there is an inherent error in such a measurement.

independence. Studies have shown that regular exercise, even for individuals in their 60s, can increase maximal aerobic capacity and submaximal work capacity (Cunningham and Paterson, 1990; Cress et al, 1999; Green and Crouse, 1995; Lemura et al, 2000; Thompson, 2000) (Fig. 15–7).

Exercise programming for the older adult should emphasize the functional needs of the individual. A person's level of fitness and interests must be kept in mind (Thomas and Rutledge, 1985). Both aerobic exercise (to strengthen the cardiovascular system) and low-intensity exercise (to control weight and loss of bone mineral, to improve flexibility, and to retain muscle endurance) should

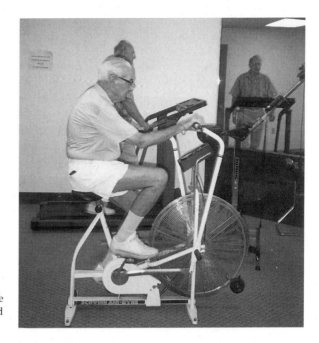

Figure 15-7

Maintaining an active exercise program through older adulthood improves physical function.

be included. It has been found that even older adults who exercise at less than 50% aerobic capacity show an improvement in submaximal exercise response (DeVito, et al, 1997). To increase $\dot{V}O_2$max, exercise intensity should be at 50% to 85% of $\dot{V}O_2$max. Thirty minutes of exercise, three times a week is recommended to improve fitness levels.

Summary

We continue to emphasize a premise that is discussed throughout this book: Exercise and training programs can improve our health and fitness. Quality of life is improved when we feel better, do more, and develop a positive self-image. Exercise helps us attain and maintain body efficiency, allowing us to function optimally within the environment. This is why health promotion and fitness activities are increasingly important in today's health care arena.

Our level of health and physical fitness is related to our level of physical activity. Many body systems work together to produce efficient, effective physical activity. Each of these systems develops uniquely, and this development can be enhanced by participation in physical fitness programs.

Because optimal health and fitness reflect our ability to maintain a physically active and independent lifestyle, fitness programming is an important focus of health care. Exercise planning and programming form a complex process. Detailed assessment of a person's ability to participate in an exercise program is necessary. Exercise programs differ according to age, health, level of fitness, and interests. As health care providers, we should become familiar with the age-related aspects of exercise and training programs to help our clients attain lifelong fitness as well as to maintain a healthy lifestyle for ourselves.

References

American College of Sports Medicine. *ACSM's Guidelines for Exercise Testing and Prescription*, 6th ed. Philadelphia: Lippincott Williams & Wilkins, 2000.

Armstrong N, Welsman JR. Development of aerobic fitness during childhood and adolescence. *Pediatr Exerc Sci* 12:128–149, 2000.

Bailey DA, Mirwald RL. The effects of training on the growth and development of the child. In Malina RM (ed). *Young Athlete's Biological, Psychological and Educational Perspectives*. Springfield, IL: Human Kinetics, 1988, pp 33–47.

Bar-Or O. *Pediatric Sports Medicine for the Practitioner*. New York: Springer Verlag, 1983.

Bar-Or O. The growth and development of children's physiologic and perceptional responses to exercise. In Ilmannen J, Valimaki I (eds). *Children and Sport—Pediatric Work Physiology*. New York: Springer Verlag, 1984, pp 3–17.

Bar-Or O. The prepubescent female. In Shangold MM, Mirken G (eds). *Women and Exercise: Physiology and Sports Medicine*. Philadelphia: FA Davis, 1988, pp 109–119.

Biegel L. *Physical Fitness and the Older Person: A Guide to Exercise for Health Care Professionals*. Rockville, MD: Aspen Publishing, 1984.

Bouchard C, Shepard RJ, Stephens T, et al. *Exercise Fitness and Health: A Consensus of Current Knowledge*. Champaign, IL: Human Kinetics, 1990.

Brooks CM. Leisure time physical activity assessment of American adults through an analysis of time diaries collected in 1981. *Am J Public Health* 77:455–460, 1987.

Buskirk ER. Exercise, fitness and aging. In Bouchard C, Shepard RJ, Stephens T, et al (eds). *Exercise, Fitness and Health: A Consensus of Current Knowledge*. Champaign, IL: Human Kinetics, 1990, pp 687–697.

Caspersen CJ, Christenson GM, Pollard RA. Status of the 1990 physical fitness and exercise objectives—evidence from NHIS 1985. *Public Health Rep* 101:587–592, 1986.

Cress ME, Buchner DM, Quiestad KA, et al. Exercise effects on physical functional performance in older adults. *J Gerontol* 54A:M242–M237, 1999.

Cunningham DA, Paterson DH. Discussion: Exercise, fitness and aging. In Bouchard C, Shepard RJ, Stephens T, et al (eds). *Exercise, Fitness and Health: A Consensus of Current Knowledge*. Champaign, IL: Human Kinetics, 1990, pp 699–704.

Cunningham DA, Paterson DH, Blimke CJR. The development of the cardiorespiratory system with growth and physical activity. In Bouleau RA (ed). *Advances in Pediatric Sport Science, vol 1: Biological Issues*. Champaign, IL: Human Kinetics, 1984, pp 85–116.

DeVito G, Hernandez R, Gonzalez V, et al. Low intensity physical training in older subjects. *J Sports Med Phys Fitness* 37:72–77, 1997.

Faulkner JA, White TP. Adaptation of skeletal muscle to physical activity. In Bouchard C, Shepard RJ, Stephens T, et al (eds). *Exercise, Fitness and Health: A Consensus of Current Knowledge*. Champaign, IL: Human Kinetics, 1990, pp 256–279.

Folinsbee LJ. Discussion: Exercise and environment. In Bouchard C, Shepard RJ, Stephens T, et al (eds). *Exercise, Fitness and Health: A Consensus of Current Knowledge*. Champaign, IL: Human Kinetics, 1990, pp 179–183.

Francis K. Status of the year 2000 health goals for physical activity and fitness. *Phys Ther* 79:405–414, 1999.

Frontera WR, Evans WJ. Exercise performance and endurance training in the elderly. *Top Geriatr Rehabil* 2:17–32, 1986.

Green HJ. Discussion: Adaptation of skeletal muscle to physical activity. In Bouchard C, Shepard RJ, Stephens T, et al (eds). *Exercise, Fitness and Health: A Consensus of Current Knowledge*. Champaign, IL: Human Kinetics, 1990, pp 281–291.

Green JS, Crouse SF. The effects of endurance training on functional capacity in the elderly: A meta analysis. *Med Sci Sports Exerc* 27:920–926, 1995.

Holman W, Klemt F, Rost R, et al. Comparative studies of physical work capacity of children in 1964 and 1984 and adaptations during competitive training. In Malina RM (ed). *Young Athlete's Biological, Psychological, and Educational Perspectives.* Springfield, IL: Human Kinetics Publishers, 1988, pp 49–59.

Jackson AS, Beard EF, Wier LT, et al. Changes in aerobic power of men, ages 25–70 years. *Med Sci Sports Exerc* 27:113–120, 1995

Jackson AS, Wier LT, Ayers GW, et al. Changes in aerobic power of women, ages 20–64 years. *Med Sci Sports Exerc* 28:884–891, 1996.

Katch FI, Katch VL. Optimal health and body composition. In Shangold MM, Mirkin G (eds). *Women and Exercise: Physiology and Sports Medicine.* Philadelphia: FA Davis, 1988, pp 23–39.

Kemper HC. Skeletal development during childhood and adolescence and the effects of physical activity. *Pediatr Exerc Sci* 12:198–216, 2000.

Knortz KA. Muscle physiology applied to geriatric rehabilitation. *Top Geriatr Rehabil* 2:1–12, 1987.

Krakenbuhl GS, Skinner JS, Kohrt WM. Developmental aspects of maximal aerobic power in children. *Exerc Sport Sci Rev* 13:503–538, 1985.

Lemura LM, VonDuvillard SO, Mookerjee S. The effects of physical training of functional capacity in adults ages 46–90: A meta analysis. *J Sports Med Phys Fitness* 40:1–10, 2000.

Mahon AD, Vaccaro T. Ventilatory threshhold and Vo_2 max changes in children following endurance training. *Med Sci Sports Exerc* 21:425–431, 1989.

Malina RM. Growth, performance, activity and training during adolescence. In Shangold MM, Mirken G (eds). *Women and Exercise: Physiology and Sports Medicine.* Philadelphia: FA Davis, 1988, pp 120–128.

Malina RM. Growth, exercise fitness and later outcomes. In Bouchard C, Shepard RJ, Stephens T, et al (eds). *Exercise, Fitness and Health: A Consensus of Current Knowledge.* Champaign, IL: Human Kinetics, 1990, pp 637–653.

McArdle WD, Katch FI, Katch VL. *Exercise Physiology: Energy, Nutrition and Human Performance*, 3rd ed. Philadelphia: Lea & Febiger, 1991.

Morrow JR, Freedson PS. Relationship between habitual physical activity and aerobic fitness in adolescents. *Pediatr Exerc Sci* 6:315–329, 1994.

Noble BJ. *Physiology of Exercise and Sport.* St. Louis: Times Mirror/Mosby College Publishing, 1986.

O'Toole ML, Douglas PS. Fitness: Definition and development. In Shangold MN, Mirkin G (eds). *Women and Exercise: Physiology and Sports Medicine.* Philadelphia: FA Davis, 1988, pp 3–19.

Pate RR, Shepard RJ. Characteristics of physical fitness in youth. In Grisolfi CV, Lamb DR (eds). *Perspectives in Exercise Science and Sports Medicine: Youth Exercise and Sport*, vol 2. Indianapolis: Benchmark Press, 1989, pp 1–45.

Payne VG, Isaacs LD. *Human Motor Development: A Life Span Approach.* Mountain View, CA: Mayfield Publishing, 1987.

Peel C. Cardiopulmonary changes with aging. In Irwin S, Tecklin JS (eds). *Cardiopulmonary Physical Therapy*, 2nd ed. St. Louis: CV Mosby, 1990, pp 477–489.

Pollock ML, Mengelkoch LJ, Graves JE, et al. Twenty-year follow-up of aerobic power and body composition of older track athletes. *J Appl Physiol* 82:1508–1516, 1997.

Powell K, Blair S. The public health burdens of sedentary living habits: Theoretical but realistic estimates. *Med Sci Sports Exerc* 26:857–865, 1994.

Rowland TW, Boyajian A. Aerobic response to endurance exercise training in children. *Pediatrics* 96: 654–663, 1995.

Saltin B. Cardiovascular and pulmonary adaptation to physical activity. In Bouchard C, Shepard RJ, Stephens T, et al (eds). *Exercise, Fitness and Health: A Consensus of Current Knowledge.* Champaign, IL: Human Kinetics, 1990, pp 187–203.

Sarkisian CA, Liu H, Gutierrez PR, et al. Modifiable risk factors predict functional decline among older women: A prospectively validated clinical prediction tool. *JAGS* 48:170–176, 2000.

Shepard RJ. *Exercise Physiology.* Toronto: BC Decker, 1987.

Smith AD. Children and sport. In Scoles P (ed). *Pediatric Orthopedics in Clinical Practice,* 2nd ed. Chicago: Year Book, 1988, pp 269–285.

Stout JL. Physical fitness during childhood and adolescence. In Campbell SK, Vander Linden DW, Palisano RJ (eds). *Physical Therapy for Children,* 2nd ed. Philadelphia: WB Saunders, 2000, pp 141–169.

Sutton JR, Farrell PA, Harber VJ. Hormonal adaptation to physical activity. ' Bouchard C, Shepard RJ, Stephens T, et al (eds). *Exercise, Fitness and Health: A Co ensus of Current Knowledge.* Champaign, IL: Human Kinetics, 1990, pp 217–257.

Talbot LA, Metter EJ, Fleg JL. Leisure time physical activities and their relati ship to cardiorespiratory fitness in health men and women, 18–95 years old. *Med Sci S rts Exerc* 32:417–425, 2000.

Thomas GS, Rutledge JH. Fitness and exercise for the elderly. In Dych' ald K (ed). *Wellness and Health Promotion for the Elderly.* Rockville, MD: Aspen Publishing, 85, pp 165–177.

Thompson L. Physiologic changes associated with aging. In Guccione A. *Geriatric Physical Therapy,* 2nd ed. St. Louis: Mosby, 2000.

U.S. Department of Health and Human Services. *Healthy People 2010: Understanding and Improving Health,* 2nd ed. Washington, DC: U.S. Government Printing Office, 2000.

U.S. Department of Health and Human Services. *Promoting Health-Preventing Disease: Year 2000 Objectives for the Nation.* Washington, DC: U.S. Public Health Services, National Institutes of Health, 1990.

Van Praagh E. Development of anaerobic function during childhood and adolescence. *Pediatr Exerc Sci* 12:150–173, 2000.

Wei JY. Cardiovascular anatomic and physiologic changes with age. *Top Geriatr Rehabil* 2:10–16, 1986.

World Health Organization. *The First Ten Years of the World Health Organization.* Geneva: World Health Organization, 1958.

Zernicke RF, Salem GJ, Alejo RK. Endurance training. In Reider B (ed). *Sports Medicine: The School Age Athlete.* Philadelphia: WB Saunders, 1991, pp 3–17.

Index